AF479153

Renal and Urologic Aspects of HIV Infection

CONTEMPORARY ISSUES IN NEPHROLOGY

VOLUME 29

Series Editor
Jay H. Stein, M.D.

Series Editors, Vols. 1-21
Barry M. Brenner, M.D.
Jay H. Stein, M.D.

Volumes Already Published

VOLUME 15
Modern Techniques of Ion Transport

VOLUME 18
Immunopathology of Renal Disease
Curtis B. Wilson, M.D., Guest Editor

VOLUME 20
The Kidney in Diabetes Mellitus

VOLUME 21
Atrial Natriuretic Peptides

VOLUME 22
Peritoneal Dialysis
Zbylut J. Twardowski, M.D., Karl D. Nolph, M.D., F.R.C.P.S.
(Glasgow), and Ramesh Khanna, M.D., Guest Editors

VOLUME 23
Hormones, Autacoids, and the Kidney
Stanley Goldfarb, M.D., and Fuad N. Ziyadeh, M.D., Guest Editors

VOLUME 24
Lipids and Renal Disease
William F. Keane, M.D., Guest Editor

VOLUME 25
Diagnostic Techniques in Renal Disease
Robert G. Narins, M.D., Guest Editor

VOLUME 26
The Progressive Nature of Renal Disease, 2nd Ed.
William E. Mitch, M.D., Guest Editor

VOLUME 27
Hemodialysis: High-Efficiency Treatments
Juan P. Bosch, M.D., F.A.C.P., F.A.C.N., Guest Editor

VOLUME 28
Pharmacology and Management of Hypertension
*William M. Bennett, M.D. and David A. McCarron, M.D.,
Guest Editors*

Forthcoming Volumes in the Series

VOLUME 30
Acute Renal Failure: Emerging New Concepts and Therapeutic
Strategies
Michael S. Goligorsky, M.D., Ph.D., Guest Editor

Renal and Urologic Aspects of HIV Infection

Guest Editors

PAUL L. KIMMEL, M.D.
Professor
Division of Renal Diseases and Hypertension
Department of Medicine
George Washington University School of Medicine and
  Health Sciences
Attending Physician
Department of Medicine
George Washington University Hospital
Washington, DC

JEFFREY S. BERNS, M.D.
Clinical Assistant Professor
Department of Medicine
University of Pennsylvania School of Medicine
Nephrologist
Division of Nephrology and Hypertension
Department of Medicine
The Graduate Hospital
Philadelphia, Pennsylvania

Series Editor
JAY H. STEIN, M.D.
Provost and Senior Vice President for Health Sciences
University of Oklahoma College of Medicine
Oklahoma City, Oklahoma

CHURCHILL LIVINGSTONE
New York, Edinburgh, London, Melbourne, Tokyo

Library of Congress Cataloging-in-Publication Data

Renal and urologic aspects of HIV infection / guest editors,   Paul L.
   Kimmel, Jeffrey S. Berns.
         p. cm. — (Contemporary issues in nephrology ; v. 29)
      Includes bibliographical references and index.
      ISBN 0-443-08952-3
      1. Kidneys—Diseases—Pathogenesis. 2. HIV infections—
   Complications. 3. Genitourinary organs—Diseases—Pathogenesis.
    I. Kimmel, Paul L.   II. Berns, Jeffrey S.   III. Series: Contemporary
   issues in nephrology ; vol. 29.
         [DNLM: 1. HIV Infections—complications. 2. HIV Infections—
   physiopathology. 3. HIV Infections—transmission. 4. Kidney
   Diseases—complications. 5. Kidney Diseases—therapy.
   6. Urogenital Diseases—complications.   W1 CO769MR v. 29 1995 / WC
   503.5 R393 1995]
   RC903.R476 1995
   616.97′92—dc20
   DNLM/DLC
   for Library of Congress   94-48435
                                                                      CIP

© Churchill Livingstone Inc. 1995

Distributed in the United Kingdom by Churchill Livingstone, Robert
Stevenson House, 1–3 Baxter's Place, Leith Walk, Edinburgh EH1
3AF, and by associated companies, branches, and representatives
throughout the world.

Accurate indications, adverse reactions, and dosage schedules for drugs
are provided in this book, but it is possible that they may change. The
reader is urged to review the package information data of the manufac-
turers of the medications mentioned.

The Publishers have made every effort to trace the copyright holders for
borrowed material. If they have inadvertently overlooked any, they will
be pleased to make the necessary arrangements at the first opportunity.

Acquisitions Editor: *Allan Ross*
Production Editor: *Dorothy J. Birch*
Production Supervisor: *Sharon Tuder*

Printed in the United States of America

First published in 1995   7 6 5 4 3 2 1

*We dedicate this book to our patients,
and our families—
Donna, Matthew, and Adam Berns and
Prudence Kline and Laura Kimmel—
and to the memory of
Karen Ann Kimmel-Slavin.*

P.L.K. and J.S.B.

Contributors

Carolyn Abitbol, M.D.
Associate Professor, Department of Pediatrics, University of Miami School of Medicine; Attending Physician, Division of Nephrology, Department of Pediatrics, Jackson Memorial Hospital, Miami, Florida

William M. Bennett, M.D.
Professor, Department of Medicine and Pharmacology, Oregon Health Sciences University School of Medicine; Co-Director, Division of Nephrology, Hypertension, and Clinical Pharmacology, Department of Medicine, University Hospital, Portland, Oregon

Mitchell C. Benson, M.D.
Associate Professor, Department of Urology, Columbia University College of Physicians and Surgeons; Director, Urologic Oncology, Department of Urology, Columbia-Presbyterian Medical Center, New York, New York

Jeffrey S. Berns, M.D.
Clinical Assistant Professor, Department of Medicine, University of Pennsylvania School of Medicine; Nephrologist, Division of Nephrology and Hypertension, Department of Medicine, The Graduate Hospital, Philadelphia, Pennsylvania

Juan P. Bosch, M.D.
Professor, Department of Medicine, George Washington University School of Medicine and Health Sciences; Director, Division of Renal Diseases and Hypertension, Department of Medicine, George Washington University Hospital, Washington, DC

Jacques J. Bourgoignie, M.D.
Professor and Director, Division of Nephrology, Department of Medicine, University of Miami School of Medicine; Chief, Nephrology Service, Department of Medicine, Jackson Memorial Hospital, Miami, Florida

Arthur H. Cohen, M.D.
Professor, Departments of Medicine and Pathology and Laboratory Medicine, University of California, Los Angeles, UCLA School of Medicine; Attending Pathologist, Department of Pathology and Laboratory Medicine, Cedars-Sinai Medical Center, Los Angeles, California

Raphael M. Cohen, M.D.
Clinical Assistant Professor, Department of Medicine, University of Pennsylvania School of Medicine; Director, Peritoneal Dialysis, Nephrologist, Division of Nephrology and Hypertension, Department of Medicine, The Graduate Hospital, Philadelphia, Pennsylvania

Michael C. Hill, M.D.
Professor, Department of Radiology, George Washington University School of Medicine and Health Sciences; Director, Cross-Sectional Imaging Section, Department of Radiology, George Washington University Hospital, Washington, DC

Michael H. Humphreys, M.D.
Professor, Department of Medicine, University of California, San Francisco, School of Medicine; Chief, Division of Nephrology, San Francisco General Hospital, San Francisco, California

Diane K. Huntington, M.D.
Assistant Professor, Department of Radiology, George Washington University School of Medicine and Health Sciences, Washington, DC

Steven A. Kaplan, M.D.
Herbert H. Irving Assistant Professor, Department of Urology, Columbia University College of Physicians and Surgeons; Director, Neurourology and the Prostate Center, Department of Urology, Columbia-Presbyterian Medical Center, New York, New York

William A. Kennedy II, M.D.
National Kidney Foundation Fellow, Department of Urology, Columbia University College of Physicians and Surgeons; Chief Resident, Department of Urology, Columbia-Presbyterian Medical Center, New York, New York

Abraham L. Kierszenbaum, M.D., Ph.D.
Chairman and Professor, Department of Cell Biology and Anatomical Studies, The City University of New York Medical School/Sophie Davis School of Biomedical Education, New York, New York

Paul L. Kimmel, M.D.
Professor, Division of Renal Diseases and Hypertension, Department of Medicine, George Washington University School of Medicine and Health Sciences; Attending Physician, Department of Medicine, George Washington University Hospital, Washington, DC

Paul E. Klotman, M.D.
Chief, Division of Nephrology, Professor, Department of Medicine, Mount Sinai School of Medicine of the City University of New York, New York, New York

Jeffrey B. Kopp, M.D.
Senior Research Investigator, Laboratory of Oral Medicine, National Institute of Dental Research, National Institutes of Health, Bethesda, Maryland

Ajit Kumar, Ph.D.
Professor, Department of Biochemistry and Molecular Biology, George Washington University School of Medicine and Health Sciences, Washington, DC

Joel Neugarten, M.D.
Associate Professor, Department of Medicine, Albert Einstein College of Medicine of Yeshiva University; Associate Director, Renal, Electrolyte, and Hypertension Division, Department of Medicine, Montefiore Medical Center, Bronx, New York

Victoriano Pardo, M.D.
Professor, Department of Pathology, University of Miami School of Medicine; Director, Electron Microscopy Laboratory, Veterans Affairs Medical Center, Miami, Florida

David M. Parenti, M.D.
Associate Professor, Department of Medicine, George Washington University School of Medicine and Health Sciences; Clinical Director, AIDS Clinical Trials Unit, Division of Infectious Diseases, Department of Medicine, George Washington University Hospital, Washington, DC

Terry M. Phillips, D.Sc.
Professor, Immunochemistry Laboratory, Division of Renal Diseases and Hypertension, Department of Medicine, George Washington University School of Medicine and Health Sciences; Director, Immunochemistry Laboratory, Division of Renal Diseases and Hypertension, Department of Medicine, George Washington University Hospital, Washington, DC

T. K. Sreepada Rao, M.D.
Professor, Department of Medicine, State University of New York Health
Science Center at Brooklyn College of Medicine; Director, Hemodialysis,
the University Hospital of Brooklyn, Brooklyn, New York

Michael R. Rudnick, M.D.
Clinical Professor, Department of Medicine, University of Pennsylvania
School of Medicine; Chief, Division of Nephrology and Hypertension,
Department of Medicine, The Graduate Hospital, Philadelphia,
Pennsylvania

Patricia Schoenfeld, M.D.
Professor, Department of Medicine, University of California, San
Francisco, School of Medicine; Medical Director, University of California
Renal Center, San Francisco General Hospital, San Francisco, California

Ram R. Shukla, Ph.D.
Assistant Research Professor, Department of Biochemistry and Molecular
Biology, George Washington University School of Medicine and Health
Sciences, Washington, DC

Gary L. Simon, M.D.
Director, Division of Infectious Diseases, Professor, Departments of
Medicine and Biochemistry and Molecular Biology, George Washington
University School of Medicine and Health Sciences; Director, Division of
Infectious Diseases, Associate Chairman, Department of Medicine, George
Washington University Hospital, Washington, DC

Jose Strauss, M.D.
Professor, Department of Pediatrics, University of Miami School of
Medicine; Attending Physician and Division Director, Division of
Nephrology, Department of Pediatrics, Jackson Memorial Hospital,
Miami, Florida

Rashmi Vijayvargiya, M.D.
Clinical Assistant Professor, Department of Medicine, West Virginia
School of Osteopathic Medicine, Lewisburg, West Virginia; Director and
Attending Physician, Hemodialysis Unit, Department of Medicine,
Veterans Administration Medical Center, Beckley, West Virginia

Gaston Zilleruelo, M.D.
Professor, Department of Pediatrics, University of Miami School of
Medicine; Attending Physician, Division of Nephrology, Department of
Pediatrics, Jackson Memorial Hospital, Miami, Florida

Preface

A link between acquired immunodeficiency syndrome (AIDS) and kidney disease was first established by several investigators about a decade ago. Initially, controversy raged regarding whether the renal disease encountered in patients with human immunodeficiency virus (HIV) infection was intimately associated with the syndrome, was perhaps a direct effect of the retroviral infection, or was related more to risk factors for the development of focal segmental glomerulosclerosis in other settings, such as the use of intravenous drugs. Since that time, HIV infection and its attendant complications and therapies have been associated with a wide variety of clinical renal, urologic, fluid, and electrolyte disorders. HIV infection has raised new ethical and medical issues concerning dialysis, transplantation, and the occupational safety of dialysis staff. A veritable explosion in the areas of immunology and molecular biology of HIV infection has revolutionized our understanding of human cell biology, immunology, and molecular genetics. Presently, the study of the virology of HIV has not only increased our knowledge regarding the pathogenesis and pathophysiology of HIV-associated renal diseases, but has also tremendously augmented our understanding of more common diseases, such as immune complex glomerulonephritis, focal segmental glomerulosclerosis, and orchitis.

Renal and Urologic Aspects of HIV Infection, the latest volume in the *Contemporary Issues in Nephrology* series, assembles in a single book an overview of the renal aspects of HIV infection for the clinical nephrologist, internist, pediatrician, urologist, transplant surgeon, infectious disease specialist, radiologist, pathologist, and basic scientist, as well as other health care workers who may be involved in the care of patients with renal disease and HIV infection. A group of authors has been assembled to provide expertise, clinical experience, and an investigative focus on their discipline. Each chapter has been peer reviewed by experts in their fields.

The book begins with a general consideration of the pathogenesis and clinical features of HIV infection, followed by several chapters devoted to various clinical manifestations of HIV infection, including fluid and electrolyte disturbances, acute renal failure, glomerulopathies, urologic disorders, renal aspects of treatment of HIV and related opportunistic infections, and pediatric renal diseases, as well as renal pathology and radiology. Next, implications of HIV infection for dialysis and transplantation are presented, including a review of occupational and medicolegal issues. Finally, recent advances in the molecular biology and basic sciences of HIV-related renal and genitourinary tract diseases are delineated.

Several chapters, such as those on the molecular pathogenesis of HIV infection and nephropathy, immune complex renal disease, and pathogenesis of testicular disease, are particularly intended to provide a comprehensive bibliography and serve as an impetus for future research directions in these exciting fields.

We hope this volume will be of value to the scientist studying HIV in the laboratory as well as the clinician caring for adults and children with AIDS. We have been impressed with both the exponential growth of knowledge and the suffering that has followed the outbreak of the HIV epidemic. This viral illness has affected nephrology as it has all other areas of medicine, and has indelibly changed clinical practice. We hope the advances outlined in this volume will help the readers gain insight into the nature of the disease, and most importantly, enhance the care of patients with HIV infection now and in the future.

Paul L. Kimmel, M.D.
Jeffrey S. Berns, M.D.

Contents

1

Molecular Pathogenesis and Natural History of HIV Infection: An Overview

David M. Parenti

Gary L. Simon

EPIDEMIOLOGY

The acquired immunodeficiency syndrome (AIDS) was first recognized in 1981 by clinicians in New York and San Francisco who described outbreaks of *Pneumocystis carinii* pneumonia and Kaposi sarcoma in homosexual men who had no identifiable risk factors for these unusual clinical disorders.[1] The human immunodeficiency virus (HIV) was identified as the etiologic agent of this immune disorder by several groups of investigators in 1983 and 1984. This virus was identified as a retrovirus by demonstrating reverse transcriptase in the supernatant of tissue cultures of lymphocytes obtained from patients with AIDS. Since the beginning of the epidemic over 340,000 cases of AIDS have been reported to the Centers for Disease Control and Prevention (CDC).[2] By the end of 1992, HIV infection had become the most important cause of attributable mortality in men 25 to 44 years of age, and the fourth most important cause of death in women in that age group.[3]

Studies of the biology and epidemiology of this infection indicated that HIV belonged to the lentivirus family of retroviruses. Lentiviruses tend to have a long incubation period, cause latent infection, and have a cytopathic effect on some infected cells. In addition, involvement of the hematopoietic and central nervous systems (CNS) are characteristic features of lentiviral infection.

TRANSMISSION

Transmission of HIV is dependent on several factors: the nature of the contact (sexual contact, needle sharing, blood transfusion), the stage of HIV infection of the donor, and the body fluid involved. The efficiency of sexual transmission varies between populations with different HIV risk factors, although it is often difficult to control for either the number or types of sexual encounters when attempting to analyze these factors. The risk of transmission to male or female partners of HIV-infected patients who acquired their infection via blood transfusion is approximately 10 to 20 percent.[4,5] By contrast, the rate of male-to-female transmission following sexual contact with bisexual males may be as high as 40 percent. It is not clear why the efficiency of heterosexual transmission in Africa is so high, reaching 40 to 60 percent by some estimates.

Cofactors such as the presence of coinfection with herpes simplex virus (HSV) or other causes of genital ulcers play a role in determining the "efficiency" of transmission.[6–8] Epidemiologic data from Africa have shown higher rates of HIV infection in patients with coexistent syphilis, chancroid, HSV, and *Chlamydia* infection. In the infected individual concomitant infection with other viruses may upregulate HIV production, thus increasing viral load and favoring HIV transmission. Antiretroviral therapy can decrease viral load and could conceivably make transmission less likely, although there are little data to support this hypothesis.

VIROLOGY

The structure of HIV is similar to that of other retroviruses.[9–11] HIV has a viral core consisting of two identical strands of RNA, replicative enzymes including reverse transcriptase and core proteins, and an envelope protein (gp120) with a transmembrane component (gp41). The viral genome consists of both structural and, unlike other retroviruses, regulatory genes. The structural gene, *gag*, encodes for core proteins p15, p17, and p24, which are initially synthesized as a precursor molecule, p55, and which is cleaved by viral protease. The *pol* gene encodes for reverse transcriptase (RNA-dependent DNA polymerase), protease, integrase, and RNase H. RNase H degrades RNA in a DNA-RNA complex. The *env* gene encodes for gp160, which is cleaved to form the outer membrane protein gp120 and the transmembrane component gp41. Other portions of the viral genome include the long-terminal repeat sequences (LTRs) located at either end of the RNA molecule and at least six additional genes: *tat, rev, vif, nef, vpr,* and *vpu.* These genes encode for regulatory and accessory functions and play key roles in the viral life cycle.

PATHOGENESIS
Intracellular Events

Infection with HIV is initiated by the binding of virus to host cells. This binding is mediated through the CD4 receptor on the cell surface of T lymphocytes, macrophages, Langerhans cells, and follicular dendritic cells. A specific interaction exists between viral gp120 and the CD4 receptor. Binding of gp120 with CD4 is not the only mechanism of infection, however, because viral infection of cells lacking CD4 antigen has also been demonstrated. HIV infection of nerve tissue cell lines is mediated by the binding of gp120 to a galactosyl ceramide cell surface receptor.[12,13] Renal glomerular endothelial and perhaps mesangial cells may also be infected in vitro.[14] Cells that lack the CD4 receptor may also be infected by HIV through antibody-Fc receptor facilitated attachment and entry[15–17] or via the complement receptor.[18]

After binding of HIV to the CD4 surface receptor, viral entry into the cell appears to be facilitated by viral gp41, the transmembrane protein.[19] Evidence to support this concept includes the finding that viral infection can be prevented in vitro by the administration of antibodies to gp41.[20] Once inside the cell, reverse transcription of viral RNA results in the production of double-stranded DNA.[11,17,21] This proviral DNA undergoes circularization, migrates to the nucleus, and is subsequently integrated into the host cell chromosome via viral integrase. Following integration there may be a prolonged state of latency in which there is no detectable expression of viral products. Alternatively, viral replication may occur with transcription of proviral DNA, production of viral RNA and viral proteins, and release of viral progeny. Both the viral RNA-dependent DNA polymerase and the cellular RNA polymerase that forms the new viral genome lack an error-correction mechanism and therefore mutations are frequent.[10] Mutations involving the *env* gene are frequently larger ones involving insertions or deletions, whereas the *gag* and *pol* genes are most commonly affected by point mutations.[22]

A multiplicity of factors such as coinfection with other viruses and local and systemic cytokine levels may influence the development of productive infection. Studies in several laboratories have shown that HIV replication does not readily occur in resting cells. Reverse transcription, integration, and spread of virus occurs much more efficiently in activated T cells, and T lymphocytes with latent HIV infection do not express virus unless there is cellular activation.[17,23] Cellular expression of HIV may be upregulated by transfection with other viruses, especially HSV and cytomegalovirus (CMV).[17,23–25]

Examination of peripheral blood mononuclear cells (PBMCs) for expression of HIV mRNA or viral proteins by immunofluorescence or in situ hybridization has shown that only 1 in 10,000 to 1 in 100,000 lymphocytes are infected with HIV.[26,27] Utilization of the polymerase chain reaction (PCR) has allowed more precise enumeration of all cells with incorporation of HIV genetic material into the host cell genome. Using the PCR, the number of infected cells is higher in patients with AIDS (1/100)[27] compared with the number in patients with asymptomatic infection (1/100 to 1/100,000).[28] An increase in the proportion of infected cells may parallel immunologic and clinical disease progression.[29] HIV-infected circulating monocytes can be detected in less than 10 percent of asymptomatic individuals.[30]

Viral replication is governed by a combination of host factors and the products of viral regulatory genes.[10,11,31] Two of the most well-characterized viral regulatory genes are *tat* (transactivator of transcription) and *rev* (regulator of viral protein expression). These genes encode for polypeptides that upregulate viral replication. Both of these genes are trans-acting genes because their polypeptide products exert their effects on genes that are located some distance away from the *tat* and *rev* elements on the genome.

The binding of the *tat* polypeptide to the *tat* response element (TAR, *tat* acceptor region) on the LTR of the viral genome is critical for viral gene expression. Mutants that lack *tat* produce undetectable or minimal amounts of viral RNA. The primary role of *tat* is that of a transcriptional activator. Binding of *tat* to TAR increases the efficiency of initiation of transcription and stabilizes elongation of mRNA, whereas the absence of *tat* results in attenuated transcription.[31] The *tat* protein not only enhances the production of structural genes, but also acts to further augment its own production and that of other positive regulatory genes such as *rev*, thus acting as a potent amplifier of viral replication.[11]

The effects of *tat* may not be limited only to transactivation of HIV replication. *Tat* may also transactivate genes unrelated to HIV, such as those of the JC virus.[32] DNA viruses such as CMV and HSV may act as cofactors in HIV replication by activating T cells which will promote HIV replication.[17,23] In addition, exposure to *tat* results in increased production of cytokines such as tumor necrosis factor-α (TNF-α), interleukin-4 (IL-4), and transforming growth factor-β (TGF-β). In vitro data also suggest that *tat* may stimulate spindle cell proliferation and facilitate the development of Kaposi sarcoma.[33]

The *rev* element regulates the composition of viral cytoplasmic RNA.[10,31] Mutants that lack *rev* produce RNA that is distinctly different from the wild virus. There appears to be a sequential expression of RNA in cells infected with HIV. The RNA synthesized initially contains elements that encode for regulatory proteins, whereas the RNA that is produced later codes for structural elements of the virus. *rev* promotes the production of late-stage RNA that codes for structural proteins, which means that it also downregulates the production of viral progeny by reducing its own production and that of other regulatory products such as *tat*.

Another protein that enhances viral replication is viral protein R (*VPR* gene). This protein may be important at an early step in viral replication as it is packaged with other proteins during viral assembly.[34] Possible mechanisms involved in the action of viral protein R include stabilization of viral RNA, facilitation of reverse transcriptase, facilitation of migration of proviral DNA into the nucleus and integration into genomic DNA, or enhancement of expression of HIV-1 promoters.

Gene products that downregulate viral expression have also been identified. The *nef* gene product is a phosphoprotein associated with cytoplasmic membrane structures and may be important in signal transduction,[10,31] although its precise mechanism of action is unclear. Viruses constructed with mutations in the *nef* gene replicate more readily in in vitro culture systems.[35]

Host cellular proteins are also critical elements in the viral life cycle. Binding of host proteins to the LTR region may accelerate or inhibit viral replication. YC-1 is a cellular protein that binds to the LTR region and reduces transcription. Another cellular protein, nuclear factor κB (NF-κB), binds to a specific binding site on the HIV LTR and increases the rate of transcription initiation. NF-κB is a transcription factor that is induced during the T-cell response to infection by cytokines such as TNF-α, interleukin-1 (IL-1), interleukin-6 (IL-6), and granulocyte-macrophage colony stimulating factor (GM-CSF).[31]

Viral RNA is used as the template to make two types of precursor proteins: viral capsid proteins and replicative enzymes. These are assembled beneath the plasma membrane where a myristic acid attached to the viral capsid precursor protein facilitates their insertion into the host cell membrane.[21] gp120 is expressed on the surface of the host cell and during budding is incorporated into the outer membrane of the virus. There is a gene site specified as PSI, which may be involved in packaging of the virus.

Cellular Events

Following mucosal exposure to HIV the virus disseminates to lymphoid organs such as lymph nodes, spleen, and liver. In these organs the virus is trapped by follicular dendritic cells that may then present the virus to CD4+ lymphocytes and other cells.[36] The follicular dendritic cells have CD4 surface receptors and are permissive for replication of HIV. There is also evidence that intestinal M cells may allow transcellular migration of HIV with subsequent presentation to lymphocytes or macrophages at submucosal sites.[37] Early in the course of infection HIV is sequestered in lymphoid tissues trapped extracellularly by the follicular dendritic cells and is found in only small amounts in peripheral blood.[23,36,38] The virus actively replicates in lymph nodes even in this early asymptomatic "latent" period. Histopathologic studies have recently demonstrated that as time progresses the virus becomes localized primarily within lymphocytes within the germinal centers. There is progressive destruction of the follicular dendritic cell network, loss of trapping ability of the lymphoid organs, and spillage of virus into peripheral blood. Destruction of the follicular dendritic network may also impair the ability of the lymphoid system to trap other microorganisms.

There is strain variability in HIV with respect to surface structure and host cell/tissue tropism. Some strains replicate well in macrophages only, others in both lymphocytes and macrophages. Strains that are tropic for macrophages predominate early in infection, and can preferentially replicate by as much as 10,000-fold compared with their rate of replication in CD4+ lymphocytes.[39] Such macrophage-infecting strains may represent as many as 50 percent of clinical isolates.[30] Isolates that grow preferentially in macrophages are isolated more often from the CNS.[40] Switching from macrophage tropism to lymphocyte tropism has been well described,[41] and may be associated with disease progression.[11,42,43] Regulation of this type of cellular tropism has been recently localized to the gp120 surface glycoprotein in a non-CD4 binding region.[40,44,45]

HIV is not cytopathic for macrophages and can accumulate in intracellular compartments.[39,46] HIV-infected macrophages may represent a reservoir for delivery of virus to protected sites such as the CNS. Infected macrophages are believed to be located primarily in the tissues as less than 10 percent of patients have detectable HIV DNA in circulating monocytes, even in patients infected with macrophage tropic strains.[30] Specific subsets of macrophages such as those with a higher density of CD4 receptors may be at higher risk of infection or may be differentially affected by cytokines such as TNF-α or IL-6.

Immunopathogenesis

Because at most only 1 in 100 CD4+ lymphocytes is infected with HIV, it has been difficult to explain the profound decline in CD4+ lymphocyte numbers that is the hallmark of HIV infection. Potential mechanisms of lymphocyte destruction include direct lysis from budding virus, "innocent bystander" lysis of noninfected cells, or syncytia formation.[11] Apoptosis or programmed cell death is another recently postulated mechanism for cell depletion.[11,23,47] Apoptosis is a normal process in T-cell development whereby specific stimuli lead to death of immature thymocytes rather than cell proliferation and cytokine secretion. In HIV infection cell-associated or circulating gp120 may trigger this process in uninfected cells by cross-linking surface structures such as the CD4 receptor.[36,47] Lytic mechanisms in other cell types are less well understood. In neural cells lysis may occur through increases in intracellular calcium and effects on calcium channels.[48,49]

The immune response to HIV involves both the humoral and cellular immune system, although the relative impact of each of these components of the immune system in terms of protection or modification of infection is unclear. A specific antibody may be protective either through direct neutralization or via antibody-dependent cellular cytotoxicity (ADCC). Neutralizing antibodies have been detected to both core and envelope proteins, particularly the hypervariable (V3) loop of gp120. Unfortunately there is substantial antigenic variability in viral envelope proteins and the antigenic epitopes change frequently.[10]

The hallmark of AIDS is progressive loss of CD4 cells, with disruption of cellular immune responses. A specific population of T "memory" cells (CD29 + CD45RO +) appears to be preferentially infected with HIV.[50] These "memory" cells are responsible for the response to recall antigens and augmentation of B-cell function, and their functional impairment explains much of the immunologic dysfunction associated with HIV infection. HIV products such as gp120, tat protein, and gp41 can also suppress T-lymphocyte function.[51] Monocyte-macrophage function remains relatively intact during HIV infection, although abnormalities of chemotaxis have been reported.[52,53]

HIV infection is also associated with chronic immune activation.[54] There is spontaneous hyperactivation of B lymphocytes, monocyte activation, lymph node hyperplasia, and increased cytokine production. This is most evident during the early stages of HIV infection when there is a vigorous host response. HIV products may cause chronic stimulation of the immune response by acting as superantigens.[23] Superantigens are antigens that need only bind to the variable-β region of the T-cell antigen receptor and are not required to bind to the mixed histocompatibility (MHC) class II receptor or other sites on the T-cell antigen receptor to stimulate an immune response. This relatively nonspecific binding allows stimulation of a much larger fraction of T cells than would occur with more specific antigens.

A variety of cell-mediated lytic mechanisms have been well described in the host response to HIV infection, including ADCC, lysis by natural killer cells, and MHC class I restricted cytotoxic T-lymphocyte (CTL) mediated lysis.[23] Unfortunately HIV infection is associated with impairment of these lytic activities. Although most patients make antibodies capable of mediating ADCC, its value as a protective mechanism in HIV infection has not been established. Natural killer cell activity has also been shown to be impaired in patients with HIV infection.[55]

HIV-specific CD8+ CTLs may be one of the most critical cellular mechanisms for control of HIV infection. These cells have been detected in peripheral blood, cerebrospinal fluid, and bronchoalveolar lavage (BAL) fluid.[56-62] HIV-specific CD8+ CTLs inhibit viral replication in CD4+ cells in vitro.[63-65] The activity of the CTLs is directed against structural[56-62] and regulatory proteins,[56-62,66] both of which may be displayed on the cell surface in MHC class I restricted fashion. HIV infection results in a reduced capacity of CD8+ T cells to undergo clonal expansion[67] with resultant loss of HIV-specific cytolytic activity.[68,69] This decreased cellular immune function may be caused by atypical activation of CD8+ T cells or expansion of specific subsets of CD8+ cells, such as CD8+DR+ clones.[69]

Cytokines

The role of cytokines in the regulation of HIV expression is complex and is still being unraveled. Cytokines produced by both T cells and B cells may operate in both positive and negative feedback loops and may act at transcriptional and post-transcriptional levels.[11,23,36,54] Different cytokines produce markedly different effects on HIV expression and may vary depending on whether lymphocytes or monocytes are being studied. For example, IL-4 and interferon-γ (IFN-γ) increase HIV replication in lymphocytes, but decrease HIV expression in monocytes.[36] IFN-α decreases expression in both lymphocytes and monocytes, and may also interfere with the budding of HIV from the surface of the infected cell.[70] IL-1 (lymphocytes and monocytes), IL-6 (monocytes), and GM-CSF (monocytes) all increase HIV expression and replication.

Another cytokine, TNF-α, may be of special importance in the pathogenesis of HIV infection, and may be responsible in part for the wasting syndrome that is often seen in the late stages of HIV infection.[36] Elevated plasma levels of TNF-α have been noted in HIV-infected patients,[71,72] and in vitro studies with B lymphocytes obtained from HIV-infected subjects demonstrate increased spontaneous production of TNF-α.[73,74] TNF-α can also increase HIV expression in both lymphocytes and monocytes in vitro. The intracellular action of TNF-α is effected by NF-κB-mediated augmentation of gene transcription in the promoter region of HIV.[75]

Clones of CD4+ T-helper cells have been identified that facilitate cellular immunity and produce IL-2 and interferon-α (T_{H1} lymphocytes), with other clones facilitating humoral immunity and producing primarily IL-4, IL-6, and IL-10 (T_{H2} lymphocytes). A decrease in recall antigen stimulated IL-2 production with an associated rise in IL-4 synthesis has been noted during the course of progression of HIV infection, and may be detected prior to a decline in the CD4 count.[76] The cause of this "switch" from T_{H1} to T_{H2} cytokine production (IL-2 to IL-4 production) has been postulated to result from cross regulation by other cytokines such as IL-10. Alternatively, selective infection and depletion of T_{H1} lymphocytes may be responsible. This process may be facilitated by HIV-infected macrophages acting as the antigen-presenting cells for the T_{H1} response. This switch might be responsible for the immunologic sequelae of HIV infection, including loss of cell-mediated immune function and hyperactivation of antibody-producing cells.

The important role of cytokines in modulating viral replication is further evidenced by preliminary investigations in which viral expression and replication can be inhibited by selective cytokine blockade. Thalidomide reduces TNF-α production in vitro and reduces serum TNF-α levels in patients with lepromatous leprosy.[77] In vitro studies with PBMCs obtained from HIV-infected patients have shown that thalidomide reduces viral expression.[78] Other immunomodulators such as pentoxifylline,[79] which blocks secretion of TNF-α, and IL-1 receptor antagonist,[36] which competitively binds to the IL-1 receptor, inhibit replication of HIV in vitro.

CLINICAL MANIFESTATIONS

Classification of HIV Infection

The term *AIDS* was initially designated by the CDC in order to establish an epidemiologic framework to study the immunodeficiency syndrome. The clinical stages of HIV infection have been subject to several classification schemes, including adult and pediatric classifications by the CDC[80–82] and the Walter Reed schema.[83] In the early 1980s, AIDS was narrowly defined for epidemiologic purposes; however, over the past 10 years an appreciation of the spectrum and continuum of disease caused by HIV has developed. The most recent CDC classification focuses on HIV as a viral infection with a broad spectrum of clinical manifestations and a continuum of immunologic and clinical deterioration.[82] The 1993 revised classification also focuses on the importance of the CD4 lymphocyte in the natural history of HIV infection. All individuals with less than 200 CD4 cells/μl are classified as having AIDS, as well as those with more progressive symptoms, opportunistic infections, or related neoplasms.

Acute Infection

Symptoms of primary or acute infection may occur in 50 to 90 percent of seroconverters, typically 2 to 4 weeks after exposure.[84,85] Data concerning acute infection have accumulated from transfusion recipients, infected health care workers, and others with definite dates of HIV exposure. The syndrome is manifested as a nonspecific viral illness similar to acute mononucleosis.[84,86] Symptoms include fever, myalgias, arthralgias, a maculopapular or morbilliform rash, and lymphadenopathy. A viral or "aseptic" meningitis may also develop during this period. High levels of HIV viremia can be detected by viral cocultivation or measurement of p24 antigen in

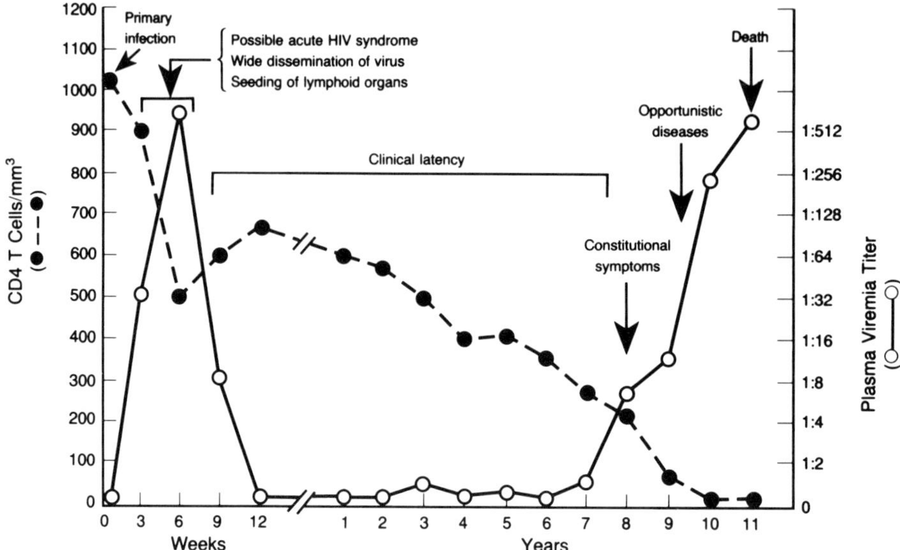

Fig. 1-1. The natural history of HIV infection. (From Pantaleo et al.,[23] with permission.)

serum[23,85,87,88] (Fig. 1-1). Serum antibodies are detectable by enzyme-linked immunosorbent assay (ELISA) or Western blot 1 to 2 months after the onset of the clinical syndrome. As serum p24 antibody is detected, the serum p24 antigen level will decline and not reappear until later in the course of the illness. The impact of therapy at this early stage of HIV infection has not yet been clarified.[85]

Asymptomatic Infection

The asymptomatic interval is quite variable and may last for several years. Despite the absence of clinical symptoms, gradual deterioration of the immune system ensues. This group is meant to include only individuals with early HIV infection and would not include someone who is asymptomatic following an opportunistic infection.

Progressive Generalized Lymphadenopathy

As HIV infection progresses many patients will develop persistently enlarged lymph nodes. This phase has been termed persistent generalized lymphadenopathy (PGL) or the lymphadenopathy syndrome (LAS). PGL has been defined as lymph nodes larger than 1 cm in diameter involving two or more extrainguinal sites, in the absence of any other etiology. Certain lymph node groups appear to be preferentially involved, particularly the posterior cervical and occipital nodes.[89] Histopathologic examination reveals nonspecific lymphoid hyperplasia. Viral replication continues in lymph nodes throughout the asymptomatic period, and the viral load within these enlarged lymph nodes may be much higher than that found in peripheral blood.[36] Involution of enlarged lymph nodes is a poor prognostic sign and reflects lymphocyte depletion.

Advanced Disease

As the CD4 count declines during the course of HIV infection, a variety of HIV-associated symptoms can develop (Fig. 1-1). These include "minor" infections such as oral or vaginal candidiasis or herpes zoster, bacillary angiomatosis, oral hairy leukoplakia, listeriosis, and pelvic inflammatory disease.[82] Constitutional symptoms such as fever, weight loss, night sweats, and unexplained diarrhea may also be present; this combination of symptoms was previously termed AIDS-related complex (ARC). Other clinical manifestations of HIV infection such as idiopathic thrombocytopenic purpura, HIV cardiomyopathy, and cervical dysplasia would also be included in this category.

A number of conditions developing late in the course of HIV infection are reflective of more severe impairment of host immune function. Patients with all levels of CD4 lymphocyte counts and conditions in this category are designated as having AIDS. HIV encephalopathy, the HIV wasting syndrome, HIV-related neoplasms, and major secondary opportunistic infections are included.

Neurologic Disease

Evidence of HIV infection of the CNS can be detected very early after infection, manifested by pleocytosis, elevated cerebrospinal fluid protein levels, positive HIV culture, and oligoclonal protein bands on cerebrospinal fluid examination.[90,91] These laboratory abnormalities may be difficult to distinguish from other processes such as neurosyphilis or tuberculous meningitis. Later in the course of HIV infection HIV encephalopathy may develop.[92] It may be gradual in onset and inapparent unless sophisticated neuropsychiatric testing is performed. Progression to psychomotor retardation and coma is not uncommon. A vacuolar myelopathy may develop as well. Peripheral neuropathy, either sensory or inflammatory motor, is common in patients with moderately advanced or severely advanced disease. Differentiation from neuropathy as a complication of antiretroviral therapy may be difficult.

Opportunistic Infections

A large set of major infections represent those established as "AIDS defining conditions": *P. carinii* infection; cryptococcosis; disseminated histoplasmosis; coccidioidomycosis; disseminated CMV infection or CMV retinitis; cerebral toxoplasmosis; *Mycobacterium avium-intracellulare, M. kansasii,* or *M. tuberculosis* infection; esophageal or tracheobronchial candidiasis; chronic ulcerative HSV infection; progressive multifocal leukoencephalopathy (PML); cryptosporidiosis; isosporiasis; strongyloidiasis; recurrent *Salmonella* bacteremia; and recurrent bacterial pneumonias. These infections are thought to represent evidence of more significant immunosuppression.

Malignancies

Several neoplasms have been associated with HIV infection. These include B-cell tumors such as Hodgkin's and non-Hodgkin's lymphoma, Burkitt's lymphoma, and primary CNS lymphoma.[93] The development of these tumors is believed to be related to Epstein-Barr virus infection. Other HIV-related tumors include Kaposi sarcoma,[33,94] squamous cell carcinoma of the rectum, and human papillomavirus-related invasive cervical cancer.[95–97]

HIV Infection in Women

The incidence of HIV infection in women is increasing and HIV is now the fourth most frequent cause of death in women 25 to 44 years of age.[3] The natural history of HIV infection in women may be somewhat different from that of HIV infection in men. Candidiasis is a common problem, particularly chronic or recurrent vaginal candidiasis. Vaginal candidiasis was seen in 70 percent of 24 Rhode Island women studied over a several year period.[98] Oral and esophageal candidiasis were also prominent problems. The incidence of *Pneumocystis* infection was quite low, occurring in only 30 percent, compared with 60 to 70 percent in HIV-infected homosexual men. There is no clear explanation for these differences in clinical presentation.

Human papilloma-virus-associated cervical dysplasia and neoplasia are also more commonly associated with HIV infection. Several studies have now demonstrated higher rates of cervical dysplasia, high-grade dysplasia, and multifocal lesions.[95–97] Papilloma virus infection is therefore more prevalent, and when it occurs, it tends to be more severe. In order to detect cervical neoplasia and atypia earlier, Papanicolaou smears are recommended every 6 months in HIV-infected women.[99]

HIV in Pregnancy

HIV infection occurs most commonly in sexually active women, who may become pregnant. In fact, routine screening during pregnancy often leads to an initial diagnosis of HIV infection. It has been suggested that pregnancy may accelerate the deterioration of immune function seen in HIV infection, although there are currently little clinical data to support this notion. Several studies have demonstrated that transmission to the fetus occurs in 20 to 30 percent of pregnancies.[100–104] Vertical transmission of HIV infection from mother to fetus may take place during pregnancy, or at delivery if transmission is similar to the mode of transmission of hepatitis B. Ninety-five percent of perinatal hepatitis B infections are estimated to occur at the time of delivery. In some cases fetal material recovered following interruption of pregnancy has been culture or PCR positive for HIV, supporting the concept of vertical transmission prior to delivery.[105–107] Risk factors for transmission during pregnancy include severe maternal disease, significant immunosuppression, viral load, and premature delivery.[100,108–111] There is evidence that antibodies against gp120, or particularly the V3 loop, may be protective.[112,113] Controversy exists as to whether cesarean section can decrease HIV transmission at the time of delivery.[109,114,115]

Clinical trials of antiretroviral therapy of HIV infection during pregnancy are currently being analyzed. A large multicenter study sponsored by the AIDS Clinical Trials Group (ACTG 076) was recently halted by the Data Safety Monitoring Board because zidovudine (ZDV) therapy substantially reduced the transmission of HIV during pregnancy.[116] ZDV was given to pregnant women with CD4 counts greater than $200/\mu l$ who were enrolled between 14 and 34 weeks of pregnancy. They also received intravenous ZDV during labor and the neonates received ZDV elixir. There was no increase in birth defects; however, potential long-term sequelae are unknown.

DISEASE PROGRESSION

Time to Progression

The latent period between the time of infection and the development of CDC-defined AIDS is the time to progression. Since the beginning of the HIV epidemic, considerable variability in time to development of clinical progression has been noted. This is undoubtedly multifactorial in origin, but may be related to host factors such as age,[117–119] coinfection with other viruses, or to viral virulence factors such as the ability to form syncytia in vitro.[120] The most informative studies are those in which the date of infection can be precisely determined. Cohort studies of homosexual men such as the San Francisco series or the Multicenter AIDS Cohort Study (MACS), and blood transfusion recipients have been studied in the most detail.[121–124] The median time for progression in these studies is approximately 10 years. Children and transfusion recipients may progress more rapidly.

Symptoms and Signs

Clinical progression of HIV infection has been associated with a number of symptoms and signs. The "constitutional" symptoms of persistent fever, weight loss, diarrhea, and night sweats have been associated with immunologic deterioration and identified as markers of poor prognosis.[89,124] Involution of lymph nodes, oral candidiasis, and oral hairy leukoplakia may be associated features. The risk of clinical progression also appears higher in individuals who had symptomatic rather than asymptomatic primary infection episodes.[125–128]

Laboratory Features

Immunologic deterioration is best measured by declining T-cell numbers with an estimated loss of 60 CD4 + cells/mm^3/y[129,130] (Fig. 1-1). Other "surrogate" markers of disease progression are elevated serum β_2-microglobulin and neopterin levels, and the presence of serum p24 antigen.[122,124,131] Serum p24 antigen is detectable early after infection prior to the development of p24 antibody, and again in the later stages of infection as viral burden increases. Elevated serum concentrations of soluble receptors for TNF-α may also correlate with progression.[132] Although the CD4 count is a valuable predictor of disease progression, it may be less useful as a surrogate marker of immunologic response to antiretroviral therapy.[133,134] A significant decline in CD4 numbers may herald the development of viral resistance.[135]

Recently, the ability of viral isolates to form syncytia in vitro has been linked to more rapid clinical progression, as is a switch from a nonsyncytium to syncytium-inducing phenotype.[120,136–138] A switch from macrophage tropic to lymphocyte tropic strains has also been linked to clinical progression.[11,42,43] Finally, recent results from an antiretroviral trial suggest that the development of resistance to ZDV is associated with more rapid progression of HIV infection.[139] The risk of development of *P. carinii* pneumonia is directly correlated with circulating CD4 lymphocyte number, the risk rising substantially when absolute CD4 counts drop below 200/μl.[140] This has been useful in identifying subgroups of patients that might benefit from anti-*Pneumocystis* prophylaxis.

Measures of Viral Load

Use of clinical endpoints (opportunistic infection, death) in clinical trials is being replaced by surrogate markers or more direct measurements of viral load. Indicators of viral load include serum acid-dissociated p24 antigen, plasma HIV viremia by in vitro culture, quantitation of DNA or RNA by PCR, or measurement of RNA by branched DNA (bDNA) assay.[141] Quantitative measurement of plasma viremia as an indicator of viral burden has been examined in several studies.[142,143] Using this technique virtually all patients with advanced disease will have detectable virus in plasma.[144,145] The amount of virus also is correlated with the stage of HIV infection.[137,143,146]

Quantitation of viral DNA by PCR has also been investigated as a measure of viral load and is closely correlated with the proportion of infected cells.[29] Patients who remain clinically stable over time have lower amounts of HIV as detected by quantitative DNA PCR. Substantially more virus is detectable in patients who undergo rapid clinical deterioration. Quantitation of HIV DNA is a measure of the number of infected cells, whereas RNA is a better measure of viral replicative activity. Recently, quantitation of viral RNA by bDNA assay has also correlated with clinical stage of disease.[141] Several of these techniques are currently being used to evaluate the response to antiretroviral therapy.

ANTIRETROVIRAL THERAPY

The advent of antiretroviral chemotherapy has made a significant impact on the care of individuals with HIV infection. Antiretroviral therapy has been shown to delay the fall in CD4 numbers, delay the development of opportunistic infection, and to improve survival in some populations.[147–151] The benefits of antiretroviral therapy have been best demonstrated in individuals with advanced disease, and the value of therapy early in the natural history of HIV infection remains controversial. In order to arrive at a more rapid evaluation of drug efficacy, recent clinical trials have focused on the use of surrogate markers as measures of therapeutic response. Increases in the absolute CD4 cell count have been noted with several agents; however, the increases are modest and may only partially account for the clinical benefit noted.[133,134,151] Current clinical trials are also focusing on measurement of viral load to determine response to antiretroviral therapy.

The drugs most studied to date are in the class of nucleoside analogs or chain terminating reverse transcriptase (RT) inhibitors. Included in this class are the FDA-approved agents zidovudine (ZDV, also known as azidothymidine [AZT]), didanosine (ddI), zalcitabine (ddC), stavudine (d4T), and investigational agents such as 3TC. Therapy is limited by substantial toxicity, waning efficacy, and the development of resistance. Resistance to ZDV can be detected as early as 3 months into therapy, and resistance develops more rapidly in individuals with lower CD4 counts and more advanced disease.[152,153] After 12 months of therapy with ZDV, 89 percent of isolates from individuals with advanced disease and 31 percent of those with early stage infection will have some level of resistance.[152] Mutations in the RT gene conferring resistance to ZDV and other nucleoside analogs have been mapped to multiple sites.[154–157]

The lack of sustained benefit of ZDV monotherapy and evidence for the development of resistance have led to trials of combination regimens using nucleoside analogs. Combination therapy has been postulated to improve efficacy, allow lower dosages leading to decreased toxicity, and to prevent the development of resistance. The combinations best studied to date are ZDV/ddC[158] and ZDV/ddI.[159,160] Combination therapy with ZDV/ddI appears to be more effective than alternating or sequential therapy with ZDV and ddI.[160] Non-nucleoside RT inhibitors have also been developed that bind to alternative sites and presumably act by altering the conformation of RT. Several of these compounds (nevirapine, atevirdine, delavirdine) are currently being studied in clinical trials. They rapidly select for resistance and therefore will only be used in combination regimens. Clinical trials with agents directed against alternative targets in the HIV life cycle, such as protease and *tat* inhibitors, are currently underway.

Optimal therapy requires an individualized approach based on clinical stage, prior antiretroviral exposure, and the presence of clinical or laboratory evidence of disease progression. ZDV is recommended as initial therapy for symptomatic individuals with less than 200 CD4 cells/µl. Most clinicians recommend ZDV for asymptomatic individuals between 200 cells/µl and 500 cells/µl, although this is controversial. For those with less than 200 CD4 cells/µl, combination therapy with ZDV/ddI or ZDV/ddC should be considered. Patients who are intolerant of ZDV or who demonstrate clinical progression on ZDV may be switched to ddI or ddC, or given combination therapy with ZDV/ddI or ZDV/ddC.

SUMMARY

HIV is a retrovirus capable of latency in a variety of human cells. A number of viral genes have been identified that code for structural proteins and enzymes necessary for viral replication, viral integration into the host genome, and post-translational protein modification. Viral regulatory proteins either increase or decrease viral gene expression in different cell types. The pathogenesis of infection involves a complicated series of intracellular and extracellular events leading to depletion of CD4 + T lymphocytes and substantial alterations in immune function. The interactions between cellular cytokines and viral activation are complex and are still being elucidated.

After exposure to the virus most individuals develop a primary infection syndrome followed by a long asymptomatic or latent period. During this period there is continued replication of HIV in the lymphoid tissue with gradual destruction of the lymph node architecture. Associated with declining immune function are a number of infectious complications, neurologic manifestations, and HIV-associated malignancies. Clinical progression is directly related to declining CD4 cell numbers, increase in measures of viral load, and change to syncytium-inducing phenotypes. Single-agent or combination antiretroviral therapy may alter the natural history of HIV infection.

REFERENCES

1. Centers for Disease Control and Prevention: Kaposi's sarcoma and *Pneumocystis* pneumonia among homosexual men—New York City and California. MMWR 30:305, 1981
2. Centers for Disease Control and Prevention: HIV/AIDS surveillance report. Vol. 5. p. 3. US Department of Health and Human Services, Public Health Service, Atlanta, 1993
3. Centers for Disease Control and Prevention: Mortality attributable to HIV

infection among persons aged 25–44 years—United States 1991 and 1992. MMWR 42:869, 1993

4. Peterman TA, Stoneburner RL, Allen JR et al: Risk of human immunodeficiency virus transmission from heterosexual adults with transfusion-associated infections. JAMA 259:55, 1988

5. Anderson RM, May RM: Epidemiological parameters of HIV transmission. Nature 333:514, 1988

6. Plummer FA, Simonsen JN, Cameron DW et al: Cofactors in male-female sexual transmission of human immunodeficiency virus type 1. J Infect Dis 163:233, 1991

7. Hook EW, Cannon RO, Hanmias AJ et al: Herpes simplex virus infection as a risk factor for human immunodeficiency virus infection in heterosexuals. J Infect Dis 165:251, 1992

8. Telzak EE, Chiasson MA, Bevier PJ et al: HIV-1 seroconversion in patients with and without genital ulcer disease. Ann Intern Med 119:1181, 1993

9. Vaishnav YN, Wong-Staal F: The biochemistry of AIDS. Annu Rev Biochem 60:577, 1991

10. Bryant ML, Ratner L: Biology and molecular biology of human immunodeficiency virus. Pediatr Infect Dis J 11:390, 1992

11. Levy JA: Pathogenesis of human immunodeficiency virus infection. Microbiol Rev 57:183, 1993

12. Harouse JM, Bhat S, Spitalnik SL et al: Inhibition of entry of HIV-1 in neural cell lines by antibodies against galactosyl ceramide. Science 253:320, 1991

13. Bhat S, Spitalnik SL, Gonzalez-Scarano F: Galactosyl ceramide or a derivative is an essential component of the neural receptor for human immunodeficiency virus type 1 envelope glycoprotein gp120. Proc Natl Acad Sci USA 88:7131, 1991

14. Green DF, Resnick L, Bourgoignie JJ: HIV infects glomerular endothelial and mesangial but not epithelial cells in vitro. Kidney Int 41:956, 1992

15. Takeda A, Tuazon CU, Ennis FA: Antibody-enhanced infection by HIV-1 via Fc receptor-mediated entry. Science 242:580, 1988

16. Homsy J, Meyer M, Levy JA: Serum enhancement of HIV infection correlates with disease in HIV-infected individuals. J Virol 64:1437, 1990

17. Rosenberg ZF, Fauci AS: Immunopathogenesis of HIV infection. FASEB J 5:2382, 1991

18. Robinson WE, Kawamura T, Gorny MK et al: Human monoclonal antibodies to the human immunodeficiency virus type 1 (HIV-1) transmembrane glycoprotein gp41 enhance HIV-1 infection in vitro. Proc Natl Acad Sci USA 87:3185, 1990

19. Kowalski M, Bergeron K, Dorfman T et al: Attenuation of human immunodeficiency virus type 1 (HIV-1) cytopathic effect by a mutation affecting the transmembrane envelope glycoprotein. J Virol 65:281, 1991

20. Ho DD, Sarngadharan MG, Hirsch MS et al: Human immunodeficiency virus neutralizing antibodies recognize several conserved domains on the envelope glycoproteins. J Virol 61:2024, 1987

21. Haseltine WA: Molecular biology of the human immunodeficiency virus type 1. FASEB J 5:2349, 1991

22. Dougherty JP, Temin HM: Determination of the rate of base-pair substitution and insertion mutation in retrovirus replication. J Virol 62:2817, 1988

23. Pantaleo G, Graziosi C, Fauci A: The immunopathogenesis of human immunodeficiency virus infection. N Engl J Med 328:327, 1993

24. Gendelman HE, Phelps W, Feigenbaum L et al: Trans-activation of the human immunodeficiency virus long terminal repeat sequence by DNA viruses. Proc Natl Acad Sci USA 83:9759, 1986

25. Mosca JD, Bednarik DP, Raj NB et al: Activation of human immunodeficiency virus by herpesvirus infection: identification of a region within the long terminal repeat that responds to a trans-acting factor encoded by herpes simplex virus 1. Proc Natl Acad Sci USA 84:7408, 1987

26. Harper ME, Marselle LM, Gallo RC et al: Detection of lymphocytes expressing human T-lymphotropic virus type III in lymph nodes and peripheral blood from infected individuals by in situ hybridization. Proc Natl Acad Sci USA 83:772, 1986

27. Schnittman SM, Psallidopoulos MC, Lane HC et al: The reservoir for HIV-1 in human peripheral blood is a T cell that maintains expression of CD4. Science 245:305, 1989

28. Psallidopoulos MC, Schnittman SN, Thompson LM et al: Integrated proviral human immunodeficiency virus type 1 is present in CD4 + peripheral blood lymphocytes in healthy seropositive individuals. J Virol 63:4626, 1989

29. Schnittman SM, Greenhouse JJ, Psallidopoulos MC et al: Increasing viral burden in CD4 + T cell from patients with human immunodeficiency virus (HIV) infection reflects rapidly progressive immunosuppression and clinical disease. Ann Intern Med 113:438, 1990

30. Poli G: The role of mononuclear phagocytes in the pathogenesis of HIV infection. p. 683. In Fauci AS (moderator): Immunopathogenic mechanisms in human immunodeficiency virus (HIV) infection. Ann Intern Med 114:678, 1991

31. Cullen BR: Regulation of HIV-1 gene expression. FASEB J 5:2361, 1991

32. Tada H, Rappaport J, Lashgari M et al: Trans-activation of the JC virus late promoter by the tat protein of type 1 human immunodeficiency virus in glial cells. Proc Natl Acad Sci USA 87:3479, 1990

33. Ensoli B, Barillari G, Zaki Salahuddin S et al: Tat protein of HIV-1 stimulates growth of cells derived from Kaposi's sarcoma lesions of AIDS patients. Nature 345:84, 1990

34. Cohen EA, Terwilliger EF, Jalinoos Y et al: Identification of HIV-1 vpr product and function. J AIDS 3:11, 1990

35. Cheng-Mayer C, Iannello P, Shaw K et al: Differential effects of nef on HIV replication: implications for viral pathogenesis in the host. Science 246:1629, 1989

36. Fauci AS: Multifactorial nature of human immunodeficiency virus disease: implications for therapy. Science 262:1011, 1993

37. Amerongen HM, Weltzin R, Farnet CM et al: Transepithelial transport of HIV-1 by intestinal M cells: a mechanism for transmission of AIDS. J AIDS 4:760, 1991

38. Pantaleo G, Graziosi C, Demarest JF et al: HIV infection is active and progressive in lymphoid tissue during the clinically latent stage of disease. Nature 362:355, 1993

39. Gartner S, Markovits P, Markovitz DM et al: The role of mononuclear phagocytes in HTLV-III/LAV infection. Science 233:215, 1986

40. Westervelt P, Gendelman HE, Ratner L: Identification of a determinant within the human immunodeficiency virus 1 surface envelope glycoprotein critical for productive infection of primary monocytes. Proc Natl Acad Sci USA 88:3097, 1991

41. Weiss SH, Goedert JJ, Gartner S et al: Risk of human immunodeficiency virus (HIV-1) infection among laboratory workers. Science 239:68, 1988
42. Schuitemaker H, Koot M, Kootstra NA et al: Biological phenotype of human immunodeficiency virus type 1 clones at different stages of infection: progression of disease is associated with a shift from monocytotropic to T-cell-tropic virus populations. J Virol 66:1354, 1992
43. Cheng-Mayer C, Weiss C, Seto D et al: Isolates of human immunodeficiency virus type 1 from the brain may constitute a special group of the AIDS virus. Proc Natl Acad Sci USA 80:8575, 1989
44. Liu Z, Wood C, Levy J et al: The viral envelope gene is involved in macrophage tropism of a human immunodeficiency virus type 1 strain isolated from brain tissue. J Virol 64:6148, 1990
45. O'Brien WA, Koyanagi Y, Namazie A et al: HIV-1 tropism for mononuclear phagocytes can be determined by regions of gp120 outside the CD4-binding domain. Nature 348:69, 1990
46. Gendelman HE, Orenstein JM, Martin MA et al: Efficient isolation and propagation of human immunodeficiency virus on recombinant colony-stimulating factor 1-treated monocytes. J Exp Med 167:1428, 1988
47. Gougeon ML, Montagnier L: Apoptosis in AIDS. Science 260:1269, 1993
48. Brenneman DE, Westbrook GL, Fitzgerald SP et al: Neuronal cell killing by the envelope protein of HIV and its prevention by vasoactive intestinal peptide. Nature 335:639, 1988
49. Dreyer EB, Kaiser PK, Offermann JT et al: HIV-1 coat protein neurotoxicity prevented by calcium channel antagonists. Science 248:364, 1990
50. Schnittman SM, Lane HC, Greenhouse J et al: Preferential infection of CD4 + memory T cells by human immunodeficiency virus type 1: evidence for a role in the selective T-cell functional defects observed in infected individuals. Proc Natl Acad Sci USA 87:6058, 1990
51. Krowka J, Stites D, Mills J et al: Effects of interleukin 2 and large envelope glycoprotein (gp120) of human immunodeficiency virus (HIV) on lymphocyte proliferative responses to cytomegalovirus. Clin Exp Immunol 72:179, 1988
52. Poli G, Bottazzi B, Acero R et al: Monocyte function in intravenous drug abusers with lymphadenopathy syndrome and in patients with acquired immunodeficiency syndrome: selective impairment of chemotaxis. Clin Exp Immunol 62: 136, 1985
53. Rosenberg ZF, Fauci AS: The immunopathogenesis of HIV infections. Adv Immunol 47:377, 1989
54. Fauci AS: The relation between HIV and the human immune system. p. 678. In Fauci AS (moderator): Immunopathogenic mechanisms in human immunodeficiency virus (HIV) infection. Ann Intern Med 114:678, 1991
55. Bonavida B, Katz J, Gottlieb M: Mechanism of defective NK cell activity in patients with acquired immunodeficiency syndrome (AIDS) and AIDS-related complex. I. Defective trigger on NK cells for NFKB production by target cells and partial restoration by IL 2. J Immunol 137:1157, 1986
56. Walker BD, Charrabarti S, Moss B et al: HIV-specific cytotoxic T lymphocytes in seropositive individuals. Nature 328:345, 1987
57. Plata F, Autran B, Martins LP et al: AIDS virus-specific cytotoxic T lymphocytes in lung disorders. Nature 328:348, 1987
58. Sethi KK, Naher H, Stroehmann I: Phenotypic heterogeneity of cerebrospinal fluid-derived HIV-specific and HLA-restricted cytotoxic T-cell clones. Nature 335:178, 1988

59. Koenig S, Earl P, Powell D et al: Group-specific, major histocompatibility complex class I-restricted cytotoxic responses to human immunodeficiency virus 1 (HIV-1) envelope proteins by cloned peripheral blood T cells from an HIV infected individual. Proc Natl Acad Sci USA 85:8638, 1988

60. Nixon DF, Townsend AR, Elvin JG et al: HIV-1 gag-specific cytotoxic T lymphocytes defined with recombinant vaccinia virus and synthetic peptides. Nature 336:484, 1988

61. Koup RA, Sullivan JL, Levine PH et al: Detection of major histocompatibility complex class 1-restricted, HIV-specific cytotoxic T lymphocytes in the blood in infected hemophiliacs. Blood 73:1909, 1989

62. Riviere Y, Tanneau-Salvadori F, Regnault A et al: Human immunodeficiency virus-specific cytotoxic responses of seropositive individuals: distinct types of effector cells mediate killings of targets expressing gag and env proteins. J Virol 63:2270, 1989

63. Tsubota H, Lord CI, Watkins DI et al: A cytotoxic T lymphocyte inhibits acquired immunodeficiency syndrome virus replication in peripheral blood lymphocytes. J Exp Med 169:1421, 1989

64. Walker CM, Moody DJ, Sites DP et al: CD8+ T lymphocyte control of HIV replication in cultured CD4+ cells varies among infected individuals. Cell Immunol 119:470, 1989

65. Koenig S: HIV-specific immunity and the pathogenesis of AIDS. p. 685. In Fauci AS (moderator): Immunopathogenic mechanisms in human immunodeficiency virus (HIV) infection. Ann Intern Med 114:678, 1991

66. Koenig S, Fuerst TR, Wood LV et al: Mapping the fine specificity of a cytolytic T cell response to HIV-1 nef protein. J Immunol 145:127, 1990

67. Margolick JB, Volkman DJ, Lane HC et al: Clonal analysis of T lymphocytes in the acquired immunodeficiency syndrome. Evidence for an abnormality affecting individual helper and suppressor T cells. J Clin Invest 76:709, 1985

68. Hoffenbach A, Langlade-Demoyen P, Dadaglio G et al: Unusually high frequencies of HIV-specific cytotoxic T lymphocytes in humans. J Immunol 142:452, 1989

69. Pantaleo G: Mechanisms of CD8+ cell dysfunction in HIV infection. p. 687. In Fauci AS (moderator): Immunopathogenic mechanisms in human immunodeficiency virus (HIV) infection. Ann Intern Med 114:678, 1991

70. Poli G, Orenstein JM, Kinter A et al: Interferon-alpha but not AZT suppresses HIV expression in chronically infected cell lines. Science 224:575, 1989

71. Lahdevitra J, Maury CP, Teppo AM et al: Elevated levels of circulation cachectin/tumor necrosis factor in patients with acquired immunodeficiency syndrome. Am J Med 85:289, 1988

72. Poli G, Fauci AS: Cytokine modulation of HIV expression. Semin Immunol 5:165, 1993

73. Rieckmann P, Poli G, Kehrl JH et al: Activated B lymphocytes from human immunodeficiency virus-infected individuals induce virus expression in infected T cells and a promonocytic cell line, U1. J Exp Med 173:1, 1991

74. Boue F, Wallon C, Goujard C et al: HIV induces IL-6 production by human B lymphocytes: role of IL-4. J Immunol 148:3761, 1992

75. Duh EJ, Maury WJ, Folks TM et al: Tumor necrosis factor alpha activates human immunodeficiency virus type 1 through induction of nuclear factor binding to the NF-kappa B sites in the long terminal repeat. Proc Natl Acad Sci USA 86:5974, 1989

76. Clerici M, Hakim FT, Venzon DJ et al: Changes in interleukin-2 and interleukin-4 production in asymptomatic, human immunodeficiency virus-positive individuals. J Clin Invest 91:759, 1993
77. Sampaio EP, Moreira AL, Sarno EN et al: Prolonged treatment with recombinant interferon γ induces erythema nodosum leprosum in lepromatous leprosy patients. J Exp Med 175:1729, 1992
78. Makonkawkeyoon S, Limson-Pobre RN, Moreira AL et al: Thalidomide inhibits the replication of human immunodeficiency virus type 1. Proc Natl Acad Sci USA 90:5974, 1993
79. Fazely F, Dezube BJ, Allen-Ryan J et al: Pentoxifylline (Trental) decreases the replication of the human immunodeficiency virus type 1 in human peripheral blood mononuclear cells and in cultured T cells. Blood 77:1653, 1991
80. Centers for Disease Control and Prevention: Classification system for human T-lymphotropic virus type III/lymphadenopathy-associated virus infections. MMWR 35:334, 1986
81. Centers for Disease Control and Prevention: Revision of the CDC surveillance case definition for acquired immunodeficiency syndrome. MMWR 36:1S, 1987
82. Centers for Disease Control and Prevention: 1993 revised classification system for HIV infection and expanded surveillance case definition for AIDS among adolescents and adults. MMWR 41(RR-17):1, 1992
83. Redfield RR, Wright DC, Tramont EC: The Walter Reed staging classification for HTLV-III/LAV infection. N Engl J Med 314:131, 1986
84. Ho DD, Sarngadharan MG, Resnick L et al: Primary human T-lymphotropic virus type III infection. Ann Intern Med 103:880, 1985
85. Niu MT, Stein DS, Schnittman SM: Primary human immunodeficiency virus type 1 infection: review of pathogenesis and early treatment intervention in humans and animal retrovirus infections. J Infect Dis 168:1490, 1993
86. Fox R, Eldred LJ, Fuchs EJ et al: Clinical manifestations of acute infection with human immunodeficiency virus in a cohort of gay men. AIDS 1:35, 1987
87. Clark SJ, Saag MS, Decker WD et al: High titers of cytopathic virus in plasma of patients with symptomatic primary HIV-1 infection. N Engl J Med 324:954, 1991
88. Daar ES, Moudgil T, Meyer RE et al: Transient high levels of viremia in patients with primary human immunodeficiency virus type 1 infection. N Engl J Med 324:961, 1991
89. Kaslow RA, Phair JP, Friedman HB et al: Infection with the human immunodeficiency virus: clinical manifestations and their relationship to immune deficiency. Ann Intern Med 107:474, 1987
90. Ho DD, Rota TR, Schooley RT et al: Isolation of HTLV-III from cerebrospinal fluid and neural tissues of patients with neurologic syndromes related to the acquired immunodeficiency syndrome. N Engl J Med 313:1493, 1985
91. Hollander H, Stringari S: Human immunodeficiency virus-associated meningitis: clinical course and correlations. Am J Med 83:813, 1987
92. McArthur JC: Neurologic manifestations of AIDS. Medicine 66:407, 1987
93. Kaplan LD: HIV-associated lymphoma. AIDS Clin Rev 145, 1993–94
94. Mitsuyasu RT: Clinical aspects of AIDS-related Kaposi's sarcoma. Curr Opin Oncol 5:835, 1993
95. Feingold AR, Vermund SH, Burk RD et al: Cervical cytologic abnormalities and papillomavirus in women infected with human immunodeficiency virus. J AIDS 3:896, 1990

96. Maiman M, Fruchter RG, Serur E et al: Human immunodeficiency virus infection and cervical neoplasia. Gynecol Oncol 38:377, 1990
97. Centers for Disease Control and Prevention: Risk for cervical disease in HIV-infected women—New York City. MMWR 39:846, 1990
98. Carpenter CC, Mayer KH, Fisher A et al: Natural history of acquired immunodeficiency syndrome in women in Rhode Island. Am J Med 86:771, 1989
99. Minkoff HL, DeHovitz JA: Care of women infected with the human immunodeficiency virus. JAMA 266:2253, 1991
100. Goedert JJ, Drummond JE, Minkoff HL et al: Mother-to-infant transmission of human immunodeficiency virus type 1: association with prematurity or low anti-gp120. Lancet 2:1351, 1989
101. Blanche S, Rouzioux C, Guihard Moscato ML et al: A prospective study of infants born to women seropositive for human immunodeficiency virus type 1. N Engl J Med 320:1643, 1989
102. Andiman WA, Simpson BJ, Olson B et al: Rate of transmission of human immunodeficiency virus type 1 infection from mother to child and short-term outcome of neonatal infection. Am J Dis Child 144:758, 1990
103. Halsey N, Boulos R, Holt E et al: Transmission of HIV-1 infections from mothers to infants in Haiti. JAMA 264:2088, 1990
104. Ryder R, Nsa W, Hassig S et al: Perinatal transmission of the human immunodeficiency virus type 1 to infants of seropositive women in Zaire. N Engl J Med 320:1637, 1992
105. Jovaisas E, Koch MA, Schafer A et al: LAV/HTLV-III in a 20 week fetus. Lancet 2:1129, 1985
106. Sprecher S, Soumenkoff G, Puissant F et al: Vertical transmission of human immunodeficiency virus (HIV) in a 15-week fetus. Lancet 2:228, 1986
107. Lyman WD, Kress Y, Kure K et al: Detection of HIV in fetal central nervous system tissue. AIDS 4:917, 1990
108. Gabiano C, Tovo PA, de Martino M et al: Mother to child transmission of HIV: risk of infection and correlates of transmission. Pediatrics 90:369, 1992
109. Newell ML, Dunn D, Peckham CS et al: Risk factors for mother-to-child transmission of HIV-1: European Collaborative Study. Lancet 339:1007, 1992
110. Mofenson LM: Preventing mother to infant HIV transmission: what we know so far. The AIDS Reader, March/April 1992
111. St. Louis ME, Brown C, Kamenga M et al: High maternal CD8+ lymphocyte counts predict increased risk for perinatal HIV-1 transmission. Ninth International Conference on AIDS, Berlin, 1993, p. 83. abstract no. WS-CO2-5
112. Scarlatti G, Albert J, Rossi P et al: Mother-to-child transmission of human immunodeficiency virus type 1: correlation with neutralizing antibodies against primary isolates. J Infect Dis 168:207, 1993
113. Markham RB, Coberly J, Ruff AJ et al: Maternal IgG1 and IgA antibody to V3 loop consensus sequence and maternal-infant HIV-1 transmission. Lancet 343:390, 1994
114. Goedert JJ, Duliege AM, Amos CI et al: High risk of HIV-1 infection for first born twins. Lancet 338:1471, 1991
115. Tovo PA: Caesarean section and perinatal HIV transmission: what next? Lancet 342:630, 1993
116. Connor EM, Sperling RS, Gelber R et al: Reduction of maternal-infant transmission of human immunodeficiency virus type 1 with zidovudine therapy. N Engl J Med 331:1173, 1994

117. Eyster ME, Gail MH, Ballard JO et al: Natural history of human immunodeficiency virus infections in hemophiliacs: effects of T-cell subsets, platelet counts, and age. Ann Intern Med 107:1, 1987

118. Blaxhult A, Granath F, Lidman K et al: The influence of age on the latency period to AIDS in people infected by HIV through blood transfusion. AIDS 4: 125, 1990

119. Phillips AN, Lee CA, Elford J et al: More rapid progression to AIDS in older HIV-infected people: the role of CD4+ T-cell counts. J AIDS 4:970, 1991

120. Koot M, Keet IP, Vos AH et al: Prognostic value of HIV-1 syncytium-inducing phenotype for rate of CD4+ cell depletion and progression to AIDS. Ann Intern Med 118:681, 1993

121. Medley GF, Anderson RM, Cox DR et al: Incubation period of AIDS in patients infected via blood transfusion. Nature 328:719, 1987

122. Moss AR, Bachetti P, Osmund D et al: Seropositivity for HIV and the development of AIDS or AIDS-related condition: three-year follow-up of the San Francisco cohort. BMJ 296:745, 1988

123. Giesecke J, Scalla-Tomba G, Berglund O et al: Incidence of symptoms and AIDS in 146 HIV-infected Swedish hemophiliacs and blood-transfusion recipients. BMJ 297:99, 1988

124. Moss AR, Bachetti P: Natural history of HIV infection. AIDS 3:55, 1989

125. Pedersen C, Lindhardt BO, Jensen BL et al: Clinical course of primary HIV infection: consequences for subsequent course of infection. BMJ 299:154, 1989

126. Pedersen C, Gerstoft J, Lundgren J et al: Development of AIDS and low CD4 cell counts in a cohort of 180 HIV seroconverters. Ninth International Conference on AIDS, Berlin, 1993 p. 279, abstract PO-B01-0862

127. Bachmeyer C, Boufassa F, Sereni D et al: Prognostic value of acute symptomatic HIV-1 infection. Ninth International Conference on AIDS, Berlin, 1993, p. 280, abstract PO-B01-0870

128. Keet IP, Krijnen P, Koot M et al: Predictors of rapid progression to AIDS in HIV-1 seroconverters. AIDS 7:51, 1993

129. Lang W, Perkins H, Anderson RE et al: Patterns of T lymphocyte changes with human immunodeficiency virus infection: from seroconversion to the development of AIDS. J AIDS 2:63, 1989

130. Levy JA: The transmission of HIV and factors influencing progression to AIDS. Am J Med 95:86, 1993

131. Fahey JL, Taylor JM, Detels R et al: The prognostic value of cellular and serologic markers in infection with human immunodeficiency virus type 1. N Engl J Med 322:166, 1990

132. Godfried MH, van der Poll T, Weverling GJ et al: Soluble receptors for tumor necrosis factor as predictors of progression to AIDS in asymptomatic human immunodeficiency virus type 1 infection. J Infect Dis 169:739, 1994

133. Choi S, Lagakos SW, Schooley RT et al: CD4+ lymphocytes are an incomplete surrogate marker for clinical progression in persons with asymptomatic HIV infection taking zidovudine. Ann Intern Med 118:674, 1993

134. Lagakos SW: Surrogate markers in AIDS clinical trials: conceptual basis, validation, and uncertainties. Clin Infect Dis, suppl. 1, 16:S22, 1993

135. Mayers DL, Wagner KF, Chung RC et al: Zidovudine (AZT) resistance is temporally associated with clinical failure in patients on AZT therapy. First National Conference on Human Retroviruses, Washington, DC, 1993, p. 55, abstract no. 3

136. Tersmette M, Gruters RA, de Wolf F et al: Evidence for a role of virulent human immunodeficiency virus (HIV) variants in the pathogenesis of acquired immunodeficiency syndrome: studies on sequential HIV isolates. J Virol 63: 2118, 1989

137. St. Clair MH, Hartigan PM, Andrews JC et al: Zidovudine resistance, syncytium-inducing phenotype, and HIV disease progression in a case-control study. J AIDS 6:891, 1993

138. Bozzette SA, McCutchan JA, Spector SA et al: A cross-sectional comparison of persons with syncytium- and non-syncytium-inducing human immunodeficiency virus. J Infect Dis 168:1374, 1993

139. D'Aquila RT, Johnson VA, Welles S et al: Zidovudine resistance at entry to ACTG protocol 116B/117 predicted HIV-1 disease progression. First National Conference on Human Retroviruses, Washington, DC, 1993, p. 136, abstract no. 460

140. Phair J, Munoz A, Detels R et al: The risk of *Pneumocystis carinii* pneumonia among men infected with human immunodeficiency virus type 1. N Engl J Med 322:161, 1990

141. Pachl C, Saxer M, Elbeik T et al: Quantitation of HIV-1 RNA in plasma using a branched DNA (bDNA) signal amplification assay: evaluation of specimen collection and stability. First National Conference on Human Retroviruses and Related Infections, Washington, DC, 1993, p. 110, abstract no. 312

142. Ho DD, Moudgil T, Alam M: Quantitation of human immunodeficiency virus type 1 in the blood of infected persons. N Engl J Med 321:1621, 1989

143. Coombs RW, Collier AC, Allain JP et al: Plasma viremia in human immunodeficiency virus infection. N Engl J Med 321:1626, 1989

144. Saag M, Crain MI, Decker WD et al: High-level viremia in adults and children infected with human immunodeficiency virus: relationship to disease stage and CD4 lymphocyte levels. J Infect Dis 164:72, 1991

145. Katzenstein DA, Holodniy M, Israelski DM et al: Plasma viremia in human immunodeficiency virus infection: relationship to stage of disease and antiviral treatment. J AIDS 5:107, 1992

146. Corey L, Coombs RW: The natural history of HIV infection: implications for the assessment of antiretroviral therapy. Clin Infect Dis, suppl. 1, 16:S2, 1993

147. Fischl MA, Richman DD, Grieco MH et al: The efficacy of azidothymidine (AZT) in the treatment of patients with AIDS and AIDS-related complex: a double-blind placebo-controlled trial. N Engl J Med 317:185, 1987

148. Volberding PA, Lagakos SW, Koch MA et al: Zidovudine in asymptomatic human immune deficiency virus infection: a controlled trial in persons with fewer than 500 CD4-positive cells per cubic millimeter. N Engl J Med 322:941, 1990

149. Graham NM, Zeger SL, Park LP et al: Effect of zidovudine and *Pneumocystis carinii* pneumonia prophylaxis on progression of HIV-1 infection to AIDS. Lancet 338:265, 1991

150. Moore RD, Hidalgo J, Sugland BW et al: Zidovudine and the natural history of the acquired immunodeficiency syndrome. N Engl J Med 324:1412, 1991

151. Cooper DA, Gatell JM, Kroon S et al: Zidovudine in persons with asymptomatic HIV infection and CD4+ cell counts greater than 400 per cubic millimeter. N Engl J Med 329:297, 1993

152. Richman D, Grimes JM, Lagakos SW: Effect of stage of disease and drug dose on zidovudine susceptibilities of isolates of human immunodeficiency virus. J AIDS 3:743, 1990

153. Richman DD: Resistance of clinical isolates of human immunodeficiency virus to antiretroviral agents. Antimicrobial Agents Chemother 37:1207, 1993
154. Larder BA, Kemp SD: Multiple mutations in HIV-1 reverse transcriptase confer high-level resistance to zidovudine (AZT). Science 246:1155, 1989
155. Kellam P, Boucher CA, Larder BA: Fifth mutation in human immunodeficiency virus type 1 reverse transcriptase contributes to the development of high-level resistance to zidovudine. Proc Natl Acad Sci USA 89:1934, 1992
156. Gu Z, Gao Q, Li X et al: Novel mutation in the human immunodeficiency virus type 1 reverse transcriptase gene that encodes cross-resistance to 2',3'-dideoxyinosine and 2',3'-dideoxycytidine. J Virol 66:7128, 1992
157. Fitzgibbon JE, Howell RM, Haberzettl CA et al: Human immunodeficiency virus type 1 pol gene mutations which cause decreased susceptibility to 2',3'-dideoxycytidine. Antimicrobial Agents Chemother 36:153, 1992
158. Skowron G, Bozette SA, Lim L et al: Alternating and intermittent regimens of zidovudine and dideoxycytidine in patients with AIDS or AIDS-related complex. Ann Intern Med 118:321, 1993
159. Collier AC, Coombs RW, Fischl MA et al: Combination therapy with zidovudine and didanosine compared with zidovudine alone in HIV-1 infection. Ann Intern Med 119:786, 1993
160. Yarchoan R, Lietzau JA, Nguyen BY et al: A randomized pilot study of alternating or simultaneous zidovudine and didanosine therapy in patients with symptomatic human immunodeficiency virus infection. J Infect Dis 169:9, 1994

2

Electrolyte, Acid-Base, and Endocrine Disturbances in Patients with HIV Infection

Michael H. Humphreys
Patricia Schoenfeld

INTRODUCTION

Human immunodeficiency virus (HIV) infection is associated, directly or indirectly, with involvement of every organ system in the body. The kidneys are no exception, as this volume attests. Although most interest has focused on the occurrence of specific patterns of glomerular disease, it has also become recognized that characteristic fluid, electrolyte, and acid-base disturbances occur with regularity in HIV-infected patients. Related to these are endocrinologic abnormalities. This chapter reviews the nature of these disturbances.

ELECTROLYTE DISTURBANCES

Disorders of Serum Sodium Concentration

Hyponatremia

The most common electrolyte disturbance in HIV-infected patients is hyponatremia, occurring in 28 to 56 percent of patients.[1-5] Most of these have been inpatients with symptomatic acquired immunodeficiency syndrome (AIDS), although a high incidence was also observed in outpatients in one series.[3] The major mechanisms responsible for the development of hyponatremia have been hypovolemia, usually resulting from gastrointestinal fluid losses, and euvolemic conditions resembling the syndrome of inappropriate secretion of antidiuretic hormone (SIADH)[1-3,5] (Table 2-1). In the former circumstance, the hyponatremia reflects the loss of sodium and water, with partial replacement of water; to the extent that the renal response to the hypovolemia has been assessed, appropriate sodium conservation has been observed.[1,5] However, in one study a nonrenal route of fluid loss could not be detected in a group of hyponatremic patients believed on clinical grounds to be hypovolemic[3]; measured urine sodium concentration averaged 49.9 mEq/L, leading these authors to speculate that the patients may have had underlying renal sodium wasting as the basis for the hypovolemia.[3] The lack of more detailed documentation requires that this possibility be viewed with caution.

In AIDS patients who are hyponatremic in the setting of euvolemia, most functional data support the diagnosis of SIADH, with inappropriately elevated urine osmolality and high urine sodium concentration. In most cases overt endocrine, cardiac, hepatic, or renal disease have been absent.[1,2,5] In some patients an elevated plasma vasopressin concentration has been documented.[1,2] These patients have a high prevalence of pulmonary or central nervous system (CNS) opportunistic infections known to be associated with SIADH in other settings. Occasional patients with HIV infection and hyponatremia have had adrenal dysfunction, thought to be the basis for the hyponatremia because it rapidly corrected after administration of glucocorticoid hormone.[1,2,5] In view of the frequent involvement of the adrenal glands with

Table 2-1. Hyponatremia in AIDS

Author	No. of Patients	$[Na]_s$ (mEq/L)	Hyponatremia (%)	Hypovolemic	Euvolemic
Agarwal et al.[1]	103	≤130	35	13/36	23/36
Vitting et al.[2]	71	≤132	52	—	—
	48		56	10/16	6/16
Cusano et al.[3]	96	≤130	31	21/24	3/24
Peter[4]	81	<135	28	—	—
Tang et al.[5]	210	<135	39	25/57	26/57

various disease processes in HIV-infected patients (see below), the possibility that hyponatremia reflects adrenal insufficiency must always be considered.

As is the case in other settings of hyponatremia, morbidity and mortality of hyponatremic HIV-infected patients is greater than in such patients without hyponatremia.[2,3,5]

Hypernatremia

Hypernatremia is much less common in AIDS patients and usually reflects the development of drug-induced nephrogenic diabetes insipidus. Foscarnet, rifampin, and amphotericin B have been incriminated in producing this abnormality.

Disorders of Serum Potassium Concentration

Hypokalemia

Hypokalemia is also commonly seen in AIDS patients; one series observed it in 17 percent of inpatients reviewed retrospectively over a 3-year period.[4] Most frequently, the hypokalemia results from gastrointestinal (GI) fluid and electrolyte losses as a result of infections; in one case diarrheal potassium loss was so profound that it masked the hyperkalemia normally expected in adrenal crisis.[6] Some drugs associated with hypokalemia in AIDS patients[7] are listed in Table 2-2.

Hyperkalemia

Hyperkalemia has attracted more interest. An initial report by Kalin and associates[8] described hyperkalemia in four AIDS patients; the authors attributed the hyperkalemia to hyporeninemic hypoaldosteronism on the basis

Table 2-2. Agents Used in the Treatment of AIDS That Are Associated With an Abnormal Serum Potassium Concentration

Hypokalemia
Didanosine
Foscarnet
Rifampin
Amphotericin B
Itraconazole
Hyperkalemia
Trimethoprim
Dapsone (when used with trimethoprim)
Ketoconazole
Pentamidine

(Data from Bern et al.[7])

of subnormal renin and aldosterone stimulation by furosemide, and a beneficial therapeutic response to exogenous mineralocorticoid hormone.[8] However, each of these patients was receiving intravenous trimethoprim/sulfamethoxazole therapy for opportunistic infections. It has subsequently been shown that trimethoprim in the high doses employed for such treatment (20 mg/kg) reaches levels in tubular fluid in the distal nephron sufficient to mimic the action of a potassium-sparing diuretic and inhibit collecting duct potassium secretion.[9] Trimethoprim shares structural similarity with amiloride and triamterene, and, like these agents, also inhibits short-circuit current, a measure of sodium transport, in cultured cells derived from the toad distal nephron.[10] Potassium secretion in the distal nephron is closely linked to sodium reabsorption; these compounds inhibit sodium reabsorption through luminal sodium channels, and thereby produce hyperkalemia. The incidence of this form of hyperkalemia may be quite high; in one study, 20 percent of patients treated with oral trimethoprim/sulfamethoxazole developed moderate hyperkalemia (serum potassium 5.1 to 6.1 mEq/L),[11] and based on prospective studies, the average serum potassium may increase from 0.6 to 1.1 mEq/L with this treatment.[9,12]

Hyperkalemia can also occur from the use of other drugs used in the treatment of AIDS patients[7] (Table 2-2). In the case of pentamidine, hyperkalemia almost always occurs in association with renal insufficiency caused by this agent.[13] In one study, the incidence of hyperkalemia was greater when trimethoprim was used in conjunction with dapsone rather than with sulfamethoxazole (53 percent versus 20 percent).[11] Drug-induced hyperkalemia almost always resolves with removal of the responsible agent. Hyperkalemia can also reflect adrenal insufficiency, or, as argued by Kalin and associates,[8] isolated aldosterone deficiency. However, systematic testing of adrenal reserve in a large number of HIV-infected patients failed to reveal a gross abnormality in aldosterone secretion,[14] and therefore isolated mineralocorticoid deficiency is likely an uncommon occurrence in these patients.

Other Disturbances

Abnormalities in serum calcium and phosphorus concentrations have been observed as drug-related complications in HIV-infected patients. Foscarnet has been observed to cause both hypercalcemia with hyperphosphatemia and hypocalcemia with hypophosphatemia.[7] One case also linked hypokalemia, hypocalcemia, hypophosphatemia, and hypomagnesemia to foscarnet administration.[15] In a series of in vitro experiments, Jacobson et al.[16] found that foscarnet causes a dose-dependent reduction in the ionized calcium concentration without changes in total calcium or phosphate concentration. These investigators also commented on the clinical observation that transient hyperphosphatemia often occurs in the second week of foscarnet induction therapy, for which there is currently no explanation. Pentamidine also can cause hypocalcemia and hypomagnesemia. A number of agents increase serum uric acid concentration, including didanosine (ddI), rifampin, etham-butol, and pyrazinamide.[7] Foscarnet has also been reported to cause nephro-genic diabetes insipidus.[17] Hypercalcemia has also been reported in patients with AIDS and CMV infection[17a], *Mycobacterium avium-intracellulare* infec-tion[17b], and lymphoma.[17c]

ACID-BASE DISTURBANCES

AIDS patients are at risk of the development of respiratory alkalosis and respiratory acidosis because of pulmonary or CNS involvement with oppor-tunistic infections or other disease processes. Recent attention has also been drawn to the occurrence of metabolic acidosis. This can result from three different mechanisms. The first is hyperchloremic metabolic acidosis occur-ring from loss of alkali in diarrheal stool in patients with intestinal infec-tions. The second reflects renal tubular acidosis, also hyperchloremic, in-duced by drugs such as rifampin and amphotericin B[7]; the acidification defect is associated with potassium wasting and resides in the distal neph-ron. As mentioned previously, there is a possibility of hypoaldosteronism in AIDS patients, which can also lead to hyperchloremic metabolic acidosis.

Less well understood is the occurrence of lactic acidosis in AIDS patients. Two recent reports[18,19] described a total of eight patients with severe meta-bolic acidosis accompanied by a high anion gap. Blood lactate levels were markedly elevated and contributed to the increased anion gap, but there was no evidence of hypoxemia, tissue hypoperfusion, malignancy, or sepsis. The possibility was suggested that a "mitochondrial myopathy"[18] caused by zidovudine could be responsible[18,19] even though not all patients were taking this drug at the time they had lactic acidosis.[19] Subsequently, three more anecdotal cases have been reported as Letters to the Editor[20–22] that also suggested a link to zidovudine therapy, although autopsy findings of Wer-nicke's encephalopathy led to the suggestion that thiamine deficiency could be responsible.[22] Although the occurrence of this form of severe metabolic acidosis is rare, it is of grave clinical import;[18,19] patients with this entity should be given thiamine in addition to other supportive measures. Further clinical investigation is necessary to characterize the cause(s) and manage-ment of AIDS-related lactic acidosis.

ENDOCRINE ABNORMALITIES

Modes of Endocrine Involvement

Pathology of all the endocrine organs has been observed in patients with HIV infection, and abnormal endocrine function occurs at all stages of the disease. Clinically important endocrine dysfunction or overt glandular fail-ure occurs less frequently, but may play a critical role in the management of

Table 2-3. Drug-Induced Endocrine Abnormalities

Foscarnet
    Ionized hypocalcemia
    Transient hyperphosphatemia
    Nephrogenic diabetes insipidus

Rifampin
    Increased hepatic metabolism of steroid hormones
    Adrenal insufficiency
    Decreased serum thyroxine and free thyroxine index

Ketoconazole
    Gonadal function
        Transient blockade of testosterone synthesis and sustained decrease in serum testosterone levels
        Oligospermia and azoospermia
        Impotence and decreased libido
        Gynecomastia
    Adrenal function
        Decreased serum cortisol response to corticotropin stimulation
        Decreased urine cortisol excretion

Pentamidine
    Hypoglycemia due to cytotoxic inflammation of pancreatic B cells
    Diabetes mellitus secondary to pancreatic B-cell destruction

some patients. The mechanisms by which these abnormalities occur include invasion of the endocrine gland by tumor or infectious agents resulting in tissue destruction, alterations in hormonal production and secretion due to the HIV infection directly or because of cytokine or other immune abnormalities that interfere with normal hormone function, and the effects of acute and chronic illness, as well as therapeutic agents that interfere with normal hormone secretion and actions (Table 2-3).

Some endocrine glands are affected more commonly than others in patients with HIV infection and the frequency of such involvement has varied among autopsy series. Some of these variations may be due to stage of illness or to the nature and severity of the complications of HIV infection.

Adrenal

The adrenal is the endocrine gland most frequently affected by the consequences of HIV infection. Infiltration and destruction of adrenal tissue by infectious agents has been documented in many autopsy series; responsible agents have included CMV, *Mycobacterium tuberculosis, M. avium-intracellulare, Cryptococcus, Toxoplasma,* and *Pneumocystis carinii.*[23,24] Tumor invasion with Kaposi sarcoma and lymphoma has also been documented, as well as adrenal hemorrhage and cortical lipid depletion.[25] The frequency of infection and the extent of adrenal destruction or impairment with these pathologic processes is variable in reported series. Although CMV adrenalitis has been reported in 40 to 92 percent of patients dying of AIDS, the degree of tissue destruction does not usually exceed 50 to 60 percent, which is less than the 90 percent tissue loss required to produce adrenal insufficiency.[26,27] However, studies of adrenal function, including circulating levels of adrenal hormones, and provocative tests of adrenal gland responsiveness have shown that there are well-defined biochemical abnormalities in adrenal steroid metabolism that may lead to clinical impairment in some patients.[14,25,28–30b]

Membreno et al.[14] studied 74 patients with AIDS and 19 patients with earlier disease designated as AIDS-related complex (ARC), using fasting cosyntropin and prolonged adrenocorticotropic hormone (ACTH) infusions.[14] Baseline data showed that the mean basal plasma cortisol level was significantly higher in AIDS patients than in normal controls. By contrast, the patients with ARC were not different from normal. One hour after cosyntropin stimulation, 86 percent of the patients had a normal cortisol response; however, 17-deoxysteroid levels were significantly lower than normal controls and all patients had reduced 18-hydroxydeoxycorticosterone levels. After 3 days of supraphysiologic ACTH stimulation, 10 of 14 patients with AIDS achieved a normal stimulated cortisol level, but were still significantly lower than in normal subjects. The 17-deoxysteroid responses were uniformly below normal values in this AIDS group. In contrast to the patients with clinical AIDS, the patients with ARC or a chronically ill control group achieved normal cortisol levels after ACTH stimulation, as well as normal 17-deoxysteroid responses. Four patients from these studies had adrenal insufficiency that was characterized by inappropriately low ACTH levels despite reduced cortisol and aldosterone levels, hyperkalemia, and hypotension. The cause of adrenal insufficiency in those patients was not defined, but might reflect a primary pituitary abnormality as described below. Adrenal insufficiency has also been reported in a patient treated with rifampin, which can increase hepatic metabolism of glucocorticoids.[31]

Other adrenal function studies in patients with early, asymptomatic HIV infection by Merenich et al.[28] showed that peak ACTH stimulation resulted in cortisol values in the normal range but consistently lower than in controls. This group of patients did not have elevated baseline cortisol levels, in contrast to the findings of Membreno et al., suggesting that this occurs later in the illness, perhaps in response to the stress of infectious and malignant complications.

The results of these studies suggest that the zona fasciculata (ZF) is the target tissue in patients with HIV infection and that the 17-hydroxysteroid pathway and later cortisol levels are most commonly impaired in these patients.[14] In contrast, the zona glomerulosa and plasma renin activity were normal despite abnormal ZF function. This pattern of abnormalities suggests a pituitary defect, which is also supported by the fact that ACTH levels were not elevated in some patients with frank adrenal insufficiency.[14]

Deficient mineralocorticoid function has been observed in patients who are clinically ill with AIDS, and has been implicated in abnormalities of sodium and potassium metabolism, and acid-base disturbances as described above.[8] When these common abnormalities occur, the clinician should look for the more subtle abnormalities of ZF adrenal dysfunction as well as the possible presence of marginal or frank adrenal insufficiency, especially in the patient with a history of tuberculosis or CMV infection.

Hypothalamic-Pituitary-Gonadal Function

Clinical symptoms and morphologic evidence of gonadal dysfunction have been commonly described in men with HIV infection.[32] Symptoms of decreased libido, impotence, hair loss and change in hair texture, and muscle wasting are frequently encountered, and autopsy studies have shown severe testicular atrophy in the absence of local infection or inflammation in men dying with AIDS. Croxson et al.[32] studied 59 homosexual men with various stages of HIV infection and 26 homosexual men who were HIV negative to evaluate the hypothalamic-pituitary-gonadal (HPG) axis and serum hormone levels. These investigators found a decrease in serum testosterone in men with AIDS compared with noninfected controls, accompanied by elevated luteinizing hormone (LH) and follicle stimulating hormone (FSH) levels, indicating primary gonadal dysfunction. Serum testosterone levels rose after stimulation with human chorionic gonadotropin, suggesting that the defect is functional and reversible and may be related to underlying immune system abnormalities and cytokine function. Data from Dobs et al.[33] and Raffi et al.[30b] agreed with these findings of depressed testosterone levels in men with AIDS. However, some of their patients exhibited normal or low serum gonadotropin levels, which they interpreted to represent hypogonadotropic hypogonadism rather than primary gonadal disease as proposed by Croxson and associates. The patient group studied by Dobs et al. included intravenous drug users as well as heterosexual and homosexual men. Because the use of opiates is known to cause hypogonadotropic hypogonadism, this factor may have resulted in some of the differences in those two studies. Serum prolactin levels were normal or elevated in patients with clinical AIDS, and computed tomography (CT) scans and autopsy data have not provided clear evidence of hypothalamic disease. There is an autopsy report that documented direct infectious involvement of the pituitary with CMV, *Pneumocystis,* and possibly *Toxoplasma* in six patients and questionable neurohypophyseal lesions in two others dying with CNS infections.[34] Thus, it remains unclear whether gonadal dysfunction in men is the result of functional hypogonadotropic hypogonadism or primary testicular failure due to other HIV infection-related abnormalities. Drug therapy with ketoconazole can inhibit steroidogenesis in the testes as well as the adrenal, and can contribute to oligospermia, impotence, and gynecomastia.[35]

Gynecologic and gonadal dysfunction in women with HIV infection has been less well documented and serious investigation has been lacking in this area. Increased rates of cervical disease, protracted gynecologic infections, and menstrual irregularities have been reported frequently by clinicians for many years.[36] It is also clear that gynecologic disease becomes more frequent as the stage of HIV illness progresses. The relationship between human papillomavirus (HPV) and malignant cervical disease needs to be addressed in infected women. The resultant issue of safe sexual practices in women with HIV infection should be stressed to prevent not only HPV but also other sexually transmitted diseases. It is recommended that HIV-infected women be screened with papilloma smears every 6 months and all gynecologic infections be treated aggressively and with follow-up exams. There is currently no clear policy on the use of hormonal therapy for menopause or for birth control or menstrual irregularities in HIV-infected women. The potential medical and psychological benefits of hormonal therapy in these women are numerous and, because there is no clear contraindication to their use, they should be prescribed where standard indications exist.

Thyroid

Both infection and malignancy have been documented in the thyroid of patients with HIV infection.[37–39] CMV inclusions and thyroiditis caused by *P. carinii* have been reported as well as tumor invasion by Kaposi sarcoma with complete destruction of the gland and resultant hypothyroidism.[40] The frequency of such thyroid involvement is not known, but clinical disorders of thyroid function appear to be uncommon. Most asymptomatic HIV-infected patients have normal thyroid function, but some have increased total T_4 and T_3 concentrations, which are thought to be due to increased serum levels of thyroid binding globulin.[41] It has also been noted that some patients with HIV infection do not have as large an elevation in reverse T_3 (rT_3) levels or low T_3 with acute illness as occurs in other patients with equivalent degrees of illness.[30b,41] This inappropriate response of rT_3 production may contribute to the prominent wasting and cachexia that are observed in many patients with AIDS. It has been hypothesized by Fujii et al.[42] that this abnormality may be due to increased levels of cytokines including tumor necrosis factor-α (TNF-α) and interleukin-1 (IL-1). Injection of these cytokines into animals results in increased hepatic levels of type 1 iodothyronine 5′-deiodonase, which synthesizes T_3 from T_4 and breaks down rT_3.

In summary, clinically evident hyperthyroidism or hypothyroidism do not occur more often in HIV-infected patients than in normal subjects. Drug therapy with rifampin has been reported to decrease serum thyroxine levels and the free thyroxine index, so this needs to be kept in mind when ordering thyroid function studies.[43]

Pancreas

The pancreas can be involved with opportunistic organisms and malignancies, such as Kaposi sarcoma and lymphoma.[44] Specific clinical symptoms resulting from this involvement have not been well defined. Pancreatic endocrine dysfunction has been well documented as a result of drug therapy with pentamidine, which initially causes acute toxic injury to the β-cells, resulting in increased insulin release and hypoglycemia.[27,45] Sustained use of this agent may cause permanent damage or destruction of the islet cells and result in diabetes mellitus.

Acute pancreatitis has also been reported with pentamidine and other medications, including ddI.[44]

Parathyroid

Evidence for impaired secretion of parathyroid hormone (PTH) in HIV-infected patients has been noted by Hellman et al.,[45a] who found that serum intact PTH levels were lower in HIV-1 infected patients than in normal controls. Patients with no or mild immunodeficiency had lower PTH levels than patients with more advanced immunodeficiency. By contrast to normal controls and patients with advanced immunodeficiency, there was no correlation between serum calcium and PTH levels in the patients with no or mild immunodeficiency, who were normocalcemic despite having significantly lower intact PTH levels. The authors speculated that since parathyroid cells express a protein recognized by antibodies directed against CD4, the HIV-1 receptor, these cells may react with circulating antibody, resulting in impaired release of PTH. A reduction in CD4 antibodies later in the disease may then lead to an increase in PTH secretion and normalization of the relationship between serum calcium and PTH levels.[45a]

The AIDS Wasting Syndrome and Metabolic Disorders

All patients with HIV infection lose weight during the course of their disease and in some patients this process is so severe that it defines an AIDS complication known as wasting disease or "slim disease" in Africa. Patients with both HIV infection and end-stage renal disease seem particularly prone to weight loss, perhaps because of the combined metabolic abnormalities associated with uremia and HIV infection. Because of the devastating nature of this complication for which little effective therapy has been found, the pathogenesis, mediators, and other metabolic abnormalities that lead to wasting in HIV-infected patients have been investigated rather extensively.

The clinical presentation of wasting is that of progressive weight loss, often associated with acute illness. In many cases patients do not regain all the lost weight after recovery from the acute insult.[46] A relationship between weight loss and survival has been demonstrated, showing that death tends to occur when body weight has dropped to 66 percent of ideal weight.[47] These studies imply that survival in some patients may be a function of loss of lean body mass rather than the presence of infection and malignancy.[47] Patients with AIDS have depletion of lean body mass or body cell mass as measured by total body potassium.[46] Body fat content may be normal despite the presence of decreased lean mass.[46]

Many possible mediators of wasting and cachexia in patients with AIDS as well as other diseases like cancer have been identified and include immunologic abnormalities, altered cytokine and lipid metabolism, impaired energy balance, abnormal protein metabolism, and nutritional factors such as anorexia and malabsorption. A unified hypothesis that connects all these factors has not been developed; wasting in AIDS probably results from a complex interaction of many factors.

Metabolic Abnormalities

Disturbances in immune function and cytokine metabolism and have been implicated in the pathogenesis of wasting in acute infection as well as AIDS. Early studies in AIDS patients reported elevated TNF levels, and implicated this substance in the pathogenesis of cachexia. However, subsequent studies have shown that TNF is not always elevated in patients with AIDS, that elevated levels do not invariably lead to wasting, and that there is no clear relationship between circulating TNF levels and the degree of weight loss.[47] TNF does affect lipid metabolism by stimulating an increase in hepatic lipogenesis and very-low-density lipoprotein production, leading to an increase in triglyceride levels.[48] This ability to increase fatty acid synthesis is also shared by other cytokines including IL-1, IL-6, and interferon-α. Although 50 percent of AIDS patients have elevated triglyceride levels, there is no correlation between the TNF concentration in the serum and hypertriglyceridemia. However, serum interferon-α is significantly correlated with elevated triglyceride levels as well as effects on lipid metabolism in fat cells and the liver.[48,49]

Increased metabolic activity can also lead to weight loss. Resting energy expenditure (REE) is increased in patients with HIV infection and increases with progression to clinical AIDS.[50] This increase in REE may not be accompanied by accelerated weight loss until patients reach advanced stages of AIDS complicated by the presence of severe infection. Protein degradation and synthesis are also increased with sepsis and infection, and negative nitrogen balance occurs in these situations as well. In the absence of opportunistic infection, protein turnover in HIV-infected patients is decreased and resembles the adaptation seen in starvation.

Nutritional Abnormalities

GI disease is common in patients with HIV infection, and is often caused by opportunistic infections, malignancies, and perhaps direct HIV involvement of the bowel. These abnormalities can cause diarrhea, malabsorption, pain, and other symptoms that interfere with normal nutrient intake and contribute to increased nutrient and electrolyte losses in the stool. In addition, nausea, anorexia, and vomiting are frequent symptoms associated with many illnesses and further impair nutritional intake. Many patients are on numerous medications including chemotherapy, which contribute to GI symptoms and anorexia. In the presence of increased REE and the energy requirements of acute infection and malignancy, most patients cannot keep their calorie and protein intake high enough to avoid weight loss and progressive wasting.

Therapy for Wasting

Because most weight loss occurs during acute illness, early diagnosis and treatment of such complications are of great benefit in reducing the magnitude of nutritional depletion and weight loss. Increased alimentation during prolonged illness has been used, but may result in an increase in body fat rather than lean tissue mass.[51] As mentioned above, recovery from these episodes of illness is often incomplete and may lead to stepwise reductions in lean body mass.

Treatment of anorexia is difficult, but can occasionally be ameliorated with appetite stimulants such as megace and marinol. Oral protein-calorie supplements are effective ways to provide extra nutrition, but are often limited by diarrhea and palatability. Recently, short-term studies with growth hormone in patients with HIV infection have shown that positive nitrogen balance can be achieved along with increases in body weight.[52] Long-term use of this agent alone or with insulin-like growth factor-1 may provide additional therapeutic options for nutritionally impaired patients with HIV infection and AIDS.

REFERENCES

1. Agarwal A, Soni A, Ciechanowsky M et al: Hyponatremia in patients with the acquired immunodeficiency syndrome. Nephron 53:317, 1989
2. Vitting KE, Gardenswartz MH, Zabetakis PM: Frequency of hyponatremia and nonosmolar vasopressin release in the acquired immunodeficiency syndrome. JAMA 263:973, 1990
3. Cusano AJ, Thies HL, Siegal FP et al: Hyponatremia in patients with acquired immune deficiency syndrome. J AIDS 3:949, 1990
4. Peter SA: Electrolyte disorders and renal dysfunction in acquired immunodeficiency syndrome patients. J Nat Med Assoc 83:889, 1991
5. Tang WW, Kaptein EM, Feinstein EI et al: Hyponatremia in hospitalized patients with the acquired immunodeficiency syndrome (AIDS) and the AIDS-related complex. Am J Med 94:169, 1993
6. Guerra I, Kimmel PL. Hypokalemic adrenal crisis in a patient with AIDS. South Med J 84:1265, 1991
7. Berns JS, Cohen RM, Stumacher RJ et al: Renal aspects of therapy for human immunodeficiency virus and associated opportunistic infections. J Am Soc Nephrol 1:1061, 1991
8. Kalin MF, Poretsky L, Seres DS et al: Hyporeninemic hypoaldosteronism associated with acquired immune deficiency syndrome. Am J Med 82:1035, 1987
9. Velazquez H, Perazella MA, Wright FS et al: Renal mechanism of trimethoprim-induced hyperkalemia. Ann Intern Med 119:296, 1993
10. Choi MJ, Fernandez PC, Patnaik A et al: Brief report: trimethoprim-induced hyperkalemia in a patient with AIDS. N Engl J Med 328:703, 1993
11. Medina I, Mills J, Leoung G et al: Oral therapy for *Pneumocystis carinii* pneumonia in the acquired immunodeficiency syndrome. A controlled trial of trimethoprim-sulfamethoxazole versus trimethoprim-dapsone. N Engl J Med 323:776, 1990
12. Greenberg S, Reiser IW, Chou SY et al: Trimethoprim-sulfamethoxazole induces reversible hyperkalemia. Ann Intern Med 119:291, 1993
13. Lachaal M, Venuto RC: Nephrotoxicity and hyperkalemia in patients with acquired immunodeficiency syndrome treated with pentamidine. Am J Med 87:260, 1989

14. Membreno L, Irony I, Dere W et al: Adrenocortical function in acquired immuno-deficiency syndrome. J Clin Endocrinol Metab 65:482, 1987
15. Gearhart MO, Sorg TB: Foscarnet-induced severe hypomagnesemia and other electrolyte disorders. Ann Pharmacother 27:285, 1993
16. Jacobson MA, Gambertoglio JG, Aweeka FT et al: Foscarnet-induced hypocal-cemia and effects of foscarnet on calcium metabolism. J Clin Endocrinol Metab 72:1130, 1991
17. Farese RV, Schambelan M, Hollander H et al: Nephrogenic diabetes insipidus associated with foscarnet treatment of cytomegalovirus retinitis. Ann Intern Med 112:955, 1990
17a.Zaloga GP, Chernow B, Eil C: Hypercalcemia and disseminated cytomegalovirus infection in the acquired immunodeficiency syndrome. Ann Intern Med 102:331, 1985
17b.Delahunt JW, Romeril KE: Hypercalcemia in a patient with the acquired immu-nodeficiency syndrome and *Mycobacterium avium intracellulare* infection, letter. J AIDS 7:871, 1994
17c.Adams JS, Fernandez M, Gacad MA et al: Vitamin D metabolite-mediated hyper-calcemia and hypercalciuria in patients with AIDS and non-AIDS-associated lymphoma. Blood 73:235, 1989
18. Gopinath R, Hutcheon M, Cheema-Dhadli S et al: Chronic lactic acidosis in a patient with acquired immunodeficiency syndrome and mitochondrial myopa-thy: biochemical studies. J Am Soc Nephrol 3:1212, 1992
19. Chattha G, Arieff AI, Cummings C et al: Lactic acidosis complicating the ac-quired immunodeficiency syndrome. Ann Intern Med 118:37, 1993
20. Coyle T, Abel E: Lactic acidosis and AIDS, letter. Ann Intern Med 119:344, 1993
21. Chariot P, Dubreuil-Lemaire ML, Gherardi R: Lactic acidosis and AIDS (letter). Ann Intern Med 119:344, 1993
22. Baram D, Cooke J: Lactic acidosis and AIDS (letter). Ann Intern Med 119:345, 1993
23. Welch K, Finkbeiner W, Alpers CE et al: Autopsy findings in the acquired im-mune deficiency syndrome. JAMA 252:1152, 1984
24. Reichert CM, O'Leary TJ, Levens DL et al: Autopsy pathology in the acquired immune deficiency syndrome. Am J Pathol 112:357, 1983
25. Donovan DS Jr, Dluhy RG: AIDS and its effect on the adrenal gland. Endocrinol 1:227, 1991
26. Grinspoon SK, Bilezikian JP: HIV disease and the endocrine system. N Engl J Med 327:1360, 1992
27. Masharani U, Schambelan M: The endocrine complications of acquired immuno-deficiency syndrome. Adv Int Med 38:323, 1993
28. Merenich JA, McDermott MT, Asp AA et al: Evidence of endocrine involvement early in the course of human immunodeficiency virus infection. J Clin Endocri-nol Metab 70:566, 1990
29. Boushey HA, Warnock DG, Smith LH Jr: Adrenocortical function in the acquired immunodeficiency syndrome. West J Med 148:70, 1988
30. Greene LW, Cole W, Greene JB et al: Adrenal insufficiency as a complication of the acquired immunodeficiency syndrome. Ann Intern Med 101:497, 1984
30a.Oberfield SE, Kairam R, Bakshi S et al: Steriod response to adrenocorticotropin stimulation in children with human immunodeficiency virus infection. J Clin Endocrinol Metab 70:578, 1990
30b.Raffi F, Brisseau JM, Planchon B et al: Endocrine function in 98 HIV-infected patients: a prospective study. AIDS 5:729, 1991
31. Ediger SK, Isley WL: Rifampicin-induced adrenal insufficiency in the acquired

immunodeficiency syndrome: difficulties in diagnosis and treatment. Postgrad Med J 64:405, 1988
32. Croxson TS, Chapman WE, Miller LK et al: Changes in the hypothalamic-pituitary-gonadal axis in human immunodeficiency virus-infected homosexual men. J Clin Endocrinol Metab 68:317, 1989
33. Dobs AS, Dempsey MA, Ladenson PW et al: Endocrine disorders in men infected with human immunodeficiency virus. Am J Med 84:611, 1988
34. Sano T, Kovacs K, Scheithauer BW et al: Pituitary pathology in acquired immunodeficiency syndrome. Arch Pathol Lab Med 113:1066, 1989
35. Pont A, Graybill JR, Craven PC et al: High-dose ketoconazole therapy and adrenal and testicular function in humans. Arch Intern Med 144:2150, 1984
36. Denenberg R: Female sex hormones and HIV. AIDS Clin Care 5:69, 1993
37. Frank TS, Livolsi VA, Connor AM: Cytomegalovirus Infection of the thyroid in immunocompromised adults. Yale J Biol Med 60:1, 1987
38. Gallant JE, Enriquez RE, Cohen KL: *Pneumocystis carinii* thyroiditis. Am J Med 84:303, 1988
39. Krauth PH, Katz JF: Kaposi's sarcoma involving the thyroid in a patient with AIDS. Clin Nucl Med 12:848, 1987
40. Mollison LC, Mijch A, McBride G: Hypothyroidism due to destruction of the thyroid by Kaposi's sarcoma. Rev Infect Dis 13:826, 1991
41. Lopresti JS, Fried JC, Spencer CA: Unique alterations of thyroid hormone indices in the acquired immunodeficiency syndrome (AIDS). Ann Intern Med 110:970, 1989
42. Fujii T, Sato K, Ozawa M: Effects of interleukin-1 on thyroid metabolism in mice: stimulation by IL-1 of iodothyronine 5'-deiodinating activity (IL-1) in the liver. Endocrinol 124:167, 1989
43. Isley WL: Effect of rifampin therapy on thyroid function tests in a hypothyroid patient on replacement L-thyroxine. Ann Intern Med 107:517, 1987
44. Schwartz MS, Brandt LJ: The spectrum of pancreatic disorders in patients with acquired immune deficiency syndrome. Am J Gastroenterol 84:459, 1989
45. Waskin H, Stehr-Green JK, Helmick CG et al: Risk factors for hypoglycemia associated with pentamidine therapy for pneumocystis pneumonia. JAMA 260:345, 1988
45a.Hellman P, Albert J, Gidlund M et al: Impaired parathyroid hormone release in human immunodeficiency virus infection. AIDS Res Human Retrovir 10:391, 1994
46. Kotler DP, Wang J, Pierson RN Jr: Body composition studies in patients with the acquired immunodeficiency syndrome. Am J Clin Nutr 42:1255, 1985
47. Grunfeld C, Kotler DP: The wasting syndrome and nutritional support in AIDS. Sem Gastrointestinal Dis 2:25, 1991
48. Grunfeld C, Feingold KR: Metabolic disturbances and wasting in the acquired immunodeficiency syndrome. N Engl J Med 327:329, 1992
49. Grunfeld C, Pang M, Doerrler W et al: Lipids, lipoproteins, triglyceride clearance, and cytokines in human immunodeficiency virus infection and the acquired immunodeficiency syndrome. J Clin Endocrinol Metab 74:1045, 1992
50. Hommes MJT, Romijn JA, Godfried MH et al: Increased resting energy expenditure in human immunodeficiency virus-infected men. Metabolism 39:1186, 1990
51. Kotler DP, Tierney AR, Ferraro R et al: Enteral alimentation and repletion of body cell mass in malnourished patients with acquired immunodeficiency syndrome. Am J Clin Nutr 53:149, 1991
52. Mulligan K, Grunfeld C, Hellerstein MK et al: Anabolic effects of recombinant human growth hormone in patients with wasting associated with human immunodeficiency virus infection. J Clin Endocrinol Metab 77:956, 1993

3

Acute Renal Failure in Patients with HIV Infection

T. K. Sreepada Rao
Jeffrey S. Berns

INTRODUCTION

ARF DUE TO PRERENAL AZOTEMIA AND INTRINSIC
RENAL DISEASE
    Incidence
    Differential Diagnosis
    Clinical Course and Management

ARF DUE TO URINARY TRACT OBSTRUCTION

CONCLUSION

INTRODUCTION

Clinical manifestations in persons infected with the human immunodeficiency virus (HIV) may be conspicuously absent (asymptomatic seropositive individuals) or there may be severe constitutional symptoms, opportunistic infections, unusual malignancies, and cachexia associated with the acquired immunodeficiency syndrome (AIDS). It has also become evident that HIV infection results in systemic diseases involving virtually all organs, including the kidneys. In 1983, about three years after the initial recognition of AIDS as a new clinical entity, a unique form of renal disease, AIDS-associated nephropathy (AAN), now often termed HIV-associated nephropathy (HIVAN), was described.[1–3] HIVAN is characterized by proteinuria, normal blood pressure, enlarged kidneys, focal and segmental glomerulosclerosis (FSGS), and an often rapid progression to end-stage renal disease (ESRD).[4–7] A wide variety of fluid-electrolyte disorders and other renal diseases have also been described in association with HIV infection and AIDS[5–12] (Table

Table 3-1. Renal Disorders and HIV Infection

Coincidental renal disorders
    Acute renal failure (see Table 3-2)
    Fluid-electrolyte and acid-base disorders
        Hyponatremia
        Hypokalemia and hyperkalemia
        Hypouricemia and hyperuricemia
        Hypomagnesemia
        Hypocalcemia and hypercalcemia
        Lactic acidosis
        Renal tubular acidosis
        Diabetes insipidus
        Inappropriate antidiuretic hormone secretion
    Renal infections
    Infiltrative and malignant disorders
        Lymphoma
        Kaposi sarcoma
        Renal cell carcinoma, metastatic malignancies
        Nephrocalcinosis, renal calcifications
Specific HIV-related disorders
    Focal segmental glomerular sclerosis (HIV-associated nephropathy)
    Other glomerulopathies: minimal change, mesangial proliferative GN, membranoproliferative GN, proliferative immune-complex GN, IgA nephropathy

Table 3-2. Acute Renal Failure and HIV Infection

Prerenal azotemia
    Hypovolemia: diarrhea, vomiting, fluid losses (fever)
    Hypotension: septic shock, hemorrhage
    Hypoalbuminemia: cachexia, malnutrition, nephrotic syndrome
Intrinsic renal diseases
    Acute tubular necrosis: hypotension, ischemia, nephrotoxins
    Rhabdomyolysis and myoglobinuric renal failure
    Allergic interstitial nephritis
    Nonsteroidal anti-inflammatory drugs
    Hemolytic uremic syndrome
    Thrombotic thrombocytopenic purpura
    Glomerulonephritis: IgA, postinfectious, immune-complex
    Plasmacytic interstitial nephritis
    Light-chain deposition disease, multiple myeloma
Obstructive uropathy
    Crystal-induced tubular obstruction: acyclovir, sulfadiazine, acute uric acid nephropathy
    Retroperitoneal fibrosis
    Extrinsic ureteral compression: lymph nodes, tumors
    Intrinsic obstruction: fungus balls, blood clots
    Bladder and urethral obstruction: neurogenic bladder, Kaposi sarcoma

3-1). Among the more common of these is acute renal failure (ARF), which is often due, either directly or indirectly, to infectious or neoplastic complications of HIV infection, or therapeutic and diagnostic agents employed in the management of patients with AIDS. In addition, a variety of glomerular, tubulointerstitial, and vascular diseases of the kidneys may present with ARF. This chapter focuses primarily on the spectrum of ARF, which occurs in patients with HIV infection and AIDS (Table 3-2). Patients with HIV infection and AIDS are also still susceptible to the myriad other causes of ARF that occur in uninfected patients.

ARF DUE TO PRERENAL AZOTEMIA AND INTRINSIC RENAL DISEASE

Incidence

The causes of ARF in patients with AIDS are in many respects similar to those encountered in the usual acute-care nephrology consultative practice, although the relative frequency of certain types of ARF may be different in HIV-infected patients than in uninfected patients. In addition, a variety of renal injuries seen rarely, if at all, in patients without HIV infection may also be encountered (Table 3-2). Rao and colleagues[4] reported that of 750 patients with AIDS treated at two institutions in Brooklyn, New York, between 1982 and 1986, 23 patients (3 percent) developed ARF secondary to nephrotoxic injury, ischemic insults, or both. During about the same period, renal failure (serum creatinine ≥ 5 mg/dl) was found in approximately 4 percent of 1,635 patients (1,090 with AIDS, 545 with AIDS-related complex [ARC]) seen in Miami; of 100 consecutive patients seen by their nephrology service, 72 had azotemia (both acute and chronic), with or without azotemia, as the main indication for nephrology consultation.[6] The renal failure was reversible in only 26 percent of these cases (i.e., 1 percent of the total population). Others have reported incidences of severe ARF of up to 20 percent, with mild azotemia occurring much more commonly.[2,7,13–16] For instance, Valeri and Neusy,[14] defining ARF as a rise in the serum creatinine of at least 2 mg/dl, found a 20 percent incidence of ARF among 449 patient records reviewed retrospectively. Over 50 percent of the patients had developed some degree of azotemia if defined as a 0.3 mg/dl or greater increase in serum creatinine above baseline. Studies in hospitalized patients without HIV infection have found the incidence of ARF to be about 2 to 5 percent.[17,18]

Differential Diagnosis

Patients with AIDS often suffer from hypovolemia caused by vomiting, diarrhea, malabsorption, and central nervous system (CNS) involvement with obtundation. Hypotension may complicate hypovolemia and septic shock. Opportunistic infections, sepsis, and multiorgan dysfunction with associated metabolic disturbances and compromised cardiorespiratory status are often treated with multiple potentially nephrotoxic agents. It is not surprising, therefore, that many investigators have found prerenal azotemia and acute tubular necrosis (ATN) to be relatively common in patients with AIDS.[4,7,14–16,19,20] Data from the large retrospective series of Valeri and Neusy[14] are shown in Table 3-3; similar findings have been reported by others. Cantor et al.,[16] for example, among 39 patients with AIDS and ARF, reported the cause to be nephrotoxic drugs in 59 percent, intravascular volume depletion in 18 percent, urinary tract obstruction in 8 percent, sepsis in 5 percent, and interstitial nephritis, rhabdomyolysis, and acute uric acid nephropathy in 2.5 percent (1 patient each).

Not infrequently, patients present initially with some degree of azotemia, which then progresses relatively rapidly. When this occurs in association with heavy proteinuria in the absence of any apparent inciting or complicating factors such as hypotension or administration of nephrotoxic agents, a diagnosis of HIVAN is often entertained. HIVAN, as noted above, may be characterized by a very rapid loss of renal function, with a clinical course consistent with ARF.[1–7] Histologic examination of renal biopsy specimens in uncertain cases may help to clarify the proper diagnosis in these patients. Another glomerulopathy developing in intravenous drug addicts and that, like HIV-associated nephropathy, tends to occur in young black males, is heroin-associated nephropathy.[21–25] This entity, similarly to HIVAN, is characterized histopathologically by changes of focal and segmental glomerulosclerosis, although without other features of HIVAN such as marked tubular ectasia and ultrastructural inclusions. Heroin-associated nephropathy usually progresses more slowly than HIVAN, with ESRD developing over a period of years rather than weeks to months.

Table 3-3. Frequency of Causes of ARF in Patients with AIDS

	All Cases[a] (%)	Severe ARF[b] (%)
Volume depletion	38	30
Drug-related	47	42
TMP-SMX	10	7
Pentamidine	18	14
Amphotericin B	11	9
Contrast	4	6
Others	4	6
Hemodynamic/shock	8	17
Rhabdomyolysis	0.2	1
Urinary retention	0.2	1
Unknown	7	9

Abbreviation: TMP-SMX, trimethoprim-sulfamethoxazole.

[a] Increase in serum creatinine of $\geq$0.3 mg/dl above baseline. n = 425.

[b] Increase in serum creatinine of $\geq$2 mg/dl above baseline. n = 88.

(Data from Valeri and Neusy.[14])

Table 3-4. ARF Due to Drugs Used to Treat HIV
and Related Infections

Nephrotoxic ATN
    Foscarnet
    Amphotericin B
    Pentamidine
    Rifampin
    Capreomycin
    Acyclovir (?)
Crystal-induced
    Acyclovir
    Sulfadiazine
    TMP-SMX (rare)
    Ciprofloxacin (?)
Tubulointerstitial nephritis
    Foscarnet
    Interferon-α
    TMP-SMX
    Acyclovir (?)
    Sulfadiazine
    Rifampin
    Ciprofloxacin
    Ethambutol (?)
    Pyrazinamide (rare)
    Azithromycin (rare)
Other causes
    Rhabdomyolysis: itraconazole (rare)
    Glomerular diseases: interferon-α, rifampin
    Hemoglobinuria: dapsone (rare)
    Vasculitis: TMP-SMX (rare)
"Pseudo-ARF" due to inhibition of creatinine secretion
    Trimethoprim (TMP-SMX)
    Pyrimethamine

Abbreviation: TMP-SMX, Trimethoprim-sulfamethoxazole.

Administration of nephrotoxic antimicrobial and antiviral drugs (Table 3-4) is a major iatrogenic cause of ARF in patients with HIV infection and AIDS[4,14,16,26] (see Ch. 10). Some of the agents most commonly employed in the management of patients with AIDS-associated opportunistic infection that can result in renal impairment are pentamidine, amphotericin B, trimethoprim-sulfamethoxazole (TMP-SMX), sulfadiazine, acyclovir, and foscarnet. Because intravascular volume depletion appears to increase the risk of nephrotoxicity of many of these drugs, and as discussed above, is very common among hospitalized HIV-infected patients, close attention to the intravascular volume status of these patients is important. Supplemental isotonic saline solutions should be administered if appropriate.

Pentamidine is used for the treatment and prophylaxis of *Pneumocystis carinii* infections. ARF occurs in about 25 percent of patients receiving intravenous pentamidine, is usually mild and nonoliguric, and is reversible upon stopping the drug.[27,28] Severe ARF requiring dialysis is much less common, and usually is associated with the concomitant use of other nephrotoxic drugs. ARF after inhaled pentamidine use has been reported,[29,30] although this is very rare compared with intravenous use of the drug. ARF with myoglobinuria has also been reported in association with use of pentamidine.[31] A variety of fluid and electrolyte disturbances, such as hyperkalemia, hypomagnesemia, and hypocalcemia have also occurred in patients treated with pentamidine.

The nephrotoxicity of amphotericin B, used in treatment of systemic fungal infections, is well recognized.[32,33] ARF, which is usually mild, occurs in as many as 85 percent of patients receiving this drug, especially with large cumulative doses, but often responds to increased sodium supplementation, discontinuation of diuretics, and reduction in the dose or frequency of administration.[34–36] Severe or irreversible ARF is rare. Renal tubular acidosis, hypokalemia, hypomagnesemia, nephrogenic diabetes insipidus, and renal salt wasting may also complicate use of amphotericin B.

TMP-SMX, used in AIDS patients to treat and prevent *P. carinii* and *Toxoplasma gondii* infections, may cause ARF due to interstitial nephritis, associated with fever, rash, eosinophilia, and eosinophiluria.[37] Vasculitis and ARF due to crystalluria may also occur rarely. Trimethoprim, an organic cation that inhibits renal tubular secretion of creatinine, may cause acute elevation of the serum creatinine that mimics nonoliguric ARF (although the blood urea nitrogen [BUN] will not increase), but is not due to an actual reduction in glomerular filtration rate (GFR).[38,39] Trimethoprim also appears to be responsible for hyperkalemia, which has recently been recognized to occur in some patients with use of TMP-SMX, by exerting a K^+-sparing amiloridelike effect on distal nephron apical sodium transport.[40–43]

Sulfadiazine is a sulfonamide used along with pyrimethamine for the management of CNS toxoplasmosis in patients with AIDS. Renal failure secondary to sulfadiazine-induced crystalluria has been increasingly recognized in this patient population.[44–47] Predisposing factors include volume depletion and a low urinary pH. Sulfadiazine-induced ARF should be suspected in patients with signs and symptoms of nephrolithiasis, such as flank pain and hematuria, although patients may also be relatively asymptomatic. Sulfadiazine calculi are typically radiolucent, but may appear as multiple echogenic foci on ultrasonography, with or without hydronephrosis. Characteristic "shocks of wheat" crystals may be seen on urinalysis. The mainstay of treatment of sulfadiazine crystalluria is volume replacement, either parenterally or orally, and alkalinization of urine with either sodium bicarbonate or oral sodium citrate, which leads to rapid resolution of clinical symptoms and renal dysfunction. It may not be necessary to discontinue sulfadiazine therapy because of ARF in all patients, as crystalluria and ARF may not recur if adequate fluid intake is maintained. ARF due to tubulointerstitial nephritis may also occur rarely with sulfadiazine. Pyrimethamine, like trimethoprim, can also reduce creatinine clearance by inhibition of renal tubular secretion of creatinine.[48] Thus, there may be an increase in the serum creatinine concentration, although the GFR remains unchanged.

Acyclovir is an antiviral agent effective against herpes simplex and varicella-zoster infections. Intravenous use, particularly in high doses, may be associated with ARF secondary to crystalluria and obstructive nephropathy.[49–52] Intravascular volume depletion, preexisting renal insufficiency, and large bolus doses of the drug predispose to crystallization of acyclovir in renal tubules and collecting ducts, causing reversible ARF. Oral acyclovir therapy has only very rarely resulted in renal dysfunction.[53] Histologic features of acyclovir-induced ARF include crystal deposits, tubulointerstitial nephritis, and acute tubular necrosis. Treatment consists of correction of any volume depletion and stopping the drug.

ARF may develop in over half of patients receiving foscarnet.[54–57] Although usually mild and reversible, foscarnet-induced ARF may be severe and require treatment with dialysis. Direct cytotoxic effects, tubulointerstitial nephritis and ATN, and foscarnet crystal deposition in glomerular capillaries may contribute to the development of ARF with this drug.[57–59]

Most of the antimycobacterial drugs are only very rarely nephrotoxic, if at all, although rifampin can cause ARF, particularly when used in an interrupted or discontinuous manner.[60,61] Patients may present with the abrupt onset of oliguric ARF accompanied by fever, hypotension, abdominal pain, and other systemic symptoms. In these patients, ARF has typically been associated with tubulointerstitial nephritis and ATN. Crescentic glomerulonephritis, mesangial proliferative glomerulonephritis, and thrombotic thrombocytopenic purpura have also been uncommonly reported in association with administration of rifampin.[62–64]

Other agents used to treat HIV infection or HIV-related opportunistic infections that have been reported to cause ARF are ciprofloxacin,[65] interferon-α,[66,67] and dapsone. Fortunately, the antiretroviral agents zidovudine (ZDV, also know as azidothymidine [AZT]), didanosine (ddI), and zalcitabine (ddC) have as yet not been associated with nephrotoxic ARF. Numerous other drugs commonly used in patients with HIV infection and AIDS can also cause ARF, including the nonsteroidal anti-inflammatory agents (NSAIDs), radiographic contrast material, antineoplastic chemotherapeutic agents, and the aminoglycoside antibiotics.

The use of unorthodox drug therapies by HIV-infected patients may also produce severe nephrotoxicity. Intravenous injection of hydrogen peroxide as a "treatment" of HIV infection was recently described in a patient who developed hemoglobinemia and ARF accompanying a fatal reaction to this self-medication.[68] Germanium lactate citrate, taken by some HIV-infected patients as an "immunostimulant," has been reported to cause ARF associated with mild proteinuria (<1 g/d).[69] Renal biopsy in two patients revealed a focal lymphoplasmacytic tubulointerstitial nephritis with vacuolar cell degeneration and periodic acid-Schiff (PAS)-positive intracellular deposits, mainly in the distal renal tubules.[69] The glomeruli were normal except for mild mesangial proliferation. By electron microscopy, electron-dense deposits were seen in the mitochondria of distal tubular cells. Using neutron activation analysis, very high germanium concentrations were found in renal biopsy and liver tissues. Renal insufficiency in both of these patients persisted despite discontinuation of the drug. Other reports of inorganic and organic germanium compound nephrotoxicity have similarly highlighted the potential severity of the renal failure associated with ingestion of these compounds.[70,71] Other clinical features seen in these patients include lactic acidosis, pancreatitis, and liver failure with hepatic steatosis.

Many forms of glomerular diseases have been reported to present with ARF in HIV-infected patients, including postinfectious glomerulonephritis (GN),[72] membranoproliferative GN,[73] IgA nephropathy,[74–76] and proliferative immune-complex glomerulonephritis[77] (see Ch. 5). Rare cases of multiple myeloma and light-chain deposition disease have also been reported in association with ARF in patients with AIDS.[78,79]

Thrombotic thrombocytopenic purpura (TTP) and hemolytic uremic syndrome (HUS) have also been reported in association with ARF in HIV-infected patients[80–83] (see Ch. 6). HIV-associated HUS/TTP may occur in patients not previously known to be HIV infected, in those who are asymptomatic but seropositive, or in those with AIDS. Whether a direct causal relation between HIV infection and these disorders exists remains unclear. HIV-associated HUS/TTP is often associated with a grave prognosis, and early treatment with plasmapheresis may be indicated.

Lymphomas and other malignancies involving the kidneys and urinary tract are rare causes of obstructive renal failure in patients with HIV infection (see below and Ch. 9), but may also cause ARF due to direct infiltration of the renal parenchyma.[84,85] A rare but treatable cause of ARF in HIV-positive patients is plasmacytic interstitial nephritis,[86] which is characterized histopathologically by a marked interstitial infiltrate of plasma cells and small and large lymphocytes (Fig. 3-1). This disorder may respond to corticosteroid therapy.

Renal failure due to complications of illicit parenteral drug abuse may also be encountered in HIV-infected patients[21,25] (Table 3-5). Myoglobinuric ARF secondary to nontraumatic rhabdomyolysis may occur due to muscle compression in drug users following drug overdoses and coma, or as a direct effect of cocaine.[87,88] Necrotizing vasculitides have been reported in abusers of amphetamines, heroin, and other drugs, and with hepatitis B and C virus infection.[89,90] Proliferative glomerulonephritides, which may be associated with cryoglobulinemia, have also been reported in association with hepatitis B and C infection.[90–92] Intravenous drug abusers may develop acute glomerulonephritis due to bacterial endocarditis or chronic cutaneous infection, and allergic interstitial nephritis as a complication of treatment of these infections.

Clinical Course and Management

The clinical features of ARF in patients with AIDS are similar to those observed in other acutely ill patients. Unlike the tendency for HIVAN to

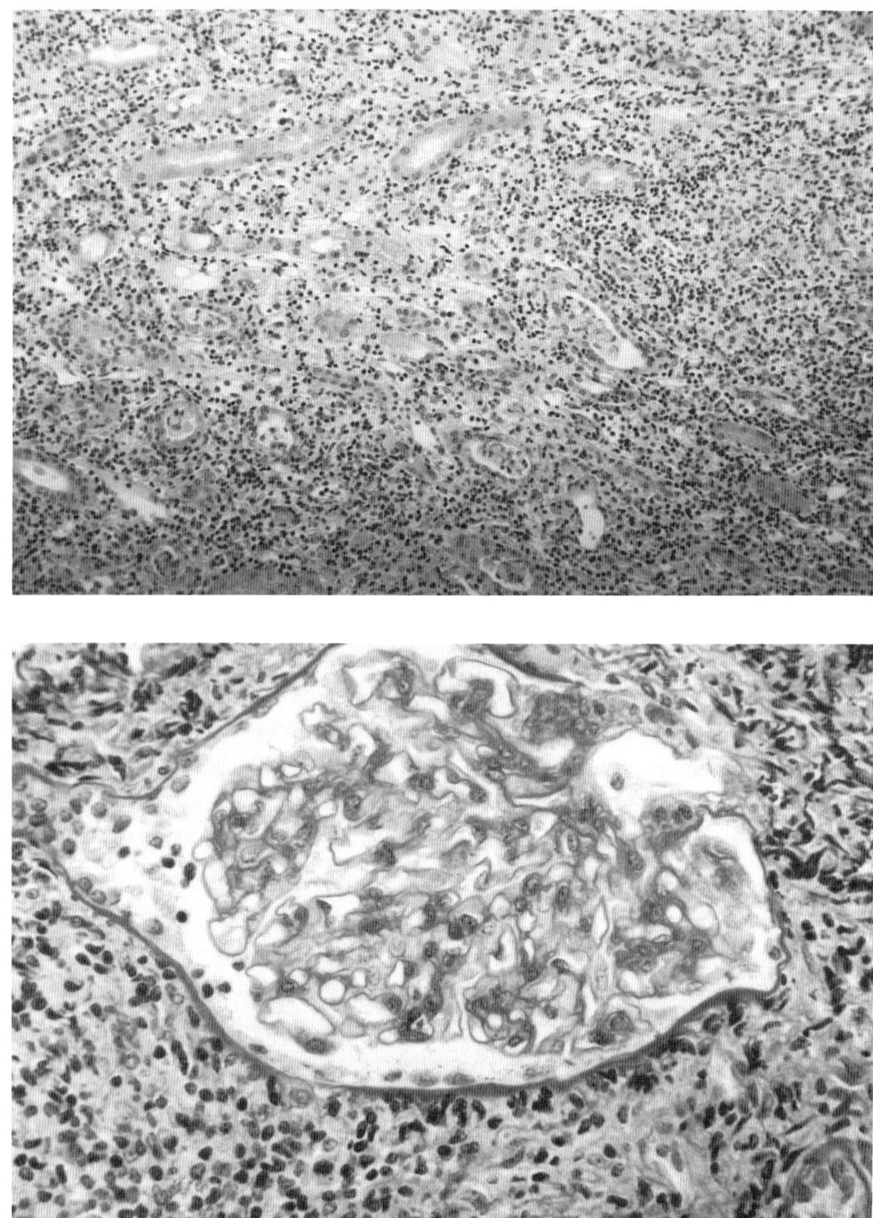

Fig. 3-1. Plasmacytic interstitial nephritis. **(A)** Extensive interstitial inflammatory infiltrate with leukocytes and plasma cells. **(B)** Normal-appearing glomerulus with dense surrounding mononuclear cell infiltrate. (H&E.)

Table 3-5. Acute Renal Failure Related to Parenteral Drug Abuse

Rhabdomyolysis with myoglobinuria
    Muscle injury due to coma and external muscle compression
    Toxic effect of heroin or contaminants
    Toxic effect of cocaine
Necrotizing vasculitis, polyarteritis nodosa
    Associated with hepatitis B or C infection
    Associated with use of methamphetamine, other drugs
Acute glomerulonephritis
    Bacterial endocarditis
    Hepatitis B or C infection: cryoglobulinemia, membranoproliferative glomerulo-
        nephritis
Allergic interstitial nephritis
Sepsis

occur predominantly in black patients, ARF appears to occur equally commonly in black and white patients.[16] The clinical management of prerenal azotemia in patients with HIV infection and AIDS is no different from uninfected patients, and depends largely upon correction of any intravascular volume deficits and reversal of hypotension. Both oliguric and nonoliguric forms of renal failure may be seen. The clinical outcome of ARF is variable, ranging from a mild self-limited course of nonoliguric or oliguric ARF with azotemia of short duration, to severe uremia that may require dialysis, intensive medical care, and other life support. In many instances, ATN is a terminal event in patients with other severe and often multisystem primary illnesses, and in whom dialysis support would not significantly alter the prognosis. Nevertheless, some gravely ill patients who receive dialysis will recover sufficient renal function and survive the acute event.

In an early study of 23 patients by Rao and colleagues,[4] all 6 subjects with ATN in whom the highest serum creatinine level attained was 6 mg/dl or less recovered without needing dialytic support. In the 17 remaining patients who had serum creatinine levels 6 mg/dl or greater, 11 terminally ill and hemodynamically unstable patients who could not be dialyzed died with renal failure. Five of the remaining 6 patients who were repeatedly hemodialyzed regained renal function, whereas only one of these patients did not recover. Of these 6 patients, none of whom survived more than 2 years, 2 died within less than 1 month, and 2 others died in less than 1 year. Marques et al.,[19] in a study from Brazil, reported a 72 percent mortality of ARF within 4 weeks among 38 HIV-infected patients. Cantor and colleagues[16] found a 23 percent short-term mortality with HIV-related ARF, with 61 percent of their patients recovering to a serum creatinine level of 2 mg/dl or less. In the report of Valeri and Neusy[14] describing 425 episodes of ARF of varying severity, dialysis was required in 4 of 17 patients in whom the serum creatinine increase was 6 mg/dl or greater; 9 of these 17 patients died.[14] The highest mortality was seen in patients with ATN due to hemodynamic instability (70 percent) and with aminoglycoside-related ARF (50 percent). Others have likewise found that ATN and severe ARF is often a preterminal event in patients with AIDS, but that many patients recover fully after supportive care. However, persistent renal insufficiency that progressively worsens with each additional insult is not uncommon,[14,15] and occasional patients with ARF remain permanently dependent on chronic dialysis.

Whether the prognosis of AIDS-associated ARF is different from that encountered in the general nephrologic practice has not been well studied. Rao and Friedman[93] have compared the outcome of severe ARF (serum creatinine >6 mg/dl) in 146 HIV-positive patients with a group of 306 uninfected subjects. Despite being younger, the AIDS patients with ATN were felt to be much more critically ill overall, such that 36 percent of the patients were agonal or too hemodynamically unstable for dialysis to be performed, whereas only 18 percent of the uninfected patients were thought to be untreatable. Eighty percent of stable nonoliguric patients who could be managed conservatively without dialysis (14 percent of the total in both HIV-infected and uninfected groups) regained renal function. In patients with ATN treated with dialysis and other supportive care, recovery of renal function occurred in only 56 percent of the patients with HIV infection and 47 percent of those without HIV infection, reflecting the overall mortality rates of 60 percent in patients with AIDS and 56 percent in the uninfected group. These differences were not statistically significant and are indicative of the grave prognosis of ARF from any cause. In summary, ATN occurred in a younger group of AIDS patients, but rates of recovery of renal function and survival were comparable to those encountered in other hospitalized patients with ARF,[94,95] and were influenced by underlying primary illness(es) and hemodynamic status of patients, rather than HIV infection per se.

The choice between peritoneal dialysis, hemodialysis, or continuous dialysis treatments such as continuous arteriovenous hemofiltration and continuous venovenous hemofiltration is somewhat arbitrary depending on the medical status of the patient and the availability of institutional resources. A full discussion of all of the medical and ethical issues of dialysis in HIV-infected patients is beyond the intended scope of this chapter (see Chs. 12 and 13). At times, dialysis may be unsuitable because of hemodynamic instability, whereas in others, an aggressive supportive approach to allow time for recovery of renal function may allow patients to survive the acute insult, as discussed above. A decision to withhold dialysis or other interventional care should only be made after mutual discussions with the primary and other consulting physicians, taking into consideration the wishes of patient, family members, and significant others.

ARF DUE TO URINARY TRACT OBSTRUCTION

ARF due to obstruction of the urinary tract in patients with HIV infection is uncommon (see Ch. 9), perhaps in part reflecting the relatively young age of this patient population, which tends therefore to be free of some of the more common causes of obstructive uropathy such as benign prostatic hypertrophy.[96–98] Sulfadiazine and acyclovir-induced crystalluria, discussed above, and acute uric acid nephropathy from chemotherapy-induced tumor lysis, may produce obstructive uropathy from intratubular crystal precipitation. Extrarenal causes of obstruction include fungus balls, retroperitoneal fibrosis, ureteropelvic infiltration with tumors, ureteral compression from retroperitoneal lymphadenopathy, as well as bladder outlet obstruction, which may be on a neurogenic basis or due to urethral obstruction caused by penile Kaposi sarcoma or other lesions.[99,100] Genitourinary tuberculosis can also cause urinary tract obstruction.[101] Vigorous attempts should be made to exclude urinary tract obstruction in patients with AIDS and undiagnosed renal failure. Diagnostic and therapeutic approaches to such patients, in conjunction with radiologists and urologists, are similar to that of non-HIV-infected patients.

CONCLUSION

In summary, ARF is a common complication in patients with AIDS that may be directly due to HIV-related disease processes or as a consequence of diagnostic and therapeutic interventions. Clinicians should recognize that many forms of ARF in these patients may be treatable or reversible, but that ARF may also accompany terminal stages of the disease. Irrespective of the etiology, ARF contributes significantly to morbidity and mortality in AIDS patients. Early diagnosis and intervention with dialysis, and other vigorous supportive maneuvers may be indicated in some AIDS patients with ARF. On the other hand, clinical and ethical dilemmas arise frequently in the care of these often young patients with multiorgan terminal disease.

REFERENCES

1. Rao TKS, Filippone EJ, Nicastri AD et al: Associated focal and segmental glomerulosclerosis in the acquired immunodeficiency syndrome. N Engl J Med 310:669, 1984
2. Gardenswartz MH, Lerner CW, Seligson GR et al: Renal disease in patients with AIDS: a clinicopathologic study. Clin Nephrol 21:197, 1984
3. Pardo V, Aldana M, Colton RM et al: Glomerular lesions in the acquired immunodeficiency syndrome. Ann Intern Med 101:429, 1984
4. Rao TKS, Friedman EA, Nicastri AD: The types of renal disease in the acquired immunodeficiency syndrome. N Engl J Med 316:1062, 1987
5. Bourgoignie JJ, Meneses R, Ortiz C et al: The clinical spectrum of renal disease associated with human immunodeficiency virus. Am J Kidney Dis 12:131, 1988
6. Glassock RJ, Cohen AH, Danovitch G, Parsa P: Human immunodeficiency virus infection and the kidney. Ann Intern Med 112:35, 1990
7. Seney FD Jr, Burns DK, Silva FG: Acquired immunodeficiency syndrome and the kidney. Am J Kidney Dis 16:1, 1990

8. Humphreys MH, Schoenfeld PY: Renal complications in patients with the acquired immunodeficiency syndrome. Am J Nephrol 7:1, 1987
9. Schoenfeld PY, Humphreys MH: Acquired immunodeficiency syndrome and renal disease: report from the National Kidney Foundation–National Institutes of Health task force on AIDS and kidney disease. Am J Kidney Dis 16:14, 1990
10. Carbone L, D'Agati V, Suh JI et al: Course and prognosis of human immunodeficiency virus associated nephropathy. Am J Med 87:389, 1989
11. Bourgoignie JJ: Renal complications of human immunodeficiency virus type 1. Kidney Int 37:1571, 1990
12. Vitting KE, Gardenswartz MH, Zabetakis PM et al: Frequency of hyponatremia and nonosmolar vasopressin release in the acquired immunodeficiency syndrome. JAMA 263:973, 1990
13. Vaziri ND, Barbari A, Licorish K et al: Spectrum of renal abnormalities in acquired immune-deficiency syndrome. J Nat Med Assoc 77:369, 1985
14. Valeri A, Neusy AJ: Acute and chronic renal disease in hospitalized AIDS patients. Clin Nephrol 35:110, 1991
15. Soni A, Agarwal A, Chander P et al: Evidence for an HIV-related nephropathy: a clinico-pathologic study. Clin Nephrol 31:12, 1989
16. Cantor ES, Kimmel PL, Bosch JP: Effect of race on expression of acquired immunodeficiency syndrome-associated nephropathy. Arch Intern Med 151:125, 1991
17. Shusterman N, Strom BL, Murray TG et al: Risk factors and outcome of hospital-acquired acute renal failure. Clinical epidemiologic study. Am J Med 83:65, 1987
18. Hou SH, Bushinsky DA, Wish JB et al: Hospital-acquired renal insufficiency: a prospective study. Am J Med 74:243, 1983
19. Marques LPJ, Rioja LS, Basilio-de-Oliveira CA et al: Kidney and HIV-infection. Clin Nephrol 37:269, 1992
20. Gnionsahe DA, Kadio A, Boka BM: Renal lesions observed in 240 black African patients infected by the human immunodeficiency virus, abstracted. Kidney Int 44:466, 1993
21. Rao TK, Nicastri A, Friedman E: The nephropathies of drug addiction and acquired immunodeficiency syndrome. p. 340. In Tisher CG, Brenner BM (eds): Renal Pathology with Clinical and Functional Correlations. JB Lippincott, Philadelphia, 1989
22. Rao TKS, Nicastri AD, Friedman EA: Natural history of heroin-associated nephropathy. N Engl J Med 290:19, 1974
23. Llach F, Descoeudres C, Massry SG: Heroin-associated nephropathy. Clinical and histological studies in 19 patients. Clin Nephrol 11:7, 1979
24. Dubrow A, Mittman N, Ghali V, Flamenbaum W: The changing spectrum of heroin-associated nephropathy. Am J Kidney Dis 5:36, 1985
25. Baldwin D, Gallo G, Neugarten J: Drug abuse with narcotics and other agents. p. 1219. In Schrier RW, Gottschalk GW (eds): Diseases of the Kidney. 5th Ed. Little Brown, Boston, 1993
26. Berns JS, Cohen RM, Stumacher RJ, Rudnick MR: Renal aspects of therapy for human immunodeficiency virus and associated opportunistic infections. J Am Soc Nephrol 1:1061, 1991
27. Andersen R, Boedicker M, Ma M, Goldstein EJC: Adverse reactions associated with pentamidine isethionate in AIDS patients: recommendation for monitoring therapy. Drug Intell Clin Pharm 20:862, 1986

28. Wharton JM, Coleman DL, Wofsy CB et al: Trimethoprim-sulfamethoxazole or pentamidine for *Pneumocystis carinii* pneumonia in the acquired immunodeficiency syndrome: a prospective randomized trial. Ann Intern Med 105:37, 1986

29. Chapelon C, Raguin G, DeGennes C: Renal insufficiency with nebulised pentamidine (letter). Lancet 2:1045, 1989

30. Miller RF, Delany S, Semple SJG: Acute renal failure after nebulised pentamidine (letter). Lancet 1:1271, 1989

31. Sensakovic J, Suarez M, Perez G et al: Pentamidine treatment of *Pneumocystis carinii* pneumonia in the acquired immunodeficiency syndrome. Association with acute renal failure and myoglobinuria. Arch Intern Med 145:2247, 1985

32. Bell NH, Andriole VT, Sabesin SM, Utz JP: On the nephrotoxicity of amphotericin B in man. Am J Med 33:64, 1962

33. Butler WT, Bennett JE, Alling DW et al: Nephrotoxicity of amphotericin B: early and late effects in 81 patients. Ann Intern Med 61:175, 1964

34. Branch RA: Prevention of amphotericin induced renal impairment: a review of the use of sodium supplementation. Arch Intern Med 148:2389, 1988

35. Llanos A, Cieza J, Bernardo J et al: Effect of salt supplementation on amphotericin B nephrotoxicity. Kidney Int 40:302, 1991

36. Heidemann HT, Gerkins JF, Spickard WA et al: Amphotericin B nephrotoxicity in humans decreased by salt repletion. Am J Med 75:476, 1983

37. Smith EJ, Light JA, Filo RS, Yum MN: Interstitial nephritis caused by trimethoprim-sulfamethoxazole in renal transplant recipients. JAMA 244:360, 1980

38. Berglund F, Killander J, Pompeius R: Effect of trimethoprim-sulfamethoxazole on the renal excretion of creatinine in man. J Urol 114:802, 1975

39. Shouval D, Ligansky M, Ben-Ishary D: Effect of cotrimoxazole on normal creatinine clearance. Lancet 1:244, 1978

40. Greenber S, Reiser IW, Chou S-Y, Porush JG: Trimethoprim-sulfamethoxazole induces reversible hyperkalemia. Ann Intern Med 119:291, 1993

41. Velazquez H, Perazella MA, Wright FS, Ellison D: Renal mechanism of trimethoprim-induced hyperkalemia. Ann Intern Med 119:296, 1993

42. Choi MJ, Fernandez PC, Patnaik A et al: Trimethoprim-induced hyperkalemia in a patient with AIDS. N Engl J Med 328:703, 1993

43. Schlanger LE, Kleyman TR, Ling BN: K^+-sparing diuretic actions of trimethoprim: inhibition of Na^+ channels in A6 distal nephron cells. Kidney Int 45:1070, 1994

44. Goadsby PJ, Donaghy AJ, Lloyd AR, Wakefield D: Acquired immunodeficiency syndrome and sulfadiazine-associated acute renal failure. Ann Intern Med 107:783, 1987

45. Carbone LG, Bendixen B, Appel GB: Sulfadiazine-associated obstructive nephropathy occurring in a patient with the acquired immunodeficiency syndrome. Am J Kidney Dis 12:72, 1988

46. Simon DI, Brosius FC III, Rothstein DM: Sulfadiazine crystalluria revisited. Arch Intern Med 150:2379, 1990

47. Oster S, Hutchison F, McCabe R: Resolution of acute renal failure in toxoplasmic encephalitis despite continuance of sulfadiazine. Rev Infect Dis 12:618, 1990

48. Opravil M, Keusch G, Luthy R: Pyrimethamine inhibits renal secretion of creatinine. Antimicrob Agents Chemother 37:1056, 1993

49. Brigden D, Rowling AE, Weeds NC: Renal function after acyclovir intravenous injection. Am J Med suppl. 1A, 73:182, 1982

50. Keeney RF, Kirk LE, Brigden D: Acyclovir tolerance in humans. Am J Med suppl. 1A, 73:171, 1982
51. Sawyer MH, Webb DE, Balow JE, Straus SE: Acyclovir induced renal failure; course and histology. Am J Med 84:1067, 1988
52. Becker BN, Fall P, Hall C et al: Rapidly progressive acute renal failure due to acyclovir: case report and review of the literature. Am J Kidney Dis 22:611, 1993
53. Eck P, Silver SM, Clark EC: Acute renal failure and coma after a high dose of oral acyclovir (letter). N Engl J Med 325:1178, 1991
54. Jacobson MA, O'Donnell JJ, Mills J: Foscarnet treatment of cytomegalovirus retinitis in patients with the acquired immunodeficiency syndrome. Antimicrob Agents Chemother 33:736, 1989
55. Gaub J, Pedersen C, Poulsen AG et al: The effect of foscarnet (phosphonoformate) on human immunodeficiency virus isolation, T-cell subsets and lymphocyte function in AIDS patients. AIDS 1:27, 1987
56. Cacoub P, Deray G, Baumelou A et al: Acute renal failure induced by foscarnet: 4 cases. Clin Nephrol 29:315, 1988
57. Deray G, Martinez F, Katlama C et al: Foscarnet nephrotoxicity: mechanism, incidence and prevention. Am J Nephrol 9:316, 1989
58. Beaufils H, Deray G, Katlama C et al: Foscarnet and crystals in glomerular capillary lumens (letter). Lancet 336:755, 1990
59. Yusufi ANK, Szczepanska-Konkel M, Kempson SA et al: Inhibition of human renal epithelial Na + /P$_i$ cotransport by phosphonoformic acid. Biochem Biophys Res Commun 139:679, 1986
60. Nessi R, Bonoldi GL, Redaelli B, DiFilippo G: Acute renal failure after rifampicin: a case report and survey of the literature. Nephron 16:148, 1976
61. Davis CE, Carpenter JL, Ognibene AJ, McAllister CK: Rifampin-induced acute renal failure. South Med J 79:1012, 1986
62. Neugarten J, Gallo G, Baldwin DS: Rifampin induced nephrotic syndrome and acute interstitial nephritis. Am J Nephrol 3:38, 1983
63. Hirsch DJ, Bia FJ, Kashgarian M, Bia MJ: Rapidly progressive glomerulonephritis during antituberculous therapy. Am J Nephrol 3:7, 1983
64. Fahal IH, Williams PS, Clark RE, Bell GM: Thrombotic thrombocytopenic purpura due to rifampicin (letter). BMJ 304:882, 1992
65. Lo WK, Rolston KVI, Rubenstein EB, Bodey GP: Ciprofloxacin-induced nephrotoxicity in patients with cancer. Arch Intern Med 153:1258, 1993
66. Quesada JR, Talpaz M, Rios A et al: Clinical toxicity of the interferons in cancer patients: a review. J Clin Oncol 4:234, 1986
67. Averbuch SD, Austin HA, Sherwin SA et al: Acute interstitial nephritis with the nephrotic syndrome following recombinant leukocyte A interferon therapy for mycosis fungoides. N Engl J Med 310:32, 1984
68. Hirschtick RE, Dyrda SE, Peterson LC: Death from an unconventional therapy for AIDS (letter). Ann Intern Med 120:694, 1994
69. Hess B, Raisin J, Zimmermann A et al: Tubulointerstitial nephropathy persisting 20 months after discontinuation of chronic intake of germanium lactate citrate. Am J Kidney Dis 21:548, 1993
70. Sanai T, Okuda S, Onoyama K et al: Germanium dioxide-induced nephropathy: a new type of renal disease. Nephron 54:53, 1990
71. Krapf R, Schaffner T, Iten PX: Abuse of germanium associated with fatal lactic acidosis. Nephron 62:351, 1992

72. Korbet SM, Schwartz MM: Human immunodeficiency virus infection and nephrotic syndrome. Am J Kidney Dis 20:97, 1992
73. Kim KK, Factor SM: Membranoproliferative glomerulonephritis and plexogenic pulmonary arteriopathy in a homosexual man with acquired immunodeficiency syndrome. Hum Pathol 18:1293, 1987
74. Jindal KK, Trillo A, Bishop G et al: Crescentic IgA nephropathy as a manifestation of human immunodeficiency virus infection. Am J Nephrol 11:147, 1991
75. Katz A, Bargman JM, Miller DC et al: IgA nephritis in HIV-positive patients: a new HIV-associated nephropathy. Clin Nephrol 38:61, 1992
76. Kimmel PL, Phillips TM, Ferriera-Centeno A et al: Brief report: idiotypic IgA nephropathy in patients with human immunodeficiency virus infection. N Engl J Med 327:702, 1992
77. Kimmel PL, Phillips TM, Ferreira-Centeno A et al: HIV-associated immune-mediated renal disease. Kidney Int 44:1327, 1993
78. Thomas MA, Ibels LS, Wells JV et al: IgA kappa multiple myeloma and lymphadenopathy syndrome associated with AIDS virus infection. Aust NZ J Med 16:402, 1986
79. Shimamura T, Weiss LS, Walker JA et al: Light chain nephropathy in a 19-month-old boy with AIDS. Acta Pathol Jpn 42:500, 1992
80. Berns JS, Tomaszewski JE: Hemolytic-uremic syndrome and thrombotic thrombocytopenic purpura associated with human immunodeficiency virus infection and acquired immunodeficiency syndrome. p. 299. In Kaplan BS, Trompeter RS, Moake JL (eds): Hemolytic-Uremic Syndrome and Thrombotic Thrombocytopenic Purpura. Marcel Dekker, New York, 1992
81. Boccia RV, Gelmann EP, Baker C et al: A hemolytic-uremic syndrome with the acquired immunodeficiency syndrome. Ann Intern Med 101:716, 1984
82. Jokela J, Flynn T, Henry K: Thrombotic thrombocytopenic purpura in a human immunodeficiency virus (HIV) seropositive homosexual man. Am J Hematol 25:341, 1987
83. Thompson CE, Damon LE, Ries CA, Linter CA: Thrombotic microangiopathies in the 1980s: clinical features, response to treatment, and the impact of the human immunodeficiency virus epidemic. Blood 80:1890, 1992
84. Navarro JF, Liano F, Garcia Larana J et al: Lymphomatous infiltration of the kidneys as presentation of acquired immunodeficiency syndrome. Nephrol Dial Transplant 9:174, 1994
85. Tuso PJ: Renal failure associated with lymphoma in acquired immunodeficiency syndrome. Conn Med 56:291, 1992
86. Hom J, Venuto RC, Murray BM: Plasmacytic interstitial nephritis in a HIV+ patient. Abstracts, 19th Annual Meeting of the National Kidney Foundation, Washington, DC, Dec. 1989, p. A11
87. Pogue VA, Nurse HM: Cocaine-associated acute myoglobinuric renal failure. Am J Med 86:183, 1989
88. Roth D, Alarcon FJ, Fernandez JA et al: Acute rhabdomyolysis associated with cocaine intoxication. N Engl J Med 319:673, 1988
89. Citron BP, Halpern M, McCarron M et al: Necrotizing angiitis associated with drug abuse. N Engl J Med 283:1003, 1970
90. Johnson RJ, Couser WG: Hepatitis B infection and renal disease: clinical, immunopathogenetic and therapeutic considerations. Kidney Int 37:663, 1990
91. Johnson RJ, Gretch DR, Yamabe H et al: Membranoproliferative glomerulonephritis associated with hepatitis C virus infection. N Engl J Med 328:465, 1993

92. Agnello V, Chung RT, Kaplan LM: A role for hepatitis C virus infection in type II cryoglobulinemia. N Engl J Med 327:1490, 1992
93. Rao TKS, Friedman EA: Outcome of acute renal failure (ARF) in patients with HIV infection, abstracted. J Am Soc Nephrol 5:403, 1994
94. Finn WF: Recovery from acute renal failure. p. 553. In Lazarus JM, Brenner BM (eds): Acute Renal Failure. 3rd Ed. Churchill Livingstone, New York, 1993
95. Spiegel DM, Ullian ME, Zerbe GO, Berl T: Determinants of survival and recovery in acute renal failure patients dialyzed in intensive-care units. Am J Nephrol 11:44, 1991
96. O'Reagan S, Russo P, Lapointe N, Rousseau E: AIDS and the urinary tract. J AIDS 3:244, 1990
97. Kaplan MS, Wechsler M, Benson MC: Urologic manifestations of AIDS. Urology 30:441, 1987
98. Miles BJ, Melser M, Farah R et al: The urological manifestations of the acquired immunodeficiency syndrome. J Urol 142:771, 1989
99. Comiter S, Glasser J, Al-Askarie S: Ureteral obstruction in a patient with Burkitt's lymphoma. Urology 39:277, 1992
100. Spector DA, Katz RSS, Fuller H et al: Acute nondilating obstructive renal failure in a patient with AIDS. Am J Nephrol 9:129, 1989
101. Shafer RW, Kim DS, Weiss JP, Quale JM: Extrapulmonary tuberculosis in patients with human immunodeficiency virus infection. Medicine 70:384, 1991

4

Glomerulosclerosis Associated with HIV Infection

Jacques J. Bourgoignie

INTRODUCTION

Focal and segmental glomerulosclerosis (FSGS) is the most common glomerulopathy encountered in patients with human immunodeficiency virus (HIV) infection. There are over 350 patients with histologically proven FSGS, more than 75 patients with diffuse mesangial proliferation, and about 100 patients with other glomerulopathies and HIV infection reported in the literature. FSGS, however, was not part of the pathologic manifestations described early in the acquired immunodeficiency syndrome (AIDS) epidemic.[1] Indeed, FSGS was not mentioned in autopsy series of patients dying of AIDS in the early 1980s. Moreover, several reports in the late 1980s,[2–4] and even as recently as 1992 from Hanover, Germany,[5] do not report an increased incidence of FSGS in patients with AIDS. This paradox stems from the evolution of the AIDS epidemic, which initially involved mainly white homosexual patients, and the demography of the populations under study at various medical centers.

An increased incidence of nephrotic syndrome and FSGS in patients with AIDS was first reported in 1984 from New York and Miami. In New York,

Rao et al.[6] reported 9 patients with the nephrotic syndrome and 10 patients with FSGS among 92 patients with AIDS. Gardenswartz et al.[7] observed 7 patients with proteinuria greater than 2 g/d, 2 patients with FSGS, and 2 patients with diffuse mesangial hypercellularity among 32 patients with AIDS. In Miami, Pardo et al.[8] followed 75 patients with AIDS prospectively; 9 percent had proteinuria in excess of 3 g/d. FSGS was found in 5 and diffuse mesangial proliferation in 4 of 36 patients autopsied or biopsied. Since then, Rao and Friedman, and Pardo and Bourgoignie have extended their observations, and several investigators from various parts of the world have confirmed these findings. Nevertheless, the overall incidence of HIV-associated glomerulosclerosis and other chronic involvement of the kidney is rare relative to other organ systems involved in patients with HIV infection.

EPIDEMIOLOGY

The possibility was raised that intravenous drug use was responsible for the glomerulosclerosis seen in patients with AIDS because intravenous drug use is a definite risk factor for AIDS and can itself result in FSGS. In each of the original reports cited above, however, less than 50 percent of patients were intravenous drug users. Moreover, it rapidly became evident that AIDS-associated glomerulosclerosis also occurred in patients who did not use intravenous drugs,[9] as well as in children with perinatal AIDS.[10] These observations, together with characteristic clinical manifestations and renal histologic and ultrastructural features in patients with AIDS, as well as in HIV-infected individuals who had not yet developed AIDS, indicated that the nephropathy was different from that seen in intravenous drug users.[9–13]

The conflicting reports about the prevalence of HIV-associated glomerulosclerosis in different areas of the United States appear to reflect geographic differences in the demography of the populations studied.[14,15] Although isolated cases of HIV-associated glomerulosclerosis have been described in white and Hispanic patients,[13,16–21] a demographic analysis of patients with HIV infection and renal disease indicates a high prevalence of glomerulosclerosis in series where intravenous drug users and black patients prevail. By contrast, series with a low prevalence of glomerulosclerosis include a higher proportion of white individuals.

The predilection of the disease for blacks is striking. At the University of Miami/Jackson Memorial Medical Center where the ratio of white to black patients with AIDS was 3:1, HIV-associated nephropathy was found 10 times more frequently in black patients than in white patients.[22] By contrast, the prevalence of glomerulosclerosis in the literature was less than 1 percent among 690 predominantly white, autopsied patients with AIDS;[23] a report from Europe, in 1992, denies the existence of the glomerulopathy on the basis of an absence of clinical findings in a series of 203 prospectively studied white patients with HIV infection.[5] Such negative findings support the contention that race, for whatever reason, is an important cofactor in the expression of HIV-associated glomerulosclerosis. Other reports from ethnically mixed populations in San Francisco,[24] Rio de Janeiro,[25] and Paris[17] confirm the vulnerability of blacks to HIV-associated glomerulosclerosis. In Washington, DC, although no difference in the incidence of acute renal failure was identified among white and black patients with AIDS, the overwhelming proportion of patients with HIV infection developing chronic renal failure were black.[26]

Essentially all cases of HIV-associated glomerulosclerosis reported from Europe are described in black patients originating from countries of Central Africa or the Caribbean basin.[17,27–29] A recent report from Paris is particularly enlightening.[17] In this study, 60 patients with HIV infection were biopsied because of symptoms of renal disease. Thirty-one patients were white and 3 had FSGS. By contrast, 29 patients were black and 23 had FSGS ($P < 0.001$). Nevertheless, an outstanding incidence of the nephropathy has not yet been reported from tropical Africa; autopsies and renal biopsies, however, are rarely performed. The occurrence of HIV-associated glomerulosclerosis also has not been reported from countries of Southeast Asia where the epidemic flourishes.

The usual risk factors and modes of HIV contamination have been recognized among patients with HIV-associated glomerulosclerosis, that is, transfer of the virus by intravenous drug use or contaminated blood products as well as homosexual or heterosexual modes of transmission. Thus, in the United States, the majority of adults with HIV-associated glomerulosclerosis are young (20 to 40 years old) and 90 percent are black. Thirty to 50 percent have a history of intravenous drug use. The remainder include homosexual or bisexual men, immigrants from countries of the Caribbean basin who deny intravenous drug use or homosexuality, recipients of contaminated blood products, and heterosexual partners of HIV-infected individuals. The male-to-female distribution is not different than that reported for AIDS patients without renal disease.[11,30]

Not all patients have AIDS at the time glomerulosclerosis is diagnosed. Indeed, an important number of patients with HIV-associated glomerulosclerosis are asymptomatic HIV-infected individuals or patients with only constitutional symptoms without evidence of opportunistic infection or malignancy characterizing AIDS when they present with renal disease and are subjected to a diagnostic renal biopsy. Of the 173 patients in the literature for whom the stage of HIV infection at the time of renal biopsy was identifiable, 95 (55 percent) had AIDS and 78 (45 percent) were asymptomatic or had only constitutional symptoms.[4,7,9–13,17,18,20,26,28,31–42] Thus, the glomerulosclerosis has been labeled "HIV-associated" rather than "AIDS-associated" nephropathy.

The description by Kimmel et al.[43] of an IgA nephropathy in patients with HIV infection suggests that there may be more than one type of HIV-associated nephropathy. Therefore, the nomenclature of HIV-associated nephropathies should be amended to include the associated qualifying histologic feature such as minimal change, diffuse mesangial proliferation, glomerulosclerosis, or IgA nephropathy. The nephrotic syndrome is not a prominent manifestation of HIV-associated IgA nephropathy. Unlike HIV-associated glomerulosclerosis, HIV-associated IgA nephropathy has been reported exclusively in white patients with early HIV infection presenting with microscopic or macroscopic hematuria, absent or modest azotemia, and slowly progressive renal disease.[44]

CLINICAL COURSE

Patients with HIV-associated glomerulosclerosis present with a nephrotic syndrome and/or renal insufficiency. Hypoalbuminemia and serum creatinine concentration in excess of 2 mg/dl are usual at initial presentation. Ten to 20 percent of patients may have normal renal function.[20] The onset of the nephropathy is often abrupt with massive, nonselective proteinuria, sometimes in excess of 20 g/d, and uremia. These fulminant lesions may present as acute renal failure in patients who were well only a few weeks or months before hospital admission.[45]

In a minority of patients with AIDS, minimal proteinuria and azotemia at presentation increase insidiously over a period of several months to 1 year until a nephrotic syndrome becomes evident, with rapid evolution thereafter to uremia and end-stage renal failure.[45]

In contrast with other types of nephrotic syndrome, patients with AIDS and glomerulosclerosis frequently have little or no peripheral edema, and blood pressure is often normal even with advanced renal failure. Dehydration and low blood pressure as a consequence of constitutional symptoms, chronic diarrhea, and/or malnutrition or malabsorption may result in intravascular volume depletion and prevent the accumulation of fluid in the interstitial tissue in patients with AIDS. Serum albumin concentration is decreased, often without reciprocal increase in serum cholesterol concentration. In patients who have not developed the complications of AIDS, the absence of edema suggests that functional manifestations of tubulointerstitial involvement may result in salt wasting and prevent sodium retention.

The diagnosis of HIV-associated glomerulosclerosis is not difficult in patients with AIDS. In the absence of clinical AIDS, the diagnosis should be suspected when risk factors are elicited. Investigations of these patients fail to detect other known causes of nephrotic syndrome. Serum complement proteins are normal as are the usual serologic tests for collagen vascular disease, hepatitis, or syphilis. There may be a polyclonal increase in serum immunoglobulins. CD4 cell count is usually low but may be normal.[17] HIV infection should be confirmed by the finding of circulating HIV antibodies. Sometimes a renal biopsy performed in the work-up of a patient with apparently idiopathic nephrotic syndrome leads to an unexpected diagnosis of glomerulosclerosis with features suggesting HIV-associated nephropathy. Thus, all patients with a nephrotic syndrome should be tested for possible

HIV infection. As awareness of the nephropathy increases, HIV-associated glomerulosclerosis is now often diagnosed clinically. Not all HIV-seropositive patients, however, who develop proteinuria and renal insufficiency have glomerulosclerosis.[46] Accurate and early histologic diagnosis remains essential, particularly if the effects of antiviral agents or other potential therapy on the course of the nephropathy are to be assessed.

In HIV-seropositive individuals with a nephrotic syndrome, the identification of normal-sized or large kidneys (13 to 15 cm) with increased echogenicity supports a diagnosis of HIV-associated glomerulosclerosis[10,30,47-49] because kidney size is often decreased in other types of chronic renal disease. This clinical feature correlates with pathologic reports of enlarged kidneys found at autopsy of patients with AIDS and glomerulosclerosis.[10] Amyloidosis with nephrotic syndrome and large kidneys can occur in AIDS patients and should be considered in the differential diagnosis.[9,17,33,50] The enlargement of the kidneys does not correlate with the severity of the proteinuria.[30]

The progression to renal insufficiency is rapid in nephrotic patients, with an interval from initial clinical presentation to dialysis of only weeks to a few months (median of 11 weeks).[9,20,42] The rate of progression can vary and appears slower in Hispanics than in blacks.[13] In non-nephrotic patients, kidney survival is more prolonged. The meaning of modest proteinuria (0.5 to 2.0 g/24 h), however, is uncertain in patients with HIV infection in the absence of histologic evaluation. The rapidity with which renal function deteriorates in HIV-associated glomerulosclerosis contrasts with the slower progression of renal disease observed in the idiopathic variety of FSGS and in patients with glomerulosclerosis secondary to other etiologies.[9] Patient survival is dictated by the clinical progression of the HIV infection and is independent of the renal disease.

PATHOLOGY

The pathology of HIV-associated glomerulosclerosis is detailed in Chapter 8. Distinctive findings are summarized in Table 4-1. Whereas none of these features is specific or pathognomonic, the concomitant presence of glomerular and tubulointerstitial lesions is highly suggestive of HIV-associated glomerulosclerosis.

Several instances of minimal change disease have been reported in pro-

Table 4-1. Distinctive Pathologic Findings in HIV-Associated Glomerulosclerosis

"Collapsed" glomerular capillaries
Visceral glomerular epitheliosis
Microcystic tubules with variegated casts
Focal tubular simplification
Endothelial tubuloreticular inclusions

teinuric patients with HIV infection, including two that later evolved to glomerulosclerosis.[51] The significance of minimal glomerulopathy or focal mesangial hyperplasia in the pathogenesis of glomerular sclerosis must await prospective studies that include serial renal biopsies performed in patients with minimal proteinuria.

Diffuse and global mesangial hyperplasia, on the other hand, is readily identified histologically in approximately 25 percent of children with perinatal AIDS and nephrotic proteinuria and in 13 percent of adults.[51] The characteristic tubulointerstitial histologic features and the kidney enlargement of HIV-associated glomerulosclerosis are absent in patients with diffuse mesangial lesions, and the kidneys are not enlarged at autopsy.[10] These findings support the dominant role of the tubulointerstitial lesions in the pathogenesis of the nephromegaly seen in HIV-associated glomerulosclerosis. Clinically, these patients disclose variable proteinuria with little decrease in renal function. Like minimal lesions, the hypothesis that diffuse mesangial lesions may precede HIV-associated glomerulosclerosis is attractive, but documented transition to HIV-associated glomerulosclerosis is rare.[45]

PATHOGENESIS

FSGS is not an HIV-specific nephropathy. It can develop in a variety of apparently unrelated clinical conditions and is one way for the kidney to respond to injury. In addition to an idiopathic variety or primary form, secondary forms of FSGS can be identified with aging, and in patients with obesity, unilateral renal agenesis, reflux nephropathy, heroin addiction, diabetes mellitus, hypertension, and sickle cell disease.[52] Experimentally, it can be induced by partial renal ablation.[53] Inasmuch as the pathogenesis of FSGS in the above clinical conditions is unknown,[54] the mechanisms leading from HIV infection to focal and segmental or global glomerulosclerosis are also presently unknown.

Various theories have been proposed to explain the pathogenesis of HIV-associated glomerulosclerosis (Table 4-2). Many do not appear to be primary

Table 4-2. Factors Proposed in the Pathogenesis
of HIV-Associated Glomerulosclerosis

1. Infectious or malignant complications
2. Immune complexes
3. Intrarenal hemodynamic changes
4. *Mycoplasma fermentans*
5. Immunodeficiency per se
6. Tubular necrosis
7. Tubular obstruction
8. Renotropic HIV
9. Genetic background
10. Renal localization of HIV

factors involved in the genesis of the nephropathy; rather, they may be contributory components or cofactors to explain the rapid progression to end-stage renal failure.

1. An important role cannot be ascribed to the numerous infectious or malignant complications that define AIDS, nor to the drugs used to treat AIDS, inasmuch as the nephropathy also occurs in about 40 percent of otherwise asymptomatic patients with HIV infection and patients with only constitutional symptoms.

2. The lack of immunopathologic features, usually associated with immune-complex glomerulopathies, mitigates against an immune pathogenesis. Circulating immune complexes are frequent in AIDS patients, and mesangial deposits can be present whether or not clinical renal disease is overt.[8,10]

3. An intrarenal hemodynamic component has been suggested by Langs et al.[20] because of the often striking glomerular capillary wall collapse present in renal biopsy specimens in the absence of widespread and complete glomerular obliteration by sclerosis. Such a mechanism, although speculative, could explain the disparity observed between the severe and often fulminant functional impairment and the sometimes modest structural alterations. Blood-borne cytokines or cytokines locally produced by activated resident cells might contribute to changes in glomerular hemodynamics.

4. A pathogenic role in the development of HIV-associated glomerulosclerosis has been assigned to *Mycoplasma fermentans* (incognitus strain) by Bauer et al.[19] The presence of this antigen was demonstrated by immunohistochemistry and electron microscopy in glomerular endothelial and epithelial cells, glomerular basement membrane, tubular epithelial cells and casts, and mononuclear interstitial cells of 15 patients with AIDS and glomerulosclerosis. By contrast, none of 15 patients with AIDS and normal renal histologic findings and none of 5 patients dying of non-AIDS diseases had evidence of this mycoplasma in renal parenchymal cells. Only autopsy specimens, however, were examined in this study. Others have been unable to confirm these ultrastructural findings in renal biopsy material.[51,55]

5. A type of focal glomerulosclerosis identical to that of HIV-associated glomerulosclerosis has been reported in children with severe combined immunodeficiencies or other immunodeficiencies.[56] The nephropathy was considered to result from the altered immune status. Tubuloreticular inclusions were not described and tubular dilatation was not prominent. This proposal also would not explain the occurrence of HIV-associated glomerulosclerosis in HIV patients with normal CD4 counts.[17]

6. Cohen and Nast[12] have emphasized the role of tubular necrosis in the rapid loss of renal function in HIV-associated glomerulosclerosis. This element certainly is contributory but is not a primary pathogenic factor of the nephropathy.

7. Striking tubular dilatations containing variegated casts are often seen in renal biopsies of patients with HIV-associated glomerulosclerosis. These large casts apparently are not eliminated in the urine. Therefore, tubular obstruction has been implicated as another possible mechanism in the rapid progression of the nephropathy.[45]
8. The biologic properties of the virus may be associated with a differential ability to replicate in cells from different tissues.[57] There is no evidence, however, that certain subtypes of the virus may localize preferentially to the kidney.
9. The genetic makeup of affected individuals represents an important cofactor in the expression of HIV-associated glomerulosclerosis. As described earlier, HIV glomerulosclerosis prevails in black patients, likely in relation to their genetic background, which may also be responsible for an increased expression of renal failure in black patients with hypertension or diabetes mellitus. The converse is true for the well-known predominance of IgA nephropathy in white and Asian patients, whether it be idiopathic or HIV associated.
10. Finally, there is accumulating and substantial evidence that HIV can localize in the kidney. A direct relationship, however, between the presence of HIV in renal parenchymal cells and the pathogenesis of HIV-associated glomerulosclerosis has not been established conclusively because of inconsistent observations and because of demonstration of HIV in renal cells of patients with, as well as without, nephropathy. Therefore, the mechanisms whereby HIV may lead eventually to glomerulosclerosis remain unknown.

In 1990, we speculated that infected blood-borne lymphocytes or monocytes/macrophages could disseminate HIV to the kidney or, alternatively, directly infect glomerular or tubular cells bearing the CD4 antigen receptor or subpopulations of resident monocytes/macrophages. Activation of parenchymal renal cells or resident monocytes/macrophages might spread HIV to other cell populations and produce an inflammatory response that would mediate the destruction of renal tissue.[45] If HIV were renotropic, the kidney might serve as sanctuary for the virus, as was demonstrated for cytomegalovirus.[58] This outline has increased in complexity.

Several pieces of evidence support the possible localization of HIV in the kidney (Table 4-3).

1. Indirect evidence stems from the well-documented patients who have had a renal transplant and became HIV infected by a cadaver kidney despite extensive ex vivo perfusion of the donor organ.[59–61]
2. T lymphocytes and monocytes/macrophages expressing the CD4 molecule are the primary receptor cells for HIV. In these cells, the CD4 antigen is the membrane receptor for the envelope glycoprotein (gp120). Resident bone-marrow-derived cells have been demonstrated in rodent[62] but not in human kidney.[63] Nevertheless, a preliminary report described the presence of CD4 antigen in mesangial cells of nor-

Table 4-3. Evidence Suggesting Possible Localization of HIV in the Kidney

1. Renal transplantation
2. CD4 antigen expression in mesangial cells
3. p24 HIV antigen in tubular epithelial cells
4. Identification of HIV genome by in situ hybridization in tubular and glomerular epithelial cells
5. HIV replication in glomerular cells
6. Identification of viral DNA by PCR in renal parenchymal cells
7. Simian immunodeficiency
8. Transgenic mouse with noninfectious HIV provirus

Abbreviation: PCR, polymerase chain reaction.

mal human kidney, suggesting that direct HIV infection of glomeruli was possible.[64] This finding, however, has not been confirmed by Alpers et al.[63]

3. Direct evidence of HIV localization in the kidney was provided by Cohen et al.[65] Using a monoclonal antibody, these investigators localized HIV core p24 antigen by immunohistochemistry in the cytoplasm of tubular epithelium. Replication of these findings, however, has been difficult because of problems of specificity with the various immunohistochemical probes used for virus antigen detection.[66–68]

4. Using the more sensitive in situ hybridization technique and a cDNA probe for HIV nucleic acid, the same investigators found the HIV genome not only in tubular epithelial cells, but also in glomerular epithelia in 10 of 11 patients with HIV-associated glomerulosclerosis, unlike in kidneys from HIV-seropositive patients with immune complex glomerulonephritis or HIV-seronegative patients.[65] Using alternate DNA probes, however, others have been unable to detect HIV genomic nucleic acid in renal tissue, but only in passenger leukocytes.[67,68]

5. Green et al.[69] succeeded in infecting glomerular cells by exposing homogeneous cultures of human glomerular capillary endothelial cells, mesangial cells, and epithelial cells to HIV in vitro. Infection developed fast, consistently, and was generalized with glomerular endothelial cells, whereas infection was slow, inconsistent, and limited with mesangial cells. Infectivity attempts were unsuccessful with glomerular epithelial cells. Erice and Kim[70] also succeeded in infecting human mesangial cells in culture, whereas Alpers et al.[63] could not. The methodology used by the last researchers, however, might not have been sensitive enough to detect a low level of mesangial infection, as others have found that coculture with normal peripheral blood mononuclear cells after exposure to HIV or detection of HIV DNA by polymerase chain reaction (PCR) was required.[69] Shukla et al.[71] recently transfected human mesangial cells in culture with a functional HIV gene.

6. Using the sensitive PCR technique, Kimmel et al.[72] detected HIV DNA in 28 renal biopsies of 29 HIV-infected patients with nephrotic proteinuria of various etiologies. Moreover, microdissection of glomeruli, tubules, interstitial cells, and infiltrating inflammatory cells identified

the HIV genome in all but interstitial cells.[72] The HIV genome was present in renal cells of HIV-infected patients with or without nephropathy, but not of HIV-seronegative patients. Thus, in these studies, the HIV genome appears to be ubiquitous in renal tissue of HIV-seropositive patients regardless of nephropathologic outcome, risk factor, and stage of HIV infection. The studies do not identify which cell(s) within the glomerulus contained the HIV genome.

The finding of HIV proviral DNA in renal tissue of HIV-infected patients regardless of nephropathy indicates that the presence of the HIV genome is not sufficient for the development of glomerulosclerosis. Some triggering local mechanism must be crucial for the expression of renal disease. Host factors related to immune or genetic response to HIV must be associated with the induction of the nephropathy.

7. The difficulties of unraveling the pathogenesis of HIV-associated glomerulosclerosis have been compounded by the lack of an animal model. In monkeys, simian immunodeficiency virus may produce a disease similar to AIDS in humans. In the rhesus, *Macaca mulatta*, mesangial hyperplasia as well as a sclerosing glomerulopathy may ensue. No virus, however, was identified in the kidney.[73]

8. Another animal model was recently described by Dickie et al.[74] They produced transgenic mice using a noninfectious HIV provirus transgene in which *gag* and *pol* sequences encompassing the coding sequences for p24, p15, protease, reverse transcriptase, and the amino terminus of p34 endonuclease were deleted. The transgenic animals remained healthy and transmitted the transgene to their progeny. Tissue expression and specificity was variable, and possibly dependent on host transcriptional proteins.[75] Three lines of mice in which the transgene was present in the kidney were produced from eight transgenic founders. The heterozygous mice were immunocompetent and did not experience opportunistic infections, but they eventually developed renal disease. Renal expression of proviral mRNA was transient and evident in glomeruli, but not in tubules, before the onset of proteinuria. The proteinuria was progressive, leading to a severe nephrotic syndrome, uremia, and death.[76]

The kidneys of severely proteinuric animals were enlarged (twice normal) and showed a spectrum of pathologic changes resembling HIV-associated glomerulosclerosis including microcystic dilated tubules filled with proteinaceous casts, simplification of tubular epithelium, mild mononuclear interstitial nephritis, segmental or global glomerulosclerosis with reactive epithelial cells, and marked expansion of mesangial cell matrix with increased deposition of laminin, collagen, and heparan sulfate proteoglycan.[76] Some glomeruli showed mesangial hypercellularity. Subcellular ultrastructural particles, such as tubuloreticular inclusions, were absent.[74] Renal tubular cells expressed increased amounts of tissue growth factor-β (TGF-β) and normal cell polarization for Na^+-K^+-ATPase.[77] Because the virus is not replicating in this model, these findings suggest that HIV-1 gene products alone can induce many of the features of HIV-associated glomerulosclerosis and implicate HIV genes directly in its pathogenesis.

There is increasing evidence that cytokines and growth factors play an important role in the progression of idiopathic glomerulosclerosis.[54] The tubular hyperplasia and dilatation characteristic of HIV-associated glomerulosclerosis suggest a role for cytokines and growth factors in the expression of the nephropathy. There is emerging evidence that such factors may contribute importantly to the rapid progression and possibly the pathogenesis of HIV-associated glomerulosclerosis. An increased influx of macrophages,[78] increased production of cytokines,[79] and increased expression of TGF-β[80,81] have been described in the kidneys of patients with HIV-associated glomerulosclerosis. TGF-β particularly has been implicated in the mesangial expansion and sclerosis evident in HIV-associated glomerulosclerosis. TGF-β, but not tumor necrosis factor (TNF) or platelet-derived growth factor (PDGF), has also been shown to activate HIV gene expression in human mesangial cells transfected with an HIV provirus.[71]

TREATMENT

There have been no prospective treatment trials of HIV-associated glomerulosclerosis. One reason has been the concern of treating infected patients with steroids or immunosuppressive agents. The other is that the pharmacodynamics of new antiviral agents were unknown until recently and their toxicities not established in patients with renal insufficiency.

When they have been used, corticosteroids have usually been ineffective on proteinuria or progression of renal disease.[21,45,82] A recent report, however, indicates that corticosteroids given at a dose of 60 mg/d for 2 to 6 weeks reduced mean serum creatinine in four patients with biopsy proven HIV-associated glomerulosclerosis from 9.1 to 3.3 mg/dl.[38] There was no effect on proteinuria, and two of the four patients experienced serious adverse effects during prednisone treatment. These uncontrolled observations warrant confirmation with additional controlled studies, as well as further clarification of the toxicities of this treatment.

There are anecdotal reports of clinical improvement with zidovudine at a dose of 300 to 800 mg/d, consisting of temporary remission of proteinuria and/or delayed occurrence of renal failure for several months,[18,34,35,84] including one patient who was able to discontinue maintenance hemodialysis temporarily. Zidovudine, however, was ineffective in nephrotic children,[21] and we have seen patients with HIV-associated glomerulosclerosis progress despite administration of prophylactic zidovudine. Nevertheless, our clinical impression is that HIV-associated glomerulosclerosis occurred less frequently in the last 2 years than it did 3 to 5 years ago; also, progression of the renal disease was not as explosive in patients who received prophylactic chemotherapy with zidovudine, didanosine (ddI), or trimethoprim-sulfamethoxazole than in those who did not. This clinical impression of a decreased incidence of end-stage renal failure secondary to HIV-associated glomerulosclerosis is corroborated by a decrease in HIV-associated end-stage renal failure also observed in 1992 in Brooklyn, New York.[85] Whether this decrease is due to prophylaxis with antiviral agents or to other factors is conjectural and circumstantial.

Nevertheless, three recent reports support a clinical effect of antiviral agents on HIV-associated glomerulosclerosis. One retrospective analysis of six patients with histologically proven HIV-associated glomerulosclerosis indicated no benefit of zidovudine (300 to 800 mg/d) in two patients with advanced renal disease, but indicated an important delay or the avoidance for the need of chronic hemodialysis for up to 33 months in four patients with less advanced renal dysfunction (serum creatinine 1.2 to 5.1 mg/dl).[28]

In another study, 15 patients with minimal renal dysfunction (mean serum creatinine 0.95 mg/dl) were prospectively treated with zidovudine at 400 to 800 mg/d. After 6 to 26 months of follow-up, mean serum creatinine was unchanged for the group and no patient developed an overt nephropathy or progressed to end-stage renal failure. The same study describes four patients with biopsy-proven HIV-associated glomerulosclerosis in whom azotemia stabilized or decreased, and proteinuria improved after 3 to 24 months of treatment with 400 mg/d zidovudine.[86]

In the third study, 43 of 54 patients with 2+ proteinuria received zidovudine while 11 did not. Zidovudine had little effect in patients already azotemic at the time of initiation of therapy; all patients became uremic or developed end-stage renal failure. On the other hand, only 5 of 37 nonazotemic patients who were given zidovudine developed mild azotemia after 2 years of treatment, whereas 4 of 10 nonazotemic patients who remained untreated developed end-stage renal failure.[87]

Although the evidence is soft, these observations suggest that zidovudine prophylaxis may protect the kidney, at least when used early in proteinuric patients before azotemia develops.

Cyclosporine has been used in children with HIV-associated glomerulosclerosis and reportedly induced a remission of the nephrotic syndrome for up to 1 year in three children with perinatal AIDS and normal renal function. At follow-up, two of these children were in remission and one, who had two renal biopsies, showed no progression of focal glomerulosclerosis after 12 months.[21] There is no report of the use of cyclosporine in adults with HIV-associated glomerulosclerosis.

Once end-stage renal failure develops and supportive maintenance dialysis is needed, the complications of HIV are the dominant factor in patient survival as they are in HIV-infected patients without renal involvement.[9,42,88] Prolonged survival is the rule in asymptomatic HIV-infected individuals on chronic hemodialysis or peritoneal dialysis much like it is for patients with end-stage renal failure who are HIV seronegative. Patients with constitutional symptoms are prone to bacterial infections. Whereas their mortality exceeds that of HIV-seronegative patients on chronic hemodialysis, their survival far exceeds that of patients with clinical AIDS. By contrast, based on a review of patients reported in the literature, survival of patients with clinical AIDS is short and rarely exceeds 1 year even with maintenance hemodialysis. They may develop a syndrome of unexplained malnutrition and wasting, and a "failure to thrive" that is unresponsive to intensive nutritional support.[9] The effects of antiviral agents in HIV-infected patients on chronic dialysis are unknown. With better prophylaxis of potential opportunistic infections, it appears that prolonged survival is possible in individual patients with AIDS. The decision to withhold renal replacement therapy in patients with terminal AIDS must be individualized.[89]

CONCLUSION

In conclusion, HIV-associated nephropathy is a clinical and pathologic entity that leaves many unanswered questions. Why is the incidence of renal disease relatively infrequent in relation to other organ systems affected by HIV? What systemic and local factors are involved in the expression of HIV-associated nephropathy and in its rapid progression to end-stage renal disease? What are the roles of cytokines, growth factors, and HIV per se in the pathogenesis of glomerulosclerosis? How does HIV enter renal cells and which renal cells are susceptible to HIV infection in vivo? Understanding the underlying pathogenesis is important because HIV-associated glomerulosclerosis may be an accelerated, collapsed-in-time form of glomerulosclerosis with pathogenic mechanisms that may be intrinsically similar and directly relevant to those prevailing in other forms of glomerulosclerosis.

ACKNOWLEDGMENT

The author is grateful to Mrs. Sonia Barton for editorial assistance.

REFERENCES

1. Wormser GP, Stahl RE, Bottome EG (eds): AIDS and Other Manifestations of HIV Infection. Noyes Publications, Park Ridge, NY, 1987
2. Seney FD Jr, Burns DK, Silva FG: Acquired immunodeficiency syndrome and the kidney. Am J Kidney Dis 16:1, 1990
3. Balow JE, Macher AM, Rook AH: Paucity of glomerular disease in acquired immunodeficiency syndrome (AIDS), abstracted. Kidney Int 29:178, 1986
4. Mazbar SA, Schoenfeld PY, Humphreys MH: Renal involvement in patients infected with HIV: experience at San Francisco General Hospital. Kidney Int 37:1325, 1990
5. Brunkhorst R, Brunkhorst U, Eisenbach GM et al: Lack of clinical evidence for a specific HIV-associated glomerulopathy in 203 patients with HIV infection. Nephrol Dial Transplant 7:87, 1992

6. Rao TK, Filippone EJ, Nicastri AD et al: Associated focal and segmental glomerulosclerosis in the acquired immunodeficiency syndrome. N Engl J Med 310: 669, 1984
7. Gardenswartz MH, Lerner CW, Seligson GR et al: Renal disease in patients with AIDS: a clinicopathologic study. Clin Nephrol 21:197, 1984
8. Pardo V, Aldana M, Colton RM et al: Glomerular lesions in the acquired immunodeficiency syndrome. Ann Intern Med 101:429, 1984
9. Rao TK, Friedman EA: Renal syndromes in the acquired immunodeficiency syndrome (AIDS): lessons learned from analysis over 5 years. Artif Organs 12:206, 1988
10. Pardo V, Meneses R, Ossa L et al: AIDS-related glomerulopathy: occurrence in specific risk groups. Kidney Int 31:1167, 1987
11. D'Agati V, Cheng JI, Carbone L et al: The pathology of HIV-nephropathy: a detailed morphologic and comparative study. Kidney Int 35:1358, 1989
12. Cohen AH, Nast CC: HIV-associated nephropathy: a unique combined glomerular, tubular and interstitial lesion. Mod Pathol 1:87, 1988
13. Soni A, Agarwal A, Chander P et al: Evidence for an HIV-related nephropathy: a clinicopathological study. Clin Nephrol 31:12, 1989
14. Bourgoignie JJ, Ortiz-Interian C, Green DF et al: The epidemiology of human immunodeficiency virus-associated nephropathy. p. 484. In Hatano M (ed): Nephrology. Vol. 1. Springer Verlag, Tokyo, 1991
15. Humphreys MH: Human immunodeficiency virus-associated nephropathy. East is East and West is West? Arch Intern Med 150:253, 1990
16. Valeri A, Neusy AJ: Acute and chronic renal disease in hospitalized AIDS patients. Clin Nephrol 35:110, 1991
17. Nochy D, Gotz D, Dosquet P et al: Renal disease associated with HIV infection. A multicentric study of 60 patients from Paris hospitals. Nephrol Dial Transplant 8:11, 1993
18. Babut-Gay ML, Echard M, Kleinknecht D, Meyrier A: Zidovudine and nephropathy with human immunodeficiency virus (HIV) infection (letter). Ann Intern Med 111:856, 1989
19. Bauer FA, Wear DJ, Angritt P, Lo SC: *Mycoplasma fermentans* (incognitus strain) infection in the kidneys of patients with acquired immunodeficiency syndrome and associated nephropathy: a light microscopic, immunohistochemical, and ultrastructural study. Human Pathol 22:63, 1991
20. Langs C, Gallo GR, Schacht RG et al: Rapid renal failure in AIDS-associated focal glomerulosclerosis. Arch Intern Med 150:287, 1990
21. Ingulli E, Tejani A, Fikrig S et al: Nephrotic syndrome associated with acquired immunodeficiency syndrome in children. J Pediatr 119:710, 1991
22. Bourgoignie JJ, Ortiz-Interian C, Green DF, Roth D: Race, a co-factor in HIV-1 associated nephropathy. Transplant Proc 21:3899, 1989
23. Bourgoignie JJ, Pardo V: The nephropathology in human immunodeficiency virus (HIV-1) infection. Kidney Int 35:S19, 1991
24. Frassetto L, Schoenfeld PY, Humphreys MH: Increasing incidence of human immunodeficiency virus-associated nephropathy at San Francisco General Hospital. Am J Kidney Dis 18:655, 1991
25. Lopes GS, Marques LPJ, Rioja LS et al: Glomerular disease and human immunodeficiency virus infection in Brazil. Am J Nephrol 12:281, 1992
26. Cantor ES, Kimmel PL, Bosch JP: Effect of race on expression of acquired immunodeficiency syndrome-associated nephropathy. Arch Intern Med 151:125, 1991

27. van der Reijden HJ, Schipper MEF, Danner SA, Arisz L: Glomerular lesions and opportunistic infections of the kidney in AIDS: an autopsy study of 47 cases. Adv Exp Med Biol 252:181, 1989

28. Michel C, Dosquet P, Ronco P et al: Nephropathy associated with human immunodeficiency virus: a report of 11 cases including 6 treated with zidovudine. Nephron 62:441, 1992

29. Esforzado N, Feliz T, Almirall J et al: Nephropathy in human immunodeficiency virus infection. Med Clin (Barcelona) 98:764, 1992

30. Bourgoignie JJ, Meneses R, Ortiz C et al: The clinical spectrum of renal disease associated with human immunodeficiency virus. Am J Kidney Dis 12:131, 1988

31. Chander P, Soni A, Bhagwat R et al: Renal ultrastructural markers in AIDS-associated nephropathy. Am J Pathol 126:513, 1987

32. Alpers CE, Harawi S, Rennke HG: Focal glomerulosclerosis with tubuloreticular inclusions: possible predictive value for acquired immunodeficiency syndrome (AIDS). Am J Kidney Dis 12:240, 1988

33. Baumelou A, Assogba V, Beaufils H et al: Pathologie rénale associée à l'infection à virus VIH et au syndrôme d'immunodéficience acquise. p. 42. In Chatelain C, Jacobs C (eds): Sémin Uro-Néphrologie. Masson, Paris, 1989

34. Cook PP, Appel RG: Prolonged clinical improvement in HIV-associated nephropathy with zidovudine therapy, abstracted. J Am Soc Nephrol 1:842, 1990

35. Lam M, Park MC: HIV-associated nephropathy: beneficial effect of zidovudine therapy (letter). N Engl J Med 323:1775, 1990

36. Genderini A, Bertani T, Bertoli S et al: HIV-associated nephropathy: a new entity. A study of 12 cases. Nephrol Dial Transpl, suppl. 1:84, 1990

37. Kaplan MS, Wechsler M, Benson MC: Urologic manifestations of AIDS. Urology 30:441, 1987

38. Provenzano R, Kupin W, Santiago GC: Renal involvement in the acquired immunodeficiency syndrome: presentation, clinical course and therapy. Henry Ford Hosp Med J 35:38, 1987

39. Haddoum F, Dosquet P, Mougenot B et al: Syndrôme néphrotique révélateur d'un SIDA (letter). Presse Med 16:1373, 1987

40. Meisenberg BR, Robinson WL, Mosley CA et al: Thrombotic thrombocytopenic purpura in human immunodeficiency (HIV) seropositive males. Am J Hematol 27:212, 1988

41. Coleburn NH, Scholes JV, Lowe FC: Renal failure in patients with AIDS-related complex. Urology 37:523, 1991

42. Carbone L, D'Agati V, Cheng JT, Appel GB: Course and prognosis of human immunodeficiency virus-associated nephropathy. Am J Med 87:389, 1989

43. Kimmel PL, Phillips TM, Farkas-Szallasi T et al: Idiotypic IgA nephropathy in patients with HIV infection. N Engl J Med 327:702, 1992

44. Bourgoignie JJ, Pardo V: Human immunodeficiency virus-associated nephropathies (editorial). N Engl J Med 327:729, 1992

45. Bourgoignie JJ: Renal complications of human immunodeficiency virus type 1. Kidney Int 37:1571, 1990

46. Korbet SM, Schwartz MM: Renal biopsy conference from the Rush-Presbyterian St. Luke's Medical Center: human immunodeficiency virus infection and nephrotic syndrome. Am J Kidney Dis 20:97, 1992

47. Hamper UM, Goldblum LE, Hutchins GM et al: Renal involvement in AIDS: sonographic pathologic correlation. Am J Roentgenol 150:1321, 1988

48. Schaffer RM, Schwartz GE, Becker JA et al: Renal ultrasound in acquired immune deficiency syndrome. Radiology 153:511, 1984

49. Kay CJ: Renal disease in patients with AIDS: sonographic findings. Am J Roentgenol 159:551, 1992
50. Cozzi PJ, Abu-Jawdah GM, Green RM, Green D: Amyloidosis in association with human immunodeficiency virus infection. Clin Infect Dis 14:189, 1992
51. Pardo V, Wetli CV, Strauss J et al: The renal complications of drug abuse and human immunodeficiency virus. In Tischer C, Brenner BM (eds): Pathology of the Kidney. 2nd Ed. Williams & Wilkins, New York, 1994
52. Goldzer RC, Sweet J, Cotran RS: Focal segmental glomerulosclerosis. Annu Rev Med 35:429, 1984
53. Brenner BM: Hemodynamically mediated glomerular disease and the progressive nature of renal disease. Kidney Int 23:647, 1983
54. Wolthuis A, van Goor H, Weening JJ, Grond J: Pathobiology of focal sclerosis. Curr Opin Nephrol Hypertens 2:458, 1993
55. Cohen AH: Mycoplasma infection in the kidneys of patients with acquired immunodeficiency syndrome (letter). Hum Pathol 22:932, 1991
56. Foster S, Hawkins E, Hanson CG et al: Pathology of the kidney in childhood immunodeficiency: AIDS-related nephropathy is not unique. Pediatr Pathol 11:63, 1991
57. Cheng-Mayer C, Levy LA: Distinct biological and serological properties of human immunodeficiency viruses from the brain. Ann Neurol 23:S58, 1988
58. Heieren MH, Vander Woude JF, Balfour HM Jr: Cytomegalovirus replicates efficiently in human kidney mesangial cells. Proc Natl Acad Sci USA 85:1642, 1988
59. Rubin RH, Jenkins RL, Shaw BW et al: The acquired immunodeficiency syndrome and transplantation. Transplantation 44:1, 1987
60. Lang P, Niaudet P: Update and outcome of renal transplantation patients with human immunodeficiency virus: the groupe cooperatif de transplantation de l'Ile de France. Transplant Proc 23:1352, 1991
61. Glassock RJ, Cohen AH, Danovitch G, Parsa KP: Human immunodeficiency virus (HIV) infection and the kidney. Ann Intern Med 112:35, 1990
62. Striker GE, Lange MA, Mackay K et al: Glomerular cells in vitro. Adv Nephrol 16:169, 1987
63. Alpers CE, McClure J, Bursten SL: Human mesangial cells are resistant to productive infection by multiple strains of human immunodeficiency virus types 1 and 2. Am J Kidney Dis 19:126, 1992
64. Karlsson-Parra A, Dimeny E, Fellstrom B, Klareskog L: HIV receptors (CD4 antigen) in normal human glomerular cells (letter). N Engl J Med 320:741, 1989
65. Cohen AH, Sun NCJ, Shapshak P, Imagawa DT: Demonstration of human immunodeficiency virus in renal epithelium in HIV-associated nephropathy. Mod Pathol 2:125, 1989
66. Barbiano di Belgiojoso G, Genderini A, Vago L et al: Absence of HIV antigens in renal tissue from patients with HIV-associated nephropathy. Nephrol Dial Transplant 5:489, 1990
67. Pardo V, Shapshak P, Yoshioka M, Strauss J: HIV associated nephropathy (HIVN). Direct renal invasion or indirect glomerular involvement, abstracted. FASEB J 5:907A, 1991
68. Nadasdy T, Hanson-Painton O, Davis L et al: Conditions affecting the detection of HIV in formalin-fixed paraffin-embedded sections in kidney and other organs from AIDS patients, abstracted. Lab Invest 64:98A, 1991
69. Green DR, Resnick L, Bourgoignie JJ: HIV infects glomerular endothelial and mesangial cells but not epithelial cells in vitro. Kidney Int 41:956, 1992

70. Erice A, Kim Y: In-vitro infection of human renal cells by human immunodeficiency virus; pathogenic implications for HIV-associated nephropathy, abstracted. Clin Res 39:219A, 1991

71. Shukla RR, Kumar A, Kimmel PL: Transforming growth factor beta increases the expression of HIV-1 gene in human mesangial cells. Kidney Int 44:1022, 1993

72. Kimmel PL, Ferreira-Centeno A, Farkas-Szallasi T et al: Viral DNA in microdissected renal tissue biopsy from HIV infected patients with nephrotic syndrome. Kidney Int 243:1347, 1993

73. Alpers CE, Baskin GB: Sclerosing glomerulopathy in rhesus monkeys with simian AIDS, abstracted. Kidney Int 35:339, 1989

74. Dickie P, Felser J, Eckhaus M et al: HIV-associated nephropathy in transgenic mice expressing HIV-1 genes. Virology 185:109, 1991

75. Bruggeman LA, Adler SH, Rappaport J, Klotman PE: Role of NF-Kb in the renal expression of HIV-1 transgenic mice, abstracted. J Am Soc Nephrol 4:596, 1993

76. Kopp JB, Klotman ME, Adler SH et al: Progressive glomerulosclerosis and enhanced renal accumulation of basement membrane components in mice transgenic for human immunodeficiency virus type 1 genes. Proc Natl Acad Sci USA 89:1577, 1992

77. Kopp JB, McCunie BK, Notkins AL et al: Increased expression of transforming growth factor beta in HIV-transgenic mouse kidney, abstracted. J Am Soc Nephrol 1:600, 1991

78. Bodi I, Abraham A, Kaul S, Kimmel PL: Macrophages in immune cell infiltrates in HIV focal glomerulosclerosis, abstracted. J Am Soc Nephrol 4:674, 1993

79. Kimmel PL, Bodi I, Abraham A, Phillips TM: Increased renal tissue cytokines in human HIV nephropathy, abstracted. J Am Soc Nephrol 4:279, 1993

80. Bodi I, Kimmel PL, Abraham A et al: Increased TGF-β expression in human HIV-associated nephropathy, abstracted. J Am Soc Nephrol 4:461, 1993

81. Border W, Yamamoto T, Noble N et al: HIV-associated nephropathy is linked to TGF-β and matrix protein expression in human kidney, abstracted. J Am Soc Nephrol 4:675, 1993

82. Strauss J, Abitbol C, Zilleruelo G et al: Renal disease in children with the acquired immunodeficiency syndrome. N Engl J Med 321:625, 1989

83. Smith MC, Pawar R, Carey JT et al: Effect of corticosteroid therapy on human immunodeficiency virus-associated nephropathy. Am J Med 97:145, 1994

84. Harrer T, Hunzelmann N, Stoll R et al: Therapy for HIV-1 related nephritis with zidovudine. AIDS 4:815, 1990

85. Rao TKS, Friedman EA: A decade of human immunodeficiency associated nephropathy, abstracted. J Am Soc Nephrol 4:284, 1993

86. Ifudu O, Rao TKS, Tan CC et al: Zidovudine improves prognosis in HIV-associated nephropathy, abstracted. J Am Soc Nephrol 4:277, 1993

87. Ahmed V, Kloser P, Miller MA, Lasker N: Does zidovudine slow the progression of HIV nephropathy?, abstracted. J Am Soc Nephrol 4:269, 1993

88. Ortiz C, Meneses R, Jaffe D et al: Outcome of patients with human immunodeficiency virus on maintenance hemodialysis. Kidney Int 34:248, 1988

89. Pennell JP, Bourgoignie JJ: Should AIDS patients be dialyzed? Trans Am Soc Artif Intern Organs 34:907, 1988

5

Immune Complex Glomerulonephritis Associated with HIV Infection

Paul L. Kimmel
Terry M. Phillips

PATHOGENIC MECHANISMS UNDERLYING IMMUNE-MEDIATED RENAL DISEASE

Antibody-Mediated Renal Disease

Immune mechanisms of pathogenesis are assumed to underlie most forms of clinical glomerulonephritis.[1-3] Dysregulation of both the humoral and cellular arms of the immune system may be associated with the development of glomerulonephritis. Two major humoral mechanisms have been delineated that can lead to the deposition of antibody in renal tissue. Antibodies may circulate in the vascular compartment, either as free immunoglobulin or in the form of an antigen-antibody complex (Table 5-1). Circulating immunoglobulins can also react with fixed, structural antigens within the kidney, resulting in the formation of in situ immune deposits. The endogenous antigen interacting with the pathogenic antibody may be, for example, a component of the glomerular basement membrane (GBM), a mesangial matrix protein, or a cell surface protein. The first instance is associated with the pathogenesis of Goodpasture syndrome,[3] while the latter mechanism is thought to underlie the pathogenesis of renal disease in animals with Heymann's nephritis, a model of membranous nephropathy, in which a specific glomerular epithelial antigen is involved.[4] Although in humans the antigen involved in the pathogenesis of membranous nephropathy has not been isolated, antibody-mediated interactions with endogenous antigens may be important in the pathogenesis of the disease.[3,4]

Alternatively, antibodies may form against antigens induced by tumor-related proteins or products of infectious organisms within renal tissue. Additionally, antibodies generated against other circulating or nonrenal antigens can cross-react with renal antigens. Such antibodies may become pathogenic, depositing within renal tissue, and initiating the development of disease.

In many cases, however, the antigen inducing antibody production may be exogenous, such as a protein product related to an infectious agent or drug. In such cases, the exogenous, nephritogenic antigen either may be directly deposited in the kidney, or through various pathologic processes (including inflammation or infection) may alter a host protein, thus initiating an immune response. Antibody reacting with "trapped," "planted," or altered renal antigens may lead to the initiation of localized inflammation or might facilitate the deposition of circulating immune complexes (CICs). In either case, histopathologic examination by immunofluorescent microscopy would reveal a distinct pattern of deposition (either granular or linear) that reflects the site of antigen binding.[3]

Immune Complex-Mediated Disease

After the formation of antigen-antibody complexes in the circulation, complexes may deposit within glomerular capillaries, initiating an immune complex-mediated mechanism of pathogenesis. CICs can accumulate in glomer-

Table 5-1. Pathogenic Mechanisms Involved in Immune-Mediated Renal Disease

Humoral Immune Mechanisms
 Direct antibody reactions with tissue-fixed antigens
  Antibody reactions with native renal antigens
   Basement membrane and extracellular matrix antigens
   GBM, TBM components, ?TBM/drug conjugates
  Antibody reactions with renal cell antigens
   Cell surface and other antigens
    Tamm-Horsfall protein, infectious agents, phagocytosed materials, other reactive antigens
  Antibody reactions with antigens trapped or "planted" in the kidney
   Charged or lectinlike molecules, DNA, immune deposit components, infectious products
 Antibody reactions with soluble antigens to form immune complexes
  Exogenous antigens
   Drugs, microbial antigens
  Endogenous antigens
   Nuclear and cellular materials, tumor antigens, thyroglobulin
Cellular Immune Mechanisms
 Polymorphonuclear leukocytes
  Neutrophils
  Eosinophils
 Mononuclear cells
  T cells
  Macrophages
  Natural killer cells
 Platelets
Activation of Mediator Pathways
 Immune
  Complement proteins
  Cytokines
  Chemokines
 Nonimmune
  Coagulation proteins
  Eicosanoids
  Oxidants
  Nitric oxide
  Others

Abbreviations: GBM, glomerular basement membrane; TBM, tubular basement membrane.
(Modified from Wilson,[3] with permission.)

uli, GBM, mesangium, tubular basement membrane, and the renal interstitium,[3] all being associated with the development of renal disease. The renal disease of systemic lupus erythematosus and cryoglobulinemia are classic examples of human CIC-mediated nephropathies.

Alternatively, antigens within the kidney may predispose to CIC deposition, a form of mixed CIC deposition and in situ mechanism of disease pathogenesis. In experimental models, in situ immune complex formation enhanced deposition of CICs, suggesting that the two mechanisms may occur concurrently, resulting in a linked, dual disorder.[3,5]

Antibody or immune complexes (ICs) deposited in renal tissue can initiate a cascade of inflammatory or cellular events resulting in the development of renal disease. Several mediators have been outlined that are important factors in determining renal histologic and functional outcomes[1,3] (Table 5-1).

Mediation of Tissue Injury

Antibodies and complement (C′) in the absence of circulating antigen can cause proteinuria without extensive evidence of pathologic renal damage at the light microscopic level, as delineated in models of membranous nephropathy.[1,3,4] Alternatively, antibodies may cause injury to the GBM[6] by reacting with either normal components of the membrane or molecules that become embedded or "planted" in the membrane. In the former case, GBM components are considered foreign and anti-GBM autoantibodies are formed,[7] representing a breakdown in the recognition of "self" and a loss of tolerance to one's own tissues. Injury to the GBM occurs when circulating anti-GBM antibodies attach to the membrane and bind C′, resulting in the formation of "linear" antibody deposition along the entire GBM. However, the presence of linear immunoglobulin deposits cannot be considered diagnostic of anti-GBM disease, as similar immunopathologic findings may be observed in other diseases with different pathophysiology and clinical outcome, such as diabetes mellitus. The clinical expression of anti-GBM antibody disease varies widely from glomerular lesions, which consist of widespread extracapillary proliferation and crescent formation, coupled variably with rapid diminution in renal function (rapidly progressive glomerulonephritis) and pulmonary hemorrhage, to very mild renal disease, sometimes detectable only by renal biopsy and immunopathologic studies. The reason for this variation in pathologic and functional response is unknown. Because circulating levels of anti-GBM antibody do not correlate well with the severity or nature of the clinical findings, other factors, such as the presence of mediators of inflammation, including C′, polymorphonuclear (PMN) and mononuclear cells, and cytokines may all contribute to the expression of the disease.

GBM injury occurs when C′ is activated after binding to the anti-GBM in situ formed IC. This activation leads to the generation of biologically active fragments possessing inflammatory, chemotactic, and vasoactive properties. These factors, in turn, cause the release of vasoactive amines and peptides from cellular sites. PMN[8] and mononuclear cells[9–11] may be attracted to the sites of immunoglobulin and C′ deposition, resulting in localized injury and destruction of the GBM.

The type of antibody may be an important determinant of its nephritogenicity. Different IgG subtypes may be associated with a range of different tissue responses. The ability of immunoglobulin subtypes to fix and activate complement may be important in determining the extent and course of inflammation.

Chemokines (chemoattractive cytokines),[12] may play an important role in the initiation and maintenance of cell-mediated pathologic events, by immune cellular tissue infiltration. Antibody-mediated activation of the membrane attack sequence (C5b-9) of C' effects glomerular cellular synthesis of basement membrane components resulting in structural changes and impairment of function.

Reactive antibodies may be generated when foreign materials become embedded or "planted" in renal structures, such as the GBM.[13] Once bound to the tissue, this material may be recognized as antigenic and become the target of host-derived immune responses, giving rise to secondary consequences, such as C' activation, chemotactic attraction of polymorphonuclear leukocytes (PMNs), and the development of localized tissue injury. Plant lectins, endogenous nucleic acids, chemically active drugs, cationic streptococcal antigens, and heterologous anti-GBM antibodies are examples of planted antigens.[3]

Cell-Mediated Immune Injury

The involvement of cell-mediated immunologic activity (i.e., effector T cells, and natural killer and killer cells) in renal disease is unclear, although lymphocytic infiltration is seen in several proliferative glomerular diseases. A few studies have shown that T-lymphocyte mitogenic responses can be elicited after incubation of patients' cells with glomerular or tubular antigens. Perhaps the most common clinical example is the cellular infiltration seen after renal tubular toxicity or during interstitial tubular disease.

Clinicopathologic studies have consistently demonstrated that interstitial fibrosis and cellular parameters, rather than glomerular factors, are associated with outcomes in several different types of glomerulonephritis.[14–16] The cellular infiltrate seen in various glomerulonephritides is composed largely of mononuclear cells, primarily lymphocytes.[9,10] Nephritogenic T lymphocytes have been associated with the pathogenesis of autoimmune renal disease in a murine model.[17]

Macrophages have also been implicated as effector cells in the pathogenesis of renal diseases of various etiologies[9–11] because of their secretory products (cytokines and other bioactive compounds such as proteases, eicosanoids, and oxidants),[1,3] and their function as antigen-presenting cells. The importance of platelets as mediators of glomerular inflammation, in part because of their production of platelet-derived growth factor (PDGF), has been recently highlighted.[18,19] Growth factors such as transforming growth factor-β (TGF-β) and PDGF have been intimately associated with the pathogenesis of renal disease[18–21] in animal models, whereas other growth factors and cytokines may modulate the function of various renal cells, and therefore, the course and outcome of renal disease.[19,22–25] The role of adhesion molecules in the pathogenesis of the ongoing inflammation in glomerulonephritis is currently of great interest.[23] Chemokines such as interleukin-8 (IL-8), monocyte chemoattractant protein-1, and regulated upon activation, normal T-cell expressed and presumably secreted (RANTES) may be important in determining the extent and type of renal tissue immune cell infiltration.[12] Such factors, in turn, may affect pathologic outcomes.

Host factors, such as the presence of intercurrent infection and state of the immune system, are thought to modify the renal response to an immune challenge. In addition, genetic factors may affect which patients develop clinically apparent disease, the severity and course of disease once initiated, and the relative and absolute extent of inflammation and fibrosis. Risk factors such as patients' age, gender, race, HLA type, and the use of intravenous drugs probably modify the fibrotic response and could amplify nephritogenic responses.

<h2 style="text-align:center">Nonspecific Mechanisms of Renal
Tissue Injury</h2>

Inflammation

Localized tissue injury can be mediated through activation of infiltrating PMNs. This activation is regulated by cytokines,[26] which interact with both immune and renal cells via specific cell membrane receptors. Two cytokines, IL-1 and tumor necrosis factor-α (TNF-α), can directly affect the glomerulus by inducing mesangial and vascular endothelial cells to produce prostaglandin E_2, platelet-activating factor, leukocyte adhesion molecules, and IL-8.[27] IL-1, TNF-α, and IL-6 are all involved in acute inflammatory reactions and are responsible for the induction of fever and release of acute phase proteins.[26,27] PMNs and eosinophils respond to chemotactic stimuli by infiltrating within areas of immunologic activity, phagocytosing infectious organisms or immunologic debris, and producing highly reactive oxygen radicals (such as hydrogen peroxide, superoxide anion, oxygen singlets, and hydroxyl radicals).[28] These radicals kill both infectious organisms and surrounding renal tissue by phospholipid peroxidation of cell membranes.

During localized inflammation, drug toxicity, or in settings of hypoxia or anoxia, cytokine-stimulated endothelial cells synthesize and release endothelin, which modulates renal vasoconstriction, ion transport, eicosanoid synthesis, renin secretion, and atrial natriuretic peptide release.[26,29] Increased levels of endothelin have been demonstrated in patients with postischemic renal failure, cyclosporin toxicity, and hypertension, and increased urinary excretion of the substance has been noted in patients with various glomerulonephritides.[29] The causal relationship of these findings to the pathogenesis of disease has not been determined. The possible roles of cytokines in mediating outcome in glomerulonephritides have recently been reviewed.[22,23,26]

Complement-Activation-Associated Injury

In addition to the binding of C' to CICs and their subsequent deposition in renal tissue, C' components can also be deposited after activation of the alternate or properdin pathway. This activation can be caused by interaction with a number of different biologic materials, such as particulate polysaccharides, lipopolysaccharides, and viral antibodies attached to "tissue resident" virus.[30] Renal biopsies of such patients show mesangial cell proliferation, an increase in mesangial matrix, and a thickening of the peripheral capillary wall due to the interposition of the mesangial cells. In some cases, glomerular C'3 deposition can be correlated with a reduction in plasma C'3 levels and the presence of an IgG antibody (C'3 nephritic factor), which exhibits an affinity for alternate pathway C'3 convertase, enhancing its activity.[31]

METHODS FOR DETECTING COMPLEXES

CIC detection assays are usually non-antigen-specific techniques based on either the physicochemical properties of the IC or its ability to interact with other biologic systems, such as C' or cell surface receptors. Although the nonspecific nature of CIC assays allows them to be applied to the detection of ICs in any disease, these assays cannot analyze the composition of the detected ICs.

Physicochemical techniques usually involve precipitation or isolation by centrifugation. Nephelometry, which is based on the ability of precipitated CICs to scatter an incidental light beam, is a simple and inexpensive technique for screening patient samples for the presence of ICs.[32] Although sensitive enough to compare with more standard assays such as the C'1q assay, nephelometry suffers from problems arising from interference caused by serum components such as lipids, which can produce unacceptable false-positive results.[32]

Precipitation with low-molecular-weight polyethylene glycol (PEG) can detect C'1q binding ICs on a size basis[33–37] and when combined with centrifugation on a PEG gradient is a useful technique for isolating ICs for analysis by other techniques.

Ultracentrifugation was the first analytical technique applied to the detection and isolation of CICs, using sucrose,[38] PEG,[36,37,39,40] or continuous zonal gradients.[41] These techniques yield only qualitative results and are now used for CIC isolation before further immunochemical analysis and CIC size determination. Ultracentrifugation is one of the few techniques available for recovering non-complement-binding CICs.[36]

The most utilized CIC detection systems are based on the ability of ICs to interact with other biologic systems, such as C'. The ability of C'1q to bind to complexed IgG has been paramount in the construction of many CIC assays. However, the disadvantages of these assays are (1) that CICs smaller than 19S and containing IgE, IgA, and IgG4 do not preferentially bind to C'1q, and (2) that C'1q is prone to bind substances other than CICs such as endotoxin, nucleic acids, and denatured immunoglobulin.[42] There are several variations of the C'1q assay, including agarose gel precipitation, C'1q-binding solid- and liquid-phase assays,[43] C'1q-binding inhibition,[42,43] and anti-C′1q capture assays.[44] Other assays based on C′ are the C′ consumption assay[34] and immunoaffinity-based assays using solid-phase antibodies directed against C′3. Immobilized antibodies have been used for both CIC isolation and as a detection system.[36,40] Conglutinin, a naturally occurring serum protein of cattle, has a high affinity for C′3 and can be used to detect C′3-binding CICs.[45,46]

Techniques involving interactions between CICs and cell membrane receptors are also common detection systems, although some of these systems have now been developed as cell-free immunoassays. The Raji cell assay is the most widely used cell-receptor-based technique for the nonspecific detection of CICs. Raji cells are a lymphoblastoid cell line that exhibits an abundance of high-affinity receptors for C′1q, C′3b, and C′3d; a low density of Fc receptors; and no surface IgG. CICs are detected by their ability to inhibit the binding of radiolabeled heat-aggregated IgG to cell surface receptors.[45,47] However, this assay is technically difficult and the presence of autoantibodies (antinuclear antibodies[48] and antilymphocyte antibodies) causes interference. Salinas et al.[49] described a variant of this assay using fetal liver cells, which possess high-affinity receptors on their surfaces for complement-binding CICs, as the target cells. Similarly, L1210 murine leukemia cells are another substitute for Raji cells.[50] These cells exhibit an abundance of Fc receptors on their surface membranes, which bind ICs in antibody excess. This system is unable, however, to detect C′-binding CICs, as the fixation of C′3 to the IC often interferes with the binding of complexed IgG to Fc receptors.[51]

Other cells, such as platelets and red blood cells (RBCs) are able to naturally bind ICs to their surface, and platelet aggregation assays have been adapted to CIC detection.[52] CICs can be detected by their ability to interact with receptors on the surface of freshly collected platelets, causing primary aggregation. This is a labor intensive but relatively sensitive technique that can detect CIC concentrations as low as 5 μg/ml. The human RBC possesses CR1 C′ receptors that can be used for quantitation of C′3-binding but not measurement of C′3d-binding CICs.[53]

A wide variety of other techniques such as inhibition of antibody-dependent cell-mediated cytotoxicity,[54] and flow cytometry using either Raji cells[55] or human C′1q-coated microspheres[56] have been applied to CIC detection. In addition, CICs have been isolated by various chromatographic techniques, including the use of size exclusion,[35] immobilized protein A,[33] and affinity chromatography.[36,37,40]

Analysis of the physicochemical properties of CICs cannot be performed by any one technique. In certain cases where specific antibodies are available, CICs containing the antigen can be precipitated out of solution by reaction with the specific antibody and analyzed by electrophoresis.[56] When purified antigens and reactive antibodies are available, antigenic material from isolated CICs can be used to investigate the ability of the complexed antigen to inhibit the binding of the antibody to its specific antigen.[56]

Isolated CICs usually must be dissociated by incubation in acidic or alkaline buffers[36,40,57]; chaotropic ions such as thiocyanate, iodide, and chloride[36,37,40]; or by enzymatic digestion with papain, pepsin, or pronase[58] before analysis can take place. Analysis of isolated CIC components can be performed by any of the modern analytical protein techniques, especially polyacrylamide gel electrophoresis,[59] isoelectric focusing,[60] and Western or immunoblotting techniques.[36,40,59,61] Other techniques such as countercurrent immunoelectrophoresis[36,40] and immunodiffusion[36,40] have been applied to detect specific antigens and/or antibodies in isolated CICs.

LABORATORY ASSESSMENT OF PATHOGENICITY

The concentration of circulating and tissue ICs, the size and overall charge of the IC, the ratio of and binding avidity of antibody and antigen, the likelihood of dissociation of the IC at the tissue level, the presence of tissue receptors for antigen and antibody, and the ability of tissue to process or incorporate deposited immunoreactants, including autocrine and paracrine cytokine generative responses, are all possibly important factors in mediating tissue pathologic outcomes in response to a specific IC challenge. In addition, the physiologic state of the host, including genetic predispositions to magnitude and quality of immune response and specific genetic background, including HLA expression, may be important factors associated with outcome.[3,62]

Diversity of Immune Complexes

ICs are composed of antigens and antibodies that bind specifically. Antigens vary in size, chemical composition, and expression of antigenic determinants. The physicochemical properties of antibodies also have significant influences on the pathophysiologic properties of an IC. ICs containing IgG4 have been shown to form small, nonprecipitating ICs, which are not easily removed by the reticuloendothelial system,[63] whereas IgM-containing ICs are usually large and easily removed by macrophages.

At any given time, within an organism, several different immunologic responses may occur simultaneously. Each of these reactions can potentially produce ICs in both the circulation and in situ. The fate of any IC will depend on its concentration, composition, size, complement-binding capacity, and overall charge.[3,37,62,64] ICs are also unstable and their composition changes as the conditions surrounding their formation (such as fluctuations in antigen, antibody, or C' concentrations) change. Immunoreactants in tissue may predispose to further immunoreactant deposition, or may affect tissue clearance of deposits.[3]

In addition to antigen-antibody IC, there exist other IC types that arise as a result of internal regulation. The host may recognize autologous antibody as an antigen and form anti-antibodies in response.[36,37] These anti-

Table 5-2. Variety of Immune Complexes
in Human Disease

Antigen (excess)/antibody
Antigen/antibody (equivalence)
Antigen/antibody (excess)
Antibody/anti-Fc (rheumatoid factor)
Antibody/anti-F(Ab)$_2$ (serum agglutinator)
Antibody/anti-FAb (allotype)
Antibody/anti-FAb (idiotype)
Antigen/antibody/anti-antibody

antibodies, or idiotypes, react with either the target immunoglobulin to produce antibody-anti-antibody IC[36,37] or they can react with the antibodies bound into existing ICs. The diversity of IC types is illustrated in Table 5-2.

Pathogenicity of ICs

The assessment of pathogenicity of immunoreactants can be addressed satisfactorily in experimental models. In clinical settings, however, it is unusual to be able to show a direct causal relationship between the immunologic findings and the development of nephropathy, in the absence of removing an offending antigen, depleting a specific antibody, or rechallenging the patient with a specific immunoreactant. Although suggestive of a causal relationship, the finding of ICs in the circulation or tissues of patients with disease does not prove that the ICs caused the pathologic outcome. Therefore, the clinical diagnosis of immune-mediated renal disease in humans must include the demonstration of immunoreactants, such as the specific antigen and antibody in question in glomerular capillaries or mesangium, usually by immunofluorescence or immunoperoxidase techniques.[3,62] In addition, the diagnosis of the pathogenicity of such immunoreactants is strengthened by their identification in the circulation and finding their concentrations are enriched in renal tissue deposits compared with the circulating levels. Concentration of such substances in tubules or glomeruli may enhance their pathogenicity. It is important to demonstrate that the concentrations of these deposited materials exceed those of a marker, such as albumin, which is subject to tissue concentration because of glomerular ultrafiltration, or tubular reabsorption. Finally, light microscopic and electron microscopic findings should be consistent with a diagnosis of immune-mediated renal disease. The latter includes the typical variety of light microscopic findings and the demonstration of electron dense deposits in glomerular capillaries and mesangial cells.

VIRUSES AND IMMUNE COMPLEX DISEASE

The role of viruses in the pathogenesis of immune complex glomerulonephritis has been appreciated for some time. Many acute and chronic viral infections are associated with the generation of CICs.[3,62] Renal disease, how-

Table 5-3. Pathogenesis of Immune Complex Nephropathy in Viral Diseases

1. Circulating immune complex disease involving viral antigens and host antiviral antibody
2. Circulating immune complex disease involving endogenous antigens released by viral-induced injury to cells and host autoantibody
3. In situ immune complex disease involving viral antigen binding to glomerular structures and host antiviral antibody or cell-mediated immunity
4. Autoimmune reactions to host glomerular structures induced by viruses (e.g., induction of self-reactive T or B cells, release of sequestered antigen, "molecular-mimicry," or activation of idiotype–anti-idiotype networks involving "peptidic self")
5. Virus-induced activation of cytokines and/or cell adhesion molecules
6. Direct cytopathogenic effect of virus on glomerular cells

(From Glassock,[62] with permission.)

ever, occurs in only a minority of such patients. The prevalence of glomerulonephritis in such patients will depend on the specificity and the sensitivity of the tests employed in establishing the diagnosis. Several possible pathogenic mechanisms involved in viral-induced glomerulonephritis have been delineated[62] (Table 5-3).

As a response to viral infection, ICs, composed of a viral product and host antibody, often reactive with viral envelope or core glycoproteins, may form in the circulation. Subsequently, given the proper physicochemical conditions, such ICs can deposit in the kidney and initiate a tissue response. Typical features of such a classic CIC mechanism include the presence of these immune products in variable concentrations and distribution in glomerular capillaries or mesangium, resulting in differential pathologic expression.

Viral infection of renal or other cells can also result in the synthesis of new tissue proteins. These may include normal host proteins, or abnormal viral or nonviral proteins. Previously immunologically privileged tissue proteins may be expressed on cell surfaces, or released into the circulation. Antibodies generated against such "neoantigens" in the circulation may form ICs, deposit in renal tissue, and initiate disease.

Alternatively, an immune response may be engendered by the interaction of viral antigens with renal structural proteins. Viral antigens that become deposited or "planted" in renal tissue can react with circulating antibody, culminating in the development of in situ mediated immune renal disease. Likewise, circulating antibodies may react in situ with an endogenous renal antigen that has been exposed, newly expressed, or released as a result of viral-induced injury to renal cells.

Autoimmune reactions that result in injury to host renal structures may be mediated by viral infection by several mechanisms. Viral infection may result in the specific or generalized activation of B cells, resulting in antibody production, or oligoclonal or polyclonal gammopathy.[3,65] Alternatively, activation of self or reactive circulating or tissue T cells may initiate nephropathic injury. Viral infection may activate the response of idiotype-antiidiotype networks, which can participate in the pathogenesis of some types of glomerulonephritis, and interstitial nephritis. Glassock[62] has speculated that "viral infection may induce autoimmune responses to endogenous tissue antigens including immunoglobulin, cell surface antigens, intracytoplasmic or nuclear antigens and constituents of extracellular matrix." In addition, because viral peptides may have structural similarities with host peptides (as in the case of HIV gp120 and HLA peptides),[66,67] autoantibody production may occur by molecular mimicry. Finally, antiviral IgG antibodies often activate the alternative complement pathway,[3] potentially leading to enhanced tissue injury.

HIV Infection and Immune Complex Renal Disease

Human immunodeficiency virus (HIV)-related CICs are common in HIV-infected patients at all stages of disease[68–80] and have been shown to play a role in the pathogenesis of immune-mediated thrombocytopenia in HIV-infected patients.[81] Deposition of such CICs may play a specific pathogenic role in mediating glomerulonephritis associated with HIV infection.[62] The direct role of the viral infection in mediating glomerulonephritis in humans is bolstered by findings in an equine retroviral infection. Infection with equine infectious anemia virus, a lentivirus of the retrovirus family, is often complicated by proliferative glomerulonephritis,[82] with features of immune-mediated renal disease.

As outlined above, circulating HIV antigens may be planted in the glomerulus, initiating renal pathologic outcomes. Deposition of circulating antibody that is reactive with tissue antigens may occur alone or facilitate an overlapping CIC deposition mechanism. Immunoreactive material taken up in glomerular cells (such as antigen or antibody trapped in the mesangium) may change their properties, such as charge or surface characteristics, facilitating the development of localized inflammation. Antigens related to infectious agents that can replicate in glomeruli[83–86] may be important in facilitating the interaction of glomerular immunoreactants with CIC.

Cohen et al.[83] demonstrated proviral HIV DNA in tubular and glomerular epithelial cells in renal tissue from HIV-infected patients with glomerulonephritis using in situ hybridization.[83] They also found HIV nucleic acid in renal tissue from patients with acquired immunodeficiency syndrome (AIDS) without clinically obvious kidney disease. HIV p24 antigen was demonstrated in tubules in one patient with immune complex glomerulonephritis but neither p24 nor envelope antigens were demonstrated in glomeruli with immune deposits.

The role of cellular incorporation of HIV genome products in the development of renal disease is unknown. Preliminary evidence suggests HIV infects renal tissue, specifically mesangial and endothelial cells, in vitro,[84] as well as epithelial cells.[83] It is possible that viral infection might lead to subsequent attachment of circulating anti-HIV antibodies or CICs (in antibody excess) to a "planted" or transformed antigen, presuming there are free epitopes available to the antibody.[62,87] Alternatively, HIV infection may alter renal cellular proteins leading to the development of an immune-mediated pathologic process.[62,87,88]

We recently demonstrated the ubiquitous presence of HIV genome in glomerular and tubular tissue from HIV-infected patients with and without renal disease.[85] A nested polymerase chain reaction (PCR) was performed to amplify target sequences within the *gag* and *env* regions of the HIV-1 proviral genome. In addition, a microdissection procedure was instituted to assess the anatomic location in renal tissue that might harbor the HIV genome. HIV-1 target sequences were amplified from glomeruli, tubular, and infiltrating inflammatory cells from HIV-infected patients with glomerulonephritis. In all cases in which it was assessed, HIV DNA was present in glomeruli of renal biopsies from patients with glomerulonephritis in the presence of HIV infection. HIV-1 proviral DNA in glomeruli, however, does not determine glomerulonephritis, as genomic markers were found in glomeruli of HIV-infected patients with other renal diseases, and in glomeruli in the absence of nephropathy. The presence of HIV genome in renal cells, whether a result of infection of renal cells or as a consequence of its presence in infiltrating immune cells, would seem to provide the necessary conditions for the implantation or expression of an antigen that might initiate an in situ mechanism of renal IC disease pathogenesis.[62] Such data, however, do not necessarily imply that productive infection with integration of DNA into the host genome, and renal cellular synthesis of HIV peptides has occurred. It is possible that the nephritogenic antigen might be an HIV gene product in renal tissue, a transformed cell, or a normal or aberrant cell protein (Fig. 5-1).

These studies demonstrating the presence of HIV genomic DNA in renal tissue of HIV-infected patients both with and without renal disease suggest that a triggering mechanism may be critical for the expression of renal disease.[85] Renal cellular responses, therefore, particularly if altered by viral infection, may be important determinants of the expression of disease.[2,62] Our finding of HIV antigens in glomerular cells in human biopsy tissue is consistent with pathologic[83] and in vitro studies[84] and strengthens the causal association of HIV infection and glomerulonephritis. To date, however, because HIV gene products in renal tissue could simply be markers of HIV infection, the pathogenic significance of a positive PCR still remains to be established.

It is of interest that a substantial proportion of the polyclonal immunoglobulin response in HIV-infected patients is comprised of IgA[89,90] and that IgA-containing CICs are prevalent in patients with HIV infection and AIDS.[71–80] These immune responses may partially explain the increasing recognition of IgA nephropathy in the HIV-infected population.[91–96]

Likewise, gp120–anti-gp120 antibody ICs have been shown to modulate immune cell function, perhaps contributing to pathogenic effects at the tis-

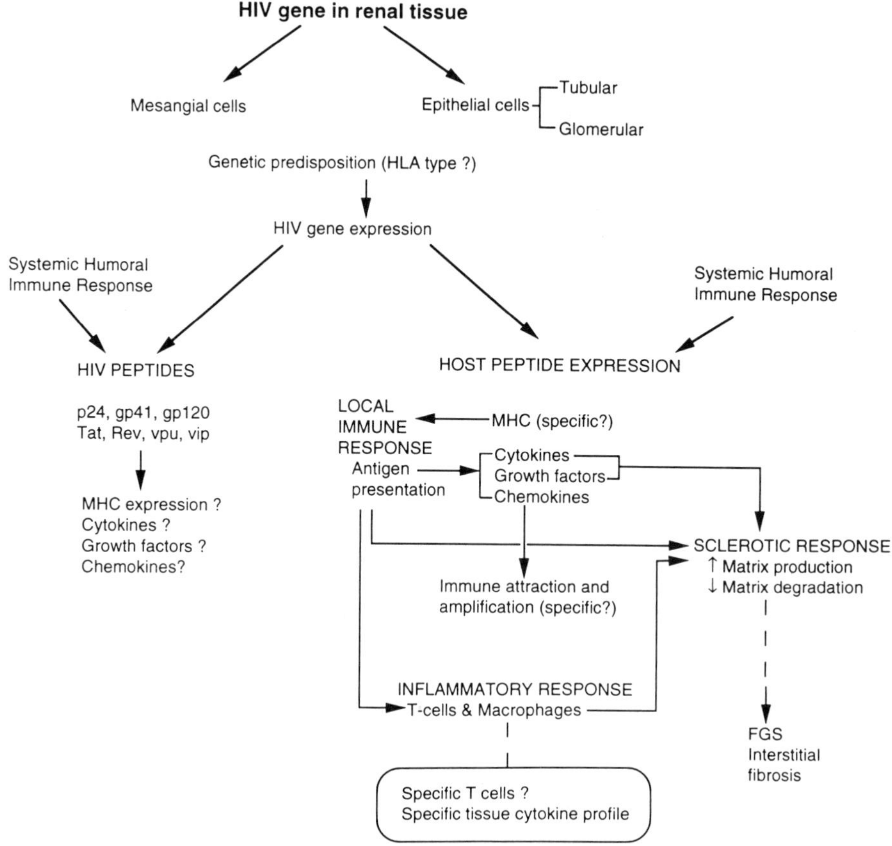

Fig. 5-1. Possible pathogenic mechanisms in the development of HIV-associated glomerulonephritis. HIV gene expression in renal tissue may result in the synthesis of HIV peptides which could facilitate deposition of circulating antibodies or immune complexes. In addition, HIV gene expression in renal tissue may initiate production of immunoreactants that may amplify local inflammatory or sclerogenic responses. See text for details.

sue level.[66,97–98] It is possible that certain specific immune responses, perhaps in response to specific modes of antigen presentation, or specific CICs are more likely to provoke an ongoing renal inflammatory response.

Recent studies have suggested that the interstitial infiltrate in HIV-associated glomerulonephritis is of similar magnitude to that seen in HIV-associated focal and segmental glomerulosclerosis (FSGS).[99] Relatively fewer macrophages constituted the interstitial inflammatory cell population in tissue from patients with glomerulonephritis when compared with interstitial renal tissue from HIV-infected patients with FSGS. However, there were relatively more interstitial B cells in the infiltrate in HIV-associated glomerulonephritis when compared with HIV-associated FSGS. The total number of interstitial immune cells correlated with serum creatinine levels and urinary protein excretion in patients with HIV-associated glomerulonephritis. Such data suggest that immune cell sequestration occurs in interstitial renal tissue of patients with HIV-associated glomerulonephritis. Specific, infiltrating B cells may also be associated with the pathogenesis of HIV-associated glomerulonephritis. The association of characteristic tissue immune parameters with specific outcomes in patients with HIV-associated glomerulonephritis suggests that cell specific factors, such as cytokine profiles, might be important in mediating tissue or disease events.

Additionally, the role of concurrent or intercurrent viral infection in affecting renal responses remains to be determined.[88,100,101] Renal parenchymal viral infection may be crucial to the pathogenesis of specific IC-mediated renal disease. The development of glomerulonephritis may be dependent on the renal parenchymal incorporation of human immunodeficiency viral antigens,[83,85,87,96] or other viral agents,[100,101] although the presence of viral genome in renal cells alone may not be a sufficient condition for disease expression. Productive renal cellular infection, on the other hand, may be an important pathogenic factor. In addition, other viral infections may cause increased expression of HIV genes in renal tissue, leading to nephropathy.

The chronicity of HIV infection, in association with the concomitant immune dysregulation, may be associated with states in which acute or chronic glomerulonephritis could develop. Epidemiologic data, however, are not yet present to support these conjectures.

GLOMERULONEPHRITIS IN PATIENTS WITH HIV INFECTION

Histopathologic findings such as membranoproliferative and diffuse proliferative glomerulonephritis,[85,102–105] membranous nephropathy,[106] and IgA nephropathy,[85,91–96] and other pathologic entities in patients with chronic renal dysfunction or nephrotic syndrome and HIV infection,[88,107–110] all possess pathologic characteristics strongly suggestive of immune-mediated etiology.

The significance of these disparate pathologic entities has been unclear. The pathologic findings described in such cases might be related to non-HIV antigen-antibody IC deposition, occurring as a consequence of immune responses against the infectious agents that complicate HIV infection, resulting in postinfectious glomerulonephritis,[104] perhaps facilitated by the polyclonal B-cell activation leading to the increased immunoglobulin production that characterizes patients with HIV infection.[65] Alternatively, specific HIV antigens and antibodies reactive with them may be involved in the pathogenesis of immune renal disease. Finally, in other cases, immune-mediated renal diseases that occur in HIV-infected patients may be only indirectly related, or unrelated to the underlying retroviral infection, or may be more closely associated with the patient's treatment.[101,111]

Recent biopsy series of patients with HIV infection and renal disease demonstrate that approximately one-quarter to one-half of the patients have glomerulonephritis.[85,109] A relatively large proportion of patients may have coexistent FSGS and IC disease.[109] The paucity of reported cases of glomerulonephritis in HIV-infected patients may be a function of sample selection, because patients with asymptomatic urinary abnormalities in the absence of nephrotic range proteinuria, transient, resolved acute renal failure, or stable, advanced renal failure and nephrotic syndrome and HIV infection may not be biopsied as frequently as uninfected patients with similar clinical features. Physicians may be reluctant to treat such patients with immunosuppressive medications. Alternatively, they may not wish to offer renal biopsy to their patients in light of the perception of lack of specific treatments, and the relatively minor importance of a mild renal disease in the context of a fatal illness, when considering the balance of risks and benefits.[96,106]

We have performed renal biopsies in 40 patients at George Washington University Medical Center with HIV infection and renal disease since 1986.[85] In this series, one-half of the patients had FSGS, but more than one-third had various forms of proliferative glomerulonephritides. In addition, two patients (5 percent) had IgA nephropathy and 5 percent had membranous nephropathy, whereas the rest had other renal diseases not obviously associated with HIV infection, such as diabetic glomerulosclerosis or minimal change disease with acute tubular necrosis (Table 5-4).

Four patients with HIV infection who presented with proteinuria and renal insufficiency were studied intensively. The renal pathologic findings in these patients were consistent with immune-mediated glomerulonephritis (Table 5-5). All the patients were black men. Three of the four had homosexuality or bisexuality as a risk factor for HIV infection. The fourth patient acquired HIV infection presumably through sex with prostitutes. None of the patients used intravenous drugs. The patients had CD4 counts ranging from near normal to markedly diminished, and were in stages II to IV of HIV infection.[112] All had diminished T-helper/suppressor ratios, and gammopathy. Three of the patients had been treated with zidovudine, and two were taking the drug at the time of biopsy. Only one patient had a slightly diminished C'3 level.

Features noted on light microscopy included mild to marked mesangial

Table 5-4. Biopsies in HIV-Infected Patients with Renal Disease, 1986–1994

No. of Patients	Clinical Pathology	%
20	Focal glomerulosclerosis	50
14	Glomerulonephritis	35
6	Focal proliferative glomerulonephritis	
2	IgA	
2	Membranous nephropathy	5
2	Acute tubular necrosis	5
2	Diabetic nephropathy	5

expansion, segmental increase of mesangial cells and matrix, diffuse mesangial expansion, and mesangial deposits. In addition, increased cellularity with lobular transformation, segmental condensation and/or simplification of the glomerular tufts and synechiae, and global or segmental proliferative and sclerosing changes were seen. Visceral epithelial cells were prominent and fibrocellular crescents were variably present.

The majority of biopsies had microcystic tubular dilatation and atrophy, interstitial fibrosis, and/or edema. The biopsies invariably exhibited interstitial infiltration with mononuclear cells, primarily macrophages and lymphocytes, and occasionally, variable amounts of plasma cells, PMNs, and/or eosinophils. The infiltrating cells in some instances permeated tubular epithelium, resulting in destruction of the tubular basement membrane.

Immunofluorescent microscopy variably showed intramembranous deposits of IgA, C'3, albumin, C'4, IgM, and C'3 as coarse granular mesangial deposits, and properdin and C'1q in mesangial granular deposits (Table 5-5). One biopsy, in addition to C'3, IgG, IgM, IgA, and C'1q, demonstrated κ and λ light chains in a mesangial distribution. IgG may be found at the periphery of tubules, or in association with C' and albumin within the proximal tubular epithelium and/or as resorption droplets.

Electron microscopy variably showed the presence of finely granular subendothelial, intramembranous, and mesangial electron dense deposits; obsolescent glomeruli with scanty electron-dense deposits; extensive segmental approximation of foot processes of visceral epithelial cells; finely granular and large electron-dense deposits within mesangial cells; and variably sized peripheral subepithelial electron-dense deposits and small and some large subendothelial deposits within capillaries obliterated by mononuclear cells (Fig. 5-2). Tubuloreticular structures were abundant within the cytoplasm of endothelial cells in three of the four cases.

CICs were detected in all patients. In one patient, an IgA-p24 HIV antigen complex, and in another an IgG antibody-gp120 HIV antigen CIC were isolated. Two patients had demonstrable levels of IgG-p24 HIV-antigen-containing CICs identified. Identical complexes were eluted from renal tissue in the first three patients. p24 HIV antigen and C' were isolated from the fourth.

In addition, HIV-related antigens were detected in all four patients' urine. The eluted antibodies reacted with the HIV antigens from the isolated CICs, the eluted renal ICs, and the isolated urinary HIV antigens (Fig. 5-3). Direct immunofluorescence for viral antigen in the eluted glomerular tissue revealed HIV antigens (Fig. 5-4). In all four patients' biopsy material, HIV antigens could be immunologically detected within glomeruli. The PCR examination confirmed the presence of HIV genome in the renal tissue in all patients.

The clinical presentation of three of the four patients was similar to that reported as typical for classic HIV-associated nephropathy.[88,107,108] The histologic findings and rate of progression were variable. There was also heterogeneity of the immunoreactants demonstrated and the electron microscopic

Table 5-5. Immunochemical Findings in Patients with HIV Infection and Glomerulonephritis[a]

Patient	Race	Risk Factor	Light Microscopy	Immuno-fluorescence Findings	Electron Microscopy	CIC	Eluates	PCR
1	W	H	FPGN Mesangial expansion	IgA, C'1q C'3	TRS Intramembranous, subepithelial, and mesangial electron-dense deposits	IgA-IgG/gp41	ND	+
2	W	H	Mesangial expansion	IgA	TRS Mesangial electron-dense deposits	IgA-IgM/p24	Identical IgA-IgM/p24	+
3	B	H	DPGN Sclerotic glomeruli Mesangial expansion	p18 p24	Subendothelial and intramembranous electron-dense deposits	IgA/p24	Identical IgA/p24	+
4	B	BIS	FPGN Sclerotic glomeruli	p18	TRS Mesangial expansion, mesangial electron-dense deposits	IgG/gp120	Identical IgG/gp120	+

5	B	HTS	FPGN Mesangial expansion	C′3, IgG IgM, C′1q p24	TRS Variably sized mesangial and subepithelial electron-dense deposits	IgG/p24	Identical IgG/p24	+
6	B	H	DPGN Sclerotic glomeruli	C′3, C′1q Properdin p18 p24	TRS Variably sized subendothelial electron-dense deposits	IgG/p24	p24	+
7	W	H	MPGN	C′3, IgG, IgM	TRS Mesangial, paramesangial, subendothelial, intramembranous, and subepithelial electron dense deposits	IgG/IFN	Identical IgG/IFN	ND
8	W	H	MPGN	ND	Variably sized subendothelial electron-dense deposits	IgG/p24; IgA/IgG (cryoprecipitable)	Identical IgA/IgG	ND

Abbreviations: W, white; B, black; H, homosexual; BIS, bisexual; HTS, heterosexual; FPGN, focal proliferative glomerulonephritis; DPGN, diffuse proliferative glomerulonephritis; MPGN, membranoproliferative glomerulonephritis; TRS, tubular reticular structures; IFN, interferon; ND, not determined.

[a] All of the patients were male.

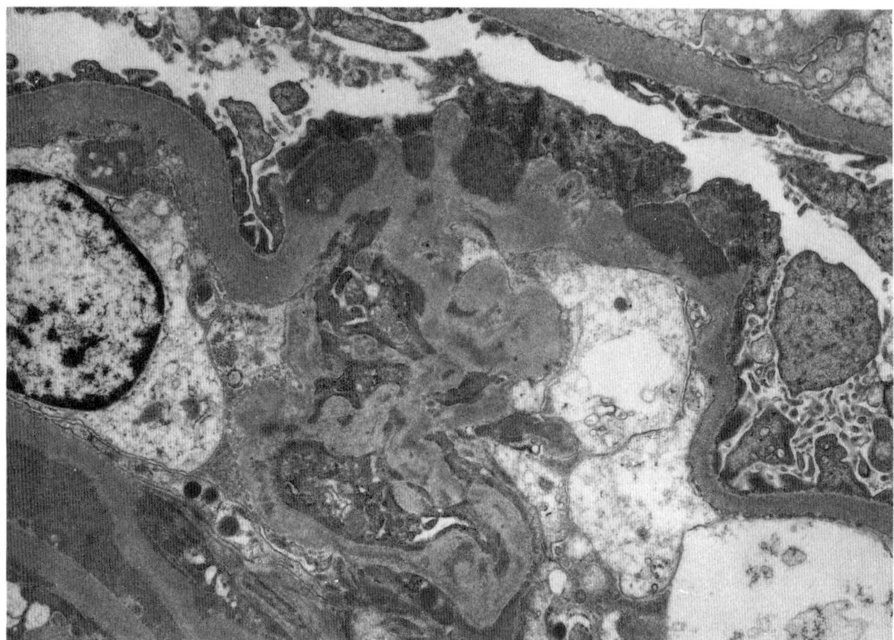

Fig. 5-2. Electron micrograph of glomerular tissue from a biopsy of a patient with postinfectious immune complex glomerulonephritis in the presence of HIV infection (see Table 5-5, patient 5) shows prominent, variably sized subepithelial deposits, and scanty mesangial electron-dense deposits. (Magnification 18,000 ×.) (From Kimmel, et al.,[87] with permission.)

distribution of deposits, suggesting different pathogenic and tissue responsive mechanisms, perhaps associated with the different immunochemical properties of the immunoreactants, systemic host responses, or with different initiating mechanisms of immune-mediated renal injury.

The presence of circulating antigen-antibody complexes, consisting of HIV p24 bound to anti-p24 IgA and anti-p24 IgG, or HIV gp120 bound to anti-gp120 IgG and elution of complexes, composed of the same material, from renal tissue from the first three patients in higher concentrations compared with plasma, suggests that one mechanism that may be responsible for the renal disease in these patients is the deposition or trapping of such complexes. The increased detection of antibody and antigen over time, and the results of enrichment studies, moreover, strengthen the likelihood that this represents true elution of tissue-deposited pathogenic ICs.

Alternatively, such disease may be associated with in situ IC formation.[1,3,62] The detection of HIV proviral DNA in renal tissue is consistent with the hypothesis that both circulating and in situ HIV antigen-specific ICs may be mechanistically associated with the development of glomerulonephritis in HIV-infected patients, and that incorporation of viral products within renal tissue may be important in the pathogenesis of HIV-associated

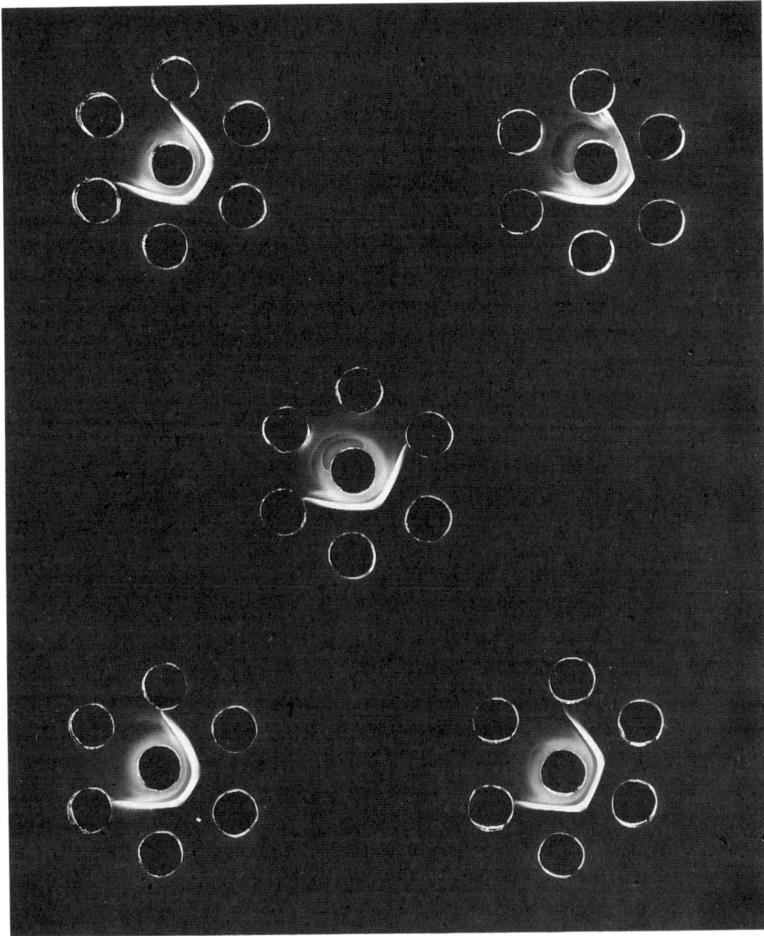

Fig. 5-3. Immunodiffusion analysis of immune complex components isolated from the circulation and renal biopsy material from three patients with HIV infection and glomerulonephritis. In the right and left upper corners, antibody from CICs was placed in the central wells and reacted with urinary antigen (well 1), CIC antigen (well 2), and antigen eluted from the renal biopsy tissue (well 3), but not with control soluble kidney extract (well 4) or phosphate-buffered saline (wells 5 and 6). Antibody from the eluate reacts in an identical manner in the right and left lower corners, establishing the identity of the immunoreactants. In the central study, renal eluate did not contain antibody in measurable quantity (patient 6, Table 5-5).

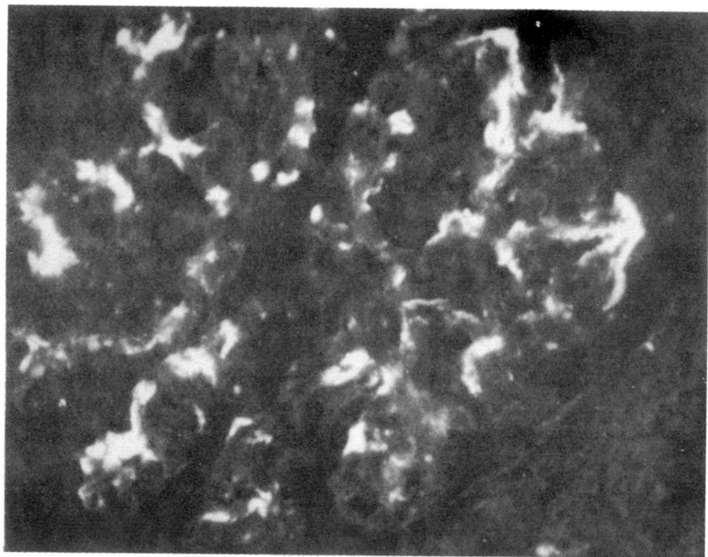

Fig. 5-4. Laser-enhanced fluorescence photomicrographs of HIV p24 localization in an acid-eluted renal biopsy section, shows localization of antigen in a glomerulus from the biopsy of an HIV-infected patient with glomerulonephritis (see Table 5-5, patient 3).

immune-mediated renal disease. The specific viral products that can mediate renal disease remain to be elucidated.

Several groups of investigators have reported cases of IgA nephropathy in patients with HIV infection.[91–96,113] Such patients often present with asymptomatic urinary abnormalities such as hematuria and proteinuria. In general the renal disease has been mild or slowly progressive,[96,113] with pathologic findings ranging from normal glomeruli to focal or diffuse mesangial proliferation, focal proliferative glomerulonephritis, and crescentic glomerulonephritis with variable interstitial fibrosis and tubular atrophy.[113] Some studies, however, have suggested that the prevalence of IgA nephropathy in HIV-infected patients may be very low.[113,114]

Both genetic factors and IC-mediated mechanisms of disease have been implicated in the pathogenesis of IgA nephropathy in the absence of HIV infection. Disordered regulation of IgA synthesis is suggested by abnormalities in the number and function of cells that produce IgA.[115] Such patients may have increased levels of shared idiotypes in antibodies both in serum and CICs.[116] Nephropathy might occur in uninfected patients with limited potential in their immunologic response repertoire, as is encountered in HIV-infected patients. Similar CICs, and IgA rheumatoid factors have been demonstrated in the circulation of uninfected patients with IgA nephropathy by other investigators as well.[117–119] The role of viral infection in the pathogenesis of IgA nephropathy in humans has been controversial. Viral infections, however, have been implicated in the pathogenesis of IgA nephropathy in patients in the absence of HIV infection.[115,120,121] Viral infection in an animal model has been demonstrated to result in the development of a form of IgA nephropathy.[115] The role of the intestine, a major site of IgA production, has been highlighted in the pathogenesis of IgA nephropathy.[115]

Increased circulating levels of IgA[65,75,76] and the presence of CICs containing IgA[73,74,78–80] have been clearly demonstrated to be a common finding in patients with HIV infection. Increased total IgA levels,[89,90] comprised of proportional augmentation in IgA1 and IgA2 levels, have been noted in a majority of HIV-infected patients. IgA1 antibodies were preferentially directed against the HIV envelope glycoproteins (gp160, gp120, and gp41), whereas there was little reactivity to *gag*-encoded peptides, especially compared with the IgG response.[90] In addition, a high proportion of patients with AIDS have increased circulating levels of IgA-containing CICs and IgA rheumatoid factors, predominantly of the IgA1 subclass.[78,79] These data suggest selective abnormalities of IgA regulation in patients with HIV infection, which may be the result of mode of antigen presentation, specifically a consequence of an intestinal response to antigen presented during anal intercourse.

Katz et al.[94] demonstrated the presence of CICs, rheumatoid factor, and anti-HIV IgA in two patients with HIV infection and IgA nephropathy. We recently described two patients with HIV infection and IgA nephropathy in whom CICs composed of IgA idiotypic antibodies reactive with anti-HIV IgG or IgM antibodies could be isolated. Both patients were young, white homosexual men, at early stages of HIV infection. Both had hematuria and proteinuria with mild renal insufficiency, polyclonal gammopathy, hypocomplementemia, and abnormal T-helper/suppressor ratios. Both had HIV antigens detected in the urine. A single CIC was isolated from plasma in each patient. The first was composed of IgA complexed to IgG, which was reactive with HIV gp41. In the second case, a complex of IgA and IgM reactive with HIV p24 was isolated. The IgA binding was antibody specific in each patient. There was no binding of IgA to IgG or IgM from either patient, or from other subjects that was not directed against the HIV peptides. In addition, the binding of the IgG and IgM in the two patients was HIV viral peptide-specific, when assessed using other HIV peptides, or other viral antigens, related to cytomegalovirus or Epstein-Barr virus. Eluates of renal biopsy tissue in the one patient in whom we had sufficient tissue for analysis contained an IC identical to that of the CIC.[96] HIV *gag* and *env* sequences were demonstrated in renal tissue from both patients by PCR.

The presence of rheumatoid factors, and idiotypic IgA antibodies reactive with anti-HIV antigen immunoglobulins, suggests immunoregulatory dysfunction associated with HIV infection, and perhaps specific or repeated modes of antigen presentation. The formation of anti-antibodies may arise as a result of polyclonal B-cell activation, or may represent a specific response to continued production of anti-HIV antibodies. The consequence of such idiotypic antibody production may be the formation of antibody/anti-

antibody CICs and their deposition in the kidney. In addition, IgA from HIV-infected patients binds to specific types of collagen in vitro.[122] Such physicochemical reactions, perhaps facilitated by alterations in tissue clearance of IgA ICs, or changes in glomerular cells secondary to interaction with viral products or immunoreactants, might therefore be critical in the development of clinical renal disease.[96,115,123]

Interestingly, all reported patients with IgA nephropathy associated with HIV infection have been white,[113] as is typically the case in patients with IgA nephropathy in the absence of HIV infection[124] in the United States. Such data add credence to the supposition that genetic factors may be important in determining renal pathologic findings in HIV-infected patients.

The role of genetic, immunologic,[1,3,62,115,124,125] and other host responses[125] may be crucial in determining renal pathologic outcomes in any type of HIV-associated glomerulonephritis. Some investigators have suggested that racial or ethnic background may be an important determinant of outcome in patients with renal disease in the presence of HIV infection.[88,107,108,125] Nochy et al.[109] demonstrated a relatively high prevalence of IC nephropathy in both black and white patients with HIV infection and renal disease. Although a majority of white patients had glomerulonephritis, there was a substantial (21 percent) prevalence of glomerulonephritis in black patients in that study. The majority of black patients, however, had IC-mediated glomerulonephritis coexistent with FSGS. Perhaps the type of antigen, its presentation, or the presence of a risk factor such as intravenous drug use may determine specific renal histologic outcomes through unknown mediating mechanisms. A sclerotic reaction accompanying glomerulonephritis may be a late consequence leading to a fibrotic response, mediated through growth factors or cytokines that may be activated in tissue, regardless of whether initiating factors engendered inflammation or an increase in matrix synthesis[87] (Fig. 5-1). Growth factor or cytokine-mediated events at the renal cellular level resulting from renal infection, paracrine effects, or as a consequence of systemic infection may mediate functional and histologic outcomes. The type of infiltrating cells or genetic factors, including HLA type, may have an important effect on outcome.

IMMUNE COMPLEX DISEASE UNRELATED TO HIV INFECTION

Alternatively, the finding of glomerulonephritis in patients with HIV infection does not necessarily imply that the two diseases are intimately related. The role of polyclonal gammopathy in the pathogenesis of glomerulonephritis has been outlined.[3] In addition, other disease entities may be present in HIV-infected patients that would result in glomerulonephritis in the absence of the viral illness.

Korbet and Schwartz[104] have delineated such issues in the case of a patient who presumably had postinfectious glomerulonephritis in the setting of HIV infection. Interestingly, this patient's biopsy was remarkable for the finding of tubular reticular structures within the endoplasmic reticulum of glomerular capillary endothelial cells. Such findings may suggest that these electron microscopic markers are either nonspecific, consistent with an activated cytokine microenvironment, or that the patient may have more than one type of nephropathy, perhaps one being subclinical. Abnormalities of glomerular epithelial and endothelial cell function may be associated with abnormal renal pathologic responses, including defective clearance of tissue ICs and aberrant antigen presentation.[104] Interestingly, this patient's serologic evidence of streptococcal infection persisted, in conjunction with lingering clinical signs of continuing renal inflammation, an uncommon course for poststreptococcal glomerulonephritis. These clinical findings, however, were amplified by the results on repeat biopsy 7 months later, which did not demonstrate resolution of disease. However, evaluation of HIV-associated immunoreactants at the tissue level, to assess their importance in this patient's clinical course, was not undertaken. This case emphasizes the disparate nature of postinfectious glomerulonephritis and HIV-associated IC renal disease, but also illustrates how the underlying immune dysregulation may modify the course of other renal diseases, rendering specific diagnosis more difficult.

We recently reported follow-up on a patient with nephrotic syndrome and membranous nephropathy in the setting of combined chronic hepatitis B virus (HBV) and HIV infection.[101,106] The renal lesion was thought to be secondary to HBV infection, on clinicopathologic grounds (including an appearance typical of secondary membranous nephropathy). The nephrotic syndrome remitted in this patient after several months, in conjunction with clearance of hepatitis B e antigen (HBeAg), consistent with HBV-associated membranous nephropathy. This case, as does the foregoing example, illustrates that nephrotic syndrome in an HIV-infected patient cannot simply be ascribed to "HIV nephropathy" without histologic evidence, and that underlying HIV infection may affect the course of another immunologically mediated renal disease.

Cryoglobulinemia has been reported in patients with HIV infection.[126–128] Although neurologic complications have been reported, in one patient with HBV and HIV infections we studied, the cryoglobulinemia was associated with membranoproliferative glomerulonephritis (Table 5-5). The patient's plasma contained two CICs: an IgG-p24 complex, and a cryoprecipitable IgA-IgG complex. The IgGs in the two CICs were identical. Renal eluate showed a single complex, identical to the circulating IgA-IgG complex. The presence of an HIV peptide in the renal eluate could not be demonstrated. This case demonstrates that even when immune-mediated renal disease is present in a patient with HIV-associated CICs, the renal disease is not necessarily directly related to the specific HIV-associated CIC.

The occurrence of such findings may be attributed to the high rate of coinfection of HBV with HIV in patients with sexual transmission or intravenous drug use as risk factors for HIV infection. Although the cryoprecipitate may be related to anti-HBV-associated antibodies, it is likely that ICs related to HIV antigens will be important in such cases as well. Hepatitis C virus infection may become an important factor in the pathogenesis of renal disease in HIV-infected patients. As such patients are studied more intensively, and the immunoreactants are better delineated through more intensive investigation of renal disease and serologic abnormalities, our understanding of the mechanisms involved in the pathogenesis of HIV-associated immune-mediated nephropathies will substantially increase.

Finally, glomerulonephritis in HIV-infected patients may be related to the treatment of the retroviral disease, or to treatment of the illnesses that complicate the underlying viral infection. We studied a patient with membranoproliferative glomerulonephritis who had been treated on a long-term basis with interferon-α for HIV infection.[111] A single CIC composed of IgG complexed to interferon-α was identified in the patient's plasma (Table 5-5). Elution studies of the renal biopsy revealed an identical IC in approximately threefold higher concentration. Although interferons have been implicated as nephrotoxins,[129,130] the use of this substance as a biologic response modifier, or the immune dysregulation caused by HIV infection may have predisposed to its pathogenic potential.

Renal biopsy is important in determining the histologic diagnosis in patients with HIV infection and renal disease.[85,87,104,106,109] One of our patients with HIV-immunoglobulin ICs, whose renal disease closely resembled post-infectious glomerulonephritis, had a spontaneous improvement in renal function over a several month observation period. Another patient with glomerulonephritis and features of FSGS had a transient beneficial response to steroid therapy. The role of such therapy could be evaluated in specific controlled trials in HIV-infected patients with renal disease with defined clinical and histologic parameters.

CONCLUSION

The type of antigen or its presentation, or the presence of intravenous drug use, an independent risk factor for the development of FSGS in the absence of HIV infection, may be important in determining renal histologic outcomes in patients with HIV infection who develop glomerulonephritis. Sclerosis in HIV-infected patients with glomerulonephritis may be a consequence of final common pathways leading to a fibrotic response, whether initiating factors originally incited an inflammatory response, or an increase in renal matrix production. In HIV-associated renal diseases, it is likely that cytokine-mediated mechanisms, associated with the common renal interstitial inflammatory cellular infiltrative response, or with renal or systemic HIV infection, may ultimately mediate fibrotic responses, regardless of the initial histologic pattern.[87]

The prevalence of inflammatory renal disease associated with HIV ICs and incorporation of both HIV genomic material and core antigen in renal tissue is unknown, but may comprise a substantial proportion of the population of patients with HIV infection and nephropathy. CIC deposition and in situ mechanisms of immune-mediated renal disease may underlie the pathogenesis of glomerulonephritis in HIV-infected patients. Renal biopsy to establish the diagnosis, and immunochemical analysis to relate the findings to the particular immune response, will ultimately expand our understanding of the pathogenesis of these diseases in particular, and immune-mediated nephropathies in general.

ACKNOWLEDGMENTS

The authors appreciate the cooperation of Istvan Bodi, M.D., Andrea Ferreira-Centeno, M.S., Tunde Farkas-Szallasi, M.D., A. Andrew Abraham, M.D., and Carleton T. Garrett, M.D., Ph.D. The authors appreciate the constructive criticisms of Dr. William Couser and Dr. Boon Ooi. The authors were supported by a grant from the NIH, NIDDK 1-RO1-DK40811.

REFERENCES

1. Couser WG: Mediation of immune glomerular injury. J Am Soc Nephrol 1:13, 1990
2. Couser WG: Mechanisms of glomerular injury in immune-complex disease. Kidney Int 28:569, 1985
3. Wilson CB: The renal response to immunologic injury. p. 1062. In Brenner BM, Rector FC (eds): The Kidney. 4th Ed. WB Saunders, Philadelphia, 1991
4. Austin HA III, Antonovich TT, MacKay K et al: NIH conference. Membranous nephropathy. Ann Intern Med 116:672, 1992
5. Ford PM, Kosatka I: The effect of in situ formation of antigen-antibody complexes in the glomerulus on subsequent glomerular localization of passively administered immune complexes. Immunology 39:337, 1980
6. Brentjens JR, Andres G: Interaction of antibodies with renal cell surface antigens. Kidney Int 35:954, 1989
7. Turner N, Lockwood CM, Rees AJ: Antiglomerular basement antibody-mediated nephritis. p. 1865. In Schrier RW, Gottschalk CW (eds): Diseases of the Kidney. Vol. 3. Little, Brown, Boston, 1993
8. Shah SV: Role of reactive oxygen metabolites in experimental glomerular disease. Kidney Int 35:1093, 1989
9. Main IW, Nikolic-Paterson DJ, Atkins RC: T cells and macrophages and their role in renal injury. Semin Nephrol 12:395, 1992
10. Schreiner GF: Role of macrophages in glomerular injury. Semin Nephrol 11:268, 1991
11. Cattell V: Macrophages in acute glomerular inflammation. Kidney Int 45:945, 1994
12. Miller MD, Krangel MS: Biology and biochemistry of the chemokines: a family of chemotactic and inflammatory cytokines. Crit Rev Immunol 12:17, 1992

13. Wilson CB: Antibody reactions with native or planted glomerular antigens producing nephrogenic immune deposits of selective glomerular cell injury. p. 1. In Wilson CB, Brenner BM, Stein JH (eds): Contemporary Issues in Nephrology. Vol. 18. Churchill Livingstone, New York, 1988

14. Shainuck LI, Striker GE, Luther RE, Benditt EP: Structural-functional correlations in renal disease. Hum Pathol 1:631, 1970

15. Risdon RA, Sloper JAC, de Wardener HE: Relationship between renal function and histological changes found in renal biopsy specimens from patients with persistent glomerular nephritis. Lancet 2:363, 1968

16. Bohle A, Mackensen-Haen S, von Gise H: Significance of tubulointerstitial changes in the renal cortex for the excretory function and concentration ability of the kidney: a morphometric contribution. Am J Nephrol 7:421, 1987

17. Neilson EG, McCafferty E, Feldman A et al: Spontaneous interstitial nephritis in kd/kd mice. An experimental model of autoimmune disease. J Immunol 133: 2560, 1984

18. Floege JF, Eng E, Young BA et al: Infusion of platelet-derived growth factor or basic fibroblast growth factor induces selective glomerular mesangial cell proliferation and cell matrix accumulation in rats. J Clin Invest 92:2952, 1993

19. Abboud HE: Growth factors in glomerulonephritis. Kidney Int 43:252, 1993

20. Isaka Y, Fujiwara N, Veda N et al: Glomerulosclerosis induced by in-vitro transfection of TGF-β or platelet derived growth factor gene into rat kidney. J Clin Invest 92:2697, 1993

21. Border WA, Okuda S, Languino LR et al: Suppression of experimental glomerulonephritis by antiserum against transforming growth factor β. Nature 346: 371, 1990

22. Floege J, Johnson RJ: Cytokines in renal inflammation. Curr Opin Nephrol Hypertens 2:449, 1993

23. Remuzzi G, Zoja C, Bertani T: Glomerulonephritis. Curr Opin Nephrol Hypertens 2:465, 1993

24. Sterzel RB, Eckhard S-L, Marx M: Cytokines and mesangial cells. Kidney Int 43:S39;S26, 1993

25. Sedor JR, Konieczkowski M, Huang S et al: Cytokines, mesangial cell activation and glomerular injury. Kidney Int 43:S39;S65, 1993

26. Phillips TM: Cytokines: relevance in the treatment of dialysis patients. p. 309. In Bosch JP (ed): Advances in Hemodialysis: High Efficiency Treatments. Vol. 19. Churchill Livingstone, New York, 1993

27. Cotran RS, Pober JS: Cytokine-endothelial interactions in inflammation, immunity, and vascular injury. J Am Soc Nephrol 1:225, 1990

28. Weiss SJ: Tissue destruction by neutrophils. N Engl J Med 320:365, 1989

29. Perico N, Remuzzi G: Role of endothelin in glomerular injury. Kidney Int 43: S39;S76, 1993

30. Burkholder PM: Immunopathology of renal disease. Clin Lab Med 6:55, 1986

31. Ng Y, Peters DK: C′3 nephritic factor (C′3NeF) dissociation of cell-bound and fluid phase stabilization of alternate pathway C′3 convertase. Clin Exp Immunol 65:450, 1986

32. Hoffken K, Schmidt CG: Quantification of immune complexes by nephelometry. Methods Enzymol 74:628, 1981

33. Siersted HC, Brandslund I, Svehag SE, Jensenius JC: Quantitation of circulating immune complexes by combined PEG precipitation and immunoglobulin specific radioimmunoassay (PICRIA). Methods Enzymol 74:538, 1981

34. Brandslund I, Siersted HC, Jensenius JC, Svehag SE: Detection and quantitation of immune complexes with a rapid polyethylene glycol precipitation complement consumption method (PEG-CC). Methods Enzymol 74:551, 1981

35. Virella G, Kilpatrick JM, Chenais F, Fudenberg HH: Isolation of soluble immune complexes from human serum: combined use of polyethylene glycol precipitation, gel filtration and affinity chromatography on protein A-sepharose. Methods Enzymol 74:644, 1981

36. Phillips TM, Queen WD, Lewis MG: The significance of circulating immune complexes in patients with malignant melanoma. p. 289. In Reisfeld RA, Ferrone S (eds): Melanoma Antigens and Antibodies. Academic Press, San Diego, 1982

37. Phillips TM, Holohan TV, Korec S et al: The pathophysiology of circulating immune complexes: their role in host-tumor interactions and removal by immunoadsorption therapy. Contemp Topics Immunobiol 15:111, 1985

38. Rodahl E, Iversen OJ, Dalen AB: Preparative isolation of immune complexes from serum by sucrose density ultracentrifugation. Scand J Immunol 20:21, 1984

39. Kauffman RH, van Es LA, Daha MR: Specific detection of IgA immune complexes. J Immunol Methods 40:117, 1981

40. Phillips TM, McDonald JS, Lewis MG: Towards tumor antibody isolation and characterization in immune complexes. p. 3. In Serrou B, Rosenfeld C (eds): Immune Complexes and Plasma Exchanges in Cancer Patients. Elsevier/North Holland, Amsterdam, 1981

41. Steensgard J, Jabobsen C: A new gradient former and simplified procedure for zonal centrifugation of immune complexes. J Immunol Methods 29:173, 1979

42. Fukuda K, Seino J, Kinoshita Y et al: Circulating immune complex-like materials which bind to heat inactivated C1q interfere with the C1q solid phase assay for immune complexes. Tohoku J Exp Med 146:449, 1985

43. Zubler RH, Carpentier N, Lambert PH: The [125I] C1q binding assay for the detection of soluble immune complexes. Methods Enzymol 74:530, 1981

44. Levinson SS, Goldman JO: Evaluation of anti-C1q capture assay for detecting circulating immune complexes and comparison with polyethylene glycol-immunoglobulin G, C'1q binding and Raji cell methods. J Clin Microbiol 25:1557, 1987

45. Theofilopoulos AN: The Raji, conglutinin, and anti-C3 assays for the detection of complement-fixing immune complexes. Methods Enzymol 74:511, 1981

46. Durand CG, Burge JJ: A new enzyme-linked immunosorbent assay (ELISA) for measuring immunoconglutinins directed against the third component of human complement. Findings in systemic lupus erythematosus. J Immunol Methods 73:57, 1984

47. Theofilopoulos AN, Wilson CB, Dixon FJ: The Raji cell radioimmune assay for detecting immune complexes in human sera. J Clin Invest 57:169, 1976

48. Horsfall AC, Venables PJW, Mumford PA, Maini RN: Interpretation of the Raji cell assay in sera containing anti-nuclear antibodies and immune complexes. Clin Exp Immunol 44:405, 1981

49. Salinas FA, Wee KH, Silver HK: Clinical relevance of immune complexes, associated antigen and antibody in cancer. Contemp Topics Immunobiol 15:55, 1985

50. Poskitt TR, Poskitt PKF: The L1210 radioimmune assay for detecting circulating immune complexes. Immunol Commun 7:543, 1978

51. Kammer GM, Schur PH: Binding of circulating immune complexes to human peripheral blood lymphocytes: effect of complement. Clin Immunol Immunopathol 10:202, 1978

52. Myllyla G: Aggregation of human blood platelets by immune complexes in the sedimentation pattern test. Scand J Hematol, suppl. 19:1, 1973

53. Tsuda F, Miyakawa Y, Mayumi M: Application of human erythrocytes to a radioimmune assay of immune complexes in serum. Immunology 37:681, 1979

54. Barkas T, Al-Khateeb SF, Irvine WJ et al: Inhibition of antibody-dependent cell-mediated cytotoxicity (ADCC) as a means of detection of immune complexes in the sera of patients with thyroid disorders and bronchogenic carcinoma. Clin Exp Immunol 25:270, 1976

55. Lightfoote M, Folkes TM, Redfield R et al: Flow-cytometric detection of circulating immune complexes. J Immunol Methods 95:107, 1986

56. Gupta RK, Morton DL: Clinical significance and nature of circulating immune complexes in melanoma patients. Contemp Topics Immunobiol 15:1, 1985

57. Hogben DN, Brown SE, Howard CR, Steward MW: HBsAg: anti HBs immune complexes. A method for separating the constituent components and assessment of the affinity of the antibody. J Immunol Methods 93:29, 1986

58. Davis JS, Godfrey SM, Winfield JB: Direct evidence for circulating DNA-anti-DNA complexes in systemic lupus erythematosus. Arthritis Rheum 21:17, 1978

59. Rodahl E, Iversen O-J: Analysis of circulating immune complexes from patients with ankylosing spondylitis by gel electrophoresis and immunoblotting using antiserum against a psoriasis associated retrovirus-like particle. Ann Rheum Dis 45:892, 1986

60. Maidment BW, Pesidero LD, Nemoto T, Chu TM: Recovery of immunologically reactive antibodies and antigens from breast cancer immune complexes by preparative isoelectric focusing. Cancer Res 41:795, 1981

61. Inman RD, Rosenberg RA, Redecha PB, Christian CL: Characterization of sequential immune complexes in infective endocarditis by Western blot analysis. J Immunol 133:217, 1984

62. Glassock RJ: Immune complex-induced glomerular injury in viral diseases: an overview. Kidney Int 40:S35;S5, 1991

63. Van der Zee JS, van Swieter P, Aalberse RC: Serological aspects of IgG_4 antibodies: II. IgG_4 antibodies form small non-precipitating immune complexes due to functional monovalency. J Immunol 137:3566, 1986

64. Mannik M: Pathophysiology of circulating immune complexes. Arthritis Rheum 25:783, 1982

65. Lane HC, Masur H, Edgar LC et al: Abnormalities of B-cell activation and immunoregulation in patients with the acquired immunodeficiency syndrome. N Engl J Med 309:453, 1983

66. Pantaleo G, Graziosi C, Fauci AS: The immunopathogenesis of human immunodeficiency virus infection. N Engl J Med 328:327, 1993

67. Zagury JF, Bernard J, Achour A et al: Identification of CD4 and major histocompatibility complex functional peptide sites and their homology with oligopeptides from human immunodeficiency virus type 1 glycoprotein gp120: role in AIDS pathogenesis. Proc Natl Acad Sci USA 90:7573, 1993

68. Nishanian P, Huskins KR, Stehn S et al: A simple method for improved assay demonstrates that HIV p24 antigen is present as immune complexes in most sera from HIV-infected individuals. J Infect Dis 162:21, 1990

69. McHugh TM, Stites DP, Busch MP et al: Relation of circulating levels of human

immunodeficiency virus antigen, antibody to p24, and HIV-containing immune complexes in HIV-infected patients. Infect Dis 158:1088, 1988

70. Portera M, Vitale F, La Licata R et al: Free and antibody-complexed antigen and antibody profile in apparently healthy HIV seropositive individuals and in AIDS patients. J Med Virol 30:30, 1990

71. McDougal SJ, Hubbard M, Nicholson JK, Jones BM: Immune complexes in the acquired immunodeficiency syndrome: relationship to disease manifestation, risk group, and immunologic defect. J Clin Immunol 5:130, 1985

72. Morrow WJW, Wharton M, Stricker R, Levy JA: Circulating immune complexes in patients with the acquired immunodeficiency syndrome contain the AIDS-associated retrovirus. Clin Immunol Immunopathol 40:515, 1986

73. Carini C, Messaroma I, Scano G et al: Characterization of specific immune complexes in HIV related disorders. Scand J Immunol 26:21, 1990

74. Ellaurie M, Calvelli T, Rubinstein A: Immune complexes in pediatric human immunodeficiency virus infection. Am J Dis Child 144:1207, 1990

75. McDougal JS, Kennedy MS, Nicholson JKA et al: Antibody response to human immunodeficiency virus in homosexual men. J Clin Invest 80:316, 1987

76. Fling J, Fischer JR, Boswell RN, Reid MJ: The relationship of serum IgA concentration to human immunodeficiency virus infection: a cross-sectional study of HIV-positive individuals detected by screening in the United States Air Force. J Allergy Clin Immunol 82:965, 1988

77. Procaccia S, Lazzarin A, Colucci A et al: IgM, IgG and IgA rheumatoid factors and circulating immune complexes in patients with AIDS and AIDS related complex with serological abnormalities. Clin Exp Immunol 67:236, 1987

78. Jackson S, Dawson LM, Kotler DP: IgA1 is the major immunoglobulin component of immune complexes in the acquired immunodeficiency syndrome. Clin Immunol 8:64, 1988

79. Jackson S, Tarkowski A, Collins JE et al: Occurrence of polymeric IgA1 rheumatoid factor in the acquired immunodeficiency syndrome. Clin Immunol 8:390, 1988

80. Lightfoote MM, Folks TM, Redfield RM et al: Circulating IgA immune complexes in AIDS. Immunol Invest 14:341, 1988

81. Karpatkin S, Nardi M: Autoimmune anti-HIV-1 gp120 antibody with antiidiotype-like activity in sera and immune complexes of HIV-1-related immunologic thrombocytopenia. J Clin Invest 89:356, 1992

82. McGuire TC, O'Rourke KI, Perryman LE: Immunopathogenesis of equine infectious anemia lentivirus disease. Dev Biol Stand 72:31, 1989

83. Cohen AH, Sun NCJ, Shapsak P, Imagawa DT: Demonstration of human immunodeficiency virus in renal epithelium in HIV-associated nephropathy. Mod Pathol 2:125, 1989

84. Green DF, Resnick L, Bourgoignie JJ: HIV infects glomerular endothelial and mesangial but not epithelial cells in vitro. Kidney Int 41:956, 1992

85. Kimmel PL, Ferreira-Centeno A, Farkas-Szallassi T et al: Viral DNA in microdissected renal biopsy tissue from HIV-infected patients with nephrotic syndrome. Kidney Int 43:1347, 1993

86. Shukla RR, Kumar A, Kimmel PL: Transforming growth factor-beta increases the expression of HIV-1 gene in transfected human mesangial cells. Kidney Int 44:1022, 1993

87. Kimmel PL, Phillips TM, Ferreira-Centeno A et al: HIV-associated immune-mediated renal disease. Kidney Int 44:1327, 1993

88. Glassock RJ, Cohen AH, Danovitch G, Parsa KP: Human immunodeficiency virus and the kidney. Ann Intern Med 112:35, 1990

89. Vincent C, Cozon G, Zittoun M et al: Secretory immunoglobulins in serum from human immunodeficiency virus infected patients. J Clin Immunol 12:381, 1992

90. Kozlowski PA, Jackson S: Serum IgA subclasses and molecular forms in HIV infection: selective increases in monomer and apparent restriction of the antibody response to IgA1 antibodies mainly directed at env glycoproteins. AIDS Res Hum Retroviruses 8:1173, 1992

91. Kenouch S, Delahousse M, Mery J-P, Nochy D: Mesangial IgA deposits in two patients with AIDS-related complex. Nephron 54:338, 1990

92. Jindal KK, Trillo A, Bishop G et al: Crescentic IgA nephropathy as a manifestation of human immunodeficiency virus infection. Am J Nephrol 11:147, 1991

93. Trachtman H, Gauthier B, Vinograd A, Valderrama E: IgA nephropathy in a child with human immunodeficiency virus type 1 infection. Pediatr Nephrol 5: 724, 1991

94. Katz A, Bargman JM, Miller DC et al: IgA nephritis in HIV-positive patients: a new HIV-associated nephropathy? Clin Nephrol 38:61, 1992

95. Schoeneman MJ, Ghali V, Lieberman K, Reisman L: IgA nephritis in a child with human immunodeficiency virus: a unique form of human immunodeficiency virus-associated nephropathy? Pediatr Nephrol 6:46, 1992

96. Kimmel PL, Phillips TM, Ferreira-Centeno A et al: Idiotypic IgA nephropathy in patients with HIV infection. N Engl J Med 327:702, 1992

97. Fauci AS: Multifactorial nature of human immunodeficiency virus disease: implications for therapy. Science 62:1011, 1992

98. Banda NK, Bernier J, Kurahara DK et al: Crosslinking CD4 by HIV gp120 primes T-cells for activation-induced apoptosis. J Exp Med 176:1099, 1992

99. Bodi I, Abraham AA, Kimmel PL: Macrophages in HIV associated renal diseases. Am J Kidney Dis 24:762, 1994

100. Seto E, Yen TSB, Peterlin BM, Ou J-H: Trans-activation of the human immunodeficiency virus long terminal repeat by the hepatitis B virus X protein. Proc Natl Acad Sci USA 85:8286, 1988

101. Schectman JM, Kimmel PL: Remission of hepatitis B-associated membranous glomerulonephritis in human immunodeficiency virus infection. Am J Kidney Dis 17:716, 1991

102. Gardenswartz MH, Lerner CW, Seligson GW et al: Renal disease in patients with AIDS: a clinicopathologic study. Clin Nephrol 21:197, 1984

103. Kenneth KK, Factor SM: Membranoproliferative glomerulonephritis and plexogenic pulmonary arteriopathy in a homosexual man with acquired immunodeficiency syndrome. Hum Pathol 18:1293, 1987

104. Korbet SM, Schwartz MM: Human immunodeficiency virus infection and nephrotic syndrome. Am J Kidney Dis 20:97, 1992

105. Reiser P, Opravil M, Pfaltz M et al: Primary pulmonary hypertension and mesangioproliferative glomerulonephritis in HIV infection. Dtsch Med Wochenschr 117:815, 1992

106. Guerra IL, Abraham AA, Kimmel PL et al: Nephrotic syndrome associated with chronic persistent hepatitis B in an HIV antibody positive patient. Am J Kidney Dis 10:385, 1987

107. Bourgoignie JJ: Renal complications of human immunodeficiency virus type 1. Kidney Int 37:1571, 1990
108. Seney FD Jr, Burns DK, Silva FG: Acquired immunodeficiency syndrome and the kidney. Am J Kidney Dis 16:1, 1990
109. Nochy D, Glotz D, Dosquet P et al: Renal disease associated with HIV infection: a multicentric study of 60 patients from Paris hospitals. Nephrol Dial Transplant 8:11, 1993
110. Ingulli E, Tejani A, Fikrig S et al: Nephrotic syndrome associated with acquired immunodeficiency syndrome in children. J Pediatr 119:710, 1991
111. Kimmel PL, Abraham AA, Phillips TM: Membranoproliferative glomerulonephritis in a patients treated with interferon alpha for HIV infection. Am J Kid Dis 24:858, 1994
112. Centers for Disease Control and Prevention: Update: acquired immunodeficiency syndrome—United States 1981–1988 MMWR 38:229, 1989
113. Bourgoignie JJ, Pardo V: HIV-associated nephropathies. N Engl J Med 327:729, 1992
114. Bebe MC, Canton P, Amiel C et al: Absence of mesangial IgA in AIDS: a postmortem study. Nephron 58:240, 1991
115. Emancipator SN: Immunoregulatory factors in the pathogenesis of IgA nephropathy. Kidney Int 38:388, 1990
116. Gonzalez-Cabrero J, Egido J, Sancho J, Moldenhauer F: Presence of shared idiotypes in serum and immune complexes in patients with IgA nephropathy. Clin Exp Immunol 68:694, 1987
117. Czersinsky C, Koopman WJ, Jackson S et al: Circulating immune complexes and immunoglobulin A rheumatoid factor in patients with mesangial immunoglobulin A nephropathies. J Clin Invest 77:1931, 1986
118. Sinico RA, Fornasieri A, Oreni N et al: Polymeric IgA rheumatoid factor in idiopathic IgA mesangial nephropathy (Berger's disease). J Immunol 137:536, 1986
119. Sinico RA, Fornasieri A, Maldifassi P et al: The clinical significance of IgA rheumatoid factor in idiopathic IgA mesangial nephropathy (Berger's disease). Clin Nephrol 30:182, 1988
120. Gregory MC, Hammond ME, Brewer ED: Renal deposition of cytomegalovirus antigen in immunoglobulin-A nephropathy. Lancet 1:11, 1988
121. Waldo FB, Britt WJ, Tomana M et al: Nonspecific mesangial staining with antibodies against cytomegalovirus in immunoglobulin A nephropathy. Lancet 1:129, 1989
122. van den Wall Bake AWL, Kirk KA, Gay RE et al: Binding of serum immunoglobulins to collagens in IgA nephropathy and HIV infection. Kidney Int 42:374, 1992
123. Hebert LA: Disposition of IgA-containing circulating immune complexes. Am J Kidney Dis 12:388, 1988
124. Jennette JC, Wall SD, Wilkman AS: Low incidence of IgA nephropathy in blacks. Kidney Int 28:944, 1985
125. Cantor ES, Kimmel PL, Bosch JP: Effect of race on the expression of AIDS-associated nephropathy. Arch Intern Med 151:125, 1991
126. Stricker RB, Sanders KA, Owen WF et al: Mononeuritis multiplex associated with cryoglobulinemia in HIV infection. Neurol 42:2103, 1992
127. Perl A, Gorevic PD, Condemi JJ et al: Antibodies to retroviral proteins and reverse transcriptase activity in patients with essential cryoglobulinemia. Arthritis Rheum 34:1313, 1991

128. Taillan B, Garnier G, Pesce A et al: Cryoglobulinemia related to hepatitis C virus infection in patients with human immunodeficiency virus infection. Clin Exp Rheumatol 11:350, 1993
129. Averbach SD, Austin HA III, Serwin SA et al: Acute interstitial nephritis with the nephrotic syndrome following recombinant leukocyte a interferon therapy for mycosis fungoides. N Engl J Med 310:32, 1984
130. Lederer E, Truong L: Unusual glomerular lesion in a patient receiving long-term interferon alpha. Am J Kidney Dis 20:516, 1992

6

Hemolytic Uremic Syndrome and Thrombotic Thrombocytopenic Purpura Associated with HIV Infection

Jeffrey S. Berns

INTRODUCTION

EPIDEMIOLOGY

CLINICAL AND LABORATORY MANIFESTATIONS

PATHOLOGY
  Kidney
  Other Tissues

ETIOLOGY AND PATHOGENESIS

CLINICAL COURSE AND TREATMENT

CONCLUSIONS

INTRODUCTION

The first report of a hemolytic uremic syndrome (HUS) in a patient with acquired immunodeficiency syndrome (AIDS) appeared in 1984, involving a homosexual man with disseminated Kaposi sarcoma and a recent episode of *Pneumocystis carinii* pneumonia.[1] In 1987 Jokela and colleagues[2] reported the development of thrombotic thrombocytopenic purpura (TTP) in a homosexual man who was seropositive for human immunodeficiency virus (HIV).

At least 15 additional cases of HUS and over 70 additional cases of TTP or unspecified thrombotic microangiopathy have since been reported in patients with HIV infection or AIDS.[3-38]

In 1925 Moschcowitz[39] reported the case of a 16-year-old girl who died after presenting with fever, petechiae, neurologic symptoms, anemia, and mild renal insufficiency with hyaline and granular casts in the urine. At autopsy there were hyaline thrombi in arterioles and capillaries of multiple organs.[39] Baehr and colleagues[40] later reported four patients with similar illnesses, highlighting the role of thrombocytopenia and further describing the associated histologic features. Subsequently, the term *thrombotic thrombocytopenic purpura* was introduced.[41] The pentad of fever, microangiopathic hemolytic anemia, thrombocytopenia, neurologic symptoms, and renal disease has since come to be associated with this disorder.[42,43]

Hämolytisch-urämische syndrome was first described in 1955 by Gasser and colleagues[44] in five patients with hemolysis, thrombocytopenia, acute renal failure, and cerebral symptoms. These original observations were subsequently extended by Habib and colleagues.[45-47] HUS is now recognized as a multisystem disorder of adults and children, of many diverse etiologies, characterized clinically by microangiopathic hemolytic anemia, thrombocytopenia, and renal disease, and histopathologically by an arteriolar and glomerular microangiopathy.[47-51] In children, HUS has been divided into two principal forms: *typical* (epidemic, enteropathic) HUS, associated with a diarrheal prodrome (D +), absence of relapses, and a good prognosis; and *atypical* (sporadic, nondiarrheal [D −]) HUS, associated with a tendency to relapse and a poorer prognosis.[50-53] Familial occurrences of both HUS and TTP have been well described.[54-56] The nature of the relationship between HUS and TTP, that is, whether these are two distinct disorders that share certain clinical and histopathologic features, or are variable expressions of a single disease process, continues to be a matter of active debate.[57,58]

The diagnosis of HUS or TTP is generally made on clinical grounds (Table 6-1). However, the distinction between these disorders may be difficult. A patient with microangiopathic hemolytic anemia and thrombocytopenia, with fever, neurologic manifestations, and mild renal involvement is likely to be diagnosed with TTP, whereas a patient with microangiopathic hemolytic anemia and thrombocytopenia with severe renal involvement after a prodromal diarrheal illness is more likely to be diagnosed with HUS. The clinical distinction between HUS and TTP in patients with HIV infection is likely to be especially imprecise. Patients with HIV infection and AIDS may present with clinical features consistent with a diagnosis of HUS or TTP, but that are instead due to other conditions (Table 6-2). They may also have multiple causes of fever, anemia, thrombocytopenia, neurologic symptoms, diarrhea, and renal disease, which together may mimic features of HUS and TTP (Table 6-2). Therefore, the term *HUS/TTP* is often used in this discussion, although diagnostic labels applied by the authors of original reports are respected.

Table 6-1. Clinical Features of HUS and TTP[a]

	HUS	TTP
Demographics		
Children	+ +	+
Adults	+	+ +
Sex	M = F	F > M
Clinical features		
Diarrheal prodrome	+ +	−
Fever	+	+ +
Bleeding manifestations	+ +	+ +
Oliguria	+ +	+
Neurologic symptoms	+	+ +
Hypertension	+ +	+
Laboratory features		
MAHA	+ +	+ +
Thrombocytopenia	+ +	+ +
Acute renal failure	+ +	+
VTEC enteric infection	+	−
Hypocomplementemia	+	−

Abbreviation: MAHA, microangiopathic hemolytic anemia.
[a] + + Most common features; + occurs but less common; − not a typical feature.

Table 6-2. Differential Diagnosis of HUS and TTP in Patients with HIV Infection or AIDS

Subacute bacterial endocarditis
Acute reaction to rifampin or dapsone
Toxemia of pregnancy
Disseminated intravascular coagulation
Malignant hypertension
Complications of cocaine abuse
Systemic vasculitis
  Idiopathic
  Related to illicit drug abuse
Collagen vascular diseases
Multiple disorders that together may mimic HUS or TTP
  Thrombocytopenia, anemia: immune thrombocytopenia, drug toxicity, bone marrow infection or neoplasm
  Neurologic disorders: cerebral toxoplasmosis, central nervous system lymphoma, progressive multifocal leukoencephalopathy, neuropathies
  Diarrhea: cytomegalovirus colitis, cryptosporidiosis, intestinal lymphoma, *Mycobacterium avium-intracellulare*
  Fever: infection, lymphoma, drug fever
  Renal failure: HIV nephropathy, hypotension, sepsis, drug-related nephrotoxicity

(Modified from Berns and Tomaszewski,[29] with permission.)

EPIDEMIOLOGY

As opposed to a female predominance in idiopathic TTP,[42,43] over 80 percent of reported cases of HUS/TTP in patients with HIV infection or AIDS have been in men (Table 6-3). While this may suggest a particular sensitivity of men for HIV-related HUS/TTP, it probably simply reflects the demographics of HIV infection. The mean age of adult patients reported with HIV-related HUS/TTP was 35 years, ranging from 20 to 65 years. The disease has also occurred in children.[28] In contrast to the apparent predilection of black patients for HIV nephropathy,[59–61] HIV-related HUS/TTP has been reported somewhat more frequently in white than in black or Hispanic patients, although race was not mentioned in many reports. A higher prevalence of TTP unrelated to HIV infection in white compared with black patients has also been noted in some series.[42] The most common risk factors for HIV infection have been male homosexuality and intravenous drug abuse. In some patients, HIV infection may have been transfusion related or heterosexually acquired, and in many reports risk factors were not stated or were unknown.

In about 25 percent of cases, patients were not previously known to be HIV positive, but instead were diagnosed with HIV infection or AIDS after presenting with HUS or TTP. In others, HIV infection was known before the onset of HUS/TTP, but the patients had been previously asymptomatic or no mention was made of prior AIDS-related illnesses. In one patient,

Table 6-3. Demographic Features of Reported Cases of HIV-Related HUS/TTP[a]

Mean age	35 y
Range	20–65 y
Sex	
Male	84%
Female	16%
HIV/AIDS stage	
A	36%
B and C	64%
HIV risk factors	
Homosexual	55%
IVDA	29%
Transfusion	9%
Heterosexual	7%
Race	
White	54%
Black	24%
Hispanic	22%

Abbreviation: IVDA, intravenous drug abuse.
[a] Not all demographic features available for all patients.

HIV infection was diagnosed 1 year after an initial presentation with HUS/ TTP.[11] Over one-half of reported patients had AIDS (Centers for Disease Control and Prevention [CDC] 1993 revised classification system category B and C[62]) when they developed HUS/TTP. Several patients were diagnosed with AIDS on clinical grounds because of the development of opportunistic infections, before the availability of HIV serologic testing, so that the association with HIV infection in these cases is not definite.[7,8,11] Helper T-lymphocyte (CD4, OKT4) counts have been highly variable, ranging from 1 to $524/mm^3$.

A patient reported by Meisenberg and colleagues[10] with a history of nephrotic syndrome and focal segmental glomerulosclerosis before the development of TTP may have had HIV nephropathy. Frem and colleagues[38] recently reported a patient with a history of intravenous drug abuse and of unknown HIV status, who received a cadaveric renal transplantation. Four years later, while receiving cyclosporine, a thrombotic microangiopathy developed leading to graft failure, and the patient was found to be HIV positive.[38] Whether HIV infection occurred pre- or post-transplant, or from the allograft is unclear in this report, as is the role of cyclosporine in the development of the thrombotic microangiopathy. Among patients known to be HIV positive, HUS/TTP developed in several who were receiving zidovudine (AZT),[18,27,29] or had recently discontinued zidovudine,[15,30,34] although in most reports the status of antiretroviral therapy was not noted. Several patients had previously been diagnosed with immune thrombocytopenic purpura (ITP),[22,32,35] a well-recognized complication of HIV infection.[63] The development of TTP in patients with chronic ITP unrelated to HIV has also been observed.[64] TTP has also occurred in patients with serologic evidence of infection with other retroviruses (human T-lymphotrophic virus [HTLV] I).[17,65]

Data are available from several centers regarding the prevalence of HIV infection among patients with HUS/TTP. Harrington and colleagues[17] retrospectively studied plasma from 50 patients with TTP seen in Miami between 1979 and 1991. Seven (14 percent) tested positive for HIV and another four tested positive for HTLV I antibodies.[17] Platanias and colleagues[11] found one patient with AIDS and another who was HIV positive among five patients seen over 3 years at the Kings County and Brooklyn Veteran's Administration hospitals. Thirty-six percent (5 of 14) of patients with TTP seen at Bellevue Hospital and the New York University Medical Center between 1985 and 1987 had AIDS- or HIV-related TTP, at a time when only 2 percent of their hospitalized patients had AIDS.[8] Thompson and colleagues[31] reviewed the records of adults with thrombotic microangiopathy at three San Francisco hospitals between 1980 and 1991. Seven out of 44 cases (16 percent) occurred in HIV-seropositive patients.[31] By contrast, only 3 percent (2 of 62) of patients with HUS/TTP at Johns Hopkins University Hospital between 1979 and 1990 were HIV positive.[24] At our institution, two patients with HIV-related HUS/TTP have been diagnosed in the last 5 years during which time another five patients were diagnosed with non-HIV-related TTP (unpublished observations). Thus, overall approximately 16 percent of cases of HUS/TTP seen at these geographically disparate institutions were related to HIV infection. HUS was reported to have developed in 0.6 percent of all HIV infected patients seen at one institution in Paris.[35a]

CLINICAL AND LABORATORY MANIFESTATIONS

The clinical features of HIV-related HUS/TTP are similar to those seen in patients with idiopathic HUS and TTP. The most common presenting symptoms are fever, headache, abdominal pain, nausea, vomiting, diarrhea, weight loss, myalgias, malaise, and lethargy. Bleeding manifestations include cutaneous petechiae, gingival bleeding, easy bruising, epistaxis, rectal bleeding, subconjunctival hemorrhage, and vaginal bleeding. Neurologic symptoms, which may be severe, include dizziness, headache, parasthesias, aphasia, blurred vision, confusion, seizures, behavioral disturbances, focal neurologic deficits, stupor, and coma.

The most common physical findings are fever, pallor, icterus, petechiae, ecchymoses, lymphadenopathy, hepatomegaly, and splenomegaly. Several patients have had Kaposi sarcoma.[1,22,27,30] Although not particularly prominent, severe hypertension has occurred, particularly in association with renal failure.[3,4,18,29,38]

Laboratory features reflect the microangiopathic process of HUS and TTP. Schistocytes, nucleated red blood cells, spherocytes, and other abnormal red blood cells are seen on the peripheral blood smear. The reticulocyte count, as expected, is often elevated, but may also be normal or low, perhaps reflecting effects of HIV infection, cancer chemotherapy, or renal failure on the bone marrow. The Coombs' negative hemolytic anemia is characterized by a hematocrit in the range of 10 to 30 percent (mean 20 percent), with a platelet count that is typically 10,000 to 20,000/ml (range 3,000 to 151,000/ml). Bilirubin and lactate dehydrogenase (LDH) levels are typically elevated. The prothrombin time (PT), partial thromboplastin time (PTT), and fibrin degradation products are usually normal, but may be mildly elevated. The urinalysis typically shows 1 to 4 + proteinuria, low-grade pyuria, microscopic hematuria, and granular casts. Nephrotic range proteinuria has also been reported,[10,18,36,38] possibly reflecting an underlying HIV nephropathy,[60,66] as was likely the case in a patient with a history of nephrotic syndrome and a kidney biopsy that showed focal and segmental glomerulosclerosis.[10] Serum creatinine levels at presentation, although not reported in all cases, were less than 2 mg/dl in over one-half of patients, between 2 and 5 mg/dl in 24 percent of patients, and greater than 5 mg/dl in 22 percent of patients. In only one patient was dialysis necessary immediately at presentation.[3] When assessing kidney function in these patients, it should be remembered that poor nutritional status and reduced muscle mass from HIV-related cachexia may lead to an underestimation of the severity of renal failure based solely on the measured blood urea nitrogen (BUN) and creatinine levels.

PATHOLOGY

Kidney

Although there are few detailed reports of renal histopathology in cases of HIV-related HUS/TTP, for the most part the findings have been similar to those seen with HUS and TTP unrelated to HIV infection.[43,47,67] These include platelet and fibrin thrombi in glomerular capillaries, small renal arterioles and interlobular arteries (Fig. 6-1), with arteriolar intimal edema, endothelial cell swelling, fibrinoid necrosis, and "onion skin" proliferation, often along with interstitial fibrosis and findings of acute tubular necrosis (ATN). Fragmented red blood cells may be seen in glomeruli and arteriolar walls.[29] On electron microscopy, glomerular capillary endothelial cells are separated from the underlying basement membrane by granular material, and collapse of the glomerular tufts with ischemic wrinkling and focal denudation of the glomerular basement membrane may be seen.[15,29,36,38] Arteriolar fibrin and fibrinogen deposits and arteriolar and glomerular deposits of fibrinogen, C1q, C3, C4, IgA, IgM, and κ and λ light chains have been found on immunofluorescent staining.[18,29,36] Tubuloreticular inclusions, as de-

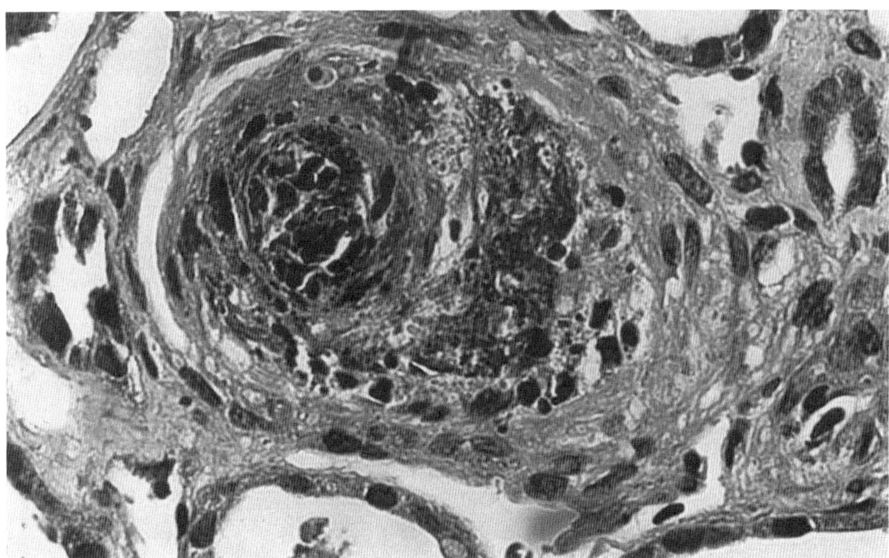

Fig. 6-1. Renal arteriole with fibrin thrombus. (From Berns and Tomaszewski,[29] with permission.)

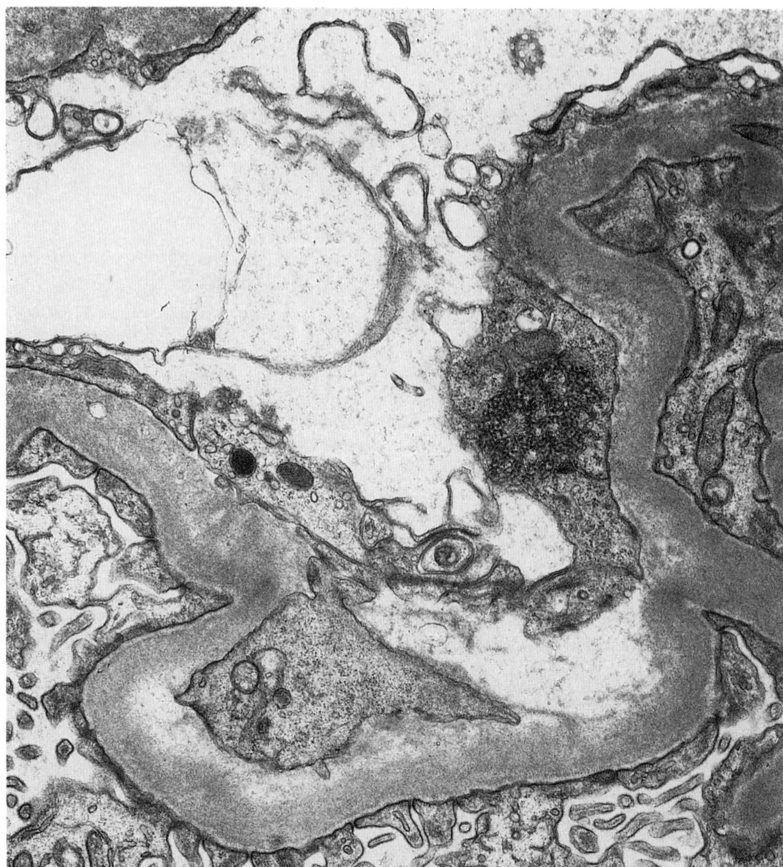

Fig. 6-2. Electron micrograph demonstrating tubuloreticular inclusions in glomerular capillary endothelial cell cytoplasm. (From Berns and Tomaszewski,[29] with permission.)

scribed in glomerular endothelial cells and other cell types in patients with HIV infection,[68,69] were seen within endothelial cell cytoplasm in three kidney biopsy specimens[29,36,38] (Fig. 6-2).

Other Tissues

Gingival biopsies showed capillary microthrombi consistent with TTP in three patients[8,10,11] but were negative in others.[7,23,29,37] Bone marrow specimens typically show erythroid hyperplasia, normal or increased numbers of megakaryocytes, and in some patients, megaloblastic changes and thrombi in bone marrow vessels. Eosinophilic thrombi and/or infarction have also been noted in the liver, heart, pancreas, thyroid, adrenal, spleen, and lymph nodes.

ETIOLOGY AND PATHOGENESIS

Although most cases of HUS/TTP are idiopathic, in that a specific cause was not identified, a variety of factors and conditions have been associated with the development of HUS and TTP. Some of the more widely recognized of these are listed in Table 6-4; many others have been less frequently reported but the significance of their association with HUS or TTP is less certain.[43,50,58,67] In several of the patients reported with HUS/TTP and HIV infection or AIDS, other possible causes of HUS/TTP, besides HIV, have also been noted.

HUS/TTP has been well described after cancer chemotherapy treatment, especially with mitomycin and, to a lesser extent, bleomycin- and cisplatin-containing regimens, but with other agents as well.[70] The patient described by Boccia et al.[1] was a homosexual man who developed HUS after a course of combination chemotherapy for disseminated Kaposi sarcoma, which included dacarbazine, doxorubicin, dactinomycin, vincristine, bleomycin, and vinblastine. Another patient, a homosexual man with Hodgkin's disease who developed *P. carinii* pneumonia while receiving chemotherapy with nitrogen mustard, vincristine, prednisone, procarbazine, doxorubicin, bleomycin, vinblastine, and dexamethasone, presented with TTP 1 year after the completion of his chemotherapy.[8] Bleomycin treatment has since been implicated in three additional patients with HIV infection and HUS/TTP.[35a,36a]

A prodromal illness with gastrointestinal symptoms of abdominal pain, vomiting, and diarrhea frequently precedes or accompanies the onset of

Table 6-4. Factors and Conditions Associated with HUS and TTP

Infections
    Verocytotoxin-producing *E. coli* O157:H7
    Shigella dysenteriae, type 1
    S. pneumoniae
    HIV
Inherited
    Autosomal recessive
    Autosomal dominant
    Congenital cobalamin (vitamin B_{12}) deficiency
Drugs
    Cyclosporin
    Mitomycin, bleomycin
    Oral contraceptives
    Quinine
Miscellaneous
    Pregnancy, postpartum
    Transplantation (kidney, liver, bone marrow)
    Carcinoma
    Complement deficiency syndromes
    Progressive systemic sclerosis (scleroderma)
    Systemic lupus erythematosus

HUS, especially in children with the classic or epidemic (D +) form. Enteric infections have also been documented in several of the patients with HIV-related HUS/TTP. Verocytotoxin-producing *Escherichia coli* (VTEC) including the 0157:H7 serotype, which has been commonly associated with classic childhood HUS,[49–51,71,72] has also been found in patients with HIV-associated HUS.[3,36a,37a] One patient with HIV-related TTP was found to have a rectosigmoiditis with stool cultures that were positive for *Shigella flexnerii*,[16] which has been associated with episodes of HUS.[73] Another patient had Salmonella group D12(9) isolated from blood and stool cultures.[21] Purpura fulminans with *Streptococcus pneumoniae* infection,[32] pancreatitis,[5] renal transplantation with use of cyclosporin,[38] cytomegalovirus (CMV),[36a] cryptosporidiosis,[35a] and pregnancy[14] have also been associated with the development of HIV- or AIDS-related HUS/TTP in individual reports. Thus, not all episodes of HUS/TTP in HIV-positive patients are necessarily related to the HIV infection, and other possible causes should be considered.

The precise pathogenetic mechanisms causing HUS and TTP are uncertain. As indicated in Fig. 6-3, endothelial injury and platelet aggregation

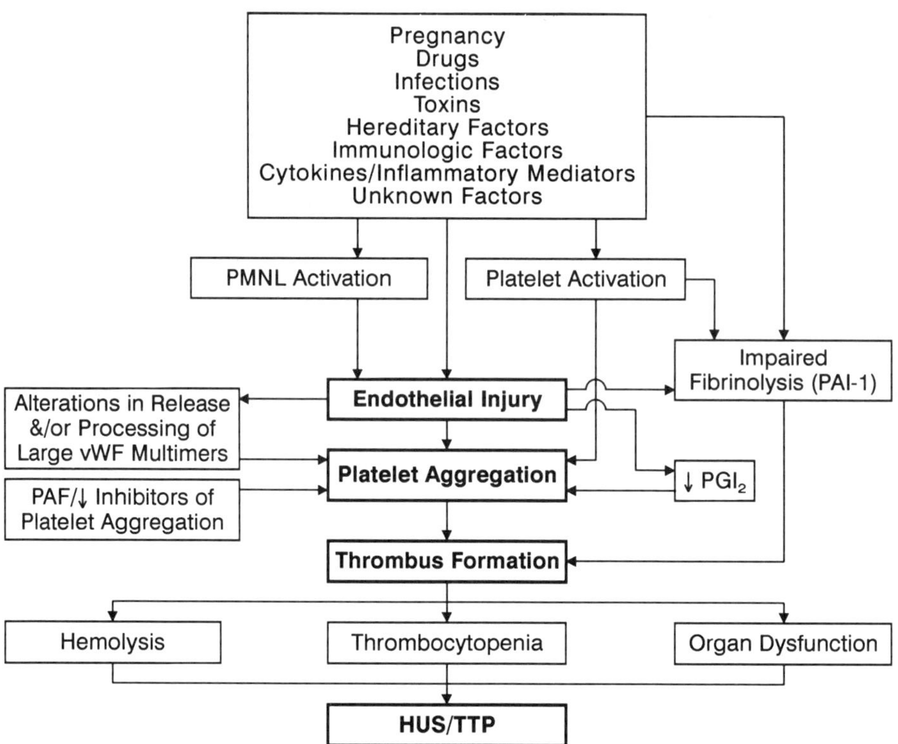

Fig. 6-3. Postulated pathogenetic mechanisms in HUS and TTP. PMNL, polymorphonuclear leukocyte; PAI-1, plasminogen activator inhibitor type 1; PAF, platelet-aggregating factor(s); vWF, von Willebrand factor; PGI₂, prostacyclin.

due to toxins, infectious agents, drugs, or hereditary, immunologic, inflammatory, or other factors may be important elements in the development of HUS and TTP.[43,50,72,74,75] A deficiency of inhibitors of platelet aggregation, such as prostacyclin (PGI$_2$); the presence of circulating plasminogen activator inhibitors, such as plasminogen-activator inhibitor type-1 (PAI-1); and abnormalities of factor VIII:von Willebrand factor (vWF) have been postulated to be important in the development of the microangiopathic process of HUS and TTP.[43,50,74-78] Moake and others have suggested that abnormalities of normally circulating vWF multimers or of "unusually large" vWF multimers resulting from disordered endothelial release or plasma processing of vWF leads to intravascular platelet aggregation by binding to the platelet membrane glycoprotein gpIIb/IIIa.[76,79-83] Platelet aggregating proteins, a deficiency of IgG molecules that normally inhibit platelet aggregation, and endothelial injury from oxygen-derived free radicals have also been suggested to play a role in some patients.[75,83-87] The above are not, of course, mutually exclusive disturbances. The clinical manifestations of HUS/TTP are thought to result from the arteriolar and capillary deposition of platelet-fibrin thrombi.

A few reports have linked HIV infection with effects on endothelial cells, circulating hemostatic factors, and platelets, possibly providing a pathophysiologic explanation for the occurrence of HUS/TTP in these patients. HIV has been shown to infect some endothelial cells,[88] including those of the human glomerulus.[89] Evidence for a possible HIV-mediated endothelial effect in the pathogenesis of HIV-related HUS/TTP was provided by the recent observation of del Arco and colleagues,[37] who detected HIV p24 antigen, using immunohistochemical staining with a monoclonal antibody, in endothelial cells of a bone marrow sample obtained from a patient with HIV-related TTP. The authors postulated that a direct cytopathic or toxic effect of endothelial cell infection with HIV could play a role in the development of TTP.[37]

Plasma levels of vWF antigen and vWF coagulant activity are markedly elevated in HIV-infected patients without HUS/TTP, particularly those with opportunistic infections,[90-93] although it is not known whether abnormalities of high-molecular-weight multimers are present. Elevated levels of fibronectin, tissue-type plasminogen activator, and plasminogen activating inhibitors, and decreased levels of protein S in some HIV-infected patients[91-93] indicate that disturbances of coagulation and fibrinolytic mechanisms may also be present. In addition, cross-reactivity of antibodies directed against HIV-glycoprotein gp160/120 with the platelet glycoprotein gpIIb/IIIa has been recently demonstrated.[94]

Several reports have examined the role of vWF in patients with HIV-related HUS/TTP. Segal and associates[15] performed immunohistologic studies of various organs from a patient who died with HIV-related TTP and found reactivity with polyclonal antibodies to factor VIII R:Ag (vWF) and a polyclonal antibody to fibrinogen/fibrin-related substances. They also demonstrated immunostaining of glomerular thrombi and capillary loops with a monoclonal antibody to platelet-specific glycoprotein gpIIb/IIIa,[15] which serves as a platelet-binding site for vWF. Beris and colleagues[16] found decreased levels of factor VIII coagulant activity and ristocetin cofactor levels and absence of high-molecular-weight vWF multimers during acute disease in one patient. With remission, factor VIII coagulant activity, vWF antigen levels, ristocetin cofactor activity, and high-molecular-weight multimer levels increased to greater than normal.[16] Leaf and colleagues,[8] however, were unable to detect abnormal vWF multimers in the plasma of two patients during their acute illness, or in the plasma of one patient who was in remission. Platelet-aggregating factors have not been found in the few patients studied.[7,8]

CMV has been shown to infect endothelial cells in vitro, resulting in a reduction of endothelial cell vWF content and induction of an endothelial-dependent procoagulant activity.[95,96] Herpes simplex virus also infects endothelial cells, resulting in a procoagulant effect and enhanced platelet aggregation and endothelial adhesion of platelets.[97,98] Therefore, it is possible (albeit purely speculative at this point) that AIDS-associated opportunistic infectious agents may be involved in the development of HUS/TTP in some patients, either alone or as a cofactor with HIV.

CLINICAL COURSE AND TREATMENT

The potentially devastating nature of HIV-related HUS/TTP is underscored by several cases of sudden death occurring within hours of presentation.[8,19,25] About one-third of patients died during the acute phase of their illness, despite aggressive therapies in most instances. Although a 67 percent (4 of 6) short-term survival rate was reported by Leaf et al.,[8] in other series the overall survival rate has been rather dismal, with mortality rates of 67 to 100 percent.[13,17,31,35a,36a] In the series reported by Thompson et al.,[31] all seven patients with HIV-related TTP died within 2 years. This contrasted with the long-term survival rate of 78 percent in their patients with HIV-negative HUS/TTP,[31] which is similar to the patient survival rate reported in other recent series of HUS and TTP in adults.[24,99,100]

Dialysis has been required in several patients. One patient with HUS, who presented with severe oliguric acute renal failure requiring acute dialysis, recovered sufficient renal function so that dialysis could be discontinued.[3] Three patients required chronic dialysis,[4,10,38] one of whom had a prior history of nephrotic syndrome with focal and segmental glomerular sclerosis on an earlier kidney biopsy and may have developed end-stage kidney disease because of HIV nephropathy,[10] and another had a failed renal allograft.[38] In others, severe renal failure developed as a terminal event or was related to other acute illnesses.

Adults with HUS/TTP unrelated to HIV are usually treated with plasma infusions and/or plasma exchange (plasmapheresis with plasma infusion).[24,43,99–101] Most patients with HIV-related HUS/TTP have also received some form of plasma therapy. The mechanisms by which plasma therapy influence the pathophysiologic processes underlying HUS/TTP remain conjectural. Plasma infusion has been postulated to replace or correct a deficiency of circulating factors that normally inhibit the platelet-aggregatory responses thought to be important in the development of HUS/TTP. Plasma exchange, on the other hand, has been suggested to also provide for the removal, by plasmapheresis, of procoagulant, platelet-aggregating, or otherwise toxic substances. A recent randomized trial by the Canadian Apheresis Study Group[99] in patients with TTP not related to HIV infection found that the remission rate and patient survival were higher in patients who were treated with plasma exchange, compared with plasma infusion. Others have also suggested that plasma exchange is superior to plasma infusion for TTP,[24,43,101] although some recommend initial treatment with plasma infusion.[57] Although supportive therapy without plasma infusion or plasmapheresis is usually recommended for children with "classic" (D+) HUS, plasma infusion or plasmapheresis using fresh frozen plasma replacement has been recommended for atypical forms of HUS.[51,53,102–105] Plasma therapy in adult patients with HUS/TTP is often combined with corticosteroids, aspirin, and dipyridamole.[106] Vincristine,[107] splenectomy, γ-globulin infusions,[108] and a variety of other therapies have also been used in patients with refractory or relapsing HUS/TTP.[43]

A direct, controlled comparison of these therapies for HIV-related HUS/TTP has not been made, so that any conclusions regarding their comparative efficacy must be tentative. Detailed descriptions of the effects of plasma exchange used as the primary therapy for HIV-related HUS/TTP have been reported in 36 patients (Table 6-5). Complete or partial remissions were obtained in 81 percent of these patients. Relapses occurred in several patients, some of whom responded to subsequent plasmapheresis, but others were refractory to further treatment.

Plasma infusion was used as the primary therapy in 19 patients, excluding 2 additional patients who received plasma infusions but died within hours of presentation[8] (Table 6-6). Only 6 of these patients developed complete remissions in response to treatment with plasma infusions. However, remissions were subsequently obtained in several patients when plasma exchange was initiated after an inadequate response to plasma infusion alone.[10,22,23,27,30,32]

Several other forms of therapy have also been used in patients with HIV-related HUS/TTP, including vincristine, zidovudine, exchange transfusions, γ-globulin, prostacyclin, vitamin E, 1-desamino-8-D-arginine (DDAVP), and splenectomy. The clinical benefit of these treatments is unclear, however. Splenectomy was not successful in the few patients in whom this treatment was reported,[31,35a,36a] and in another patient TTP developed after a splenectomy had been performed for treatment of AIDS-related ITP.[35] The development of HUS/TTP in at least two patients who were receiving zidovudine[18,29] raises questions concerning its utility, although the addition of zidovudine was thought to be important in obtaining a remission in two patients,[23,33]

Table 6-5. Plasmapheresis as Primary Treatment for HIV-Related HUS/TTP

Reference	Other Treatments	Response	Comments
Boccia et al.[1]	A, D	Remission	Relapse unresponsive to plasmapheresis; died
Jokela et al.[2]	A, F, P, D	Remission	
Farina et al.[3]		Remission	Initial hemodialysis, improved with CRI
Esforzado et al.[4]	A, P, D	Remission	Chronic hemodialysis
Nair et al.[7] (case 1)	A, P, D	Remission	
Nair et al.[7] (case 2)	A, P, D	Remission	
Leaf et al.[8] (case 1)	A, P, D	Remission	
Leaf et al.[8] (case 2)	A, F, P, D	Remission	
Leaf et al.[8] (case 3)	A, F, P, D	Remission	Relapse responded to plasmapheresis
Leaf et al.[8] (case 5)	F, P	Remission	
Botti et al.[9]	A, F, D, V	Remission	
Meisenberg et al.[10] (case 1)		Remission	
Besalduch et al.[14]	F	Remission	
Segal et al.[15]		Died	Only 4 plasmapheresis treatments
Beris et al.[16]	A, P, D, Pr, V	Remission	
Kiprov et al.[20] (4 patients)		Remission	In 2/4; 2/4 died
Pachon et al.[21]		Unknown	Left hospital after 3 treatments
Routy et al.[22] (case 2)	P, V	Remission	
Bell et al.[24] (2 patients)		Remission	In 2/2; both with treated relapses
Bullarsky et al.[26]	F, P, D	Died	
Berns and Tomaszewski[29]	A, P	Remission	Quickly relapsed, died
Rarick et al.[30] (case 1)		Remission	
Thompson et al.[31] (7 patients)		Remission	In 6/7; 1 died later with refractory relapse
Manner et al.[35]	F, P, G, V	Remission	Died of multiple pulmonary emboli
Albrecht and Stellbrink[37a]	P, G, V	No	Died 3 months later
del Arco et al.[37]	F, P	Remission	

Abbreviations: A, aspirin; P, prednisone/other steroids; D, dipyridamole; F, fresh frozen plasma; V, vincristine; Pr, prostacyclin; G, γ-globulin; CRI, chronic renal insufficiency.

Table 6-6. Plasma Infusion as Primary Therapy for HIV-Related HUS/TTP

Reference	Other treatments	Response	Comments
Cervero-Marti et al.[5]	Vitamin E	Remission	
Meisenberg et al.[10] (case 2)	P	No	Remission with plasmapheresis, A, D; quickly relapsed; responded to plasmapheresis, A, D, V
Platanias et al.[11] (case 2)	A, P, D	Remission	Relapse 14 months later responded to plasma infusion, P
Khuong et al.[13]	A, P, D	No	Partial remission with G
Routy et al.[22]	P	No	Remission with plasmapheresis; quickly relapsed; died
Salem et al.[23]	A, D, G	Remission	Relapse unresponsive to plasma infusion, responded to plasmapheresis, A, D, V, Z
Doco-Lecompte et al.[27] (case 1)		No	Died
Doco-Lecompte et al.[27] (case 2)	A, D	No	Died
Doco-Lecompte et al.[27] (case 3)	A, D, G	No (partial?)	Responded to plasmapheresis; died of respiratory failure with CRI
Rarick et al.[30] (case 2)		No	Responded to plasmapheresis
Rarick et al.[30] (case 3)		No	Died (refused further treatment)
Shivaram and Cash[32]		No	Responded to plasmapheresis
Kaloterakis et al.[33]	P, Z, V	Remission	
Chauveau et al.[36a] (6 patients)	—	Remission	In 2/6; partial response in 1 patient

Abbreviations: A, aspirin; P, prednisone/other steroids; D, dipyridamole; V, vincristine; G, γ-globulin; Z, zidovudine (AZT); CRI, chronic renal insufficiency.

and in others HUS/TTP was noted to have developed shortly after discontinuation of antiretroviral therapy.[34]

Based on these uncontrolled and limited observations, initial therapy with plasmapheresis using fresh frozen plasma replacement, if available, should be instituted as soon as a diagnosis of HIV-related HUS/TTP is made. Risks of plasma therapy may include allergic reactions, citrate toxicity, and infection.[109,110] Although an increased risk of infection was not found in a recent study of plasmapheresis treatment of lupus nephritis,[111] Wing and colleagues[112] reported the development of severe opportunistic infections, including two cases of *P. carinii* pneumonia, complicating plasmapheresis in patients with rapidly progressive glomerulonephritis.

CONCLUSIONS

An increasing number of reports appear to have now established a definite clinical association between HIV infection and the development of HUS/ TTP, with several centers finding that HIV infection seems to be relatively common among adults with HUS/TTP. Serologic testing for HIV infection would certainly appear to be appropriate for all patients who present with HUS/TTP, if they are not already known to be HIV-positive. Further epidemiologic investigation, which may require a prospective study among several centers, is needed to clarify whether the incidence of HUS/TTP is really greater among HIV-infected populations than in those without HIV infection.

Finally, a direct pathogenetic relationship between HIV infection and HUS/TTP is suggested by several pieces of pathophysiologic information, such as the finding of HIV infection of endothelial cells and disturbances of vWF, coagulation, and fibrinolysis in HIV-infected patients (both with and without HUS/TTP). Yet to be clarified is what the precise pathogenetic link between HIV infection and these disorders may be, and what the effects are of HIV infection (or infection with associated opportunistic pathogens) on the pathophysiology of the endothelium, platelets, vWF, and fibrinolytic mechanisms.

REFERENCES

1. Boccia RV, Gelmann EP, Baker C et al: A hemolytic-uremic syndrome with the acquired immunodeficiency syndrome. Ann Intern Med 101:716, 1984
2. Jokela J, Flynn T, Henry K: Thrombotic thrombocytopenic purpura in a human immunodeficiency virus (HIV) seropositive homosexual man. Am J Hematol 25:341, 1987
3. Farina C, Gavazzeni G, Caprioli A, Remuzzi G: Hemolytic uremic syndrome associated with verocytotoxin-producing *Escherichia coli* infection in acquired immunodeficiency syndrome. Blood 12:2465, 1990
4. Esforzado N, Poch E, Almirall J et al: Hemolytic uremic syndrome associated with HIV infection. AIDS 5:1041, 1991
5. Cervero Marti A, Martin J, Perez-Paya A et al: Hemolytic-uremic syndrome associated with pancreatitis in an HIV-positive patient. Ann Hematol 65:236, 1992
6. Cotte L, Preckel MP, Cahen R et al: Fatal haemolytic uraemic syndrome in an AIDS patient. Eur J Med 1:378, 1992
7. Nair JMG, Bellevue R, Bertoni M, Dosik H: Thrombotic thrombocytopenic purpura in patients with the acquired immunodeficiency syndrome (AIDS)-related complex. Ann Intern Med 109:209, 1988

8. Leaf AN, Laubenstein LJ, Raphael B et al: Thrombotic thrombocytopenic purpura associated with human immunodeficiency virus type 1 (HIV-1) infection. Ann Intern Med 109:194, 1988

9. Botti AC, Hyde P, DiPillo F: Thrombotic thrombocytopenic purpura in a patient who subsequently developed the acquired immunodeficiency syndrome (AIDS). Ann Intern Med 109:242, 1988

10. Meisenberg BR, Robinson WL, Mosley CA et al: Thrombotic thrombocytopenic purpura in human immunodeficiency (HIV) seropositive males. Am J Hematol 27:212, 1988

11. Platanias LC, Paiusco D, Bernstein S, Murali MR: Thrombotic thrombocytopenic purpura as the first manifestation of human immunodeficiency virus infection. Am J Med 87:699, 1989

12. DeNobriga J, Chu-Fong A, Elizalde A: Thrombotic thrombocytopenic purpura (TTP) in a human immune deficiency virus (HIV) positive patient: successful treatment with high dose gamma globulin (HDGG), abstracted. Proc Annu Meet Am Soc Clin Oncol 8:A21, 1989

13. Khuong MA, DeTruchis P, Oksenhendler E et al: Microangiopathie thrombotique (MAT) et infection HIV, abstracted. Int Conf AIDS 5:263, 1989

14. Besalduch J, Altes J, Morey M, Villalonga C: Purpura trombotica trombocitopenica e infeccion por virus de la inmunodeficiencia humana. Med Clin 92:795, 1989

15. Segal GH, Tubbs RR, Ratliff NB et al: Thrombotic thrombocytopenic purpura in a patient with AIDS. Cleve Clin J Med 57:360, 1990

16. Beris P, Dunand V, Osoz C, Reynard C: Association of thrombotic thrombocytopenic purpura and human immunodeficiency virus infection. Nouv Rev Fr Hematol 32:277, 1990

17. Ucar A, Fernandez HF, Byrnes JJ et al: Thrombotic microangiopathy and retroviral infections: a 13-year experience. Am J Hematol 45:304, 1994

18. Charasse C, Michelet C, Le Tulzo Y et al: Thrombotic thrombocytopenic purpura with the acquired immunodeficiency syndrome: a pathologically documented case report. Am J Kidney Dis 17:80, 1991

19. Bell M, Barnhart JS, Martin JM et al: Thrombotic thrombocytopenic purpura causing sudden, unexpected death—a series of eight patients. J Forensic Sci 35:601, 1990

20. Kiprov DD, Kwiatkowska BJ, Miller RG: Therapeutic apheresis in human immunodeficiency virus-related syndromes. p. 184. In Nydegger UE (ed): Therapeutic Hemapheresis in the 1990s. Karger, Basel, 1990

21. Pachon J, Viciana P, Espigado I, Fernandez-Alonso J: Purpura trombotica trombocitopenica en paciente con sindrome de immunodeficiencia adquirida. Rev Clin Esp 187:65, 1990

22. Routy J-P, Beaulieu R, Monte M et al: Immunologic thrombocytopenia followed by thrombotic thrombocytopenic purpura in two HIV$_1$ patients. Am J Hematol 38:327, 1991

23. Salem G, Terebelo H, Raman S: Human immunodeficiency virus associated with thrombotic thrombocytopenic purpura: successful treatment with zidovudine. South Med J 84:493, 1991

24. Bell WR, Braine HG, Ness PM, Kickler TS: Improved survival in thrombotic thrombocytopenic purpura-hemolytic uremic syndrome. N Engl J Med 325:398, 1991

25. Taff ML, Schwartz IS, Churg J, Boglioli LR: Sudden death due to thrombotic thrombocytopenic purpura and HIV infection. Am J Forensic Med Pathol 12: 89, 1991

26. Bullorsky EO, Shanley C, Napoli J et al: Purpura trombotica trombocitopenica y seropositividad para el virus de la immunodeficiencia humana adquirida. Medicina 51:241, 1991

27. Doco-Lecompte T, Molina JM, Leleu-Nahmias G, Modai J: Purpura thrombotique thrombocytopenique au cours de l'infection par le VIH. Presse Med 20: 1159, 1991

28. Church JA, Marshall G, Laug W: Thrombotic thrombocytopenic purpura (TTP) in an HIV infected child: treatment with 1-desamino-8-D-arginine (DDAVP) and intravenous immunoglobulin (IVIG), abstracted. Int Conf AIDS 5:494, 1989

29. Berns JS, Tomaszewski JE: Hemolytic uremic syndrome and thrombotic thrombocytopenic purpura associated with human immunodeficiency virus infection and acquired immunodeficiency syndrome. p. 299. In Kaplan BS, Trompeter RS, Moake JL (eds): Hemolytic Uremic Syndrome and Thrombotic Thrombocytopenic Purpura. Marcel Dekker, New York, 1992

30. Rarick MU, Espina B, Mocharnuk R et al: Thrombotic thrombocytopenic purpura in patients with human immunodeficiency virus infection: a report of three cases and review of the literature. Am J Hematol 40:103, 1992

31. Thompson CE, Damon LE, Ries CA, Linker CA: Thrombotic microangiopathies in the 1980s: clinical features, response to treatment, and the impact of the human immunodeficiency virus epidemic. Blood 80:1890, 1992

32. Shivaram U, Cash M: Purpura fulminans, metastatic endophthalmitis, and thrombotic thrombocytopenic purpura in an HIV-infected patient. NY State J Med 92:313, 1992

33. Kaloterakis A, Filiotou A, Kolnagou J et al: Thrombotic thrombocytopenic purpura in a woman with AIDS related complex: complete remission with zidovudine, abstracted. Int Conf AIDS 8:93, 1992

34. Veenstra J, van Der Lelie J, Mulder JW, Reiss P: Low-grade thrombotic thrombocytopenic purpura associated with HIV-1 infection. Br J Haematol 83:346, 1993

35. Manner CE, Gathe J Jr, Novak I et al: Thrombotic thrombocytopic purpura (TTP) in a man with AIDS and prior idiopathic thrombocytopenic purpura (ITP), abstracted. Int Conf AIDS 9:451, 1993

35a. Blanche P, Bachmeyer C, Sereni D et al: Hemolytic uremic syndrome in patients with HIV infection, abstracted. Int Conf AIDS 10:198, 1994

36. Francois A, Dhib M, Dubois D et al: Thrombotic microangiopathy (TMA) as the first manifestation of HIV infection. Clin Nephrol 39:352, 1993

36a. Chauveau D, Dessasis JF, Choukroun G et al: Hemolytic uremic syndrome and thrombotic thrombocytopenic purpura in seven HIV patients, abstracted. J Am Soc Nephrol 5:389, 1994

37. del Arco A, Martinez MA, Pena JM et al: Thrombotic thrombocytopenic purpura associated with human immunodeficiency virus infection: demonstration of p24 antigen in endothelial cells. Clin Infect Dis 17:360, 1993

37a. Albrecht H, Stellbrink HJ: Refractory Escherichia coli 0157:H7 associated hemolytic uremic syndrome and HIV-infection, abstracted. Int Conf AIDS 10:190, 1994

38. Frem GJ, Rennke HG, Sayegh MH: Late renal allograft failure secondary to

thrombotic microangiopathy-human immunodeficiency virus nephropathy. J Am Soc Nephrol 4:1643, 1994

39. Moschcowitz E: An acute febrile pleiochromic anemia with hyaline thrombosis of the terminal arterioles and capillaries. Arch Intern Med 36:89, 1925
40. Baehr G, Klemperer P, Schifrin A: An acute febrile anemia and thrombocytopenic purpura with diffuse platelet thrombosis of capillaries and arterioles. Trans Assoc Am Phys 51:43, 1936
41. Singer K, Bornstein FP, Wile SA: Thrombotic thrombocytopenic purpura: hemorrhagic diathesis with generalized platelet thromboses. Blood 2:542, 1947
42. Ridolfi RL, Bell WR: Thrombotic thrombocytopenic purpura: report of 25 cases and review of the literature. Medicine 60:413, 1981
43. Bukowksi RM: Thrombotic thrombocytopenic purpura: a review. p. 287. In Spaet TH (ed): Progress in Hemostasis and Thrombosis. Grune & Stratton, Orlando, 1982
44. Gasser C, Gautier E, Steck A et al: Hämolytisch-urämische syndrome: bilaterale nierenrindennekrosen bei akuten erworbenen hämolytischen anämien. Schweiz Med Wochenschr 85:905, 1955
45. Habib R, Mathieu H, Royer P: Maladie thrombotique arteriolocapillaire du rein chez l'enfant. Rev Fr Clin Biol 3:891, 1958
46. Mathieu H, Leclerc F, Habib R, Royer P: Etude clinique et biologique de 37 observations de syndrome hemolytique et uremique. Arch Fr Pediatr 26:369, 1969
47. Habib R: Pathology of the hemolytic uremic syndrome. p. 315. In Kaplan BS, Trompeter RS, Moake JL (eds): Hemolytic Uremic Syndrome and Thrombotic Thrombocytopenic Purpura. Marcel Dekker, New York, 1992
48. Clarkson AR, Lawrence JR, Meadows R, Seymour AE: The hemolytic-uremic syndrome in adults. Q J Med 39:227, 1970
49. Drummond KN: Hemolytic uremic syndrome—then and now. N Engl J Med 312:116, 1985
50. Kaplan BS, Cleary TG, Obrig TG: Recent advances in understanding the pathogenesis of the hemolytic uremic syndromes. Pediatr Nephrol 4:276, 1990
51. Loirat C, Baudouin V, Sonsino E et al: Hemolytic-uremic syndrome in the child. Adv Nephrol 22:141, 1993
52. Trompeter RS, Schwartz R, Chantler C et al: Haemolytic uraemic syndrome in childhood: analysis of prognostic features. Arch Dis Child 58:101, 1983
53. Fitzpatrick MM, Dillon MJ, Barratt TM, Trompeter RS: Atypical hemolytic uremic syndrome. p. 163. In Kaplan BS, Trompeter RS, Moake JL (eds): Hemolytic Uremic Syndrome and Thrombotic Thrombocytopenic Purpura. Marcel Dekker, New York, 1992
54. Kaplan BS, Chesney RW, Drummond KN: Hemolytic uremic syndrome in families. N Engl J Med 292:1090, 1975
55. Berns JS, Kaplan BS, Mackow RC, Hefter LG: Inherited hemolytic uremic syndrome in adults. Am J Kidney Dis 19:331, 1992
56. Kaplan BS, Kaplan P: Hemolytic uremic syndrome in families. p. 213. In Kaplan BS, Trompeter RS, Moake JL (eds): Hemolytic Uremic Syndrome and Thrombotic Thrombocytopenic Purpura. Marcel Dekker, New York, 1992
57. Remuzzi G: HUS and TTP: variable expression of a single entity. Kidney Int 32:292, 1987
58. Kaplan BS: Commentary on the relationships between HUS and TTP. p. 29.

In Kaplan BS, Trompeter RS, Moake JL (eds): Hemolytic Uremic Syndrome and Thrombotic Thrombocytopenic Purpura. Marcel Dekker, New York, 1992

59. Pardo V, Meneses R, Ossa L et al: AIDS-related glomerulopathy: occurrence in specific risk groups. Kidney Int 31:1167, 1987

60. Bourgoignie JJ: Renal complications of human immunodeficiency virus type 1. Kidney Int 37:1571, 1990

61. Cantor ES, Kimmel PL, Bosch JP: Effect of race on expression of acquired immunodeficiency syndrome-associated nephropathy. Arch Intern Med 151:125, 1991

62. Centers for Disease Control and Prevention: 1993 revised classification system for HIV infection and expanded surveillance case definition for AIDS among adolescents and adults. MMWR 41:1, 1992

63. Morris L, Distenfield A, Amorosi E, Karpatkin S: Autoimmune thrombocytopenic purpura in homosexual men. Part 1. Ann Intern Med 96:714, 1982

64. Krupsky M, Sarel R, Hurwitz N, Resnitzky P: Late appearance of thrombotic thrombocytopenic purpura after autoimmune hemolytic anemia and in the course of chronic autoimmune thrombocytopenic purpura: two case reports. Acta Haematol 85:139, 1991

65. Dixon AC, Kwock DW, Nakamura JM et al: Thrombotic thrombocytopenic purpura and human T-lymphotrophic virus, type 1 (HTLV-1). Ann Intern Med 110:93, 1989

66. Rao TKS, Filippone EJ, Nicastri AD et al: Associated focal and segmental glomerulosclerosis in the acquired immunodeficiency syndrome. N Engl J Med 310:669, 1984

67. Churg J, Goldstein MH, Bernstein J: Thrombotic microangiopathy including hemolytic-uremic syndrome, thrombotic thrombocytopenic purpura, and postpartum renal failure. p. 1081. In Tisher CG, Brenner BM (eds): Renal Pathology with Clinical and Functional Correlations. JB Lippincott, Philadelphia, 1989

68. Chander P, Soni A, Suri A et al: Renal ultrastructural markers in AIDS-associated nephropathy. Am J Pathol 126:513, 1987

69. Cohen AH, Nast CC: HIV-associated nephropathy. A unique combined glomerular, tubular, and interstitial lesion. Mod Pathol 1:87, 1988

70. Murgo AJ: Cancer and chemotherapy-associated thrombotic microangiopathy. p. 271. In Kaplan BS, Trompeter RS, Moake JL (eds): Hemolytic Uremic Syndrome and Thrombotic Thrombocytopenic Purpura. Marcel Dekker, New York, 1992

71. Karmali MA: The association of verocytotoxins and the classical hemolytic uremic syndrome. p. 199. In Kaplan BS, Trompeter RS, Moake JL (eds): Hemolytic Uremic Syndrome and Thrombotic Trombocytopenic Purpura. Marcel Dekker, New York, 1992

72. Obrig TG: Pathogenesis of shiga toxin (verotoxin)-induced endothelial cell injury. p. 405. In Kaplan BS, Trompeter RS, Moake JL (eds): Hemolytic Uremic Syndrome and Thrombotic Thrombocytopenic Purpura. Marcel Dekker, New York, 1992

73. Raghupathy P, Date A, Shastry JCM et al: Haemolytic-uraemic syndrome complicating shigella dysentery in south Indian children. BMJ 1:1518, 1978

74. Zoja C, Remuzzi G: The pivotal role of the endothelial cell in the pathogenesis of HUS. p. 389. In Kaplan BS, Trompeter RS, Moake JL (eds): Hemolytic Uremic Syndrome and Thrombotic Thrombocytopenic Purpura. Marcel Dekker, New York, 1992

75. Lian EC-Y: Pathogenesis of thrombotic thrombocytopenic purpura. Semin Hematol 24:82, 1987

76. Moake JL: von Willebrand factor abnormalities in thrombotic thrombocytopenic purpura and the hemolytic uremic syndrome. p. 459. In Kaplan BS, Trompeter RS, Moake JL (eds): Hemolytic Uremic Syndrome and Thrombotic Thrombocytopenic Purpura. Marcel Dekker, New York, 1992

77. Bergstein JM, Riley M, Bang NU: Role of plasminogen-activator inhibitor type 1 in the pathogenesis and outcome of the hemolytic uremic syndrome. N Engl J Med 327:755, 1992

78. Wu KK: Role of prostacyclin in the pathogenesis and therapy of thrombotic thrombocytopenic purpura. p. 483. In Kaplan BS, Trompeter RS, Moake JL (eds): Hemolytic Uremic Syndrome and Thrombotic Thrombocytopenic Purpura. Marcel Dekker, New York, 1992

79. Kelton JG, Moore JC, Murphy WG: Studies investigating platelet aggregation and release initiated by sera from patients with thrombotic thrombocytopenic purpura. Blood 69:924, 1987

80. Moore JC, Murphy WG, Kelton JG: Calpain proteolysis of von Willebrand factor enhances its binding to platelet membrane glycoprotein IIb/IIIa: an explanation for platelet aggregation in thrombotic thrombocytopenic purpura. Br J Haematol 74:457, 1990

81. Moake JL, Rudy CK, Troll JH et al: Unusually large plasma factor VIII:von Willebrand factor multimers in chronic relapsing thrombotic thrombocytopenic purpura. N Engl J Med 307:1432, 1982

82. Moake JL, Byrnes JJ, Troll JH et al: Abnormal VIII:von Willebrand factor patterns in the plasma of patients with the hemolytic-uremic syndrome. Blood 64:592, 1984

83. Kelton JG, Moore J, Santos A, Sheridan D: Detection of platelet-agglutinating factor in thrombotic thrombocytopenic purpura. Ann Intern Med 101:589, 1984

84. Lian EC-Y, Siddiqui FA, Chen SH: Platelet-agglutinating/aggregating proteins from the plasma of patients with thrombotic thrombocytopenic purpura. p. 473. In Kaplan BS, Trompeter RS, Moake JL (eds): Hemolytic Uremic Syndrome and Thrombotic Thrombocytopenic Purpura. Marcel Dekker, New York, 1992

85. Taylor CM, Powell HR: Oxygen-derived free radicals in the pathogenesis of hemolytic uremic syndrome. p. 355. In Kaplan BS, Trompeter RS, Moake JL (eds): Hemolytic Uremic Syndrome and Thrombotic Thrombocytopenic Purpura. Marcel Dekker, New York, 1992

86. Lian EC-Y, Mui PTK, Siddiqui FA et al: Inhibition of platelet-aggregating activity in thrombotic thrombocytopenic purpura plasma by normal adult immunoglobulin G. J Clin Invest 73:548, 1984

87. Siddiqui FA, Lian EC-Y: Novel platelet-agglutinating protein from a thrombotic thrombocytopenic purpura plasma. J Clin Invest 76:1330, 1985

88. Wiley CA, Schrier RD, Nelson JA et al: Cellular localization of human immunodeficiency virus infection within the brains of acquired immunodeficiency syndrome patients. Proc Natl Acad Sci USA 83:7089, 1986

89. Green DF, Resnick L, Bourgoignie JJ: HIV infects glomerular endothelial and mesangial but not epithelial cells in vitro. Kidney Int 42:956, 1992

90. Janier M, Flageul B, Drouet L et al: Cutaneous and plasma values of von Willebrand factor in AIDS: a marker of endothelial stimulation? J Invest Dermatol 90:703, 1988

91. Drouet L, Scrobohaci ML, Janier M, Baudin B: Endothelial cells: target for the HIV 1 virus? Nouv Rev Fr Hematol 32:103, 1990
92. Schved J-F, Gris J-C, Arnaud A et al: Von Willebrand factor antigen, tissue-type plasminogen activator antigen, and risk of death in human immunodeficiency virus 1-related clinical disease: independent prognostic relevance of tissue-type plasminogen activator. J Lab Clin Med 120:411, 1992
93. Lafeuillade A, Alessi MC, Poizot-Martin I et al: Endothelial cell dysfunction in HIV infection. J AIDS 5:127, 1992
94. Bettaieb A, Fromont P, Louache F et al: Presence of cross-reactive antibody between human immunodeficiency virus (HIV) and platelet glycoproteins in HIV-related immune thrombocytopenia purpura. Blood 80:162, 1992
95. Van Dam-Mieras MCE, Bruggeman CA, Muller AD et al: Induction of endothelial cell procoagulant activity by cytomegalovirus infection. Thromb Res 47:69, 1987
96. Bruggeman CA, Debie WHM, Muller AD et al: Cytomegalovirus alters the von Willebrand factor content in human endothelial cells. Thromb Haemostasis 59:264, 1988
97. Vercelloti GM: Proinflammatory and procoagulant effects of herpes simplex infection on human endothelium. Blood Cells 16:209, 1990
98. Visser MR, Tracy PB, Vercelloti GM et al: Enhanced thrombin generation and platelet binding on herpes simplex virus-infected endothelium. Proc Natl Acad Sci USA 85:8227, 1988
99. Rock GA, Shumak KH, Buskard NA et al: Comparison of plasma exchange with plasma infusion in the treatment of thrombotic thrombocytopenic purpura. N Engl J Med 325:393, 1991
100. Lichtin AE, Schreiber AD, Hurwitz S et al: Efficacy of intensive plasmapheresis in thrombotic thrombocytopenic purpura. Arch Intern Med 147:2122, 1987
101. Moake JL: An update on the therapy of thrombotic thrombocytopenic purpura. p. 541. In Kaplan BS, Trompeter RS, Moake JL (eds): Hemolytic Uremic Syndrome and Thrombotic Thrombocytopenic Purpura. Marcel Dekker, New York, 1992
102. Loirat C, Sonsino E, Hinglais N et al: Treatment of the childhood haemolytic uraemic syndrome with plasma. A multicentre randomized controlled trial. Pediatr Nephrol 2:279, 1988
103. Rizzoni G, Claris-Appiani A, Edefonti A et al: Plasma infusion for hemolytic-uremic syndrome in children: results of a multicenter controlled trial. J Pediatr 112:284, 1988
104. Gianviti A, Perna A, Caringella A et al: Plasma exchange in children with hemolytic-uremic syndrome at risk of poor outcome. Am J Kidney Dis 22:264, 1993
105. Loirat C: Treatment of hemolytic uremic syndrome with fresh-frozen plasma or with plasmapheresis. p. 431. In Kaplan BS, Trompeter RS, Moake JL (eds): Hemolytic Uremic Syndrome and Thrombotic Thrombocytopenic Purpura. Marcel Dekker, New York, 1992
106. Phillips MD: Antiplatelet agents in thrombotic thrombocytopenic purpura. p. 531. In Kaplan BS, Trompeter RS, Moake JL (eds): Hemolytic Uremic Syndrome and Thrombotic Thrombocytopenic Purpura. Marcel Dekker, New York, 1992
107. Gutterman LA: Treatment of thrombotic thrombocytopenic purpura and hemo-

lytic uremic syndrome: the role of vincristine. p. 513. In Kaplan BS, Trompeter RS, Moake JL (eds): Hemolytic uremic syndrome and thrombotic thrombocytopenic purpura. Marcel Dekker, New York, 1992

108. Raniele DP, Opsahl JA, Kjellstrand CM: Should intravenous immunoglobulin G be first-line treatment for acute thrombotic thrombocytopenic purpura? Case report and review of the literature. Am J Kidney Dis 18:264, 1991

109. Shumak KH, Rock GA: Therapeutic plasma exchange. N Engl J Med 310:762, 1984

110. Rock GA, Tricklebank GW, Kasaboski A, the Canadian Apheresis Study Group: Plasma exchange in Canada. Can Med Assoc J 142:557, 1990

111. Pohl MA, Shu-Ping L, Berl T, and the Lupus Nephritis Collaborative Study Group: Plasmapheresis does not increase the risk for infection in immunosuppressed patients with severe lupus nephritis. Ann Intern Med 114:924, 1991

112. Wing EJ, Bruns FJ, Fraley DS et al: Infectious complications with plasmapheresis in rapidly progressive glomerulonephritis. JAMA 244:2423, 1980

7

Renal Disease in Children with HIV Infection

Victoriano Pardo   *Carolyn Abitbol*
Jose Strauss   *Gaston Zilleruelo*

INTRODUCTION

Early descriptions of the clinical complications of human immunodeficiency virus (HIV) infection in children did not include reports of renal manifestations.[1] However, over the last decade a variety of electrolyte and acid-base disorders, as well as episodes of acute renal failure were subsequently noted in HIV-infected children. In addition, chronic renal diseases with varying degrees of proteinuria and renal insufficiency were identified[2-9] with clinical and pathologic features similar to those described in adults with what has been termed HIV-associated nephropathy (HIVAN).[10-15] Furthermore, some children were found to have renal disorders with clinical and pathologic features indistinguishable from other forms of idiopathic or secondary renal disease processes.[16-18]

ELECTROLYTE AND ACID-BASE DISTURBANCES AND ACUTE RENAL FAILURE

Hyponatremia and other electrolyte disturbances are common in adults with acquired immunodeficiency syndrome (AIDS)[19,20] (see Ch. 2). Strauss et al. (unpublished observations, 1981–1994) prospectively studied electrolyte disturbances among 216 children with HIV infection. Hyponatremia was documented at least once in 106 (49 percent) of these children, 77 of whom had been receiving diuretics or other drugs associated with tubular dysfunction. Hyponatremia was recurrent or persistent in 30 children (14 percent). Twenty-two of these children appeared to have HIVAN, as defined by abnormal proteinuria. Measurements of total carbon dioxide content were available from 212 children. Persistent or recurrent episodes of metabolic acidosis were documented in 23 percent of these children, most of whom also had persistent hyperkalemia suggestive of a distal renal tubular acidification defect. Most of the children with hypobicarbonatemia had abnormal proteinuria suggestive of HIVAN. In a retrospective clinicopathologic investigation of 155 children with HIV infection, 3 of 12 children who had kidney biopsies with histologically proven focal glomerulosclerosis were found to also have renal tubular acidosis.[6]

Acute renal failure (ARF) may be seen in up to 20 percent of adults with AIDS[21-24] (see Ch. 3), but appears to be much less common in children. When it does occur, ARF in children is often related to reversible prerenal azotemia. Acute tubular necrosis in children with AIDS is often related to sepsis, hemodynamic insults such as hypotension, or exposure to nephrotoxic drugs, although drug-related acute tubulointerstitial nephritis may be less common in children than in adults. ARF may also occur as a preterminal event related to opportunistic infections, central nervous system lesions, or multiple organ failure.

Asymptomatic intravascular coagulation involving the kidneys is not infrequent in HIV-infected patients, as documented by thrombosis of small renal vessels at autopsy. Also indicative of a chronic coagulopathy is the autopsy finding in some children of small segmental mesangiocapillary glomerular lesions, with glomerular capillaries displaying a fluffy, finely fibrillogranular material by electron microscopy, suggestive of fibrin deposition. Clinically significant thrombotic microangiopathy (hemolytic uremic syndrome or thrombotic thrombocytopenic purpura), which has been well described in adults with HIV infection[25–27] (see Ch. 6), has only rarely been diagnosed in HIV-infected children. One child with HIV-associated hemolytic syndrome has been reported,[28] with two additional cases identified in a review of 75 autopsies of perinatally infected children at Jackson Memorial Medical Center in Miami (unpublished observations, 1994).

HIV-RELATED CHRONIC GLOMERULAR DISEASES

Since the original descriptions of focal and segmental glomerulosclerosis in patients with AIDS in 1984,[11–13] as the number of adults with AIDS in the United States increased, a similar increase in the prevalence of HIV-related glomerular disease was observed in some geographic areas, particularly in Florida, New York, and other major cities along the East Coast. These patients presented with heavy proteinuria, rapidly progressive renal failure, and a characteristic type of focal glomerulosclerosis that was frequently associated with prominent tubulointerstitial lesions and dilated tubules. The relationships between these lesions and HIV infection, and the pathogenic role of the virus were challenged because of the apparent absence of renal involvement in patients with AIDS in other regions of the country, such as San Francisco,[29,30] and the apparent similarity between the renal lesions described in these patients and those observed in intravenous drug users without HIV infection. However, demographic differences in prevalence were largely explained by the predominant geographic distribution of large populations of black patients, who appear to be particularly susceptible to this classic form of HIVAN, along the East Coast of the United States.[31,32] In addition, renal involvement was found to occur in patients with AIDS who did not use illicit drugs, in children, and in otherwise asymptomatic HIV-infected individuals.[14]

Prevalence of Proteinuria in HIV-Infected Children

The finding of a positive urine dipstick for protein (Albustix examination of $\geq 1+$) has been considered sufficient evidence for the diagnosis of early HIVAN by Chander and colleagues,[5] who found 38 of 66 (57 percent) HIV-infected children with abnormal protein excretion. This incidence is very similar to that found by Strauss and colleagues in a prospective study of 568 children with confirmed HIV infection or perinatal exposure to HIV and dipstick-positive proteinuria used for the early identification of renal involvement (unpublished observations, 1981–1994). The presence of nephropathy was defined by the finding of dipstick proteinuria of 1 + or greater on two determinations obtained 2 weeks apart in individuals without other overt evidence of genitourinary anomalies or infection. Proteinuria was confirmed in most of these patients by an elevated urine protein/creatinine ratio (Upr/Ucr) or microalbuminuria, or both. By 18 months of age, approximately one-third of the children were found to be infected with HIV-1 through viral culture, a diagnostic polymerase chain reaction (PCR) for viral DNA, or the presence of p24 viral core protein antigenemia. On clinical evaluation, the vast majority of these children showed only mild or absent renal abnormalities. Considering the entire population of 568 children born of HIV-infected mothers, there were 84 (14.8 percent) who were diagnosed as having abnormal proteinuria. Of these, 47 (56 percent) developed nephrotic syndrome and 16 (19 percent) developed renal insufficiency; 5 of these 16 children have been treated with dialysis. Of the 298 of these children followed prospectively for up to 4.5 years, proteinuria developed in 14.8 percent. When only HIV-infected children were considered, the prevalence of proteinuria was approximately 50 percent, similar to that reported by Chander et al.[5]

On the other hand, Tarshish et al.[33] detected proteinuria in only 1.6 percent of 120 perinatally infected children during follow-up of 2.5 years. Moreover, in a retrospective investigation of 155 perinatally infected children by Strauss et al.,[6] there were only 12 with clinically apparent renal disease (8 percent). The reasons for this discrepancy remain unclear.

In some of these children found to have proteinuria, the proteinuria may have been related to complications of AIDS such as opportunistic infections, coagulation disorders, neoplasia, or the nephrotoxic effects of numerous treatments, instead of HIV-related glomerulopathies. This hypothesis receives some support from observations in adults with AIDS who have reversal of proteinuria in response to treatment of infections[34] and the virtual lack of proteinuria in a survey of 145 asymptomatic HIV-infected individuals.[35] In a study of HIV-infected patients and HIV-uninfected patients with other infectious diseases, there was an increased prevalence of proteinuria in the HIV-infected outpatients compared with seronegative subjects, but not compared with hospitalized patients with other infectious diseases.[36] On the other hand, HIVAN occurs in otherwise entirely asymptomatic HIV-infected adults, who may not have even been aware of HIV infection.

Spectrum of HIV-Related Glomerular Pathology

Although the direct pathogenetic role of HIV as a cause of glomerular or other renal disease has not been conclusively established, the entity of an HIV-associated nephropathy is generally accepted. The predominant lesion

Table 7-1. Comparison of HIV-Associated Nephropathies in Adults vs. Children

	Adults	Children
HIV transmission	IVDA, sexual contact	In utero, perinatal
AIDS incubation	Long	Short
Rate of progression to chronic renal failure	Rapid (months)	Slower (years)
Acute renal failure	Common	Uncommon
Histology	FGS: 80–90%	FGS: 50%, MH: 40%, MC: 10%
Mesangial proliferation	Focal	Diffuse

Abbreviations: IVDA, intravenous drug abuse; MH, mesangial hyperplasia; MC, minimal changes.

of HIVAN in adults, associated with the development of heavy proteinuria and a uniformly dismal prognosis, is focal glomerulosclerosis (FGS). FGS may be seen in numerous other conditions, including aging, hypertension, reflux nephropathy, steroid-resistant nephrotic syndrome, drug addiction, and glomerular hyperfiltration from numerous causes, and might be considered as a "final common pathway" in the histopathologic progression to end-stage renal disease.

Historically, the pathologic definition of HIVAN was somewhat elusive. The initial cases occurred in adults, many of whom were HIV-infected intravenous drug abusers. Therefore, it was unclear whether FGS occurring in these individuals was a distinct entity related to AIDS, or was instead related to drug abuse or other factors. Additionally, numerous reports of atypical and variant renal histopathologic features associated with possible immune-mediated stimuli added to the confusion regarding the pathogenesis of HIV-associated renal diseases. The descriptions by Strauss et al.[6] of children infected from perinatal exposure with HIVAN helped to confirm that HIVAN was related to the viral infection itself. The concept has since evolved that there is a spectrum or continuum of histopathology that occurs in children with HIV infection, including a minimal change lesion, mesangial hyperplasia, and FGS. This spectrum of glomerular pathology has also been described in adults (see Chs. 4 and 8). Whereas FGS appears to be the most clinically significant lesion in adults, mesangial hyperplasia is present nearly as often as FGS in children. The clinical manifestations and histopathologic features of glomerular involvement in children with HIV infection resemble those seen in adults. Some important features differentiating the adult and pediatric diseases are presented in Table 7-1.

HIV-ASSOCIATED FGS

Epidemiology

In children, 30 to 60 percent of cases of HIVAN occur in girls, compared with adults, in whom 80 to 90 percent of cases occur in men. Over 90 percent of cases of HIVAN in children in the United States has occurred in children of African-American or Haitian descent, reflecting the demographics of maternal HIV infection in this country. The disease also occurs in white children.[8,9] Although before 1992 the majority of mothers acquired HIV infection through intravenous drug use, more recently heterosexually acquired HIV infection has become increasingly common. There does not appear to be any demographic differences between HIV-infected mothers of infants who develop HIVAN and those who do not, other than those related to race.[4,6,8]

Clinical Course

Children with HIV-related FGS manifest renal involvement at a mean age of 3 to 4 years.[6,8] However, the initial symptoms or signs of AIDS in these children were already detectable at a mean age of about 1 year. Therefore, unlike adults, children seldom develop HIVAN as the first clinical manifestation of HIV infection. The initial renal manifestation is generally abnormal proteinuria leading to nephrotic syndrome, detected by dipstick ($\geq 2 +$), an elevated urine protein/creatinine ratio (Upr/Ucr >1), or quantitative proteinuria exceeding 1 $g/m^2/d$. Edema and ascites, when they occur, are likely multifactorial, because in addition to the nephrosis, these children also frequently have malnutrition or cardiac decompensation. Hypercholesterolemia and hypertension are rare.

Renal dysfunction may be seen at the onset, and the progression of renal insufficiency, once it begins, may often be relatively rapid, with a median interval from initial clinical presentation to end-stage renal failure of 1 year. Mean survival is about 2 years from the diagnosis of HIVAN, or about 5 years from the first clinical manifestations of AIDS. Survival is dependent on concomitant neurologic, infectious, and cardiopulmonary disease rather than renal disease, as these children typically die from nonrenal causes.

Pathology

The pathologic findings of HIVAN with FGS in children are similar to those in adults.[15,37,38] The kidneys are enlarged, with a mean weight that is usually 20 to 30 percent above age-corrected values. The parenchyma appears swollen, with a focal "parboiled" appearance related to areas of dilated tubules containing dense proteinaceous casts and interstitial mononuclear cell infiltration. Small cysts measuring up to 0.5 to 1 mm may be seen in the cortex.

By light microscopy, there is capillary collapse (Fig. 7-1), rarely as the predominant lesion, and mesangial and capillary loop sclerosis, with lobular solidification (Fig. 7-2). Focal and global or segmental mesangial proliferation is occasionally seen in some of the involved glomeruli. Even in advanced stages of the disease, glomeruli may be identified that display minimal lesions or appear normal. Caps of swollen hyperplastic visceral epithelial cells

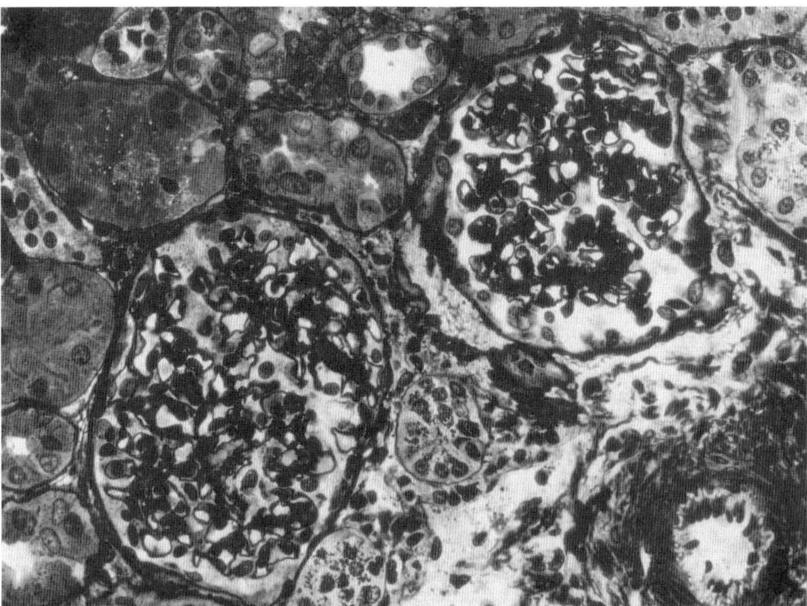

Fig. 7-1. Extensive capillary collapse in perinatal AIDS with nephrotic syndrome. (Jones periodic acid-silver methenamine, × 250.)

that contain hyaline droplets are an early feature. These are seen as circumscribing lobules, and appear to desquamate, compress glomerular capillaries, and occasionally fill the dilated uriniferous space (Fig. 7-3).

There is a prominent tubulointerstitial component that consists of a diffuse mononuclear cell infiltrate with a predominance of T8 lymphocytes[38] that may invade the tubules.[15,37,38] Tubule cells display both degenerative and regenerative changes, with flattening of the epithelium, nuclear "dropout," and irregularities in nuclear size and staining affinity (Fig. 7-2). Foci of dilated tubules attain "microcystic" proportions and contain large variegated casts. These casts consist of immunoglobulins but not Tamm-Horsfall protein. In rare instances, the tubulointerstitial component may assume an expansive nature suggesting a lymphoma, and immunohistochemical evaluation to detect clonal proliferation or use of nucleic acid probes to identify T-cell gene rearrangements may be necessary to establish a diagnosis. The tubulointerstitial component probably plays a major role in the pathogenesis of the renal dysfunction associated with HIVAN, and may also be related to the renal tubular abnormalities seen in some patients.

The features of HIV-associated FGS described above are similar to those of HIVAN in adults, although acellular and atrophic glomeruli with global sclerosis is more common in children, perhaps reflecting the more protracted course in children, who have smaller glomeruli to begin with. None of these histopathologic features are individually characteristic of HIVAN, since

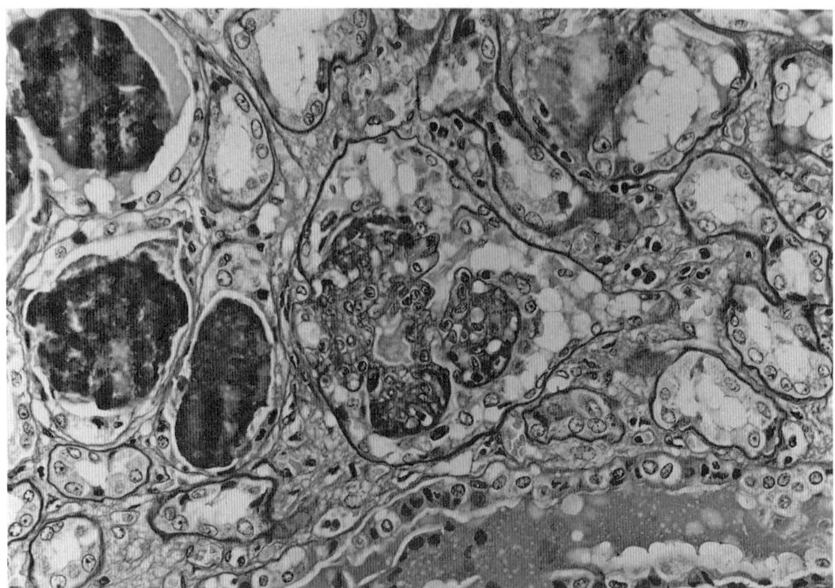

Fig. 7-2. A layer of hyperplastic visceral epithelial cells surrounds partially sclerosed lobules. Tubulointerstitial inflammation and dilated tubules containing variegated casts are seen. Tubules show degenerative and regenerative changes. (Periodic acid-Schiff, × 250.)

they may be found in other types of glomerular disease. It is rather their association and extent that characterizes and defines HIVAN.[39]

Electron microscopy confirms the presence of progressive glomerulosclerosis and discloses marked swelling of epithelial foot processes with numerous cytoplasmic vacuoles and dense bodies that represent lysosomes containing reabsorbed protein (Fig. 7-4). Most patients exhibit only occasional small mesangial deposits and/or hyaline inspissated lesions. However, Ingulli et al.[8] found extensive subepithelial loop deposits consistent with immune complexes. Tubuloreticular inclusions are apparent in the cytoplasm of endothelial cells of glomerular and interstitial capillaries[40] (Fig. 7-4). These support a diagnosis of HIV infection, but may be present in patients with systemic lupus erythematosus (SLE) or after administration of interferon-α, and may also be seen in HIV-infected patients without renal disease. A variety of nuclear inclusions (Fig. 7-4) and fibrillogranular nuclear changes as well as cytoplasmic concentric cisternae may be seen in renal parenchymal cells. However, these are not as common as tubuloreticular inclusions and are more apparent in tissues displaying autolytic changes.

Immunofluorescence microscopy findings are similar to those seen in idiopathic FGS, with IgM or C3 deposits that are predominantly mesangial or outline sclerotic lobules.

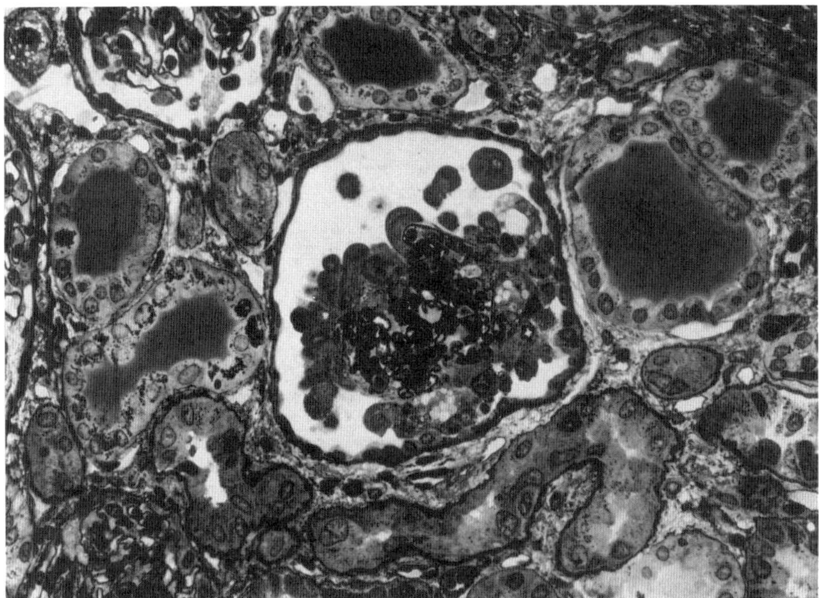

Fig. 7-3. Massive global capillary collapse. Tuft is surrounded by a crown of hyperplastic epithelial cells that appear swollen and vacuolated. (Jones periodic acid-silver methenamine, × 200.)

Other forms of glomerulosclerosis in childhood must also be considered in the differential diagnosis of HIV-associated FGS:

1. Idiopathic nephrotic syndrome with FGS usually has a prolonged course to renal insufficiency, less visceral epithelial cell involvement, and a discrete tubulointerstitial component with a higher ratio of segmentally sclerosed glomeruli and less distension of Bowman's capsule and tubules.[41]
2. Congenital glomerulosclerosis in neonates and infants, and glomerulosclerosis associated with congenital immunodeficiencies may simulate HIV-associated FGS histologically.[42–44] However, these lesions frequently involve fewer glomeruli and exhibit predominantly global and acellular sclerosis without the prominent visceral epithelial cell changes and tubulointerstitial lesions seen in HIVAN. Overt proteinuria and renal failure may be present.
3. A type of glomerulosclerosis designated "collapsing glomerulopathy" has been recently described, which is also associated with a poor prognosis.[45–47] Tubuloreticular inclusions, characteristic of HIVAN, are not seen in this disorder.

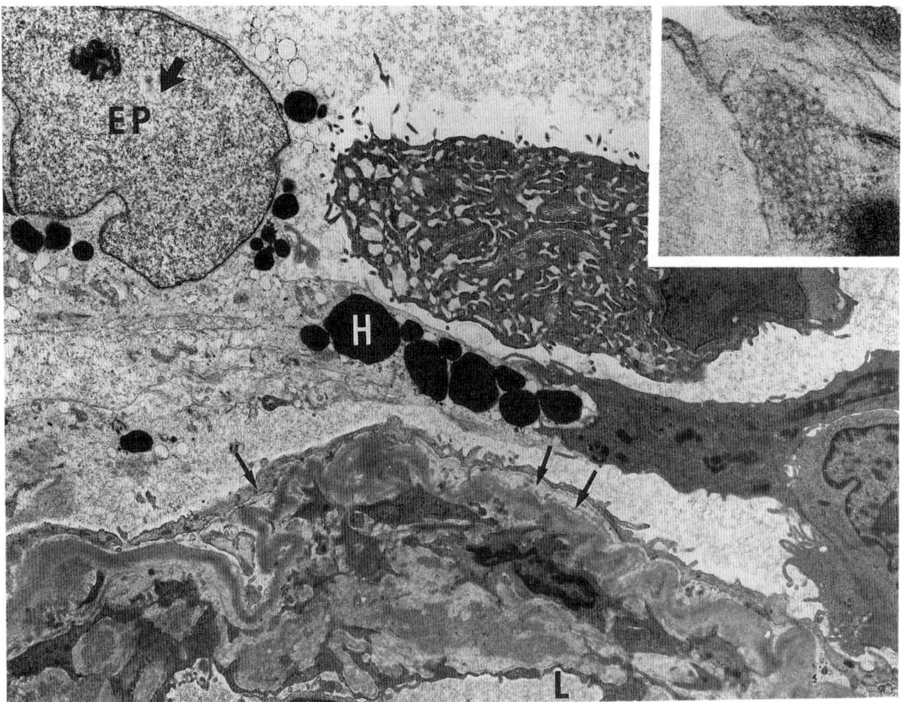

Fig. 7-4. Swollen epithelial cells containing large protein granules. Arrowhead indicates a nuclear inclusion. Remnants of visceral epithelial cells are separated from the thickened and wrinkled glomerular capillary basal lamina (*arrows*). Inset shows endothelial cell containing a tubuloreticular cytoplasmic inclusion. EP, epithelial cell; L, capillary lumen. (Uranyl acetate and lead citrate, × 11,726 [inset, × 33,480.])

Pathogenesis

The pathogenesis of FGS in patients with HIVAN remains unknown. Neither opportunistic infections nor immune complex-related processes appear to play a predominant role in most circumstances. Some of the features of HIVAN with FGS that have suggested a direct role of HIV in the development of this histopathologic lesion are shown in Table 7-2.[48–55]

Table 7-2. Evidence in Support of a Direct Role for HIV in the Pathogenesis of HIVAN With FGS

HIV replication in cultured endothelial or mesangial cells
CD4 expression in mesangial cells
p24 antigen identification in renal epithelial cells
Demonstration of HIV genome in renal parenchyma by in situ hybridization
Identification of HIV nucleoprotein by PCR in microdissected renal epithelial and interstitial cells
Similarities between simian immunodeficiency virus infection and human disease
Resemblance of HIVAN lesions in humans to those induced in transgenic mice by noninfectious HIV provirus

MESANGIAL HYPERPLASIA

The diagnostic criteria and terminology used in the literature for mesangial hyperplasia are not uniform. Furthermore, any proposed classification of these lesions is artificial because there is a spectrum of changes that extends from glomeruli that appear normal, through focal and segmental mesangial lesions, to overt diffuse and global mesangial hyperplasia/proliferation.[56–59] However, we define mesangial proliferation as the presence of more than three nuclei in a mesangial region, excluding perihilar areas, when present in more than 10 percent of glomeruli. These lesions may be further classified as focal when they are present in the minority of glomeruli, and diffuse when more than 50 percent of glomeruli are involved.

Epidemiology

Children with mesangial hyperplasia tend to be somewhat older at the time of initial detection of the nephropathy compared with those with HIVAN and FGS.[6,8] Most of the children with HIV infection and mesangial hyperplasia manifest overt proteinuria or nephrotic syndrome with pre-

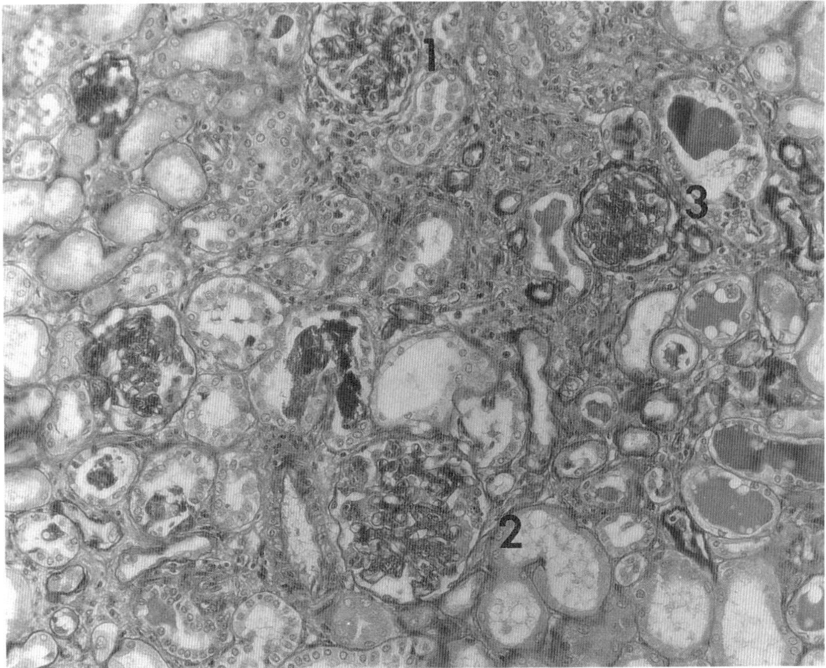

Fig. 7-5. Glomerular lesions suggesting a transition from mesangial hyperplasia to focal sclerosis (1 to 3). (Periodic acid-Schiff, × 100.)

served renal function. However, the clinical distinction between mesangial hyperplasia and HIVAN with FGS is not precise, and a biopsy may be required to establish the correct diagnosis, since some patients with FGS may also have preserved renal function. In rare instances, mesangial hyperplasia has been observed initially in children who later developed FGS with renal dysfunction[38] (Fig. 7-5). Such a transition also has been postulated in children with idiopathic nephrotic syndrome.[60] On the other hand, as a consequence of sample limitations, transitions between mesangial hyperplasia and FGS may be falsely assumed when an initial biopsy fails to detect early sclerotic changes. Thus, interpretations of these biopsies must include consideration of the clinical manifestations.

Pathology

On gross examination, the kidneys are normal in size or mildly enlarged with the notable absence of the blotchy cortical areas of tubulointerstitial involvement so characteristic of HIVAN with FGS.[6,38] Most children with mesangial hyperplasia have diffuse rather than focal mesangial hyperplasia (Fig. 7-6). The pronounced visceral epithelial cell lesions and capillary collapse seen in HIVAN with FGS are absent. Although foci of interstitial

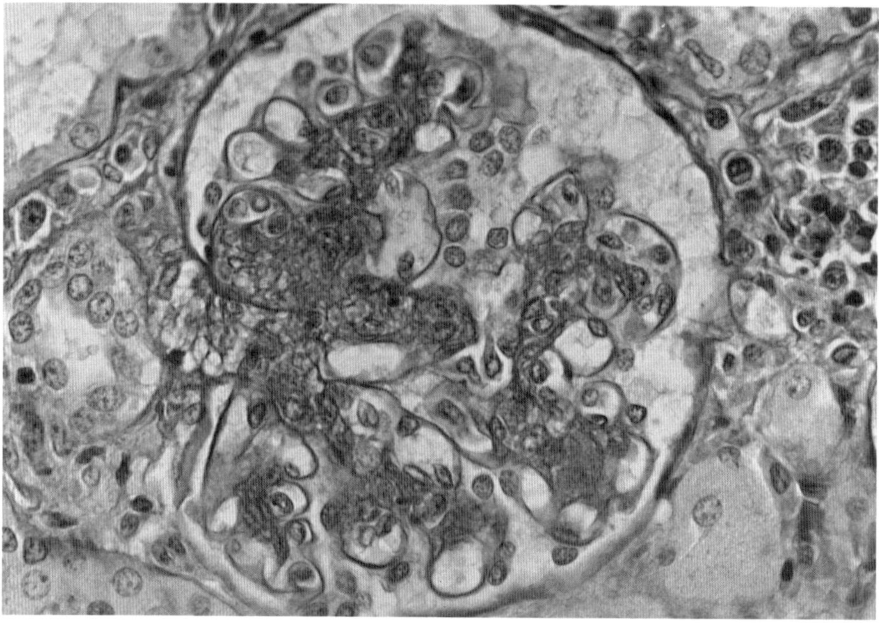

Fig. 7-6. Global mesangial hyperplasia in an HIV-infected child with proteinuria and normal renal function. Tubules appear normal. (Periodic acid-Schiff, × 500.)

mononuclear cells may be seen, the marked tubulointerstitial component with microcystic tubules encountered with FGS is usually absent. As in children with idiopathic focal sclerosis and the nephrotic syndrome, there is not a close relationship between the degree of mesangial hyperplasia and the subsequent clinical course.

Electron microscopy frequently reveals electron-dense mesangial deposits in an expanded matrix, as well as glomerular tubuloreticular inclusions. By immunofluorescence, mesangial deposits of immunoglobulins, predominantly IgG and IgM, as well as C3 may be seen.

MINIMAL GLOMERULAR LESIONS

Children with minimal glomerular lesions, representing approximately 5 to 10 percent of children with HIV nephropathy, present with clinical and demographic features indistinguishable from those with mesangial hyperplasia.[6,8] The gross appearance of the kidneys is also similar to that seen in mesangial hyperplasia. The kidneys of patients with minimal lesions, by definition, show normal glomeruli by light microscopy, although there may be mild focal and segmental mesangial hyperplasia. Clinically, these children present with proteinuria or nephrotic syndrome with normal renal function. As is the case in mesangial hyperplasia, the tubulointerstitial component typical of HIVAN with FGS is absent. Electron microscopy shows only swelling of visceral epithelial cells and foot process effacement, as well as the tubuloreticular cytoplasmic inclusions in endothelial cells seen in kidneys of HIV-infected individuals (see above). There are no electron-dense deposits. Only faint mesangial deposits of immunoglobulins and/or complement are demonstrated by immunofluorescence.

TREATMENT

Prospective trials of treatment of HIVAN in children or in adults are not available. Proteinuria has responded only transiently to steroid treatment in children with nephrotic syndrome. One instance of minimal change nephrotic syndrome in an HIV-infected child who responded to steroids has been reported.[61] Anecdotal reports of clinical improvement in proteinuria or renal insufficiency due to HIVAN with zidovudine have been observed in adults. However, this drug was found to be ineffective in nephrotic children.[8] Cyclosporine-induced remissions of up to 1 year have been noted in three children with nephrotic syndrome due to HIVAN.[8] In support of a possible therapeutic role of cyclosporine are observations that AIDS seemed to develop less commonly in HIV-infected patients who received immunosuppression with cyclosporine after renal transplantation compared with those who received azathioprine.[62,63]

Intravenous infusions of γ-globulin, used for the treatment of pediatric

AIDS, may exacerbate glomerular involvement in HIVAN, since the incidence of nephrotic syndrome was increased in children who received this treatment.[8]

Once end-stage renal failure develops, and hemodialysis or peritoneal dialysis are required, the complications of HIV infection are the determinant factors in patient survival, much as they are in patients without renal involvement. However, renal replacement therapy may increase the quality of life and rarely, particularly in children who are HIV-infected but otherwise asymptomatic, may allow for prolonged survival, as in other children with end-stage renal disease who are uninfected.

GLOMERULAR LESIONS THAT MAY NOT BE DIRECTLY RELATED TO HIV INFECTION

A variety of glomerulonephritides considered to be immune mediated have been documented in HIV-infected adults, which do not appear to differ from those seen in uninfected patients. These include postinfectious glomerulonephritis, IgA nephropathy, and lupuslike syndromes. Identification of the antigens and pathophysiologic processes responsible for these glomerular lesions is important because of potential therapeutic and prognostic implications. The hypothesis that some of these lesions may be induced by HIV-containing immune complexes rather than other antigen-antibody complexes has been validated by Kimmel and colleagues,[64] who identified HIV-containing immune complexes in the circulation and kidney eluates from adult patients with HIV infection and IgA nephropathy.[65] Two HIV-infected children with IgA mesangial deposits and glomerular hyperplasia have been reported.[16,17] Both were older children, white, and presented with hematuria, in contrast to children with HIVAN who are more typically infants, black, and present with overt proteinuria. One child with perinatal AIDS and high antinuclear antibody (ANA) and anti-double-stranded DNA (ds-DNA) titers developed a proliferative necrotizing glomerular lesion resembling that seen with SLE.[6] Membranous glomerulopathy has also been reported in a child with similar serologic findings.[18] Glomerular lesions resembling those of SLE have also been seen in HIV-infected adults.[66] Proliferative postinfectious glomerulonephritis is rare in children with perinatal AIDS.

LESIONS DETECTABLE AT AUTOPSY THAT ARE USUALLY ASYMPTOMATIC

Small foci of calcium deposits are frequently found at autopsy in the kidneys of children with AIDS. These calcifications are not associated with clinical renal abnormalities. Similar findings have been related to disseminated *Pneumocystis carinii* or mycobacterial infections in adults, and may occasionally be detectable radiographically.[15,67–69] In HIV-infected children, cytomegalovirus (CMV) and *Candida albicans* are the most frequent opportunistic agents localizing in the kidneys. Lesions related to these infections are usually focal and clinically silent. Renal infection with mycobacteria, including *M. tuberculosis*, frequently demonstrates little or no granuloma formation. Renal mycobacterial infection is usually seen in association with miliary systemic dissemination.

Acute pyelonephritis is rare in HIV-infected children, although urinary tract infections are common. Focal interstitial nephritis, used in a strict anatomic sense to indicate foci of acute or chronic inflammation, is more common in adults than children, and may be related to foci of opportunistic infections, sometimes associated with areas of tubular atrophy or ischemia.

Lymphomas are the most frequent AIDS-associated neoplasms in adults, but are quite rare in children. Kaposi sarcoma involving the kidneys and renal cell carcinoma have not yet been reported in children with AIDS.

CONCLUSION

Many of the clinical renal disorders described initially in adults with HIV infection and AIDS have also been recognized in HIV-infected children. Numerous clinical and histopathologic similarities are found in children and adults with HIV-related renal diseases, despite different routes of HIV infection in these two populations. Certain differences have been noted, particularly in the range of histopathologic presentations, although in adults as well the spectrum of HIV-associated nephropathies has broadened since the initial reports describing HIV-related FGS appeared. Little is known yet of the pathophysiology of HIV-related renal diseases in children, and whether there are differences compared with adults.

ACKNOWLEDGMENTS

Supported in part by a grant (1RO1 DK-40838-05) from the National Institutes of Diabetes and Kidney Disease, and a grant from the Children's Medical Services, Florida Department of Health and Rehabilitative Services.

REFERENCES

1. Scott GB, Buch BE, Letterman JG: Acquired immunodeficiency syndrome in infants. N Engl J Med 310:76, 1984
2. Connor E, Gupta S, Joshi V et al: Acquired immunodeficiency syndrome associated renal disease in children. J Pediatr 113:39, 1988

3. Horowitz L, Greco MA, Fekner HD: Renal pathology in infants and children with AIDS, abstracted. Mod Pathol 1:58A, 1988
4. Rousseau E, Russo P, Lapointe N, O'Regan S: Renal complications of acquired immunodeficiency syndrome in children. Am J Kidney Dis 11:48, 1988
5. Chander P, Sagel I, Weiss R et al: Renal disease in human immunodeficiency infected children, abstracted. Kidney Int 35:368A, 1989
6. Strauss J, Abitbol C, Zilleruelo G et al: Renal disease in children with the acquired immunodeficiency syndrome. N Engl J Med 321:625, 1989
7. Foster S, Hawkins E, Hanson CG, Shearer W: Pathology of the kidney in childhood immunodeficiency: AIDS-related nephropathy is not unique. Pediatr Pathol 11:63, 1991
8. Ingulli E, Tejani A, Fikrig S et al: Nephrotic syndrome associated with acquired immunodeficiency syndrome in children. J Pediatr 119:710, 1991
9. Malaga S, Santos F, Rey C, Oregas G: HIV associated nephropathy in children in Spain. p. 303. In Hatano M (ed): Nephrology. Vol. 1. Springer-Verlag, New York, 1991
10. Bourgoignie JJ, Meneses R, Ortiz C et al: The clinical spectrum of renal disease associated with human immunodeficiency virus. Am J Kidney Dis 12:131, 1988
11. Rao TK, Filippone EJ, Nicastri AD et al: Associated focal and segmental glomerulosclerosis in the acquired immunodeficiency syndrome. N Engl J Med 310: 669, 1984
12. Gardenswartz NH, Lerner CW, Seligson GR et al: Renal disease in patients with AIDS: a clinicopathologic study. Clin Nephrol 21:197, 1984
13. Pardo V, Aldana M, Colton RM et al: Glomerular lesions in the acquired immunodeficiency syndrome. Ann Intern Med 101:429, 1984
14. Pardo V, Meneses R, Ossa L et al: AIDS-related glomerulopathy: occurrence in special risk groups. Kidney Int 31:1167, 1987
15. D'Agati V, Cheng JI, Carbone L et al: The pathology of HIV-nephropathy: a detailed morphologic and comparative study. Kidney Int 35:1358, 1989
16. Trachtman H, Gauthier B, Vinograd A, Valderrama E: IgA nephropathy in a child with human immunodeficiency virus type 1 infection. Pediatr Nephrol 5: 724, 1991
17. Schoeneman MJ, Ghali V, Lieberman K, Reisman L: IgA nephritis in a child with human immunodeficiency virus: a unique form of human immunodeficiency virus-associated nephropathy. Pediatr Nephrol 6:46, 1992
18. D'Agati V, Siegle R: Coexistence of AIDS and lupus nephritis: a case report. Am J Nephrol 10:243, 1990
19. Agarwal A, Coni A, Ciechanowsky M et al: Hyponatremia in patients with the acquired immunodeficiency syndrome. Nephron 53:317, 1989
20. Peter SA: Electrolyte disorders and renal dysfunction in patients with acquired immunodeficiency syndrome. J AIDS 3:949, 1990
21. Seney FD Jr, Burns DK, Silva FG: Acquired immunodeficiency syndrome and the kidney. Am J Kidney Dis 16:1, 1990
22. Glassock RJ, Cohen AH, Danovitch G, Parsa KP: Human immunodeficiency virus (HIV) infection and the kidney. Ann Intern Med 112:35, 1990
23. Valeri A, Neusy AJ: Acute and chronic renal disease in hospitalized AIDS patients. Clin Nephrol 35:110, 1991
24. Genderini A, Bertoli S, Scorza D et al: Acute renal failure in patients with acquired immune deficiency syndrome. Am J Nephrol 1:45, 1991
25. Boccia RV, Gelmann EP, Baker C et al: A hemolytic-uremic syndrome with the acquired immunodeficiency syndrome. Ann Intern Med 101:716, 1984

26. Jokela J, Flynn T, Henry K: Thrombotic thrombocytopenic purpura in a human immunodeficiency virus (HIV) seropositive homosexual man. Am J Hematol 25: 341, 1987
27. Berns JS, Tomaszewski JE: Hemolytic uremic syndrome and thrombotic thrombocytopenic purpura associated with human immunodeficiency virus infection and acquired immunodeficiency syndrome. p. 299. In Kaplan BS, Trompeter RS, Moake JL (eds): Hemolytic Uremic Syndrome and Thrombotic Thrombocytopenic Purpura. Marcel Dekker, New York, 1992
28. Church JA, Marshall G, Laug W: Thrombotic thrombocytopenic purpura (TTP) in an HIV infected child: treatment with 1-desamino-8-D-arginine (DDAVP) and intravenous immunoglobulin (IVIG), abstracted. Int Conf AIDS 5:494, 1989
29. Balow JE, Macher AM, Rook AH: Paucity of glomerular disease in acquired immunodeficiency syndrome (AIDS), abstracted. Kidney Int 29:178A, 1986
30. Mazbar SA, Schoenfeld PY, Humpreys MH: Renal involvement in patients infected with HIV: experience at San Francisco General Hospital. Kidney Int 37: 1325, 1990
31. Cantor ES, Kimmel PL, Bosch P: Effect of race on expression of acquired immunodeficiency syndrome associated nephropathy. Arch Intern Med 151:125, 1991
32. Bourgoignie JJ, Ortiz-Interian C, Green DF et al: The epidemiology of human immunodeficiency virus-associated nephropathy. p. 484. In Hatano M (ed): Nephrology. Vol. 1. Springer-Verlag, Tokyo, 1991
33. Tarshish P, Lambert G, Wiznia A et al: HIV nephropathy in children, abstracted. J Am Soc Nephrol 4:288A, 1993
34. Brunkhorst R, Brunkhorst U, Eisenbach GM et al: Lack of clinical evidence for a specific HIV-associated glomerulopathy in 203 patients with HIV infection. Nephrol Dial Transplant 7:87, 1992
35. Baumelou A, Assogba V, Beaufils H et al: Pathologic renale associee a l'infection a virus VIH et au syndrome. p. 42. Semin Uro-Nephrologie. Masson, Paris, 1989
36. Kimmel PL, Umana WO, Bosch JP: Abnormal protein excretion in HIV-infected patients. Clin Nephrol 39:17, 1993
37. Cohen AH, Nast CC: HIV-associated nephropathy: a unique combined glomerular, tubular and interstitial lesion. Mod Pathol 1:87, 1988
38. Pardo V, Wetli C, Strauss J, Bourgoignie JJ: The renal complications of drug abuse and human immunodeficiency virus. p. 390. In Tischer C, Brenner BM (eds): Pathology of the Kidney. 2nd Ed. JB Lippincott, Philadelphia, 1994
39. Bourgoignie JJ, Pardo V: The nephropathology in human immunodeficiency virus (HIV-1) infection. Kidney Int 35:S19, 1991
40. Chander P, Soni A, Bhagwat R et al: Renal ultrastructural markers in AIDS-associated nephropathy. Am J Pathol 126:513, 1987
41. Broyer M, Meyrier A, Niaudet P, Habib R: Minimal changes and focal segmental sclerosis. p. 298. In Cameron S, Davidson AM, Grunfeld JP et al. (eds): Oxford Textbook of Clinical Nephrology. Blackwell, Oxford, 1992
42. Friedman HH, Greyzel DM, Lederer M: Kidney lesions in stillborn and newborn infants: congenital glomerulosclerosis. Am J Pathol 18:699, 1942
43. Emery JL, McDonald MS: Involuting and scarred glomeruli in the kidney of infants. Am J Pathol 36:713, 1960
44. Foster S, Hawkins E, Hanson CG, Shearer W: Pathology of the kidney in childhood immunodeficiency: AIDS related nephropathy is not unique. Pediatr Pathol 11:64, 1991
45. Weiss MA, Daquioag E, Margolin EG, Pollack VE: Nephrotic syndrome, progres-

sive irreversible renal failure and glomerular collapse: a new clinicopathologic entity. Am J Kidney Dis 7:20, 1986

46. Valeri A, Barisoni L, Seigle R et al: Predictors of progression in collapsing focal segmental glomerulosclerosis, abstracted. J Am Soc Nephrol 4:288, 1993

47. Detwiler RV, Falk RJ, Hogan SL, Jennette JE: Collapsing glomerulopathy: a clinical and pathological distinct variant of focal segmental glomerulosclerosis. Kidney Int 45:1416, 1994

48. Alpers CE, McClure J, Bursten SI: Human mesangial cells are resistant to productive infection by multiple strains of human immunodeficiency virus types 1 and 2. Am J Kidney Dis 19:126, 1992

49. Green DR, Resnick L, Bourgoignie JJ: HIV infects glomerular endothelial and mesangial cells but not epithelial cells in vitro. Kidney Int 41:956, 1992

50. Karlson-Parra A, Dimeney E, Fellstrom B, Klareskog L: HIV receptor (CD4 antigen) in normal human glomerular cells. N Engl J Med 320:741, 1989

51. Cohen AH, Sun NCJ, Shapshak P, Imagawa DT: Demonstration of human immunodeficiency virus in renal epithelium in HIV-associated nephropathy. Mod Pathol 2:125, 1989

52. Kimmel PL, Ferreira-Centeno A, Farkas-Szallasi T et al: Viral DNA in microdissected renal biopsy tissue from HIV infected patients with nephrotic syndrome. Kidney Int 43:1347, 1993

53. Bauer FA, Wear DJ, Angritt P, Lo SC: *Mycoplasma fermentans* (incognitos strain) infection in the kidneys of patients with acquired immunodeficiency syndrome and associated nephropathy: a light microscopic, immunohistochemical, and ultrastructural study. Hum Pathol 22:63, 1991

54. Alpers CE, Baskin GB: Sclerosing glomerulopathy in rhesus monkeys with simian AIDS, abstracted. Kidney Int 35:339A, 1989

55. Kopp JB, Klotman ME, Abler SH et al: Progressive glomerulosclerosis and enhanced renal accumulation of basement membrane components in mice transgenic for human immunodeficiency virus type 1 genes. Proc Natl Acad Sci USA 89:1577, 1992

56. Zollinger HV, Mihatsch MJ: Renal pathology in biopsy: light, electron, and immunofluorescent microscopy and clinical aspects. p. 28. Springer-Verlag, New York, 1978

57. International Study of Kidney Disease in Children. Primary nephrotic syndrome in children: clinical significance of histopathologic variants of minimal change and of diffuse mesangial hyperplasia. Kidney Int 20:765, 1981

58. Churg J, Sobin LH: Renal Disease: Classification and Atlas of Glomerular Diseases. Igaku-Shoin, Tokyo, 1982

59. Southwest Pediatric Nephrology Study Group: Childhood nephrotic syndrome associated with diffuse mesangial hypercellularity. Kidney Int 24:87, 1983

60. Walherr R, Gubler MC, Levy M et al: The significance of pure diffuse mesangial proliferation in idiopathic nephrotic syndrome. Clin Nephrol 10:171, 1978

61. Landor M, Bernstein L, Rubinstein A: A steroid-responsive nephropathy in a child with human immunodeficiency virus infection. Am J Dis Child 147:261, 1993

62. Schwartz A, Offerman G, Keller F et al: The effect of cyclosporine on the progression of human immunodeficiency virus type 1 infection transmitted by transplantation—data on four cases and review of the literature. Transplantation 55:95, 1993

63. Novak R: Immunosuppression: a counter-intuitive therapy for HIV infection? J NIH Res 5:54, 1993

64. Kimmel PL, Phillips TM, Ferreira-Centeno A et al: HIV-associated immune-mediated renal disease. Kidney Int 44:1327, 1993
65. Kimmel PL, Philips TM, Farkas-Szallasi T et al: Idiotypic IgA nephropathy in patients with HIV infection. N Engl J Med 327:702, 1992
66. Nochy D, Gotz D, Dosquet P et al: Renal disease associated with HIV infection. A multicentric study of 60 patients from Paris hospitals. Nephrol Dial Transplant 8:11, 1993
67. Feuestein IM, Francis P, Raffeld M, Pluda J: Widespread visceral calcifications in disseminated *Pneumocystis carinii* infection: CT characteristics. J Comput Assisted Tomography 14:149, 1990
68. Bargman JM, Wagner C, Cameron R: Renal cortical nephrocalcinosis: a manifestation of extrapulmonary *Pneumocystis carinii* infection in the acquired immunodeficiency syndrome. Am J Kidney Dis 17:712, 1991
69. Falkoff GE, Rigsby CM, Rosenfield AT: Partial, combined cortical and medullary nephrocalcinosis: US and CT patterns in AIDS-associated MAI infection. Radiology 162:343, 1987

8

Renal Pathology of HIV-Associated Nephropathy

Arthur H. Cohen

INTRODUCTION
GROSS PATHOLOGY
MICROSCOPIC FEATURES
PATHOGENESIS
OTHER GLOMERULOPATHIES

INTRODUCTION

Since the original descriptions of focal and segmental glomerulosclerosis in patients with acquired immunodeficiency syndrome (AIDS),[1-3] the details of the pathologic features have been further studied, modified, and expanded.[4-16] Consequently, with the demonstration that the renal lesion may occur in human immunodeficiency virus (HIV)-infected patients without clinical manifestations of AIDS or AIDS-related complex, and with the documentation that the disorder regularly affects tubules and often interstitium in addition to glomeruli, the lesion that was initially termed AIDS-associated focal and segmental glomerulosclerosis[1] is now known as HIV-associated nephropathy.[4,8,13-16] This chapter is primarily concerned with a detailed delineation of the pathologic aspects of that entity and possible pathogenic mechanisms and also considers briefly other nephropathies that may occur regularly in HIV-infected patients.

GROSS PATHOLOGY

The kidneys are usually enlarged bilaterally (Fig. 8-1) at any stage of clinical manifestation, including end-stage renal disease. Pardo and coworkers[12,17] documented mean combined kidney weights of up to 500 g in adults;

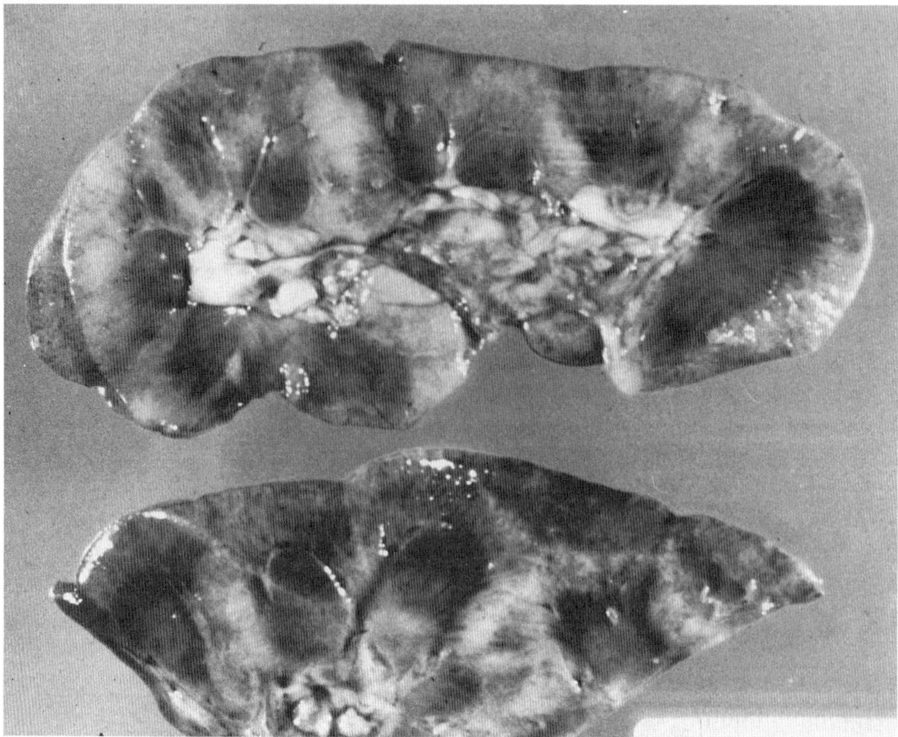

Fig. 8-1. Gross appearance of HIV-associated nephropathy. The kidney is enlarged, with pale and widened cortex.

in children, the kidneys are also usually larger than normal.[18] The capsular surface is smooth. The cortex is expanded and is more pale than the medulla (Fig. 8-1). Occasionally, small cysts are visible mainly at the corticomedullary junction; these correspond to massively dilated tubules (see below).[17,19]

MICROSCOPIC FEATURES

As mentioned above, this entity is a pan-nephropathy, with abnormalities of glomeruli, tubules, and interstitium, and with ultrastructural features affecting a variety of cells.[4,7–9,13,20–22] The glomerular abnormalities are in the broad spectrum of lesions constituting focal and segmental glomerulosclerosis. By light microscopy, perhaps the most prominent change affects visceral epithelial cells that appear to be the initial element involved in this disease process. In the affected glomerulus, epithelial cells in one or more segments are enlarged, coarsely vacuolated, contain protein reabsorption droplets, and are increased in number with mitotic figures evident in some

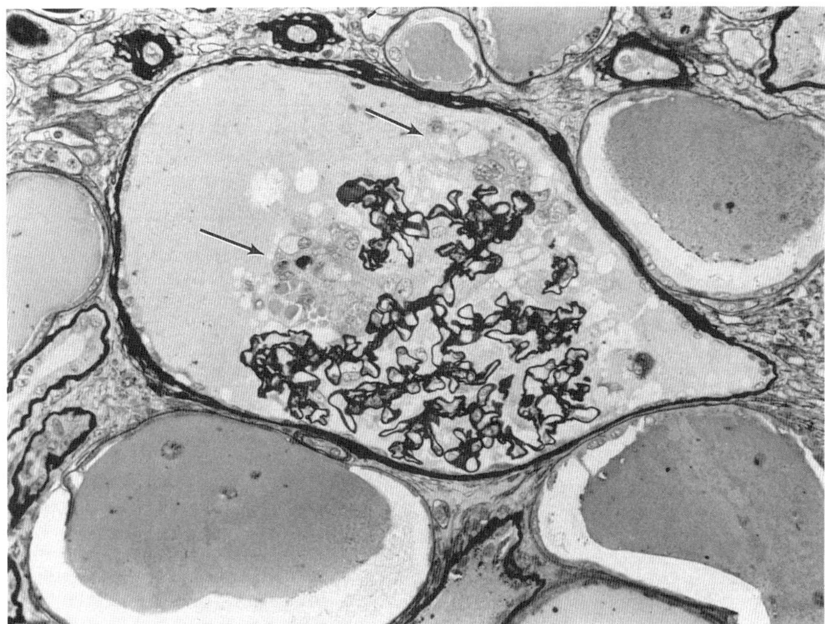

Fig. 8-2. Early lesion of glomerular involvement. There is segmental increase in size and number of visceral epithelial cells, which contain protein reabsorption droplets and vacuoles (*arrows*). Note also associated capillary wall wrinkling with narrowing of lumina and dilated Bowman's space. (Periodic acid-methenamine silver × 350.)

cells (Fig. 8-2). Less commonly, these features affect all or almost all cells of a single glomerulus and nearly obliterate the urinary space (Fig. 8-3). Capillary walls in abnormal segments are often wrinkled and/or collapsed and capillary lumina are consequently narrowed or obliterated (Fig. 8-4). Some glomeruli develop typical advanced lesions of segmental sclerosis, with capillary luminal obliteration by foam cells, insudative lesions, or increased extracellular matrix (Fig. 8-5). Many glomeruli have more extensive involvement of epithelial cells and almost complete capillary wall wrinkling and collapse (Fig. 8-6). Ultimately, there is virtual solidification of the tufts because of total capillary collapse (Fig. 8-7); the urinary spaces are dilated, often containing a precipitate of plasma protein (see below). However, even in these more advanced stages of glomerular involvement, the visceral epithelial cells maintain large size, increased numbers, protein reabsorption droplets, and large cytoplasmic vacuoles. Glomeruli without any of these alterations are somewhat enlarged, with patent capillary lumina and no increased cellularity.

Tubular abnormalities are constant but are also morphologically quite varied. Degeneration and necrosis of epithelial cells are evident early in the disorder, and occur in the absence of nephrotoxin exposure or renal ischemia.

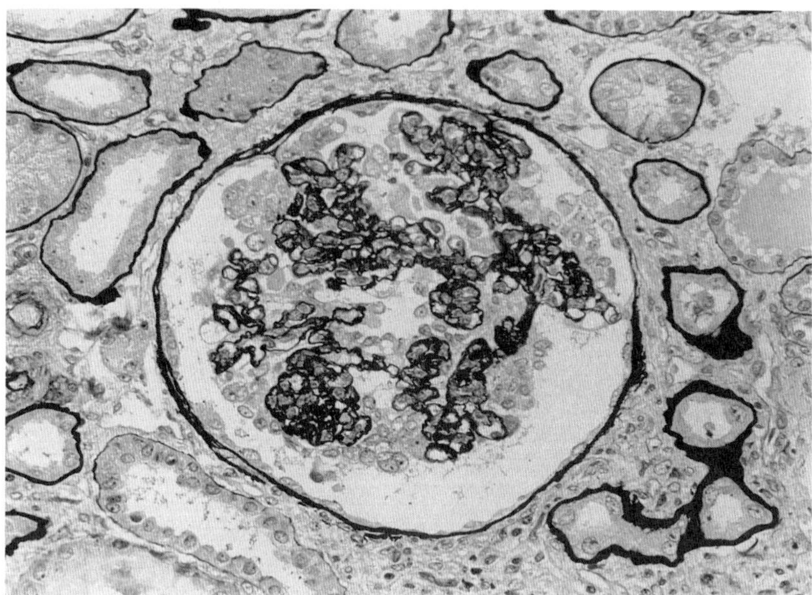

Fig. 8-3. More pronounced hyperplasia of visceral epithelium with the changes simulating a crescent. (Periodic acid-methenamine silver × 350.)

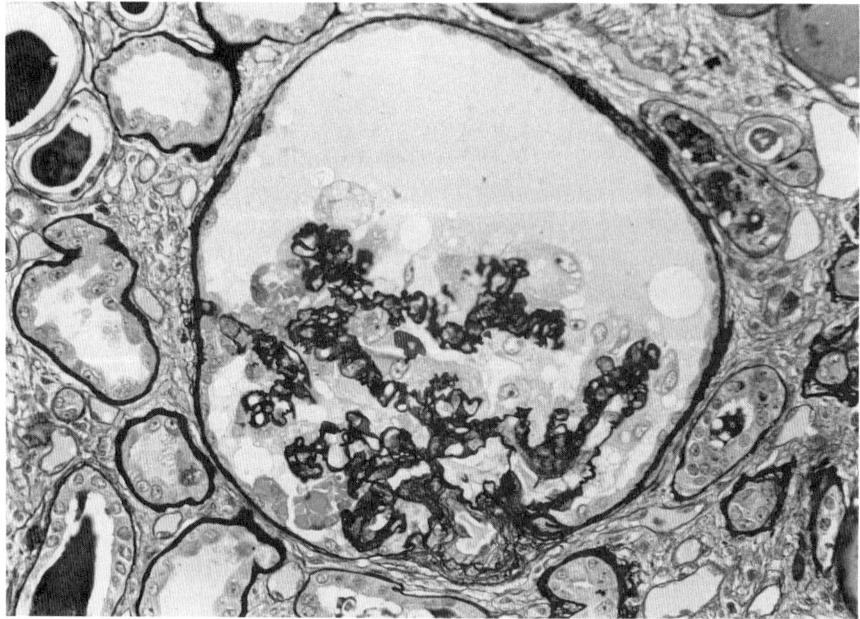

Fig. 8-4. Glomerulus with more pronounced capillary wall collapse; the urinary space is greatly dilated. The visceral epithelium displays the same changes as previously illustrated, with prominent vacuolization. (Periodic acid-methenamine silver × 350.)

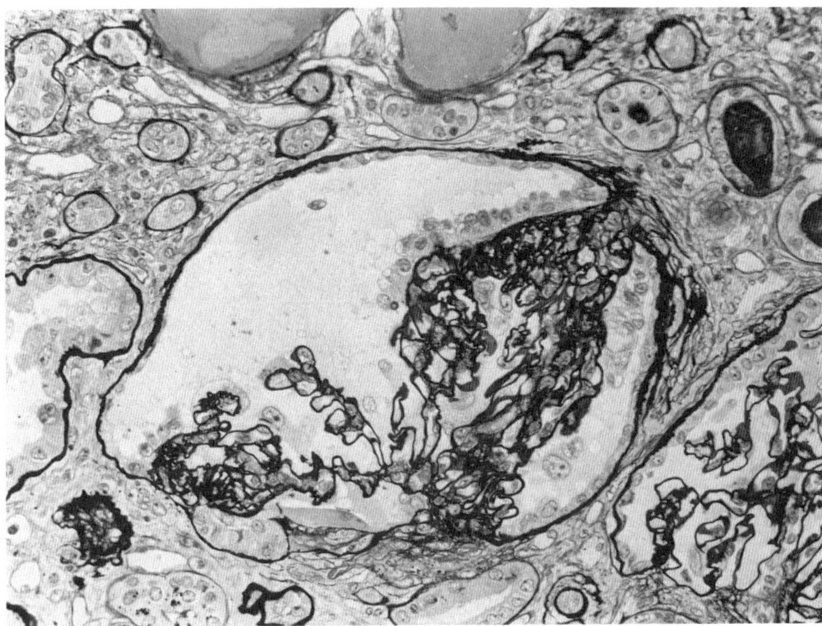

Fig. 8-5. Glomerulus with two segments of sclerosis/collapse with adherence to Bowman's capsule. There is persistence of the visceral epithelial cell abnormalities in these segments. (Periodic acid-methenamine silver × 350.)

The typical changes of acute tubular necrosis, including loss of brush border staining for proximal cells, flattening of cells of any segment of the nephron with relative dilatation of lumina, and mitotic figures, are present (Fig. 8-8). The most prominent change, however, is dilatation of tubules affecting any or all segments of the nephron (Fig. 8-9). The lumina are moderately enlarged or may be greatly so, forming structures that may be observed grossly as the small cysts described above. Indeed, the tubular diameters are often many times larger than adjacent glomeruli (Fig. 8-10). The dilated tubules are filled with a precipitate of plasma proteins as evidenced by the staining characteristics—negative to slightly positive with periodic acid-Schiff (PAS) and fuchsinophilic with Masson's trichrome stains—and by immunohistochemistry. We have documented these "casts" to be composed of all plasma proteins sought by routine immunofluorescence; these include immunoglobulins (IgG, IgA, IgM), complement components (C1q, C3), albumin, and both immunoglobulin light chains.[4] Tamm-Horsfall protein is not a component of these "casts" but is, as expected, the major or sole constituent of typical hyaline tubular casts, which are strongly PAS positive and are not generally found in the dilated tubules (Figs. 8-8B and 8-11). The plasma protein precipitate is also in Bowman's spaces of glomeruli (Fig. 8-11); the spaces are dilated and in direct continuity with dilated proximal tubules also contain-

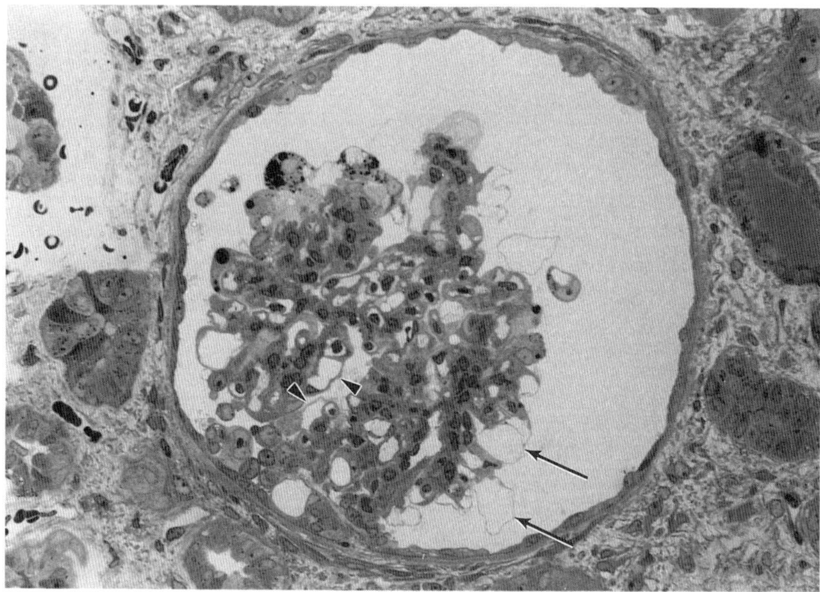

Fig. 8-6. Glomerulus with few patent capillary lumina. Visceral epithelial cells contain very large vacuoles (*arrows*) that are larger than the few patent capillaries (*arrowheads*). Protein reabsorption droplets are in many epithelial cells. (Plastic embedded, methylene blue × 350.)

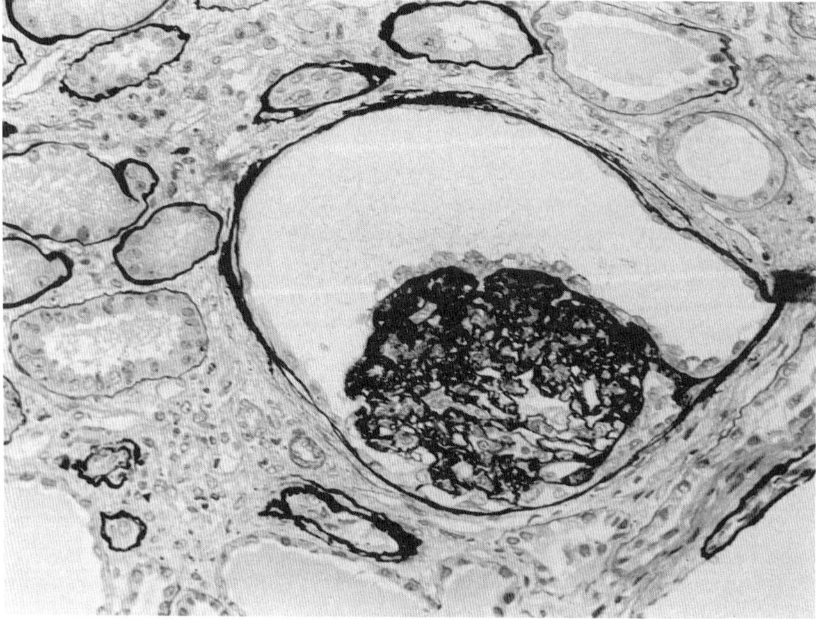

Fig. 8-7. Complete solidification of collapsed tuft with residual epithelial cell abnormalities and dilated Bowman's space. (Periodic acid-methenamine silver × 350.)

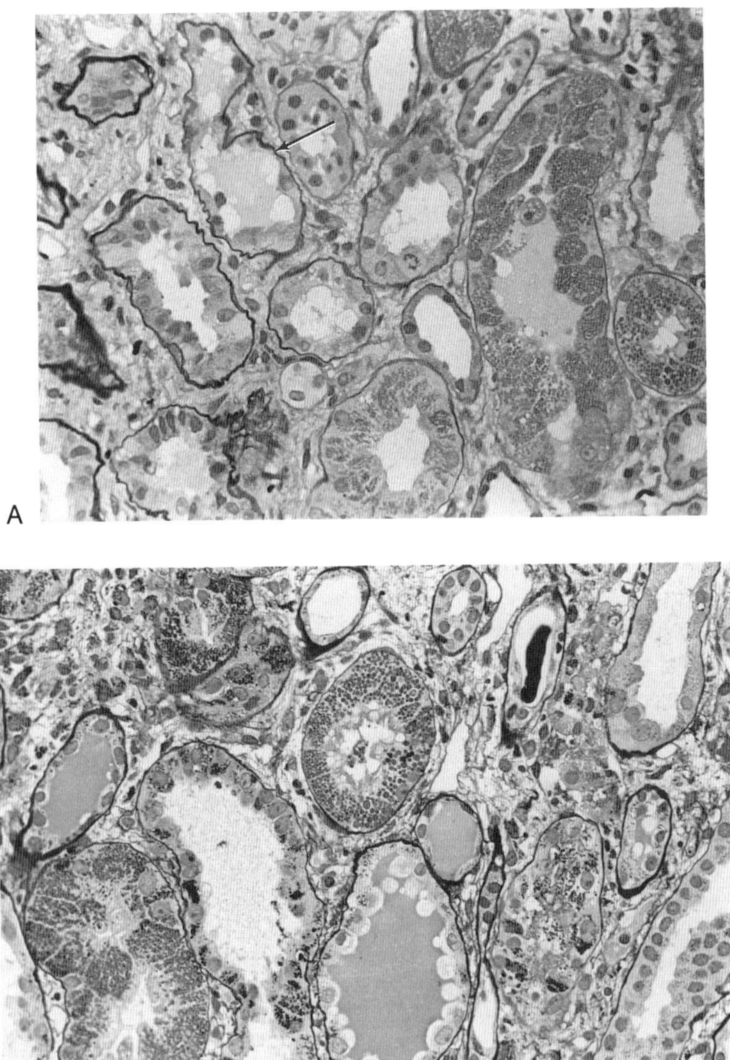

Fig. 8-8. **(A)** Tubules displaying some of the characteristic alterations. One, containing a pale luminal precipitate of plasma proteins, is lined by irregular and flattened cells with small stretches of bare basement membrane (*arrow*). Note a mitotic figure in a cell from another tubule (*center*). The cells of the proximal tubules on the right are filled with protein reabsorption droplets. There is also interstitial edema. (Periodic acid-Schiff × 350.) **(B)** Similar changes are present in this photomicrograph. In addition, the tubule at the center bottom is filled with plasma protein precipitates demonstrating the characteristic scalloped periphery at the interface with apical portions of tubular cells. A Tamm-Horsfall protein hyaline cast is in a tubule in the upper right. (Periodic acid-methenamine silver × 350.)

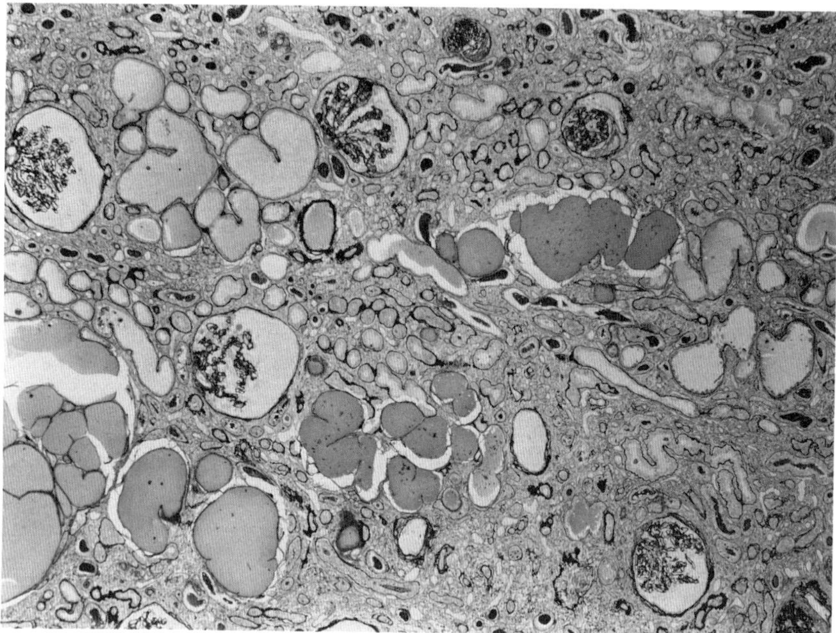

Fig. 8-9. Low-power photomicrograph discloses clusters of dilated tubules filled with pale luminal precipitates. The glomerular urinary spaces are likewise dilated. (Periodic acid-methenamine silver × 80.)

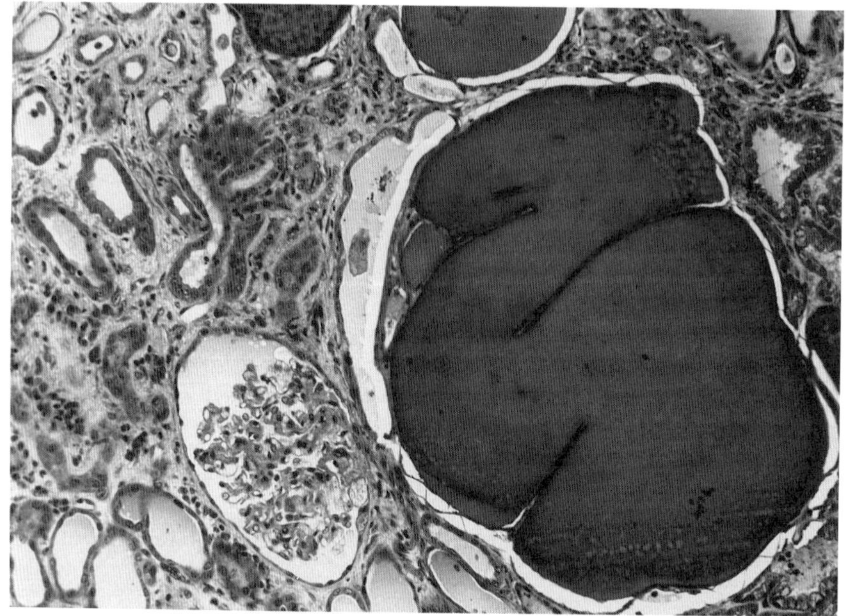

Fig. 8-10. Massively dilated tubule with plasma protein "cast" adjacent to a normal-sized glomerulus. (Masson's trichrome × 200.)

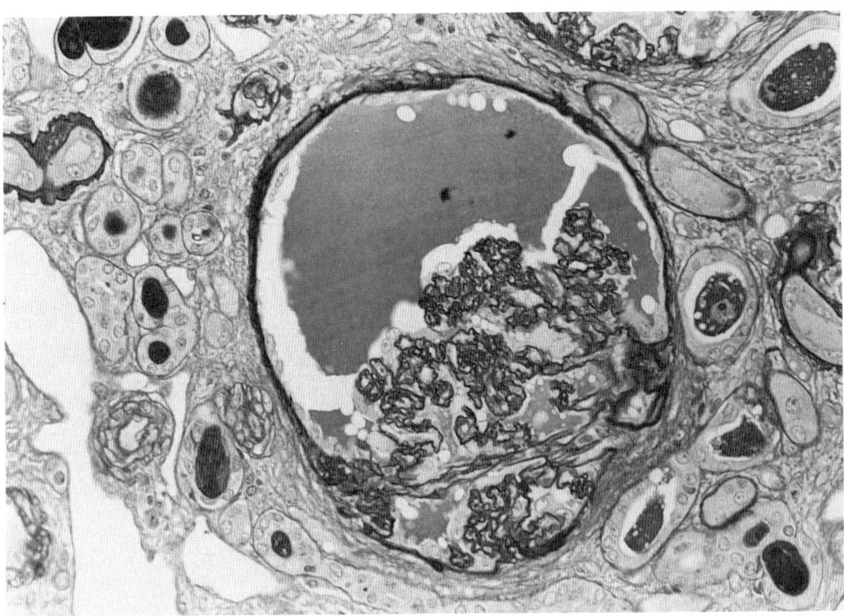

Fig. 8-11. Glomerulus with capillary tuft collapse and with dilated urinary space containing precipitate. Note the difference in staining between the contents of the urinary space and many surrounding tubules, which are filled with darker staining hyaline (Tamm-Horsfall protein) casts. (Periodic acid-Schiff × 350.)

ing the precipitate. It is very likely that the Bowman's space and tubular contents represent plasma proteins filtered by abnormal glomeruli with altered filtration barriers. It is of interest to note that it appears that the dilated "fluid-filled" tubules are virtually always in continuity with a glomerulus exhibiting abnormal visceral epithelial cells and other changes, including collapse and/or well-defined segments of sclerosis. Both in urinary spaces and in tubules, the peripheral portions of the "casts" may be scalloped, probably representing indentations produced by the apical portions of epithelial cells (Fig. 8-8B).

The interstitium is usually diffusely edematous and is variably infiltrated by lymphocytes, plasma cells, and few monocytes. As evaluated by D'Agati and coworkers,[8] lymphocyte T4/T8 ratios are less than 1.0.

Unless the patient was previously hypertensive, there are virtually no abnormalities of arteries or arterioles. Indeed, unless a prior or coexisting renal lesion is present, there is generally no evidence of chronic damage in the form of atrophied tubules with interstitial fibrosis, at least at the onset of HIV-associated nephropathy. As the disorder progresses, complete glomerular sclerosis with tubular atrophy and interstitial fibrosis ensues; however, because of persistent interstitial edema and dilated tubules, kidney

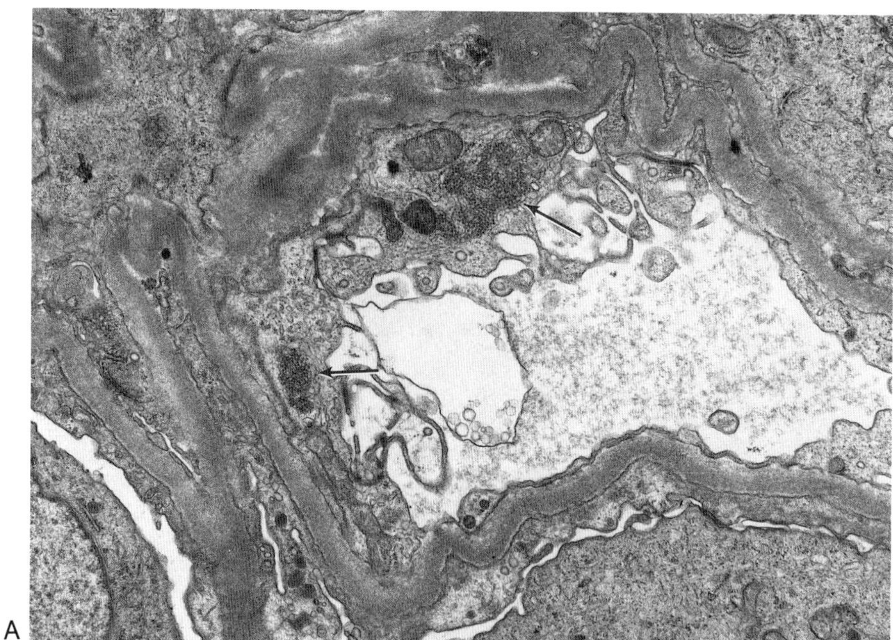

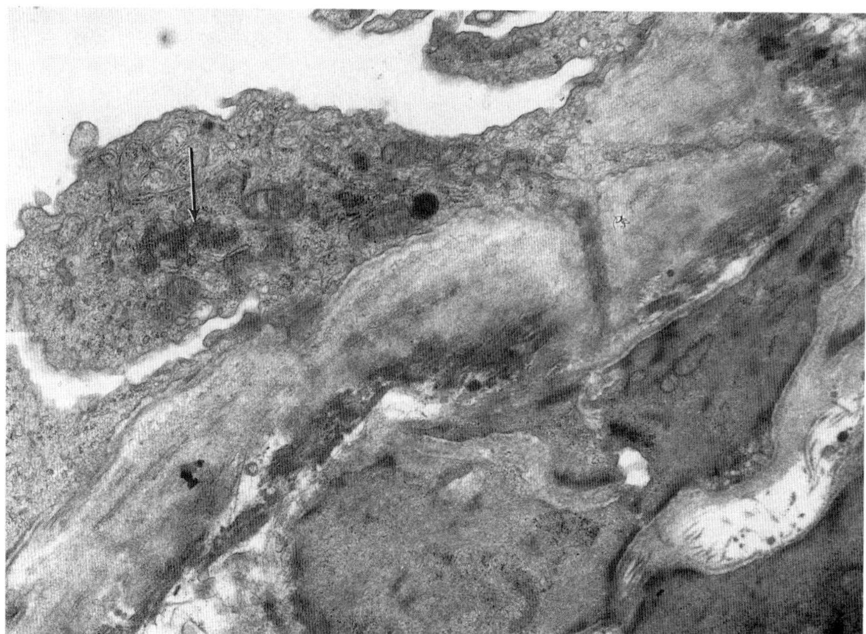

Fig. 8-12. Tubuloreticular structures. **(A)** Glomerular endothelium with two collections of tubuloreticular structures (*arrows*), one of which is much larger than the other. (× 15,000.) **(B)** Arteriolar endothelium with small tubuloreticular structure (*arrow*). (× 12,500.) (*Figure continues.*)

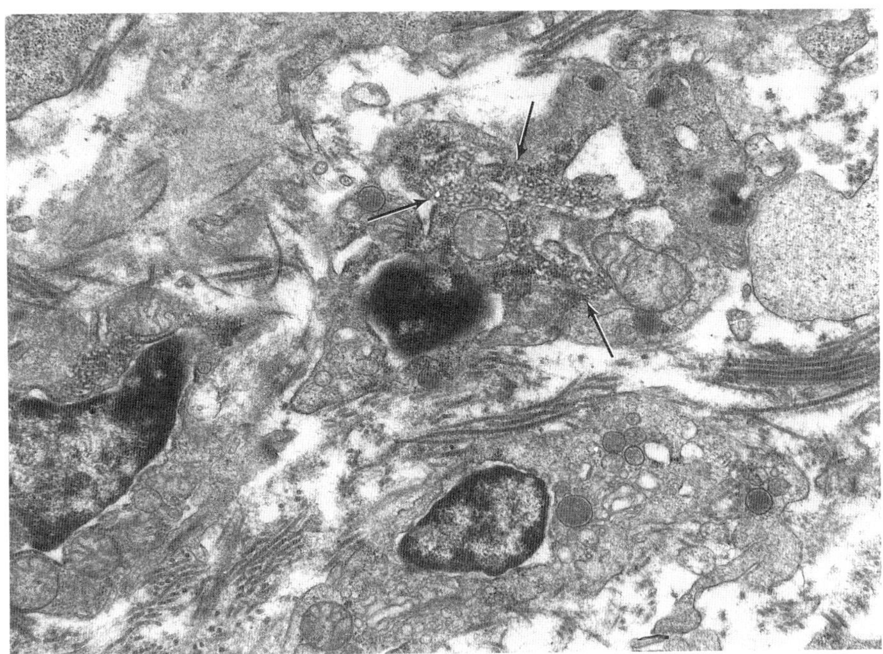

Fig. 8-12. (*Continued*). (**C**) Portion of monocyte in renal interstitium with complex and larger cytoplasmic tubuloreticular structure (*arrows*). (× 16,500.)

size remains normal, or more frequently, enlarged even as end-stage renal failure develops.[13,17,20]

Ultrastructural lesions are integral features of HIV-associated nephropathy.[4–6,8–11,13–17,19] They reflect two processes: indirect evidence of infection with HIV and the expected electron microscopic counterparts of the structural-functional renal abnormalities. Concerning HIV infection, the most prominent change is the presence of large and numerous tubuloreticular structures in the cytoplasm of endothelial cells of glomerular and peritubular capillaries as well as arteries, arterioles, and veins and less frequently in lymphocytes and monocytes[4–6,8,11,20] (Fig. 8-12). In contrast to other diseases in which these cytoplasmic modifications, considered to represent alterations induced by interferon-α, are present, they are more prominent and plentiful. Other abnormal cytoplasmic inclusions, stressed by Chander and coworkers[5,6] in the kidney and Kostianovsky and coworkers[23] and Orenstein[24] in HIV infection in many cells, include cylindrical confronting cisternae that are also known as test-tube and ring-shaped forms; they represent stacks of closely apposed membranes. They are noted most commonly in tubular and interstitial cells; in my experience, they are rather infrequent findings.

Nuclear alterations are frequently observed. Perhaps the most common are nuclear bodies, structures of dense or pale aggregates of granular or

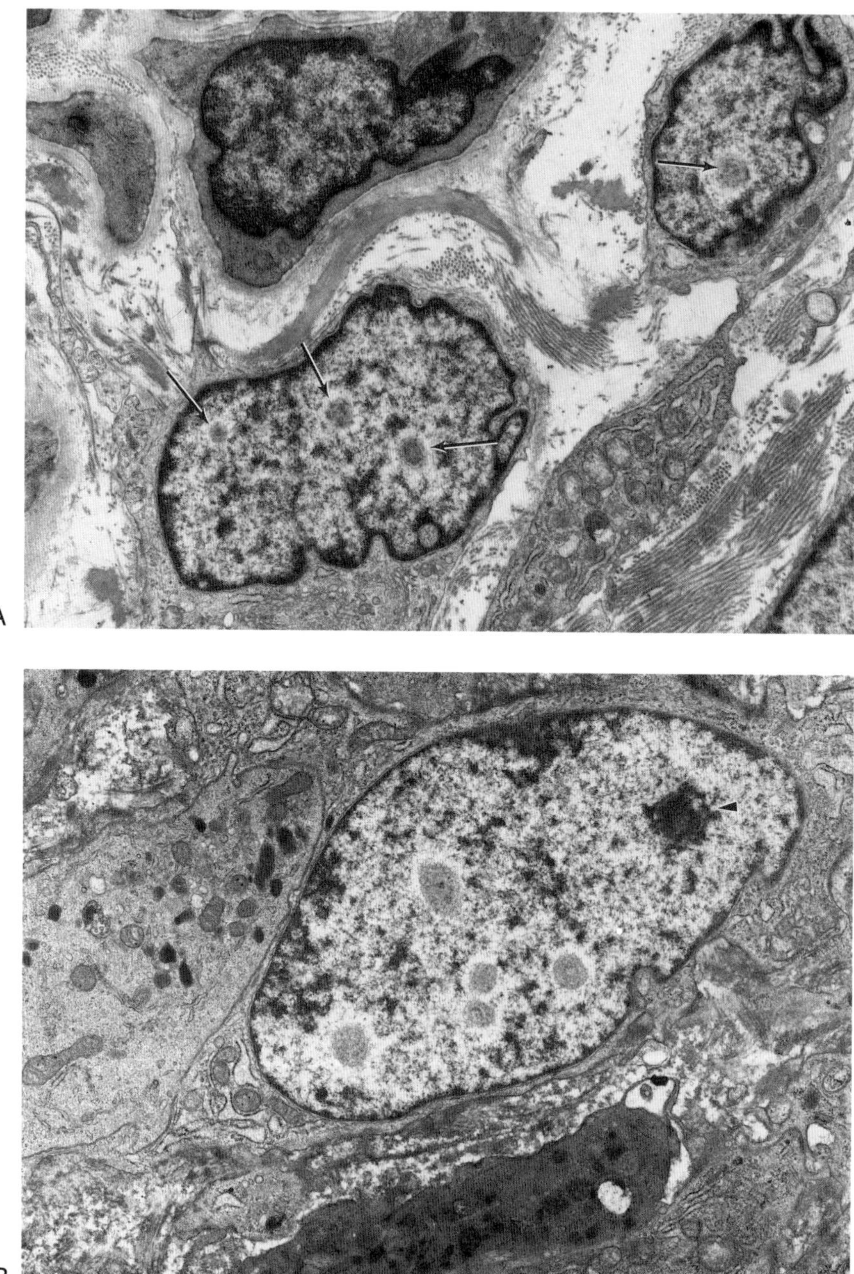

Fig. 8-13. Nuclear bodies. **(A)** Two interstitial cells with nuclear bodies (*arrows*); in one there are three with two different morphologies, whereas the second cell contains a single large body. (× 12,000.) **(B)** This interstitial cell possesses five nuclear bodies; note the clear distinction between these structures and nucleolus (*arrowhead*). (× 18,000.)

fibrillary material throughout nuclei.[25] They are classified into five different types[2,3] depending on size and structure and have been identified mainly in tubular and interstitial cells and are less frequently noted in leukocytes in the interstitium, in endothelial cells, and in glomerular visceral epithelial cells.[5,8,9,20] Most commonly, type III and, to a lesser degree, type V are increased (Fig. 8-13). These structures are clearly not specific for HIV infection and their presence has been known for many years before the era of AIDS. Their composition and function are not known, although they may be present in various viral infections. More spectacular nuclear changes include granular transformation of the chromatin, in which the normal structure is completely or partially replaced by coarse granularity, often associated with disruption of portions or all of the nuclear membrane (Fig. 8-14). This obscures the distinction between nucleus and cytoplasm. This change may be associated with swelling of cytoplasmic organelles such as mitochondria. This nuclear abnormality affects interstitial and tubular cells; in my experience, interstitial cells are far more commonly involved. It is not an artifact of fixation, because it frequently affects only one of two or more adjacent cells.[5,6,8,9,15,20,24] Another more dramatic lesion is granulofibrillar transformation of nuclei in which the normal chromatin is replaced by a combination of coarse and fine granularity with interspersed masses of pale staining filamentous structures of unknown nature. It should be pointed out that although this abnormality is known by the term *granulofibrillar,* the elon-

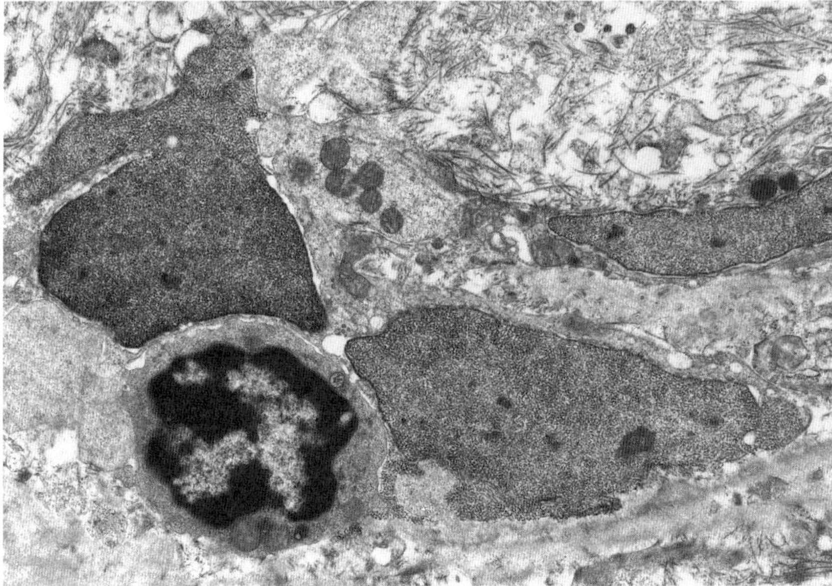

Fig. 8-14. Granular transformation of the nuclei affecting three interstitial cells; the infiltrating lymphocyte nucleus is not affected. ($\times$ 12,000.)

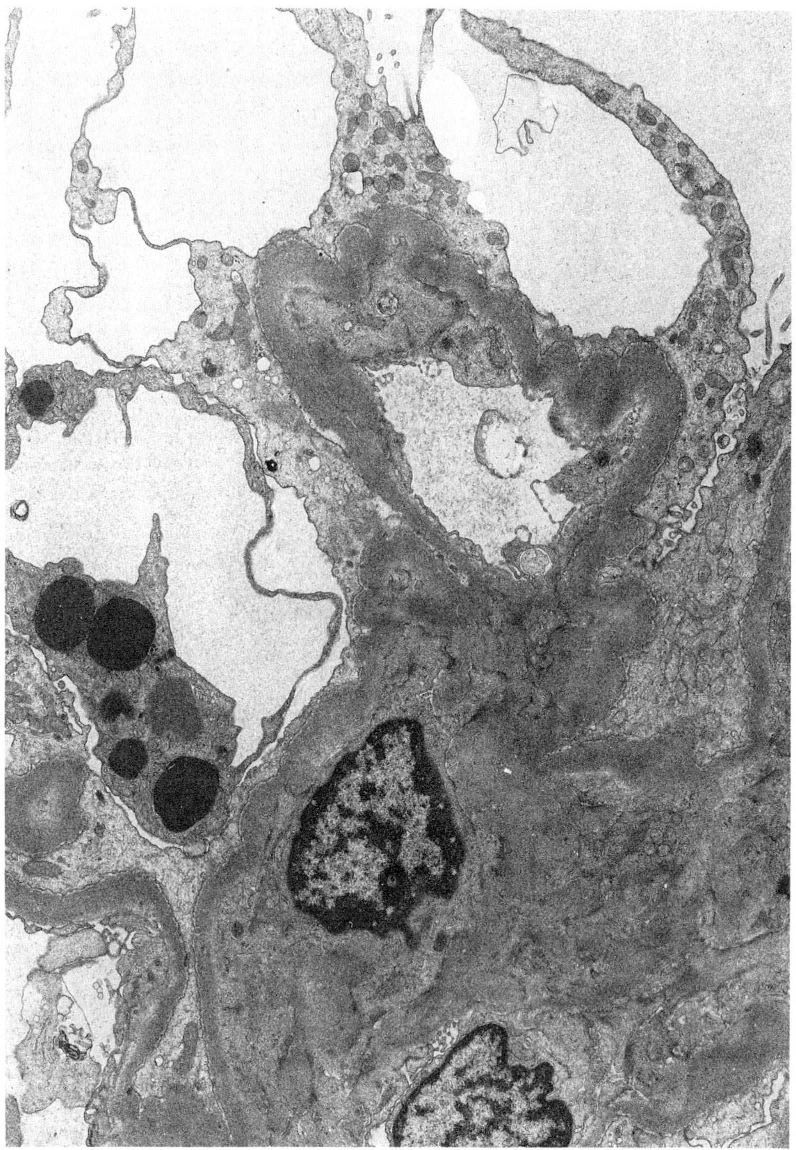

Fig. 8-15. Portions of glomerulus with wrinkled capillary wall covered by enlarged visceral epithelial cells with numerous but irregularly shaped apparently empty cytoplasmic vacuoles lined by a single membrane. The cell on the left also contains several dense lysosomes that correspond to protein reabsorption droplets. Compare to Figs. 8-2, 8-4, and 8-6. ($\times$ 8,000.)

gated structures are filaments, inasmuch as fibrils, by convention, represent extracellular structures. Perhaps more germane to a discussion of this anatomically peculiar feature is that it is noted in postmortem material and has not been described in biopsy specimens from any organ.[4–6,9]

Ultrastructural detection of HIV virions in HIV-associated nephropathy has not been reported despite careful searches.[4,5,8] Although other viruses such as cytomegalovirus (CMV) may be observed in coexisting infection, other microorganisms have not been reported as an integral lesion in the vast literature on this nephropathy. However, a single paper describes structures, interpreted as mycoplasma, in autopsy specimens[26]; other reports have not confirmed this observation (see below).[27]

The following are ultrastructural manifestations of glomerular and tubular injury. In glomeruli, the visceral epithelial cells are enlarged, contain numerous dense rounded secondary lysosomes and varying sized cytoplasmic vacuoles that appear empty, and are lined by single membranes (Fig. 8-15). In addition, some of these cells display bizarre cytoplasmic configurations, with long thin extensions attaching to the foot processes covering the capillary basement membranes. There is nearly complete effacement of the foot processes (Fig. 8-16); in the sclerotic or collapsed segments, the foot processes are separated from the original basement membrane by thin layers of new

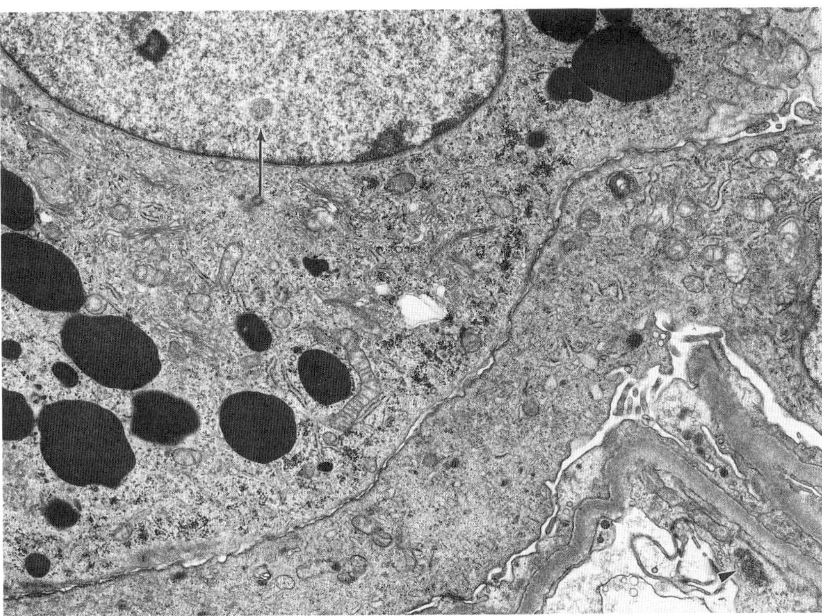

Fig. 8-16. Glomerular capillary covered by enlarged visceral epithelial cells, one of which contains dense rounded lysosomes and a single nuclear body (*arrow*). The foot processes are completely effaced. A tubuloreticular structure (*arrowhead*) is in the endothelial cell. (× 15,000.)

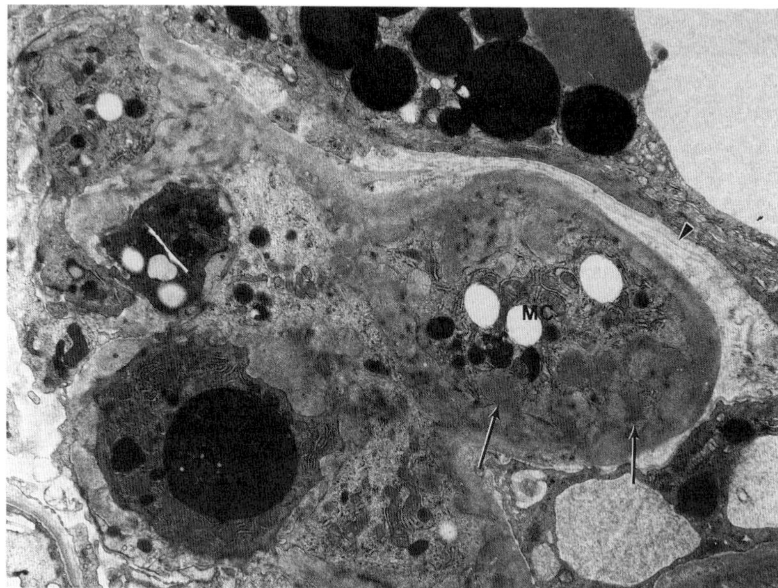

Fig. 8-17. Segment of glomerulus with sclerosis. The capillary is occluded by a combination of lipid-containing monocyte (MC) and electron-dense "deposits" (*arrows*) corresponding to insudative lesion. The visceral epithelial cell, which contains vacuoles and numerous lysosomes, is separated from the basement membrane by multiple layers of thin new basement membrane material (*arrowhead*). (× 7,000.)

basement membrane material, often with entrapped debris (Fig. 8-17). In the collapsed capillaries, endothelial cells are compressed or absent and the lumina obliterated by basement membrane material. In the wrinkled capillaries, there is infrequent peripheral migration and interposition of mesangium. Electron-dense deposits are typically absent, although rare small deposits may be observed in few mesangial regions. Capillary lumina in segments of sclerosis are obliterated by large masses of granular extracellular material ("insudative lesion"), usually with absent endothelial cells.[4,8,9,17,20] In earlier stages of this lesion, lumina are filled with lipid-containing monocytes, as in other settings in which focal and segmental glomerulosclerosis occurs.[28,29]

Aside from the features mentioned above, there are no regular or unexpected abnormalities of tubular cell morphology unique to HIV-associated nephropathy. The luminal precipitates of plasma protein described above are of medium density and are finely granular to homogeneous[4] (Fig. 8-18).

Immunofluorescence microscopy of glomeruli in HIV-associated nephropathy is not indicative of an immune-mediated lesion. As with other forms of focal and segmental glomerulosclerosis[26] and of glomerular collapse,[30] there may be segmental IgM and complement "deposits" in a coarsely granular to amorphous pattern in some glomeruli (Fig. 8-19). In some instances, mes-

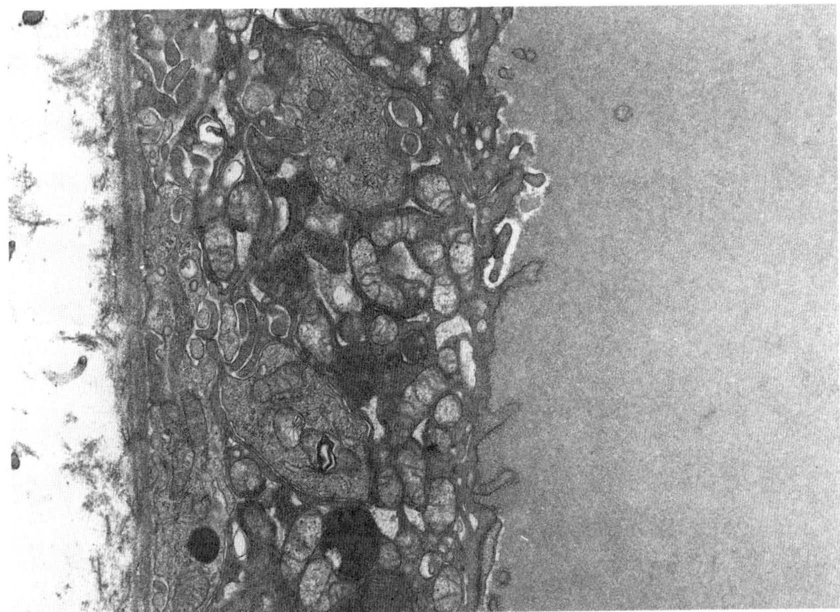

Fig. 8-18. Distal tubule with luminal pale granular material corresponding to the plasma protein precipitates illustrated in Figs. 8-8 to 8-11. (× 15,000.)

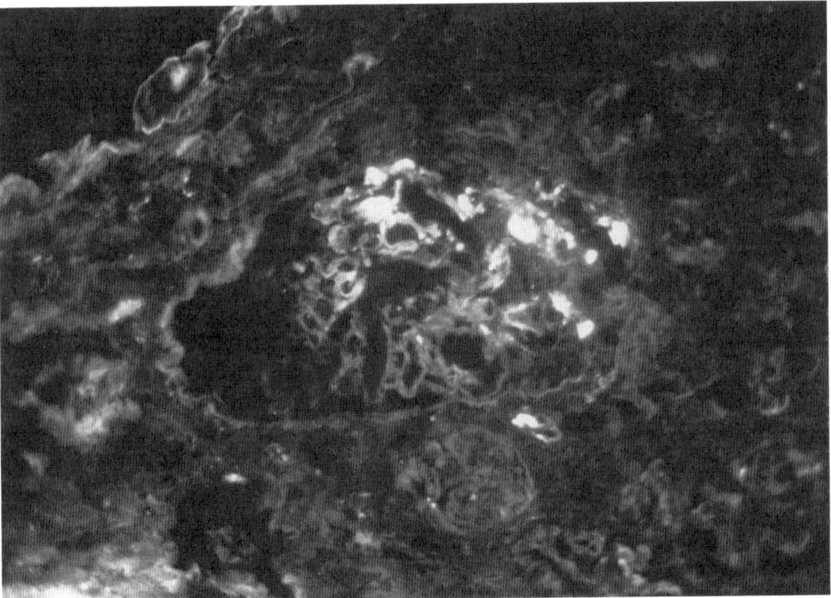

Fig. 8-19. Glomerulus with coarsely granular deposits in a segmental distribution; this corresponds to the lesion illustrated in Figs. 8-5 and 8-17. (IgM × 370.)

angial IgM and C3 may be observed.[1,2,4,5,8,12–17,20,31–33] Protein reabsorption droplets in both glomerular visceral epithelial cells and in tubular epithelial cells stain for albumin. The luminal precipitates in dilated tubules stain for all plasma proteins sought (immunoglobulins, light chains, albumin, complements); alternatively, Tamm-Horsfall protein is absent, but is demonstrated in hyaline casts as described above.[4]

The combination of findings enumerated above—focal and segmental glomerulosclerosis in early stages of evolution and/or collapsing glomerulopathy with prominent and abnormal visceral epithelial cells, tubular cell necrosis, tubular dilatation with luminal precipitates of plasma proteins, variable interstitial edema and inflammation, and ultrastructural peculiarities, especially numerous and large tubuloreticular structures—is sufficiently characteristic and distinctive, indeed unique, for HIV-associated nephropathy. A knowledgeable pathologist may be able to diagnose HIV infection on recognizing this nephropathy in a patient even if not previously known to be HIV-positive and otherwise completely asymptomatic for this virus.[4,8,11,16,20] Presently, this situation exists in many large renal biopsy services.[4,8]

PATHOGENESIS

The pathogenesis of HIV-associated nephropathy is not known for certain, although several theories, some with considerable merit, have been proposed. From a historic point of view, because the initial patients reported by Rao et al.[1] were intravenous heroin abusers, it was suggested that this renal lesion associated with AIDS actually represented heroin-associated nephropathy.[34–36] However, overwhelming epidemiologic evidence and other information concerning subsequent affected patients quickly dismissed this view.[4–6,8,10,12–16,37,38] On the other hand, the early observations that the vast majority of affected patients were black has been regularly confirmed in many reports from many centers both in the United States as well as from other parts of the world.[2,4,5,7,8,10–19,21,39–56] It has also been our impression that the course of the renal disorder is more severe in blacks than in other racial groups.[42] This marked racial predilection may well explain the relative lack of reported HIV-associated nephropathy in European centers that care for a largely white population.[21,22,47,57] The incidence or prevalence of this lesion in Africa is not known.[49] All manners of acquiring HIV infection have been associated with the development of HIV-associated nephropathy, including perinatal infection and receipt of infected blood products.[13]

Because of the mistaken belief that the glomerular lesion of HIV-associated nephropathy was similar to that induced by CMV in other settings, Heredia and coworkers[56] suggested CMV to be important in pathogenesis. This is highly unlikely. In addition to the lack of morphologic similarity between glomerular damage associated with CMV infection[58] and HIV-associated nephropathy, Nadasty and colleagues[59] were unable to identify CMV antigen or genome in tissues with HIV-associated nephropathy. As alluded to above, Bauer and colleagues[26] at the Armed Forces Institute of Pathology have suggested that another infectious agent, *Mycoplasma incognitus,* is directly responsible for the genesis of this renal lesion. They described structures that they identified as mycoplasma in virtually all locations in kidneys obtained at autopsy from patients with what they term AIDS-associated nephropathy. They also identified this organism by immunohistochemical techniques and suggested that it is pathogenically responsible for HIV-associated nephropathy. Because of morphologic considerations and the inability of other investigators[4–6,24,27] to confirm their findings, and because they did not consider that this nephropathy does not require the infectious and neoplastic features of AIDS for its genesis, their hypothesis is very unattractive. Langs and coworkers[45] have proposed that renal ischemia can account for tubular cell necrosis and glomerular collapse and, therefore, is an important pathogenic mechanism. This theory, however, does not explain the prominent structural abnormalities of glomerular visceral epithelial cells, and certainly cannot account for the massive proteinuria so characteristic of this nephropathy. Because of the well-known association of glomerulomegaly with focal and segmental glomerulosclerosis, and because enlarged glomeruli may be found in AIDS and HIV-infected patients who died without clinical renal glomerular manifestations, Pardo et al.[17,60] suggested that glomerulomegaly is pathogenically important. This does not explain the regular coexistence of tubular abnormalities.

The role of direct renal cell infection by HIV has been investigated both in biopsy tissue sections and in cell culture, often with seemingly conflicting results. Because of simultaneous structural abnormalities of glomerular and tubular epithelial cells, we wondered if a single lesion or event might affect both of these cell types and sought to identify a role for HIV in this process in biopsy specimens.[7,61] We employed immunohistochemistry using an antibody to p24 and tissue in situ hybridization using a cDNA probe. We documented HIV genome in many glomerular and tubular epithelial cells in HIV-associated nephropathy (Fig. 8-20); far less numerous tubular and no glomerular cells were positive in HIV-infected patients' kidney biopsies with immune complex-mediated glomerulonephritis and in autopsy tissue from AIDS patients without renal diseases. This suggested a direct role of HIV, either alone or in concert with other factors, in the genesis of this nephropathy. On the other hand, subsequent tissue culture studies in one laboratory have indicated that glomerular endothelial and mesangial cells, but not epithelial cells, may be infected by HIV,[62] whereas in another laboratory, mesangial cells in culture were found to be resistant to HIV infection.[63] Some further studies have also not been able to reproduce the tissue in situ hybridization results,[60] while others have documented viral DNA in renal tissue specimens, although in lymphoid rather than epithelial cells. More recent experience, however, has suggested that viral genome may indeed be found in renal tissue[64]; the difficulty of identifying virus product may be as much a matter of technical problems as with the presence or absence of

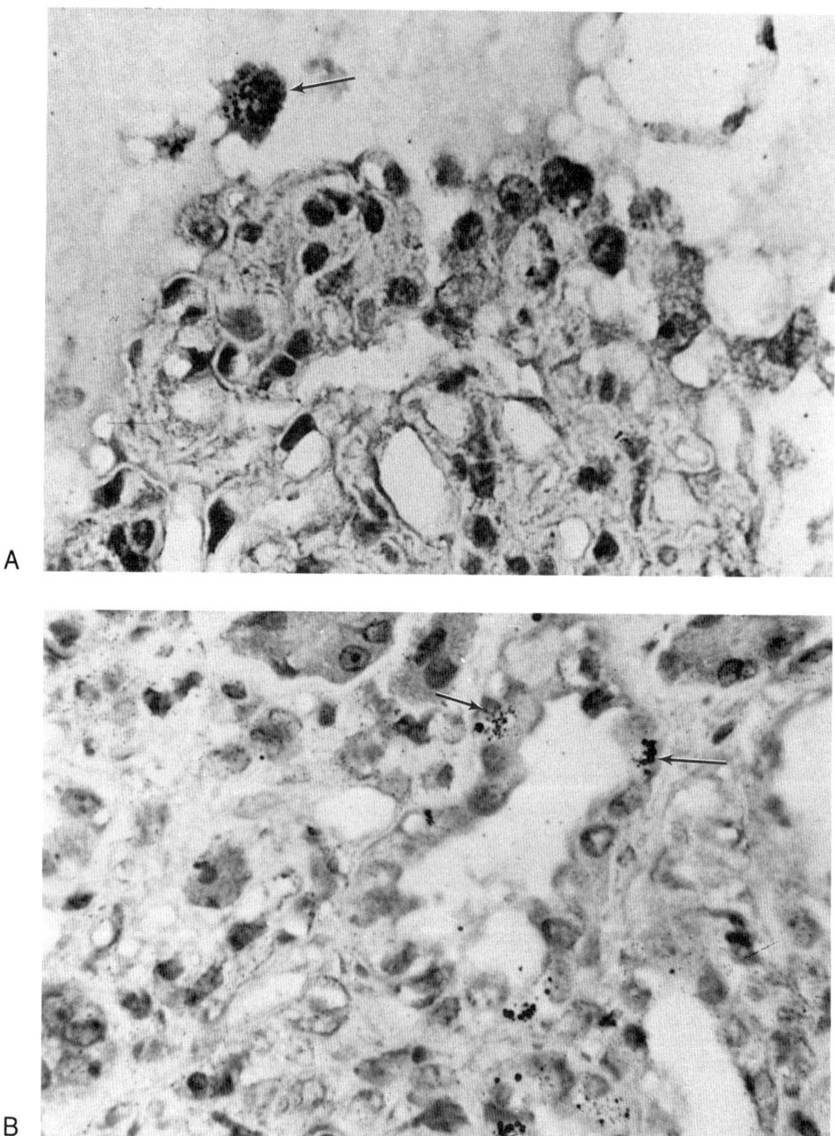

Fig. 8-20. In situ hybridization for HIV genome. **(A)** Glomerular visceral epithelial cell with multiple cytoplasmic silver grains (*arrow*). (× 800.) **(B)** Tubular epithelial cells containing numerous silver grains (*arrows*). (× 380.)

cellular infection.[65] Kimmel and coworkers,[33,64] in a series of reports, have documented HIV nucleic acid using polymerase chain reaction in portions of renal tissue microdissected from renal biopsy specimens in several disorders, including both HIV-associated nephropathy and immune complex mediated glomerulonephritis. In the few biopsies studied with HIV-associated nephropathy, HIV *gag* gene was identified in glomeruli and in tubular cells. The glomerular cell types were not indicated and, indeed, could not be using this technique.[64] In strong support of a direct or indirect role of HIV DNA or genes in the genesis of HIV-associated nephropathy is a mouse model transgenic for HIV that used a noninfectious DNA construct lacking *gag* and *pol* genes. This animal model developed a lesion that was functionally and morphologically similar to the human nephropathy.[66,67]

As noted above, we had also documented HIV p24 antigen in tubular epithelium in HIV-associated nephropathy biopsies.[61] This immunohistochemical technique was clearly not as sensitive as in situ hybridization to identify virus products. Few studies have attempted to reproduce that finding, also with mixed results.[65,68] This may be because of technical considerations[65] and/or because of the lack of diagnostic precision concerning the biopsy changes.[68]

Because of the well-known role of growth factors in the genesis of many glomerulopathies and the demonstrated effect of transforming growth factor-β (TGF-β) in the development of glomerular sclerosis,[69–73] we recently explored the role of TGF-β in HIV-associated nephropathy.[74] We found that, in contrast to HIV-infected and uninfected control biopsies, the expression of TGF-β and proteins induced by this cytokine—plasminogen activator inhibitor-1 and fibronectin containing extra domain A—was increased in glomeruli and tubulointerstitium in HIV-associated nephropathy. This suggests that TGF-β may play an important role in its pathogenesis. Further, HIV *tat* gene protein has been shown to influence some manifestations of HIV infection.[75] Alternatively, Shukla and coworkers[76] have documented that TGF-β increases expression of long terminal repeat segment (LTR) gene in transfected human mesangial cells in culture. We have also recently documented that *tat* gene protein added to cultured human mesangial cells induced expression of TGF-β mRNA and increased expression of type I collagen and biglycan, a proteoglycan specifically induced by TGF-β.[74] These findings together suggest a strong relationship between viral protein either in renal cells or directly influencing them, the production of TGF-β and its associated proteins, and the development of the glomerular and tubulointerstitial lesions of HIV-associated nephropathy. Whether this scenario or a variation is responsible, completely or in part, for this nephropathy awaits further investigation.

OTHER GLOMERULOPATHIES

There are other glomerular lesions that may be an "integral" part of HIV infection. As emphasized by Pardo, Strauss, and colleagues[2,18,19] both in adults and children with proteinuria, a relatively mild degree of mesangial hypercellularity may be present in glomeruli. Although immunofluorescence microscopy was not performed in all tissue samples in their studies, electron-dense deposits were frequently documented, indicating this to be an immune complex mediated lesion. Its relationship to HIV-associated nephropathy is unclear.

Minimal change disease with nephrotic syndrome has been occasionally described in HIV-infected patients.[8,49–52,75,77–79] Its relationship to the virus is not known, but it should be noted that that glomerulopathy may antedate the development of full-blown HIV-associated nephropathy.[8]

As discussed in detail elsewhere in this book, IgA nephropathy may well be another HIV-associated nephropathy in some patients.[21,46,47,53,80–85] This immune complex mediated glomerulonephritis, along with several other proliferative glomerulonephritides, has been shown to contain HIV antigens and respective antibodies in the glomerular immune complexes; furthermore, circulating immune complexes in some of the patients were composed of the same antigens and antibodies as the glomerular eluates.[33–85] Other entities such as membranous glomerulonephritis, membranoproliferative glomerulonephritis, and acute proliferative (postinfectious) glomerulonephritis have been described in HIV-infected patients; their relation to HIV antigens has not been well documented. Some of these glomerulopathies may be associated with other coexisting infections such as hepatitis B,[3,13,21,47,86–88] or systemic lupus erythematosus.[89] It should be pointed out that the regular tubular and interstitial changes that are an integral component of HIV-associated nephropathy are not present in these latter glomerulopathies.[4]

REFERENCES

1. Rao TKS, Filippone EJ, Nicastri AD et al: Associated focal and segmental glomerulosclerosis in the acquired immunodeficiency syndrome. N Engl J Med 310: 669, 1984
2. Pardo V, Aldana M, Colton RM et al: Glomerular lesions in the acquired immunodeficiency syndrome. Ann Intern Med 101:429, 1984
3. Gardenswartz MH, Lerner CW, Seligson GR et al: Renal disease in patients with AIDS: a clinicopathologic study. Clin Nephrol 21:197, 1984
4. Cohen AH, Nast CC: HIV-associated nephropathy: a unique combined glomerular, tubular and interstitial lesion. Mod Pathol 1:87, 1988
5. Chander P, Soni A, Sura A et al: Renal ultrastructural markers in AIDS-associated nephropathy. Am J Pathol 126:513, 1987
6. Chander P, Agarwal A, Soni A et al: Renal cytomembranous inclusions in idiopathic renal disease as predictive markers for the acquired immunodeficiency syndrome. Hum Pathol 19:1060, 1988
7. Cohen AH: Considerations of pathogenesis of HIV-associated nephropathy. p. 512. In Hatano M (ed): Nephrology: Proceedings of the Eleventh International Congress of Nephrology. Springer-Verlag, New York, 1991
8. D'Agati V, Suh JI, Carbone L et al: Pathology of HIV-associated nephropathy: a detailed morphologic and comparative study. Kidney Int 35:1358, 1989

9. Cohen AH, Nast CC: Pathology of the kidneys. p. 130. In Nash G, Said J (eds): The Pathology of AIDS and HIV Infection. WB Saunders, Philadelphia, 1992

10. Soni A, Agarwal A, Chander P et al: Evidence for an HIV-related nephropathy: a clinico-pathological study. Clin Nephrol 31:12, 1989

11. Alpers CE, Harawi S, Rennke HG: Focal glomerulosclerosis with tubuloreticular inclusions: a possible predictive value for acquired immunodeficiency syndrome (AIDS). Am J Kidney Dis 12:240, 1988

12. Pardo V, Meneses R, Ossa L et al: AIDS-related glomerulopathy: occurrence in specific risk groups. Kidney Int 31:1167, 1987

13. Glassock RJ, Cohen AH, Danovitch G, Parsa KP: Human immunodeficiency virus (HIV) infection and the kidney. Ann Intern Med 112:35, 1991

14. Seney FD, Burns D, Silva FG: Acquired immunodeficiency syndrome and the kidney. Am J Kidney Dis 26:1, 1990

15. Bourgoignie JJ: Renal complications of human immunodeficiency virus type I. Kidney Int 37:1571, 1990

16. Bourgoignie JJ, Meneses R, Ortiz-Interian C et al: The clinical spectrum of renal disease associated with human immunodeficiency virus. Am J Kidney Dis 12: 131, 1988

17. Pardo V, Bell M, Malaga S et al: Renal manifestations of human immunodeficiency virus infection. p. 137. In Damjanov I, Cohen AH, Mills SE, Young RD (eds): Progress in Reproductive and Urinary Tract Pathology. Vol. 2. Field and Wood, New York, 1990

18. Strauss J, Zilleruelo G, Abitbol C et al: Human immunodeficiency virus nephropathy. Pediatr Nephrol 7:220, 1993

19. Strauss J, Abitbol C, Zilleruelo G et al: Renal disease in children with the acquired immunodeficiency syndrome. N Engl J Med 321:625, 1989

20. Bourgoignie JJ, Pardo V: The nephropathology in human immunodeficiency virus (HIV-1) infection. Kidney Int, suppl. 35:S19, 1991

21. Nochy D, Glotz D, Dosquet P et al: Renal disease associated with HIV infection: a multicenter study of 60 patients from Paris hospitals. Nephrol Dial Transplant 8:11, 1993

22. Genderini A, Bertani T, Bertoli S et al: HIV-associated nephropathy: a new entity. A study of 12 cases. Nephrol Dial Transplant, suppl. 1:84, 1990

23. Kostianovsky M, Orenstein JM, Schaff Z, Grimley PM: Cytomembranous inclusions observed in acquired immunodeficiency syndrome: clinical and experimental review. Arch Pathol Lab Med 111:218, 1987

24. Orenstein JM: Ultrastructural pathology of human immunodeficiency virus infection. Ultrastruct Pathol 16:179, 1992

25. Bouteille M, Kalifat SR, Delarue J: Ultrastructural variations of nuclear bodies in human diseases. J Ultrastruct Res 19:474, 1967

26. Bauer FA, Wear DJ, Angritt P, Lo SC: *Mycoplasma fermentans* (incognitus strain) infection in the kidneys of patients with acquired immunodeficiency syndrome and associated nephropathy: a light microscopic, immunohistochemical, and ultrastructural study. Hum Pathol 22:63, 1991

27. Cohen AH: Mycoplasma infection in the kidneys of patients with acquired immunodeficiency syndrome (letter to the editor). Hum Pathol 22:932, 1991

28. Glassock RJ, Adler SG, Ward HJ, Cohen AH: Primary glomerular diseases. p. 1682. In Brenner BM, Rector FC Jr (eds): The Kidney. WB Saunders, Philadelphia, 1991

29. Cohen AH, Nast CC: Atlas of Renal Pathology. p. 1807. In Massry SG, Glassock RJ (eds): Textbook of Nephrology. Williams & Wilkins, Baltimore, 1989

30. Weiss MA, Daquioag E, Margolin EG, Pollak VE: Nephrotic syndrome, progressive irreversible renal failure, and glomerular "collapse:" a new clinicopathologic entity? Am J Kidney Dis 7:20, 1986
31. Rao TKS, Friedman EA: AIDS (HIV)-associated nephropathy: does it exist? An in depth review. Am J Nephrol 9:441, 1989
32. Rao TKS: Human immunodeficiency virus (HIV) associated nephropathy. Ann Rev Med 42:391, 1991
33. Kimmel PL, Phillips TM, Ferreira-Centeno A et al: HIV-associated immune-mediated renal diseases. Kidney Int 44:1327, 1993
34. Balow JE, Macher AM, Rook AH: Paucity of glomerular disease in acquired immunodeficiency syndrome (AIDS), abstracted. Kidney Int 29:178, 1986
35. Mazbar S, Humphreys MH: AIDS-associated nephropathy is not seen at San Francisco General Hospital, abstracted. Kidney Int 33:202, 1988
36. Humphreys MH, Schoenfeld PY: Renal complications in patients with acquired immunodeficiency syndrome (AIDS). Am J Nephrol 7:1, 1987
37. Humphreys MH: Human immunodeficiency virus associated-nephropathy: east is east and west is west? (editorial). Arch Intern Med 150:253, 1990
38. Frassetto L, Schoenfeld PY, Humphreys MH: Increasing incidence of human immunodeficiency virus-associated nephropathy at San Francisco General Hospital. Am J Kidney Dis 18:655, 1991
39. Bourgoignie JJ, Ortiz-Interian C, Green DF, Roth D: Race, a cofactor in HIV-I associated nephropathy. Transplant Proc 6:3899, 1989
40. Cantor ES, Kimmel PK, Bosch JP: Effect of race on expression of AIDS-associated nephropathy. Arch Intern Med 151:125, 1991
41. Carbone L, D'Agati V, Cheng JT, Appel GB: The course and prognosis of human immunodeficiency virus-associated nephropathy. Am J Med 87:389, 1989
42. Cohen AH: HIV-associated nephropathy: racial differences in severity of renal damage, abstracted. J Am Soc Nephrol 1:305, 1990
43. Dosquet P, Haddoum F, Viron B et al: Focal and segmental glomerulosclerosis (FSGS) during acquired immunodeficiency syndrome (AIDS): two observations, abstracted. Kidney Int 33:1041, 1988
44. Hory B, Bresson C, Lorge JF, Perol C: Associated focal and segmental glomerulosclerosis in the acquired immunodeficiency syndrome (letter). Am J Kidney Dis 12:169, 1988
45. Langs C, Gallo GR, Schacht RG et al: Rapid renal failure in AIDS-associated focal glomerulosclerosis. Arch Intern Med 150:287, 1990
46. Mazbar SA, Schoenfeld PY, Humphreys MH: Renal involvement in patients infected with HIV: experience at San Francisco General Hospital. Kidney Int 37:1325, 1990
47. Nochy D, Glotz D, Dosquet P et al: Renal lesions associated with human immunodeficiency virus infection: North American vs European experience. Adv Nephrol 22:269, 1993
48. Provenzano R, Kupin WW, Santiago GC: Renal involvement in the acquired immunodeficiency syndrome: presentation, clinical course and therapy. Henry Ford Hosp Med J 35:38, 1987
49. Rao TKS: Clinical features of human immunodeficiency virus associated nephropathy. Kidney Int, suppl. 35:S13, 1991
50. Rousseau E, Russo P, Lapointe N, O'Reagan S: Renal complications of acquired immunodeficiency syndrome in children. Am J Kidney Dis 11:48, 1988
51. Ingulli E, Tejani A, Fikrig S et al: Nephrotic syndrome associated with acquired immunodeficiency syndrome in children. J Pediatr 119:710, 1991

52. Lopes GS, Marques LP, Rioja LS et al: Glomerular disease and human immunodeficiency virus infection in Brazil. Am J Nephrol 12:281, 1992
53. Bourgoignie JJ, Pardo V: HIV-associated nephropathies (editorial). N Engl J Med 327:729, 1992
54. Connor E, Gupta S, Joshi V et al: Acquired immunodeficiency syndrome-associated renal disease in children. J Pediatr 113:39, 1988
55. Korbet SM, Schwartz MM: Human immunodeficiency virus infection and nephrotic syndrome. Am J Kidney Dis 20:97, 1992
56. Heredia JB, Angeles AA, Gutierrez ER et al: Nephropatia associada al sindrome di immunodeficiencia acquirida. Rev Invest Clin 39:105, 1987
57. Brunkhorst R, Brunkhorst U, Eisenback GM et al: Lack of clinical evidence for a specific HIV-associated glomerulopathy in 203 patients with HIV infection. Nephrol Dial Transplant 7:87, 1992
58. Smith RD, Wehner RW: Progressive cytomegalovirus glomerulonephritis: an experimental model. Am J Pathol 112:313, 1983
59. Nadasty T, Miller KW, Johnson LD et al: Is cytomegalovirus associated with renal disease in AIDS patients? Mod Pathol 5:277, 1992
60. Pardo V, Shapshak P, Yoshioka M, Strauss J: HIV associated nephropathy (HIVN): direct renal invasion or indirect glomerular involvement, abstracted. FASEB J 5:907A, 1991
61. Cohen AH, Sun NCJ, Shapshak P, Imagawa DT: Demonstration of human immunodeficiency virus in renal epithelium in HIV-associated nephropathy. Mod Pathol 2:125, 1989
62. Green DF, Resnick L, Bourgoignie JJ: HIV infects glomerular endothelial and mesangial but not epithelial cells in vitro. Kidney Int 41:956, 1992
63. Alpers CE, McClure J, Bursten SL: Human mesangial cells are resistant to productive infection by multiple strains of human immunodeficiency virus types 1 and 2. Am J Kidney Dis 19:126, 1992
64. Kimmel PL, Ferreira-Centeno A, Farkas-Szallasi T et al: Viral DNA in microdissected renal biopsy material from HIV infected patients with nephrotic syndrome. Kidney Int 43:1347, 1993
65. Nadasty T, Hanson-Painton O, Davis LD et al: Conditions affecting the immunohistochemical detection of HIV in fixed and embedded renal and nonrenal tissues. Mod Pathol 5:283, 1992
66. Dickie P, Felser J, Eckhaus M et al: HIV-associated nephropathy in transgenic mice expressing HIV-1 genes. Virology 185:109, 1991
67. Kopp JB, Klotman ME, Adler SH et al: Progressive glomerulosclerosis and enhanced renal accumulation of basement membrane components in mice transgenic for human immunodeficiency virus type 1 genes. Proc Natl Acad Sci USA 89:1577, 1992
68. Barbiano di Belgiojoso G, Genderini A, Vago L et al: Absence of HIV antigens in renal tissue from patients with HIV-associated nephropathy. Nephrol Dial Transplant 5:489, 1990
69. Border WA, Ruoslahti E: Transforming growth factor-β in disease: the dark side of tissue repair. J Clin Invest 90:1, 1992
70. Tomooka S, Border WA, Marshall BC, Noble NA: Glomerular matrix accumulation is linked to inhibition of the plasmin protease system. Kidney Int 42:1462, 1992
71. Border WA, Noble NA, Yamamoto T et al: Antagonists of transforming growth factor-β: a novel approach to treatment of glomerulonephritis and prevention of glomerulosclerosis. Kidney Int 41:566, 1992

72. Kagami S, Border WA, Ruoslahti E, Noble NA: Coordinated expression of B1 integrins and transforming growth factor-β-induced matrix proteins in glomerulonephritis. Lab Invest 69:68, 1993
73. Border WA, Noble NA: Cytokines in kidney disease: the role of transforming growth factor-β. Am J Kidney Dis 22:105, 1993
74. Border WA, Yamamoto T, Noble N et al: HIV-associated nephropathy is linked to TGF-beta and matrix protein expression in human kidney, abstracted. J Am Soc Nephrol 4:675, 1993
75. Zauli G, Davis BR, Re MC et al: Tat protein stimulates production of transforming growth factor-β1 by marrow macrophages: a potential mechanism for human immunodeficiency virus-1-induced hematopoietic suppression. Blood 80:3036, 1992
76. Shukla RR, Kumar A, Kimmel PL: Transforming growth factor beta increases the expression of HIV-1 gene in transfected human mesangial cells. Kidney Int 44:1022, 1993
77. Singer DR, Jenkins AP, Gupta S, Evans DJ: Minimal change nephropathy in the acquired immune deficiency syndrome. BMJ 291:863, 1985
78. Cases A, Montoliu J, Baradad M et al: Nefropatia por cambios minimos associada a un sindrome de immunodeficiencia adquirida. Med Clin (Barcelona) 86:684, 1986
79. Landor M, Bernstein L, Rubinstein A: A steroid-responsive nephropathy in a child with human immunodeficiency virus infection (letter). Am J Dis Child 147:261, 1993
80. Kenouch S, Delahousse M, Mery JP, Nochy D: Mesangial IgA deposits in two patients with AIDS-related complex. Nephron 54:338, 1990
81. Jindal KK, Trillo A, Bishop G et al: Crescentic IgA nephropathy as a manifestation of human immune deficiency virus infection. Am J Nephrol 11:147, 1991
82. Trachtman H, Gauthier B, Vinograd A, Valderrama E: IgA nephropathy in a child with human immunodeficiency virus type 1 infection. Pediatr Nephrol 5:724, 1991
83. Katz A, Bargman JM, Miller DC et al: IgA nephritis in HIV-positive patients: a new HIV-associated nephropathy? Clin Nephrol 38:61, 1992
84. Schoeneman MJ, Ghali V, Lieberman K, Reismen L: IgA nephritis in a child with human immunodeficiency virus: a unique form of human immunodeficiency virus-associated nephropathy. Pediatr Nephrol 6:46, 1992
85. Kimmel P, Phillips TM, Ferreira-Centeno A et al: Idiotypic IgA nephropathy in patients with human immunodeficiency virus infection. N Engl J Med 327:702, 1992
86. Guerra IL, Abraham AA, Kimmel PL et al: Nephrotic syndrome associated with chronic persistent hepatitis B in an HIV antibody positive patient. Am J Kidney Dis 10:385, 1987
87. Schectman JM, Kimmel PL: Remission of hepatitis B-associated membranous glomerulonephritis in human immunodeficiency virus infection. Am J Kidney Dis 17:716, 1991
88. Collins AB, Bhan AK, Dienstag JL et al: Hepatitis B immune complex glomerulonephritis: simultaneous glomerular deposition of hepatitis B surface and e antigens. Clin Immunol Immunopathol 24:137, 1983
89. D'Agati V, Seigle R: Coexistence of AIDS and lupus nephritis: a case report. Am J Nephrol 10:243, 1990

9

Urologic Manifestations of HIV Infection

William A. Kennedy II
Mitchell C. Benson
Steven A. Kaplan

INTRODUCTION

Despite the explosion of scientific literature on human immunodeficiency virus (HIV) infection and AIDS in the past decade, there has been relatively little written about the urologic manifestations of this infection.[1–3] Initially, urologic pathology related to HIV was considered unusual. This, however, was secondary to the attention directed toward the more life-threatening

Table 9-1. Urologic Manifestations of HIV Infection

Renal Disease
    Glomerulosclerosis
    Other forms of glomerulonephritis
    Acute tubular necrosis
Urologic Neoplasms
    Kaposi sarcoma
    Testicular carcinoma
    Lymphoma
        Retroperitoneal
        Testis
Urinary tract infections (see Table 9-2)
    Bacterial
    Candida albicans
    Cytomegalovirus
    Tuberculosis
Neurogenic bladder dysfunction
    Detrusor hyperreflexia
    Detrusor areflexia
Sexually transmitted diseases
    Syphilis
    Herpes Simplex
    Condyloma acuminata
    Candida albicans
    Gonorrhea
Sexual Dysfunction
    Erectile dysfunction
    Retrograde ejaculation

aspects of the disease. Recent experience has resulted in appreciation of the fact that urologic manifestations in patients with AIDS are the rule rather than the exception.[4] The purpose of this chapter is to establish how HIV infection affects both the upper and lower urinary tract. The specific areas addressed include renal disease, urologic neoplasms, urinary tract infection, neurogenic bladder dysfunction, and sexual dysfunction (Table 9-1). In addition, the medical and rehabilitative management of both urologic and neuro-urologic entities associated with HIV infection will be discussed.

RENAL DISEASE

The most common urologic manifestations of HIV infection are renal in origin.[5] Patients with HIV infection frequently present to the urologist with microscopic hematuria[5] and proteinuria.[6] These findings are present in more than 25 percent of patients with AIDS,[7] and are often due to intrinsic renal diseases such as focal and segmental glomerulosclerosis (HIV-associated nephropathy), nephrotic syndrome, or acute tubular necrosis (ATN).[7-11] Due to the frequency of microscopic hematuria and proteinuria, routine urologic evaluation of these patients, solely for this finding, is not usually recommended.[4] However, when renal failure occurs concomitantly, an evaluation is indicated and renal ultrasound is the diagnostic test of choice. A discussion of the pathophysiology of HIV-related intrinsic renal diseases is outside the scope of this chapter and is addressed extensively in other sections of this book.

Obstructive uropathy is a much less common cause of renal insufficiency than intrinsic renal diseases. When an obstructive cause is present, it is likely to be a result of urinary retention due to a neurogenic bladder. Urinary lithiasis can also occur and result in an obstructive uropathy. Presently, no data exist to suggest that urinary lithiasis is more prevalent in an HIV-infected patient population compared with the general population. If the clinical presentation is suggestive of obstructive urinary lithiasis, than a renal ultrasound is the preferred initial diagnostic test. Management of completely obstructing stones should consist of decompression of the obstructed system and subsequent treatment directed at removal of the stone. Newer noninvasive therapies such as extracorporeal shock wave lithotripsy (ESWL) may be recommended in most instances.

As the incidence of toxoplasma encephalitis in patients with AIDS has increased, combination therapy with sulfadiazine/pyrimethamine has become more frequently employed. Acute renal failure due to sulfadiazine crystal deposition in the urinary tract was well described 30 to 40 years ago[12] and has now resurfaced as a clinical entity.[12–14] Renal ultrasonography typically demonstrates a clustering of echogenic shadows within the renal collecting system, with or without hydronephrosis[15] (see also Ch. 10). Controlled alkalinization of the urine and high fluid intake, allowing for dissolution and spontaneous passage of the stones, is recommended for the treatment and prophylaxis for sulfadiazine crystalluria.

NEOPLASMS

Kaposi Sarcoma

One of the first reported manifestations of HIV infection was the appearance of Kaposi sarcoma.[2] Prior to the HIV era, Kaposi sarcoma was recognized as a relatively indolent malignancy that primarily occurred in elderly men of Mediterranean descent. It is a disease of the reticuloendothelial system presenting as solitary or diffuse neovascular tumors. The lower extremities were the primary site of involvement; however, involvement of the penis was not unusual. Today, the presence of Kaposi sarcoma in any patient less than 60 years of age is virtually diagnostic of AIDS.[16] In addition, over 90 percent of Kaposi sarcoma in HIV-infected patients has been documented in male homosexuals. The disease also has a more virulent course in the HIV-infected population.

Kaposi sarcoma has been reported to involve both the glans penis and penile shaft.[17] These may be either the classic purple papular lesion or, less commonly, an ulcerated lesion. If these lesions are large enough, they may cause obstruction and urinary retention.[4,18] Therapy is directed at the local lesion and has been especially successful in relieving urinary obstruction. External beam radiotherapy has been employed successfully to treat such lesions.[19] Surgery should only be directed at debriding severely infected and ulcerated lesions.[20] Systemic chemotherapy is reserved for patients with disseminated Kaposi sarcoma, but can be dangerous in this already immuno-suppressed population with a tendency to develop opportunistic infections.[17]

Testicular Neoplasms

Cantanese et al.[4] and Tessler and Cantanese[21] reported an association between testis tumors and the presence of HIV infection. Of 132 patients with testicular tumors, 31 (24 percent) either had AIDS, were HIV-infected, or were classified in a high-risk group. In addition, unlike the general population, nonseminomatous testicular tumors were more common than seminomatous testicular tumors.[4,21,22] HIV-infected individuals are also at increased risk of seminoma of the testis,[23] as well as bilateral synchronous testis tumors.[24] Black and Hispanic patients were also over represented in the group of HIV-infected patients with testicular tumors[4] (Fig. 9-1). This occurred despite the historically low incidence of testicular carcinoma of 1.5 percent in a nonwhite population.[25] A testicular neoplasm may be the initial

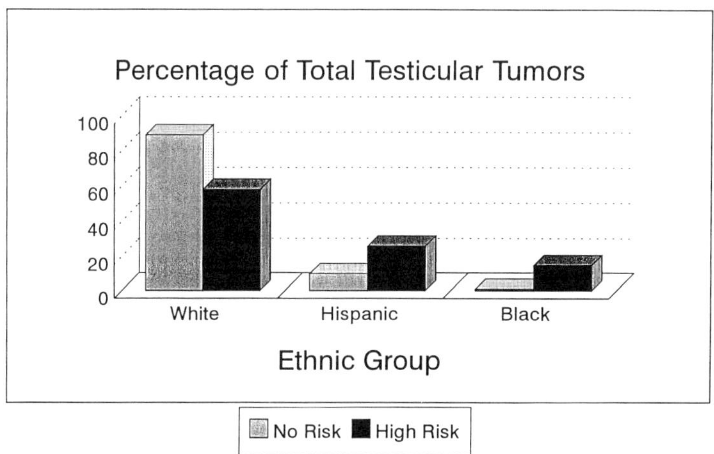

Fig. 9-1. A comparison of the racial distribution of no-risk (n = 101) and high-risk (n = 31) patients with testicular tumors. High-risk patients include those with AIDS, HIV-seropositive status, or classification in a high-risk group. (From Catanese et al.,[4] with permission.)

presenting symptom of HIV infection.[26] Consequently, HIV infection should always be in the differential diagnosis of a male presenting with a primary testicular carcinoma, particularly in nonwhite males.

Lymphoma

The concurrent presence of HIV infection and lymphoma is one of the diagnostic criteria for AIDS. In contrast with malignant lymphoma occurring in the general population, extranodal origin is common in HIV-associated non-Hodgkin's lymphomas. AIDS-related lymphoma of the genitourinary tract has been reported,[27] presenting as renal masses,[28] ureteral obstruction with resultant hydronephrosis, or lesions within the scrotum.[26] Histologically, the majority of these lymphomas are small noncleaved cell or immunoblastic lymphomas, and are B-cell phenotype as determined by immunoglobulin gene rearrangement studies.[28]

Therapy is directed at the systemic disease as well as relief of ureteral obstruction. Response rates of 52 percent have been reported with the use of intensive chemotherapeutic regimens of MACOP-B (methotrexate, Adriamycin, cyclophosphamide, vincristine, prednisone, and bleomycin). A history of concurrent opportunistic infections or Kaposi sarcoma worsens the prognosis for complete remission.[29]

URINARY TRACT INFECTION

Patients with HIV infection are at increased risk of developing infections secondary to a compromised immune system. Approximately 20 percent of patients diagnosed with AIDS will have a positive urine culture at some time during their disease.[5] Kaplan et al.,[6] in a retrospective analysis of 60 patients with AIDS, reported that although *Escherichia coli* is responsible for 80 percent of all urinary tract infections in the general population, it was the causative organism in only 25 percent of patients with AIDS. More importantly, there was an increased incidence of unusual organisms cultured as the pathogenic agent (Table 9-2), such as *Candida albicans, Acinetobacter calcoaceticus,* salmonella, and cytomegalovirus.

Uncomplicated urinary tract infections require no diagnostic studies other than a urine culture. Patients who have recurrent infection with an atypical organism or evidence of pyelonephritis should be evaluated either with an intravenous pyelogram (if the serum creatinine is within the normal range) or with an ultrasound to exclude an abscess or urinary lithiasis.

Cantanese et al.[4] reported four seropositive homosexual patients with *Staphylococcus aureus* prostatic abscesses. Fungal prostatic abscesses secondary to *Histoplasma capsulatum*[30,31] and *Cryptococcus neoformans*[32] have also been reported. Treatment consists of appropriate intravenous antimicrobial therapy, and transurethral unroofing of the prostatic abscess in the

Table 9-2. Frequency of Various Organisms
Encountered in Urinary Tract
Infections in Patients with AIDS
(n = 60)

Organism	Incidence (%)
Pseudomonas	33.3
E. coli	25.0
Klebsiella	16.7
A. calcoaceticus	8.3
Candida	8.3
Cytomegalovirus	8.3
Enterobacter	8.3
Salmonella	8.3
Serratia	8.3
S. aureus	8.3
S. epidermidis	8.3

(From Kaplan et al.,[6] with permission.)

case of antimicrobial nonresponders. In addition, renal and perinephric abscesses may occur. Renal aspergillus infections[33] and aspergillomas[34] have been diagnosed in HIV-infected patients. A combination of surgical drainage and intravenous amphotericin B administration is the recommended treatment.

The Centers for Disease Control and Prevention has established that recurrent salmonella sepsis in an HIV-seropositive patient is sufficient to diagnose AIDS.[16] There have been reports of recurrent salmonella epididymitis that are amenable to lifelong antimicrobial therapy with trimethoprim-sulfamethoxasole.[4] Cytomegalovirus may also invade the epididymis. Unlike salmonella epididymitis, patients with cytomegalovirus epididymitis usually have a negative urine culture unless specifically tested for cytomegalovirus.[35] *Toxoplasma gondii* should also be considered as a potential etiologic agent for symptomatic orchitis/epididymitis when a specific infectious agent has not been readily identified.[36] Some clinicians have advocated doing an epididymectomy for the pain associated with chronic relapsing epididymitis.[4]

Finally, there is an increased incidence of *Mycobacterium tuberculosis* in HIV-infected patients.[37] Genitourinary tuberculosis can present in many forms, including abnormalities of the kidney, ureter, bladder, prostate, and epididymis. There is an increased incidence of both renal and epididymal abscesses in patients with AIDS who have concurrent tuberculosis.

NEUROGENIC BLADDER

Patients with HIV infection often have evidence of nervous system involvement. Pathologic studies at time of autopsy on 104 patients with AIDS by Lemann et al.[38] at the New York Hospital and Memorial Sloan-Kettering

Cancer Center have demonstrated neurologic involvement in approximately 95 percent of the cases. The pathologic findings may be a direct causal effect of the HIV infection (i.e., subacute encephalitis) or secondary to concomitant infections or malignancies associated with AIDS. The nervous system involvement may be focal, generalized, peripheral, and/or central in nature.

Patients with AIDS who have neurourologic disorders pose a therapeutic dilemma for the treating physician. It is easy, and usually appropriate, to attribute most of the clinical condition to the underlying HIV infection. However, HIV-infected patients remain susceptible to other disease processes unrelated to their neurologic condition, which may be the sole or predominant cause of their voiding symptomatology. Common disorders such as urinary tract infections, prostate and bladder cancer, and benign prostatic hyperplasia (BPH) may mimic many of the symptoms of neurourologic dysfunction. To adequately treat the neurourologic symptoms in patients with AIDS, the physician must obtain a precise diagnosis. This entails a detailed understanding of the mechanics of voiding. Of greater importance is an appreciation of how different neurologic disorders affect voiding.[39]

For normal voiding to occur, there must be a systematic and coordinated integration between the neural pathways of the brain stem and spinal cord. This includes the interaction of both the somatic and autonomic nervous systems.[40–43] Whereas the parasympathetic and somatic systems are located in the sacral spinal cord, the sympathetic system is located in the thoracolumbar spinal cord. Interruption of these delicate pathways at the level of the brain, spinal cord, nerve roots, or bladder can have a deleterious effect on voiding.

Patients with HIV infection may present with the primary complaint of urinary incontinence or urinary retention. After a careful medical history, physical examination, and urodynamic evaluation, patients may be divided into two categories: those with *hyperreflexic* bladders or those with *areflexic* bladders.

Important features of the medical history should include the following: Does the patient feel himself getting wet? Is there a precipitous, uncontrollable urge to void? How long can the patient hold the urine, once the urge is experienced? Is the incontinence associated with increased intra-abdominal pressure such as coughing, sneezing or physical activity? Does the patient have both the cognitive and physical capacities to reach the bathroom? What is the fluid intake of the patient? Does the patient take any medication that may affect urine output, such as diuretics or lithium? Does the patient take other medications, such as sympathomimetics or tricyclic antidepressants, that may enhance bladder outlet obstruction? Did the patient have any previous surgery that may contribute to abnormal voiding patterns, such as transurethral resection of the prostate, radical pelvic surgery, or urethral instrumentation? Does the patient have other concomitant medical conditions, such as diabetes, which can result in impaired bladder contractility secondary to autonomic neuropathy?

A general physical examination should include assessment of the prostate in males as well as evaluation for the presence of a cystocele in females. A neurourologic examination should assess the sensory and motor condition in the perineal region. At minimum, this examination should include assessment of anal sphincter tone, perianal sensation, and presence of a bulbocavernosus reflex. Baseline laboratory studies including urine analysis, urine culture, and serum creatinine and blood urea nitrogen should also be obtained.

Urodynamic evaluation in any patient with voiding dysfunction allows simultaneous correlation of voiding symptoms with visual and/or radiographic representation.[39] This evaluation is particularly important in patients with AIDS who may have multiple etiologies for their voiding symptoms. Urodynamic studies range from simple bedside cystometrograms to sophisticated, synchronous multichannel video/pressure/flow/electromyogram studies.[39] In most patients, the etiology of the voiding dysfunction can be established using a combination of history, physical examination, and simple bedside urodynamic studies. Multichannel studies should be reserved for patients in whom these basic diagnostic maneuvers have been inconclusive, therapy has been ineffective, or in whom multifactorial etiologies for symptoms exist. Thus, patients with AIDS and cerebrovascular accidents or benign prostatic hypertrophy who are suspected of having superimposed causes for their voiding symptoms should be aggressively evaluated before instituting therapy.

Hyperreflexic Bladders

Patients with encephalitis or upper motor neuron injury who present with urinary urgency and urge incontinence are likely to have hyperreflexic bladders.[44] Anticholinergic medications can effectively treat these symptoms. In addition these patients may have severe cognitive impairment resulting in urinary incontinence because of loss of voluntary control of the external urethral sphincter. This is similar to the neurourologic impairment seen in patients with Alzheimer's or cerebrovascular disease.[44] Once urinary tract infection is excluded as an etiologic factor, these patients are best treated with condom catheter drainage or diapers.

Areflexic Bladders

Patients who have lower motor neuron involvement either primarily or secondary to concomitant infections or malignancies may develop areflexic bladders. Classically, these patients have decreased urinary stream and hesitancy and may present with frank urinary retention. Most HIV-infected patients who present with urinary retention have areflexic bladders without concomitant bladder outlet obstruction.[4] Therefore younger patients who are less likely to have bladder outlet obstruction secondary to BPH do not need a sophisticated urodynamic evaluation. These patients can be treated successfully with intermittent catheterization.

SEXUALLY TRANSMITTED DISEASES

Not surprisingly, there is an increased incidence of sexually transmitted disease in HIV-infected patients, including syphilis, herpes genitalis, condyloma acuminata, and candidiasis.

Patients with AIDS are more likely to develop tertiary syphilis despite adequate treatment of the early infection.[45] This is most likely secondary to altered and deficient cell-mediated immunity. This suggests that HIV-infected patients who present with either primary or secondary syphilis should be treated more aggressively than the general population (i.e., longer duration and multiple courses) because they respond more slowly to conventional penicillin therapy.[46]

There have been reports of increased prevalence of both genital herpes and condyloma acuminata in patients with AIDS.[47] Although amenable to treatment with acyclovir, herpetic lesions last longer in HIV-infected patients. In fact, herpetic lesions lasting longer than 30 days are suggestive of AIDS.[16] As one would expect, altered cellular immunity is the single most important factor in the systemic dissemination of herpes. Acyclovir-resistant mucocutaneous herpes simplex has also been reported in HIV-infected patients.[48,49] Intravenous administration of foscarnet[48] or topical application of trifluridine[49] has proved effective in these cases. Condyloma acuminata may appear extensively in both the genital or anal region; however, there is no evidence of systemic spread in patients with AIDS. Lasers (CO_2, KTP-532, and neodymium:YAG) have proven to be the most effective treatment for condyloma acuminatum of the external genitalia[50] and would be the treatment of choice in cases of extensive lesions.

Candidiasis is a common finding in patients with AIDS. Men who are uncircumcised are normally at increased risk of developing candida balanitis. The prevalence of balanitis is greatly increased in patients with AIDS. Although local therapy may be tried, it is usually unsuccessful and circumcision may be required.

Several studies have suggested that there may be a link between Reiter syndrome and HIV infection.[51,52] Classic Reiter syndrome consists of a triad of asymmetric oligoarthritis, conjunctivitis, and nongonococcal urethritis or cervicitis. The urethritis or cervicitis, which may often be sterile by culture, is presumed to be sexually transmitted, and usually precedes the onset of arthritis by 2 to 4 weeks. Immune dysfunction, cellular lymphokines, arthritogenic pathogens, and the direct effect of HIV have all been proposed explanations for the possible association of HIV infection and Reiter syndrome.[53]

SEXUAL DYSFUNCTION

In any debilitated patient, sexual function may be compromised. Impotence, however, may occur in HIV-infected patients who are asymptomatic or in minimally symptomatic patients with AIDS. There are a variety of psychogenic and neurogenic factors that may play a role in the sexual dysfunction of these patients. Certainly, the specter of having a disease that may be ultimately fatal has strong emotional consequences with resultant functional disabilities, including sexual dysfunction. In addition, HIV-infected patients may have primary or secondary neurologic involvement due to infection or malignancy. This may manifest as erectile dysfunction or retrograde ejaculation.[4] Success with conservative treatment of erectile dysfunction has been achieved with the use of intracavernosal injection of vasodilatory substances (i.e., papaverine or prostaglandin), or penile vacuum/constrictor devices. Irreversible measures, such as the placement of a penile prosthesis, should be avoided because of the increased incidence of infection. All patients treated for erectile dysfunction *must* be counseled on their continued infectivity and safe sexual practices.[54]

CONCLUSION

There are a variety of urologic manifestations in the HIV-infected patient. Although many are poorly documented and anecdotal, health care workers involved in the treatment of HIV-infected patients should be familiar with them. Some causal relationships are poorly understood at present. As the magnitude of the AIDS pandemic continues to increase, clinicians will be more commonly faced with the urologic manifestation of this disease.

REFERENCES

1. Centers for Disease Control and Prevention: *Pneumocystis* pneumonia—Los Angeles. MMWR 30:250, 1981
2. Centers for Disease Control and Prevention: Kaposi's sarcoma and *Pneumocystis pneumonia* among homosexual men—New York City and California. MMWR 30:305, 1981
3. Mann JM: The HIV pandemic: status and trends. In Mann JM, Tarantola DJM, Netter TW (eds): AIDS in the World. Harvard University Press, Cambridge, MA, 1992
4. Catanese AJ, Tessler AN, Morales P: AIDS and the urologist: urologic manifestations of AIDS. AUA Update Series 8:1, 1989
5. Miles BJ, Melser M, Farah R et al: The urological manifestations of the acquired immunodeficiency syndrome. J Urol 142:771, 1989
6. Kaplan MS, Wechsler M, Benson MC: Urologic manifestations of AIDS. Urology 30:441, 1987
7. Gardenswartz MH, Lerner CW, Seligson GR et al: Renal disease in patients with AIDS: a clinicopathologic study. Clin Nephrol 21:197, 1984
8. Valeri A, Neusy A-J: Acute and chronic renal disease in hospitalized AIDS patients. Clin Nephrol 35:110, 1991
9. Rao TKS, Filippone EJ, Nicastri AD et al.: Associated focal and segmental glo-

merulosclerosis in the acquired immunodeficiency syndrome. N Engl J Med 310: 669, 1984

10. Rao TKS, Friedman EA, Nicastri AD: The types of renal disease in the acquired immunodeficiency syndrome. N Engl J Med 316:1062, 1987
11. Bouroignie J: Renal complications of human immunodeficiency virus type 1. Kidney Int 37:1571, 1990
12. Simon DI, Brosius FC, Rothstein DM: Sulfadiazine crystalluria revisited. Arch Intern Med 150:2379, 1990
13. Cendron M, Garber BB: Sulfadiazine urolithiasis in a patient with AIDS. Infect Urol March/April:60, 1993
14. Carbone LG, Bendixen B, Appel GB: Sulfadiazine-associated obstructive nephropathy occurring in a patient with AIDS. Am J Kidney Dis 12:72, 1988
15. Sasson JP, Dratch PL, Shotsleeve MJ: Renal US findings in sulfadiazine-induced crystalluria. Radiology 185:739, 1992
16. Centers for Disease Control and Prevention: Revision of the CDC surveillance case definition for acquired immunodeficiency syndrome. MMWR 36:1s, 1987
17. Swierzewski SJ, Wan J, Boffini A, Faerber GJ: The management of meatal obstruction due to Kaposi's sarcoma of the glans penis. J Urol 150:193, 1993
18. Vapnek JM, Quivey JM, Carroll PR: AIDS-related Kaposi's sarcoma of the male genitalia: management with radiation therapy. J Urol 146:333, 1991
19. Bayne D, Wise GJ: Kaposi's sarcoma of penis and genitalia: a disease of our time. Urology 31:22, 1987
20. Seftel AD, Sadick NS, Waldbaum RS: Kaposi's sarcoma of the penis in a patient with the acquired immunodeficiency syndrome. J Urol 136:673, 1986
21. Tessler AN, Catanese AJ: AIDS and germ cell tumors of the testis. Urology 30: 203, 1987
22. Wilson WT, Frenkel E, Vuitch F, Sagalowsky AI: Testicular tumors in men with HIV. J Urol 147:1038, 1992
23. Palmer MC, Mador DR, Venner PM: Testicular seminoma associated with the acquired immunodeficiency syndrome and acquired immunodeficiency syndrome related complex: 2 case reports. J Urol 142:128, 1989
24. Roehrborn CG, Worrell JT, Wiley EL: Bilateral synchronous testis tumors of different histology in a patient with the immunodeficiency syndrome related complex. J Urol 144:353, 1990
25. Dixon FJ, Moore RA: Tumors of the male sex organs. In Atlas of Tumor Pathology. Armed Forces Institute of Pathology, Washington, DC, 1952
26. Sokovich RS, Bormes TP, McKiel CF: AIDS presenting as testicular lymphoma. J Urol 147:1110, 1992
27. Mohler JL, Jarow JP, Marshall FF: Unusual urologic manifestations of acquired immunodeficiency syndrome: large cell lymphoma. J Urol 138:627, 1986
28. Tsang K, Kneafsey P, Gill MJ: Primary lymphoma of the kidney in the acquired immunodeficiency syndrome. Arch Pathol Lab Med 117:541, 1993
29. Bermudez AM, Grant KM, Rodvien R, Mendes F: Non-Hodgkin's lymphoma in a population with or at risk for acquired immunodeficiency syndrome: indications for intensive chemotherapy. Am J Med 86:71, 1989
30. Zighelboim J, Goldfarb RA, Mody D et al: Prostatic abscess due to histoplasma capsulatum in a patient with the acquired immunodeficiency syndrome. J Urol 147:166, 1992

31. Marans HY, Mandell W, Kislak JW et al: Prostatic abscess due to histoplasma capsulatum in the acquired immunodeficiency syndrome. J Urol 145:1275, 1991
32. Mamo GJ, Rivero MA, Jacobs SC: Cryptococcal prostatic abscess associated with the acquired immunodeficiency syndrome. J Urol 148:889, 1992
33. Halpern M, Szabo S, Hochberg E et al: Renal aspergilloma: an unusual cause of infection in a patient with the acquired immunodeficiency syndrome. Am J Med 92:437, 1992
34. Piketty C, George F, Weiss L et al: Renal aspergilloma in AIDS. Am J Med 94:557, 1993
35. Randazzo RF, Hulette CM, Gottlieb MS: Cytomegaloviral epididymitis in a patient with the acquired immunodeficiency syndrome. J Urol 136:1095, 1986
36. Haskell L, Fusco MJ, Ares L, Sublay B: Case report: disseminated toxoplasmosis presenting as symptomatic orchitis and nephrotic syndrome. Am J Med Sci 298:185, 1989
37. Centers for Disease Control and Prevention: Tuberculosis and acquired immunodeficiency syndrome. New York City. MMWR 36:788, 1987
38. Lemann W, Cho ES, Nielsen S, Petito C: Neuropathologic findings in 104 cases of acquired immunodeficiency syndrome (AIDS): an autopsy study. J Neuropathol Exp Neurol 44:349A, 1985
39. Kaplan SA, Blaivas JG: Practical approach to the diagnosis of urinary incontinence. Semin Neurol 8:131, 1988
40. Nathan PW, Smith NC: The centripetal pathway from the bladder and urethra within the spinal cord. J Neurol Neurosurg Psychiatry 14:262, 1951
41. Nathan PW, Smith NC: The centrifugal pathway of micturation within the spinal cord. J Neurol Neurosurg Psychiatry 21:177, 1958
42. Bradley WE, Conway CJ: Bladder representation in the pontine mesencephalic reticular formation. Exp Neurol 16:237, 1966
43. Fletcher TF, Bradley WE: Neuroanatomy of the bladder-urethra. J Urol 119:153, 1978
44. Kaplan SA, Brown WC, Blaivas JG: Management of urologic dysfunction in stroke patients. Contemp Urol 2:45, 1990
45. Johns DR, Tierney M, Felsenstein D: Alterations in the natural history of neurosyphilis by concurrent infection with the human immundeficiency virus. N Engl J Med 318:1569, 1988
46. Musher DM, Hamill RJ, Baughn RE: Effect of HIV infection on the course of syphilis and on the response to treatment. Ann Intern Med 113:872, 1990
47. Kent C, Samuel M, Winkelstein W: The role of anal/genital warts in HIV infection. JAMA 258:385, 1987
48. Safrin S, Crumpacker C, Chatis P et al: A controlled trial comparing foscarnet with vidarabine for acyclovir-resistant mucocutaneous herpes simplex in the acquired immunodeficiency syndrome. N Engl J Med 325:551, 1991
49. Murphy M, Morley A, Eglin RP, Montiero E: Topical trifluridine for mucocutaneous acyclovir-resistant herpes simplex II in AIDS patient. Lancet 340:1040, 1992
50. Malloy TR, Zderic SA, Carpiniello VL: External genital lesions. p. 23. In Smith JA (ed): Lasers in Urologic Surgery. Year Book Medical Publishers, Chicago, 1989
51. Winchester R, Bernstein DH, Fischer HD et al: The co-occurrence of Reiter's

syndrome and acquired immunodeficiency syndrome. Ann Intern Med 106:19, 1987
52. Lin R: Reiter's syndrome and human immunodeficiency virus infection. Dermatologica 176:39, 1988
53. Mills OF, Saradarian KA: Reiter's syndrome and HIV infection. J Fam Pract 33:294, 1991
54. Smith JR, Forster GE, Kitchen VS et al: Infertility management in HIV positive couples: a dilemma. BMJ 302:1447, 1991

10

Renal Aspects of Antimicrobial Therapy for HIV Infection

Jeffrey S. Berns *Michael R. Rudnick*
Raphael M. Cohen *William M. Bennett*

INTRODUCTION

ANTIVIRAL AGENTS
  Zidovudine, Didanosine, Zalcitabine, Stavudine
  Foscarnet
  Acyclovir
  Ganciclovir
  Interferon-α

ANTIFUNGAL AGENTS
  Amphotericin B
  Azole Antifungal Agents: Ketoconazole, Fluconazole, Itraconazole

ANTIPROTOZOAL AGENTS
  Trimethoprim-Sulfamethoxazole
  Sulfadiazine
  Pentamidine
  Pyrimethamine
  Dapsone
  Atovaquone
  Primaquine
  Paromomycin

ANTIMYCOBACTERIAL AGENTS
  Isoniazid
  Rifampin
  Rifabutin
  Ethambutol
  Pyrazinamide

Clofazamine
Capreomycin
Ciprofloxacin and Ofloxacin

MISCELLANEOUS DRUGS
Clarithromycin and Azithromycin

CONCLUSIONS

INTRODUCTION

In patients with the acquired immunodeficiency syndrome (AIDS), acute renal failure (ARF) and fluid-electrolyte disturbances are frequent complications of drugs used to treat human immunodeficiency virus (HIV) and associated opportunistic infections (Tables 10-1 and 10-2). In this chapter, we review the renal and fluid-electrolyte complications and clinical pharmacokinetics of many of these drugs, and provide recommendations for adjusting drug doses in patients with renal insufficiency. Much of the pharmacokinetic information that is available was not obtained in HIV-infected patients. Additionally, because the use of combinations of drugs, as is so common in these patients, may alter pharmacokinetics, a certain amount of empiricism is inherent in some of these dosing suggestions. References have been limited for the most part to those that are most current, clinically oriented, related to HIV-infected patients, or update our earlier review,[1] to which the reader is referred for a more complete compilation of references. Other excellent resources for additional information are also available.[2]

Table 10-1. Drugs That May Cause Renal Insufficiency

Foscarnet
Acyclovir
Interferon-α
TMP-SMX
Sulfadiazine
Pentamidine
Dapsone[a]
Rifampin
Ethambutol[a]
Pyrazinamide[a]
Capreomycin
Ciprofloxacin
Azithromycin[a]

Abbreviation: TMP-SMX, trimethoprim-sulfamethoxazole.
  [a] Uncommon, isolated reports.

Table 10-2. Drug-Induced Fluid and Electrolyte Disturbances

Altered water balance: hyponatremia, diabetes insipidus
    Didanosine[a]
    Foscarnet[a]
    Amphotericin B
    TMP-SMX
    Rifampin
    Capreomycin
Electrolyte disorders and renal tubular abnormalities
    Zidovudine[a]
    Didanosine
    Foscarnet
    Amphotericin B
    Itraconazole[a]
    Fluconazole[a]
    TMP-SMX
    Pentamidine
    Rifampin
    Clofazamine[a]
    Ofloxacin[a]
    Capreomycin
Altered uric acid excretion or metabolism
    Didanosine
    Rifampin
    Ethambutol
    Pyrazinamide

Abbreviation: TMP-SMX, trimethoprim-sulfamethoxazole.
[a] Uncommon, isolated reports.

ANTIVIRAL AGENTS

Zidovudine, Didanosine, Zalcitabine, and Stavudine

Four antiretroviral dideoxynucleoside analogs are now available for the treatment of HIV infection: zidovudine (3'-azido-2',3'-dideoxythymidine, AZT), didanosine (2',3'-dideoxyinosine, ddI), zalcitabine (2',3'-dideoxycytidine, ddC, and stavudine (2',3'-didehydro-3'-deoxythymidine, d4T). Upon intracellular phosphorylation, these drugs exert their antiviral effect primarily by inhibiting retroviral reverse transcriptase. Despite increasingly widespread clinical use, no direct nephrotoxicity has yet been reported with these drugs.

Several cases of aerobic (type B) lactic acidosis have recently been described in patients with AIDS, some of whom were being treated with zidovudine.[3,4] A mitochondrial myopathy due to zidovudine was implicated in one patient,[3] but the biochemical basis for the lactic acidosis, and the precise role of zidovudine, as opposed to sepsis, liver disease, thiamine deficiency, or other factors, needs to be clarified. Asymptomatic hyperuricemia is common in patients treated with didanosine, particularly at higher doses, because of metabolism of this purine analog to hypoxanthine and then uric acid. Reduction of the dose and intravascular volume expansion usually correct the hyperuricemia. Hyperuricemia is not a complication of treatment with zidovudine or zalcitabine, which are pyrimidine analogs. Hypokalemia has been reported in a few patients treated with didanosine; the cause of the hypokalemia and the relative roles of didanosine itself or its citrate/phosphate/sucrose buffering vehicle are not known. Hypocalcemia, usually due to pancreatitis, may also occur in patients treated with didanosine. Symptomatic hypocalcemia has occurred, however, without clinical evidence of pancreatitis; with normal serum magnesium, phosphorus, parathyroid hormone (PTH), and vitamin D levels; and may recur upon rechallenge with didanosine.[5] A Fanconi syndrome with nephrogenic diabetes insipidus has been described in a patient who was receiving didanosine along with other medications.[6] Each didanosine tablet contains 15.7 mEq of magnesium hydroxide and 11.5 mEq of sodium, and each packet of didanosine buffered powder contains 60 mEq of sodium, which may pose problems in patients on sodium-restricted diets or with renal insufficiency. No renal toxicities of stavudine have been reported.

Clinical use of the didanosine prodrug 2′,3′-dideoxyadenosine (ddA) has been abandoned because of the potential renal toxicity of the ddA hydrolysis product adenine. When administered in high doses, adenine can lead to an obstructive uropathy and ARF due to intratubular precipitation of its metabolite 2,8-dihydroxyadenine.[7]

Approximately 15 to 20 percent of a dose of zidovudine is excreted unchanged in the urine, with 60 to 75 percent of the dose recovered as the inactive hepatic glucuronide metabolite, GAZT. Renal clearance of zidovudine exceeds glomerular filtration rate (GFR) by severalfold, indicating a contribution of tubular secretion. Probenecid, a competitive inhibitor of renal proximal tubule organic anion transport (and of hepatic glucuronidation), reduces the renal clearance of GAZT and, in some patients, zidovudine.[8] The increased area under the plasma concentration-time curve (AUC) and elimination half-life of zidovudine after probenecid administration are primarily due to inhibition of zidovudine glucuronidation by probenecid, however, because renal clearance normally accounts for only about 10 to 20 percent of total clearance. These data, as well as studies with rat renal basolateral membrane vesicles, have led to the conclusion that these compounds are secreted primarily by a proximal tubule basolateral membrane organic anion transporter. Inhibition of renal zidovudine secretion by the organic cations cimetidine and trimethoprim (TMP),[9] and studies in rat renal brush border membrane vesicles, suggest that zidovudine may also interact with an organic cation transport system.

About 25 percent of zidovudine is bound to plasma proteins. The volume of distribution, which is between 1.4 and 3.2 L/kg in normal individuals, appears to be decreased with renal failure. Renal failure reduces total body clearance and urinary excretion of zidovudine and GAZT. The elimination half-life of zidovudine in dialysis patients varies greatly, and while usually normal (about 1 hour) or only slightly prolonged, may be as much as 8 hours in some patients with end-stage renal disease (ESRD). GAZT accumulates in the presence of renal failure, without any recognized clinical effects. Zidovudine is removed by hemodialysis, although the amount removed appears to vary among patients and is probably not of great clinical significance. Little if any zidovudine is removed by peritoneal dialysis.[10,11]

The oral bioavailability of didanosine is highly variable. Between 5 and 40 percent of an oral dose appears in the urine. Renal clearance of didanosine, which exceeds GFR and is therefore thought to be in part due to tubular secretion, accounts for 30 to 35 percent of total body clearance. The drug is less than 5 percent protein bound in plasma, and has a volume of distribution of about 1 L/kg. Following a single oral dose, the mean half-life of didanosine was found to be increased from 1.5 hours in normal controls to 4.5 hours in patients with hemodialysis-dependent renal failure.[12] Advanced renal failure did not alter the volume of distribution, but the total plasma clearance was reduced by about 75 percent. Hemodialysis clearance averaged 107 ml/min, with removal of only about 20 percent of the total didanosine pool, and no significant effect on the plasma concentration. The removal of didanosine was not influenced by different dialysis membranes or hemodiafiltration.[12] No information is yet available on didanosine pharmacokinetics with peritoneal dialysis.

Little human pharmacokinetic data are available for zalcitabine and stavudine. The plasma of zalcitabine half-life ranges from about 0.5 to 3 hours, with a volume of distribution of about 0.6 L/kg. Less than 4 percent of the drug is bound to plasma proteins. About 75 percent of an oral dose is excreted unchanged in the urine, with a renal clearance of 190 ml/min/m^2, indicating that tubular secretion probably contributes to urinary excretion. The elimination half-life has been reported to be increased to as much as 8.5 hours in patients with mild to moderate renal insufficiency (data on file, Roche Laboratories). Stavudine is readily absorbed after oral administration. The volume of distribution is 0.53 L/kg, the plasma elimination half-life is 1.0 to 1.6 hours, and about 35 to 40 percent of a dose is excreted unchanged in the urine. Stavudine is thought to undergo renal tubular secretion.[12a] No information is available on zalcitabine or stavudine pharmacokinetics in patients with severe renal failure or the effects of hemodialysis and peritoneal dialysis.

Dosing recommendations for zidovudine, didanosine, and zalcitabine in patients with renal insufficiency are indicated in Table 10-3. Particularly for the latter two drugs and stavudine, additional information is needed in order to develop more precise guidelines.

Foscarnet

Foscarnet (trisodium phosphonoformate) is an inorganic pyrophosphate analog with antiviral activity against all of the human herpes viruses and HIV, which is used primarily for the treatment of serious cytomegalovirus infections and acyclovir-resistant herpes simplex infections.

Table 10-3. Dosing Recommendations: Zidovudine, Didanosine, Zalcitabine[a]

Drug/Usual Dose	Recommended Dose by GFR (ml/min)		
	50–90	10–50	<10
Zidovudine			
200 mg PO tid	Usual	Usual	100 mg tid–200 mg bid
Didanosine			
200–375 mg PO bid	Usual	200–375 mg qd	150–250 mg qd
Zalcitabine			
0.75 mg PO tid	Usual	.375–.75 mg bid	.375–.75 mg qd

[a] For hemodialysis and peritoneal dialysis: use dose recommended for GFR <10 ml/min (little or no data for didanosine and zalcitabine).

Experimentally, foscarnet acutely exerts a specific, reversible, competitive inhibition of renal proximal tubule Na^+-P_i cotransport. Inhibition of Na^+-P_i cotransport in brush border membrane vesicles from human renal cortex has been reported to be even more sensitive to foscarnet than in rat renal brush border membrane vesicles.[13] After prolonged (>0.5 hours) incubation with foscarnet an increase in Na^+-P_i cotransport has been observed, an effect attributed to an upregulatory increase in the insertion of Na^+-P_i transporters into the apical membrane.[14]

ARF has occurred in as many as two-thirds of patients treated with foscarnet and is not infrequently the dose-limiting toxicity. The urinary sediment is typically benign, although proteinuria, usually less than 1 g/d, may be present. Foscarnet-induced ARF typically begins within 1 to 3 weeks of starting the drug and is usually mild and reversible, although dialysis may be required temporarily. Recovery may be slow, particularly in patients with preexisting renal insufficiency, and the serum creatinine concentration may remain persistently elevated for several months.

Use of other nephrotoxic drugs and intravascular volume depletion may increase the risk of foscarnet-induced ARF. Intravenous infusion of 1 to 2.5 L of isotonic saline may reduce the incidence of foscarnet nephrotoxicity and allow patients with renal insufficiency to receive foscarnet without further reduction of kidney function. Intermittent infusion of foscarnet, as the drug is currently administered, may result in less nephrotoxicity than the continuous infusion protocols used initially, perhaps because of delivery of lower daily and cumulative doses or lower trough drug levels.

The mechanism of foscarnet-induced ARF is not known. The drug has been reported to exhibit dose- and time-dependent cytotoxic effects in human renal proximal tubule cells in culture. Tubulointerstitial lesions have been described in kidney biopsy and autopsy specimens from foscarnet-treated patients, with proximal tubular epithelial cell vacuolization and necrosis, an interstitial cellular infiltrate with a predominance of polymorphonuclear leukocytes, and deposition of calcium salts in areas of damaged epithelium. In a few patients, crystals described as having characteristics of crystalline foscarnet have been found in glomerular capillary lumina.

Polyuria and polydipsia in patients receiving foscarnet may be related to the sodium load of trisodium foscarnet or the large volume of fluids often administered with the drug. A single case of nephrogenic diabetes insipidus has been reported in a patient receiving foscarnet.[15] Hypocalcemia and hypercalcemia, hypophosphatemia and hyperphosphatemia, and hypomagnesemia may also occur, with hypocalcemia being the most frequent and serious disturbance. Patients who receive both foscarnet and intravenous pentamadine, which can also cause hypocalcemia, may be particularly at risk of the development of severe hypocalcemia.

Changes in the serum calcium and phosphate concentrations after foscarnet administration have been systematically studied by Jacobson and colleagues.[16] Ionized calcium levels fell below the lower limit of normal in all patients during a 2-hour infusion of 120 mg/kg, and 66 percent of those who received a 90 mg/kg dose, with symptomatic hypocalcemia developing in at least two patients. No changes in total calcium or phosphate concentrations occurred during the infusion. There were no significant changes after a 14-day course of therapy in serum phosphate, magnesium, ionized and total calcium, PTH, and 1,25-$(OH)_2$ vitamin D levels, or urinary calcium, phosphorus, magnesium, and potassium excretion.[16] In vitro studies showed an inverse relationship between serum or plasma foscarnet concentrations and ionized calcium concentration, but not with total calcium or phosphate concentrations.[16] Foscarnet did not increase protein-calcium binding, and the authors concluded that ionized hypocalcemia was probably a result of foscarnet, which is known to chelate calcium and other metal ions, complexing with ionized calcium.[16] Effects of foscarnet on bone and kidney function may also account for some of these electrolyte abnormalities.

Foscarnet is not metabolized, with elimination occurring primarily, if not exclusively, by urinary excretion. Renal clearance accounts for about 75 to 85 percent of total drug clearance. About 70 to 95 percent of a dose is excreted unchanged in the urine within 36 to 72 hours. After a highly variable initial serum half-life of 0.5 to 7 hours in patients wih normal kidney function, there is a long terminal elimination phase of several days. As much as 28 percent of a dose may be deposited into bone, from which it is probably very slowly excreted. About 15 percent of plasma foscarnet is protein bound. The hemodialytic clearance of foscarnet with cuprophane membranes has been reported to be as high as 108 ml/min.[17] In one patient on hemodialysis, the interdialytic half-life of 75 to 100 hours was reduced to 3 hours during a dialysis treatment, which resulted in a 50 percent reduction in the plasma foscarnet concentration.[17] Dose adjustments are necessary for patients with renal insufficiency and who are receiving dialysis (Table 10-4).

Acyclovir

Acyclovir (9-[(2-hydroxyethoxy)methyl]guanine) is a cyclic analog of deoxyguanosine that diffuses into cells, where its activation and accumulation is dependent on a herpes-virus-specific thymidine kinase. In vitro, acyclovir is most active against the herpes simplex viruses; varicella-zoster virus and Epstein-Barr virus are less sensitive, and cytomegalovirus, which lacks the

Table 10-4. Dosing Recommendations: Foscarnet, Acyclovir, Ganciclovir[a]

Drug/Usual Dose	Recommended Dose by GFR (ml/min)		
	50–90	10–50	<10
Foscarnet			
40–60 mg/kg IV q8h[b]	30–55 mg/kg q8h	20–30 mg/kg q8h[d]	Avoid
90–120 mg/kg IV qd[c]	60–90 mg/kg qd	50–80 mg/kg q24–48h[d]	Avoid
Acyclovir			
200–800 mg PO bid–5×/d	Usual	Usual	100–200 mg bid
5–10 mg/kg IV q8h	Usual	q12–24h	2.5–5 mg/kg qd
Ganciclovir			
5 mg/kg IV q12h[b]	1.25–2.5 mg/kg q12h	2.5 mg/kg qd	1.25 mg/kg qd
5 mg/kg IV qd[c]	2.5 mg/kg qd	1.25 mg/kg qd	0.6 mg/kg qd

[a] For hemodialysis (HD) and peritoneal dialysis (PD):
Foscarnet: 60 mg/kg IV post-HD only (limited data); no data for PD.
Acyclovir: use dose recommended for GFR <10 ml/min, give dose post-HD.
Ganciclovir: use dose recommended for GFR <10 ml/min, give dose (0.6–1.25 mg/kg) post-HD.
[b] Initiation therapy.
[c] Maintenance therapy.
[d] Avoid if GFR <30 ml/min.

thymidine kinase, is relatively resistant. Intravenous acyclovir is the drug of choice for treating serious herpes simplex or varicella-zoster infections, whereas oral acyclovir is used primarily for treatment of less severe herpes simplex infections and suppression of recurrent herpes simplex virus infection.

Evidence for significant nephrotoxicity of acyclovir was apparent from preclinical toxicologic studies, in which large parenteral doses resulted in the deposition of acyclovir crystals in distal renal tubules and collecting ducts, causing ARF due to tubular obstruction. Over the past 15 years, acyclovir nephrotoxicity has also been well documented in humans, with acute renal insufficiency developing in as many as 10 to 15 percent of patients treated with intravenous acyclovir.

Acyclovir-induced ARF usually occurs within the first few days of therapy, but may be detected after only a few doses or, more rarely, later in the course of treatment. Although patients may be asymptomatic, nausea, vomiting, and abdominal, back, or flank pain are common. Oliguria is uncommon, and the rise in the serum creatinine concentration is usually modest, in the range of 1 to 4 mg/dl, although more severe ARF may also occur. Dialysis has only rarely been necessary. Most patients recover renal function within 3 to 14 days of stopping acyclovir therapy, reducing the dose, or increasing volume repletion. Urinalysis typically shows trace proteinuria, microscopic hematuria, and variable degrees of pyuria. Birefringent needle-shaped crystals may be seen either free or within white blood cells in the urine sediment[18] (Fig. 10-1). However, it should be noted that acyclovir crystalluria has also been found in patients without ARF. The most important risk factors for acyclovir nephrotoxicity are intravascular volume contraction, preexisting renal insufficiency, and high-dose rapid bolus intravenous infusion,[19] although nephrotoxicity with oral acyclovir has also rarely been reported.[20] Volume expansion with intravenous fluids and administration of the drug over 1 hour, rather than as a bolus, reduce the risk of ARF. The risk of developing mild azotemia may be higher with high-dose intravenous therapy in outpatients than in hospitalized patients, perhaps because of less careful attention to intravascular volume status.

Crystal deposits have been seen in some, but not all, histopathologic renal specimens, which may show evidence of tubulointerstitial injury with cellular necrosis, proteinaceous tubular casts, and interstitial infiltration with lymphocytes, plasma cells, eosinophils, and occasional granulomata.[18,21] Thus, it is not clear whether acyclovir-induced ARF in humans is due entirely to an obstructive nephropathy from intratubular precipitation of acyclovir or whether a toxic, immunologic, or hypersensitivity reaction may also be involved.

In patients with underlying renal insufficiency, neurologic side effects of acyclovir, such as confusion, lethargy, coma, hallucinations, myoclonus, tremors, seizures, and psychiatric disturbances, which are usually associated with elevated blood levels of acyclovir and tend to occur in elderly patients or those on high-dose intravenous acyclovir, may occur at lower intravenous doses or even after oral administration.[22,23]

Acyclovir has limited oral bioavailability with peak serum levels after oral dosing less than 3 to 10 percent of those achieved with intravenous dosing. As implied by the findings of acyclovir crystalluria, urinary excretion is the main route of acyclovir elimination. In patients with normal renal function, the plasma half-life of an intravenous dose is approximately 2 to 3 hours, with 70 to 90 percent of a single dose excreted unchanged in the urine. The renal clearance of about 250 to 300 ml/min/m^2 greatly exceeds GFR and may result in urine concentrations of acyclovir that exceed the maximal urinary solubility of about 1.7 mg/ml, particularly after intravenous bolus administration. Probenecid, by blocking tubular secretion, reduces the renal clearance of acyclovir. Urinary excretion of the only major metabolite, 9-carboxymethoxyethylguanine, accounts for about 10 percent of a dose. As renal function declines, total plasma clearance falls, although both nonrenal clearance of acyclovir and urinary excretion of 9-carboxymethoxyethylguanine increase. In anuric patients, plasma clearance falls to approximately 10 percent of normal and the half-life increases to about 20 hours.

Acyclovir, which is only about 15 percent protein-bound and has a steady-state volume of distribution approximating total body water, is readily removed by hemodialysis, which reduces the plasma half-life to about 5.5 hours and removes about 40 to 60 percent of acyclovir body stores during a 4-hour

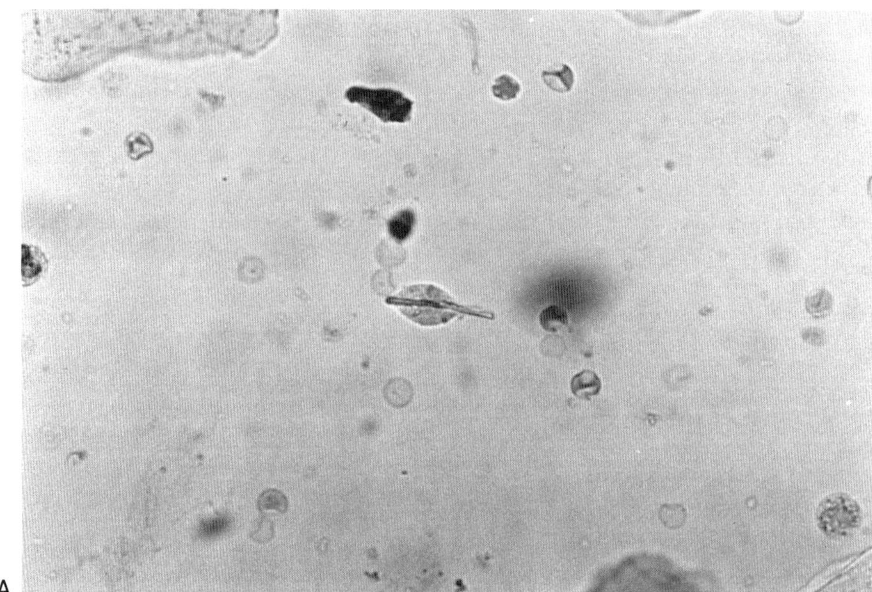

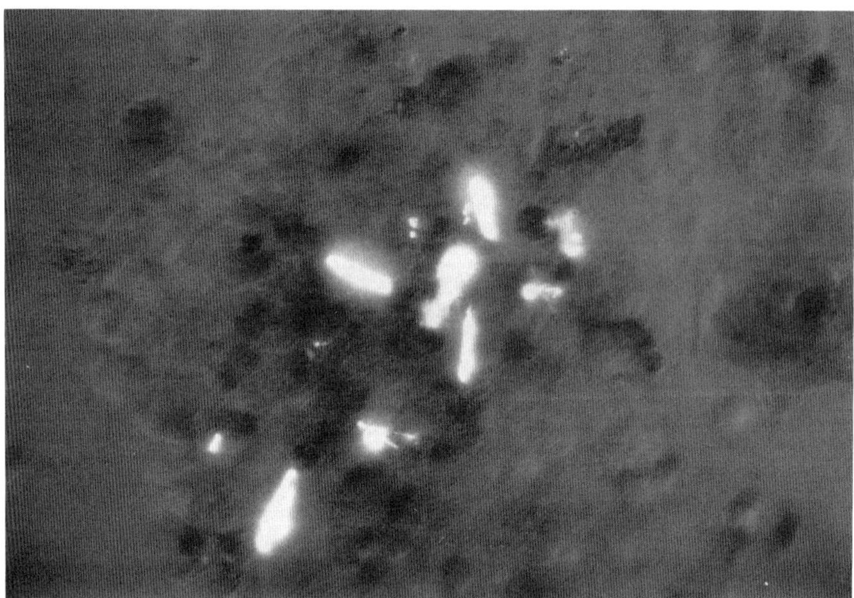

Fig. 10-1. (**A**) Needle-shaped crystal in the urine sediment of a patient with acyclovir-induced nephrotoxicity. (**B**) Birefringent crystals seen with polarizing microscopy in the urine sediment of a patient with acyclovir-induced nephrotoxicity. (From Sawyer et al.,[18] with permission.)

treatment. Although 60 to 90 percent of an intraperitoneal dose may be absorbed, both rapidly cycled peritoneal dialysis and continuous ambulatory peritoneal dialysis (CAPD) clear acyclovir from the circulation inefficiently, as does continuous arteriovenous hemodialysis (CAVHD).[24] Hemodialysis remains the therapy of choice for patients with significant acyclovir neurotoxicity and renal insufficiency, including those already treated with chronic peritoneal dialysis.[22,23] Dosing recommendations for patients with renal impairment are given in Table 10-4.

Ganciclovir

Ganciclovir (9-(1,3-dihydroxy-2-propoxymethyl)guanine, DHPG), an acyclic nucleoside analog of guanine, is structurally similar to acyclovir. As the result of a minor chemical modification, it has proven to be more effective in the treatment and prophylaxis of cytomegalovirus infection in immunocompromised hosts, including those with AIDS. Unlike acyclovir, ganciclovir has no significant nephrotoxicity.

Ganciclovir is excreted by the kidneys without metabolism, with over 90 percent of a dose appearing in the urine in 24 hours. The terminal serum half-life is approximately 2.5 to 3.5 hours in patients with normal renal function. Renal clearance is proportional to, but greater than, creatinine clearance, suggesting significant tubular secretion. The serum half-life may exceed 15 hours in patients with advanced renal failure. Ganciclovir is well-cleared by standard hemodialysis, which reduces the plasma concentration by 60 to 70 percent,[25] and continuous hemofiltration membranes.[26] Dosing guidelines for ganciclovir are provided in Table 10-4.

Interferon-α

Interferons are naturally occurring proteins released by cells in response to viruses, double-stranded RNA, foreign antigens, and mitogens. Although originally defined by their ability to interfere with viral infection, the interferons have a variety of biologic effects, and have been used extensively in cancer therapy. Three classes of interferons have been recognized: interferon-α is produced primarily by B and null lymphocytes and macrophages, interferon-β is produced primarily in epithelial cells and fibroblasts, and interferon-γ is produced mainly in T lymphocytes.[27,28] Interferon-α is available clinically as α-2a and α-2b, manufactured by recombinant DNA technology, and α-n3 derived from pooled human leukocytes. Interferon-α has been used for treatment of a variety of viral infections, such as condylomata acuminata; chronic hepatitis B and C virus infections, including hepatitis B and C virus-associated glomerulonephritis[29,30]; and HIV infection.[31] Treatment with interferons is associated with a variety of systemic toxicities including fever, flulike symptoms, hypotension (which may be severe), tachyarrhythmias, diarrhea, nausea, vomiting, leukopenia, and elevated liver function tests.[27,32]

Experimental nephrotoxicity of interferons was initially reported in studies by Gresser and colleagues.[33] Injections of newborn Swiss mice with interferon for the first 6 to 8 days of life produced a severe immune complex type of glomerulonephritis. Interferon administration may also accelerate the immune-complex glomerulonephritis that develops in New Zealand Black/New Zealand White hybrid (NZB/NZW F_1) mice. A dose-dependent inhibitory effect of interferon-α on glucose and alanine uptake in rat renal brush border membrane vesicles has also been demonstrated.

Proteinuria has been reported in as many as 65 percent of patients in some clinical trials with interferon-α, but in most series the incidence has been about 10 to 25 percent.[32,34] The proteinuria is usually less than 1 g/d, although heavier proteinuria, including the nephrotic syndrome, has been reported. Mild azotemia, which may occur in up to 10 percent of patients, may resolve despite continued treatment. More severe ARF, which may be associated with a nephrotic syndrome, has also rarely developed.

Histopathologic studies in one patient with a nephrotic syndrome and ARF showed normal-appearing glomeruli by light microscopy, with an interstitial infiltrate of leukocytes, eosinophils, and plasma cells, and diffuse epithelial cell foot process effacement without electron-dense deposits on electron microscopy.[35] In another case, a kidney biopsy revealed diffuse thickening of the glomerular basement membrane and focal segmental mesangial sclerosis without an interstitial infiltrate. Immunofluorescent studies showed focal IgM deposits along glomerular capillary loops, and focal C3 staining in blood vessel walls. Electron microscopy demonstrated electron-dense deposits and widening of the lamina rara interna by a "fluffy" material.[36] The presence of dermatologic changes and a positive antinuclear antibody (ANA) test in this patient led the authors to suggest that interferon may have induced an "autoimmune state," which caused these glomerular abnormalities. Consistent with this hypothesis is the development of systemic lupus erythematosus (SLE), with elevated ANA and anti-double-stranded DNA titers, hypocomplementemia, and low-grade proteinuria in another patient who had been receiving an extended course of interferon-α.[37]

The renal effects of recombinant leukocyte interferon-α have also been studied in renal transplant recipients.[38] In each of eight interferon-treated patients, steroid-resistant acute vascular rejection occurred, complicated by the nephrotic syndrome in three patients, which resolved when the interferon regimen was discontinued. In one of the patients with a nephrotic syndrome, a proliferative glomerulonephritis with IgM, C3, and fibrinogen deposits was present. Histologic studies showed changes of acute vascular rejection with normal glomeruli in the remaining patients.

Proteinuria and azotemia have also been reported with recombinant interferon-β and interferon-γ. In addition, several patients treated with recombinant interferon-γ for systemic sclerosis have developed acute scleroderma renal crisis, with malignant hypertension and renal failure, including one patient who had received only three small test-doses of the drug.[39] The pathogenetic role of the interferon preparation, and whether a similar problem may occur with interferon-α, is not clear.

Interferon-α is filtered by the glomerulus and then undergoes rapid proteolysis after proximal tubular reabsorption. Less than 4 percent of a dose appears in the urine.[40] Interferon-α is very rapidly cleared from the circulation, with less than 0.1 percent of a dose remaining in the circulation 24 hours after an intravenous dose. More sustained plasma levels are maintained after intramuscular or subcutaneous administration.[41] Very limited data in humans suggest that interferon-α serum levels and pharmacokinetics may be unchanged in patients with renal failure or by hemodialysis.[42] This contrasts, however, with experimental data showing elevated plasma levels and reduced clearance of interferon-α in bilaterally nephrectomized rats.[43] No specific dosing recommendations can yet be made for patients with renal insufficiency, and caution with interferon-α therapy in these patients is warranted.

ANTIFUNGAL AGENTS

Amphotericin B

Although the new azole antifungal agents discussed below are effective and safe alternatives to amphotericin B in many patients, amphotericin B remains the mainstay of treatment for deep-seated mycotic infections, especially in immunocompromised patients. This poorly soluble, lipophilic polyene macrolide antibiotic, derived as a by-product of the fermentation of a soil actinomycete, is prepared for clinical use as a colloidal suspension with sodium deoxycholate as a solubilizing agent. Because this suspension can be disrupted in an electrolyte solution, amphotericin B must be diluted in sterile water for administration. The fungicidal effect of amphotericin B is attributed to its binding to ergosterol in the cell walls of susceptible fungi, which disrupts membrane permeability, resulting in leakage of cell contents and cell death. The drug also binds to other sterols, including cholesterol, and some of the common side effects of amphotericin B such as fever, chills, local thrombophlebitis, and anemia may be due to this interaction of the drug with mammalian cell membranes.

Among the numerous toxicities of amphotericin B, renal dysfunction is one of the most frequent and troublesome, with 25 to 85 percent of patients developing azotemia or renal tubular dysfunction. Amphotericin-B-induced ARF is characteristically nonoliguric, with the urinalysis showing varying degrees of pyuria, hematuria, renal tubular cells and casts, but little proteinuria. In some patients, azotemia develops within the first few days of therapy and may resolve relatively promptly with increased sodium supplementation or discontinuation of diuretics. Many reports, however, have indicated a strong dose dependence, with renal insufficiency occurring in only 10 to 15 percent of patients who have received a cumulative dose less than 0.5 to 1 g, but in 75 to 80 percent of those who have received more than 3 to 4 g. In these patients, recovery of kidney function may occur more slowly over a period of several weeks to months after stopping the drug. Irreversible renal insufficiency has rarely been reported, particularly with cumulative doses exceeding 4 to 5 g.

Additional factors other than the cumulative dose that may increase the risk of ARF with amphotericin B include advanced age, volume depletion, underlying renal insufficiency, and concomitant use of diuretics or other nephrotoxic drugs. Intravascular volume status appears to be one of the most important determinants of amphotericin B nephrotoxicity. In animal models, sodium chloride loading has been shown to reduce the severity of amphotericin-B-induced ARF. Sodium chloride supplementation also reduces the frequency of amphotericin B nephrotoxicity in humans,[44] and may be helpful in reversing mild azotemia when it occurs early in the course of therapy. Although initial experimental observations suggested that mannitol could reduce the nephrotoxicity of amphotericin B, this has not been confirmed in humans[45] and its clinical utility remains unproven.

Experimental studies suggest that vasoconstriction, which may in part be mediated by activation of the tubuloglomerular feedback system due to increased delivery of sodium chloride to the distal tubule and macula densa, may be responsible for amphotericin-B-induced reductions in renal blood flow and GFR. Interventions that block or attenuate tubuloglomerular feedback mechanisms, such as treatment with furosemide, aminophylline, or calcium channel blockers, blunt amphotericin-B-induced renal vasoconstriction and ameliorate experimental amphotericin B nephrotoxicity. Not all studies have supported the role of the tubuloglomerular feedback system, however. Evidence for amphotericin-B-mediated vasoconstriction in other vascular beds has led to the suggestion that there may be a direct vascular effect of amphotericin B and that vasoactive mediators such as prostaglandins and cytokines may play a role in this vasoconstrictive response. An in vitro endothelium-independent vasoconstrictor effect of amphotericin B has been shown to be inhibited by aminophylline, atrial natriuretic peptide, calcium-free media, and calcium channel blockers,[46] suggesting the possibility that methylxanthine derivatives and calcium channel blockers may be effective in reducing amphotericin B nephrotoxicity. A recent in vitro study showed that histopathologic evidence of proximal tubular epithelial damage from amphotericin B could in large part be attributed to cytotoxic effects of the solubilizing component deoxycholate, that extracellular calcium played little role in this injury, and that osmotic agents, but not oxygen-free radical scavengers, were protective.[47] Thus, amphotericin B nephrotoxicity may have both an acute vascular component as well as a component due to epithelial cellular toxicity.[48] Consistent with the concept of a direct vascular effect of amphotericin B is a recent case report of malignant hypertension developing in a patient receiving the drug.[49] Human biopsy and autopsy material from patients who received amphotericin B have shown vascular changes as well as tubulointerstitial injury with acute tubular necrosis, tubular dilatation, and nephrocalcinosis with minimal glomerular changes.

Amphotericin B therapy is also frequently complicated by electrolyte disturbances. Studies with the turtle bladder and rat distal nephron elegantly demonstrated that amphotericin B increases epithelial hydrogen ion permeability without directly affecting transepithelial proton transport. The clinical manifestation of this drug-induced impairment of net hydrogen ion secretion is a "gradient-limited" distal renal tubular acidosis. The urinary acidifying defect may be subclinical (i.e., "incomplete distal renal tubular acidosis") until unmasked by diarrhea or other causes of metabolic acidosis. The accompanying hypokalemia, which has been attributed to renal potassium wasting due to increased potassium diffusion across the distal tubular epithelium, may be severe enough to cause paralysis or rhabdomyolysis and may be ameliorated by amiloride. Renal magnesium wasting with magnesium depletion may also contribute to the tendency for there to be urinary potassium wasting. Nephrogenic diabetes insipidus and renal salt wasting have also been described in patients receiving amphotericin B. Hyponatremia may develop because of the large volume of hypotonic fluids (5 percent dextrose in water) required for administration of the drug. These renal tubular abnormalities usually develop within the first few weeks of therapy, often without an impairment in the GFR, and are not prevented by measures that protect against the development of ARF. In fact, salt loading may exacerbate renal potassium wasting.[44] These tubular defects tend to resolve gradually over several months once amphotericin B is stopped.

The frequency of nephrotoxicity and other severe side effects with the standard formulation of amphotericin B has led to a search for less toxic preparations, such as liposomal amphotericin B and lipid-amphotericin B complexes. These new formulations may allow attainment of higher serum and tissue levels of the drug with less toxicity than seen with amphotericin B deoxycholate, although the clinical efficacy and toxicities of these experimental formulations remain to be established.[50]

Efforts to minimize amphotericin B nephrotoxicity, in addition to volume expansion, frequently involve manipulation of the drug-dosing regimen. Administration of twice the usual daily dose on alternate days or lowering the daily dose and extending the duration of therapy over a longer time period has been suggested, but not proven, to reduce renal toxicities of the drug. Many experts recommend temporarily stopping the drug for several days in the presence of a rising serum creatinine, with reinstitution of therapy at a reduced dose or with an alternate day regimen once the serum creatinine level stabilizes or begins to decline, although the efficacy of this approach has not been proven.

The fate of amphotericin B in the body is not well understood.[50] The drug is highly protein bound and has a steady-state volume of distribution of about 4 L/kg. No metabolites have been identified and less than 5 percent of a single dose appears in the urine after 24 hours, although up to 40 percent can be recovered in the urine after 7 days. After an initial plasma half-life of 40 hours, there is a terminal half-life of about 15 days, which presumably reflects slow release from a peripheral compartment. The drug can still be detected in blood and urine for up to 4 weeks after a single dose. Neither hepatic nor renal dysfunction appears to influence peak or trough drug levels. Other than in an attempt to reduce amphotericin-B-related ARF, dose adjustments are not necessary in patients with renal insufficiency. The large volume of distribution and extensive protein binding of amphotericin B prevent significant removal of the drug by hemodialysis or peritoneal dialysis.

Azole Antifungal Agents: Ketoconazole, Fluconazole, Itraconazole

The imidazole (ketoconazole) and triazole (fluconazole and itraconazole) agents have a broad spectrum of activity against a variety of fungi, and have been increasingly used for treatment of both superficial and systemic fungal infections. Their antifungal effects are due primarily to inhibition of the cytochrome P-450 enzyme-mediated synthesis of ergosterol, a major component of the fungal cell membrane, from lanosterol.

Compared with amphotericin B, the azoles are relatively free of significant renal toxicities. A nephrotic syndrome, which was reversible upon discontinuation of the drug, has been reported in one patient treated with itraconazole.[51] Mild hypertension, hypokalemia, and urinary frequency have also occasionally been noted in patients receiving itraconazole. In one instance, the hypokalemia was severe and associated with rhabdomyolysis.[52] Mild hypokalemia has also been seen in patients treated with fluconazole. Ketoconazole inhibits adrenal steroidogenesis and may uncommonly result in acute adrenal insufficiency. Basal serum cortisol levels and adrenal responsiveness to corticotropin have been found to be normal in patients receiving intraconazole,[53] although one case of reversible adrenal insufficiency with this drug has been reported.[52]

Ketoconazole is generally well absorbed from the gastrointestinal tract in the absence of reduced gastric acidity. It is highly bound to plasma proteins and red blood cells, with less than 1 percent free in plasma. Ketoconazole undergoes extensive hepatic metabolism with biliary excretion, and only negligible amounts of unchanged drug appear in the urine. No dose adjustments are necessary in patients with renal insufficiency. Little of the drug is removed by hemodialysis or appears in peritoneal dialysate, so supplemental doses are not necessary.[50]

Fluconazole, which may be administered either orally or intravenously, is nearly completely absorbed from the gastrointestinal tract after oral administration. It is much more water soluble than ketoconazole, and is only about 11 percent bound to plasma proteins. The elimination half-life is about 22 to 36 hours in patients with normal kidney function. Approximately 60 to 80 percent of a dose is excreted unchanged in the urine, with 10 percent appearing as metabolites.[50,54,55] Renal clearance of fluconazole is markedly reduced in patients with renal insufficiency, with an increase in the half-life to almost 60 hours in patients with a GFR of 30 to 70 ml/min and 100 to 125 hours when the GFR is less than 20 ml/min. Plasma levels fall by about 25 to 50 percent during hemodialysis treatments of 3 to 4 hours.[54,56,57] The elimination half-life of fluconazole during peritoneal dialysis is about

Table 10-5. Dosing Recommendations: Fluconazole, TMP-SMX, Sulfadiazine, Pentamidine[a]

Drug/Usual Dose	Recommended Dose by GFR (ml/min)		
	50–90	10–50	<10
Fluconazole			
100–200 mg PO/IV qd	Usual	q24–48h	q48–72h
TMP-SMX			
3–5 mg/kg PO/IV q6–8h[b,c]	12h	q18–24h	q24h or avoid
1 DS PO qd—3/wk[b,d]	Usual	Usual	Usual
Sulfadiazine			
0.5–1.5g PO q4–6h	q8–12h	q24h	q48–72h or avoid
Pentamidine			
4 mg/kg IV qd	Usual	q24–36h	q48h

[a] For hemodialysis (HD) and peritoneal dialysis (PD):
Fluconazole: 100–200 mg post-HD only, 50–100 mg qd (PD).
TMP-SMX: supplement ½ to full dose post-HD, use dose recommended for GFR <10 ml/min (PD).
Sulfadiazine: no data, avoid.
Pentamidine: use dose recommended for GFR <10 ml/min.
[b] As TMP; IV solution is TMP 16 mg/ml and SMX 80 mg/ml, DS (double-strength) tablet is 160 mg TMP/800 mg SMX.
[c] For acute infection.
[d] For prophylaxis.

70 to 85 hours, with 15 to 20 percent of an oral dose recovered in the dialysate over 48 hours. Peritoneal dialysate levels of fluconazole may reach 50 to 80 percent of the corresponding plasma level, allowing for the successful treatment of some cases of peritoneal dialysis-related fungal peritonitis. Dose adjustments for fluconazole in patients with renal failure or who are receiving dialysis are provided in Table 10-5.

Itraconazole is administered only orally, and has a rather variable gastrointestinal absorption. With chronic administration, the elimination half-life is about 30 to 40 hours, with extensive hepatic metabolism. Itraconazole is more than 99 percent bound to plasma proteins, and less than 1 percent of the active drug appears in the urine.[50,58,59] Little is known of the pharmacokinetics of itraconazole in patients with renal insufficiency. In one study, the single-dose pharmacokinetics of the drug were unchanged in patients with renal dysfunction, and neither hemodialysis nor peritoneal dialysis removed significant amounts of the drug.[60] Dose adjustments for patients with renal insufficiency or who are being dialyzed are therefore not necessary.

ANTIPROTOZOAL AGENTS

Trimethoprim-Sulfamethoxazole

Trimethoprim-sulfamethoxazole (TMP-SMX), which inhibits purine synthesis through synergistic inhibition of folate metabolism, is used in relatively high doses (TMP 15 to 20 mg/kg/d and SMX 75 to 100 mg/kg/d) to treat *Pneumocystis carinii* pneumonia (PCP) and in lower doses for PCP prophylaxis. Unexpectedly, many AIDS patients have developed significant dermatologic, hematologic, or hepatic toxicities with TMP-SMX.

Acute elevations of the serum creatinine during TMP-SMX therapy are usually due to inhibition of renal tubular creatinine secretion by TMP, an organic base, resulting in diminished creatinine clearance without a change in actual GFR. The rise in serum creatinine is roughly proportional to the baseline serum creatinine, and is usually less than 0.3 mg/dl in subjects with normal renal function. In patients with renal insufficiency, in whom creatinine secretion contributes a proportionately greater amount to the creatinine clearance, a more substantial and noticeable increase in the serum creatinine, as much as 1 to 3 mg/dl, may be seen. The serum creatinine increases within the first few days of TMP-SMX therapy, then levels off despite continuation of the drug and returns to baseline within days of TMP-SMX discontinuation. Although this effect does not reflect renal damage, it may be a source of confusion in situations where the GFR is subject to change for other reasons, as is often the circumstance in patients with AIDS.

Much less commonly, TMP-SMX may cause an acute interstitial nephritis with clinical features of systemic hypersensitivity including fever, rash, eosinophilia, and eosinophiluria. Renal histology has revealed interstitial edema, focal areas of mononuclear cell infiltration, segmental areas of tubular injury and necrosis, along with rare granuloma formation. These reactions have generally been attributed to the sulfa moiety of SMX or one of its metabolites. As with other sulfonamides, the hypersensitivity reaction may rarely present as a systemic vasculitis. Although SMX is relatively soluble in urine, its main metabolite, N^4-acetylsulfamethoxazole, is less soluble and may rarely cause crystalluria with ARF and kidney stones. Low urinary pH reduces the solubility of the drug and its metabolites, and may promote crystalluria, particularly in a highly concentrated urine.

TMP-SMX also causes alterations of tubular function resulting in electrolyte disorders. Rare cases of a renal tubular acidosis that may be associated with an inappropriately high urine pH, salt wasting, and/or hyperkalemia have been reported in patients treated with TMP-SMX. Stimulated by anecdotal observations of unexplained hyperkalemia in AIDS patients receiving TMP-SMX, several prospective studies have found elevated serum potassium concentrations in as many as 75 percent of AIDS patients receiving high-dose TMP-SMX, with potentially life-threatening hyperkalemia in up to 10 percent of cases.[61-63] The serum potassium concentration usually peaks within 7 to 10 days of initiating high-dose TMP-SMX and returns to normal within a week after discontinuation of the drug. Hyperkalemia occurs in these cases in the absence of significant reductions in the GFR and with normal renin and adrenocortical axis function, an inappropriately low or reduced urinary potassium excretion rate, and unresponsiveness to exogenous mineralocorticoid.[62-64] In experimental animals, TMP reduces renal potassium excretion and increases sodium excretion, and in rat distal tubule micropuncture studies, it reduces the lumen-negative transepithelial voltage and net potassium secretion.[63] Trimethoprim is a heterocyclic weak base that is structurally related to the potassium-sparing diuretics amiloride and triamterene, leading to the conclusion that TMP can similarly block sodium channels in distal tubular epithelium, causing a voltage-gradient defect that results in hyperkalemia, salt wasting, and renal tubular acidosis.[63,64] In vitro investigations have demonstrated that TMP, in concentration ranges that may occur in the urine of patients treated with high-dose therapy, inhibits sodium transport across frog skin epithelia and reversibly inhibits sodium-dependent amiloride-sensitive short-circuit current in the A6 cell line derived from the toad bladder.[64] Patch clamp studies in A6 cells have recently demonstrated that TMP applied to the apical but not basolateral membrane reversibly blocks amiloride-sensitive highly selective Na^+ channels.[65] It has been further speculated that an acidic urine exacerbates this complication because more urinary TMP (pK_a 7.2) will be in the protonated form that is likely to be the sodium channel blocker.[64] A higher incidence of hyperkalemia with a TMP-dapsone combination regimen compared with TMP-SMX[61] may be due to a reduction by dapsone of hepatic metabolism of TMP, leading to higher serum and urinary levels of the drug.[66] TMP-SMX in standard doses has also been reported to cause hyperkalemia in elderly patients.[67–69]

Hyponatremia, a common problem in AIDS patients, may be exacerbated by both TMP-induced salt wasting and by the large cumulative free water load necessitated by the manufacturer's recommendation that each ampule of TMP-SMX (80 mg of TMP and 400 mg of SMX) be dissolved in 75 to 125 ml of 5 percent dextrose solution. Despite its relative instability in solution, 50 ml of isotonic saline can serve as the diluent for each ampule of TMP-SMX, which would ameliorate any tendency to cause hyponatremia.

The pharmacokinetics of a combination drug such as TMP-SMX present some dosing difficulties in patients with renal failure. Both components are extensively cleared by the kidneys, with urinary acidification enhancing urinary TMP excretion and urinary alkalinization enhancing SMX excretion. Whereas 80 percent of a TMP dose is excreted unchanged in the urine, and another 20 percent is eliminated as metabolites, only 10 to 20 percent of an SMX dose is recovered unchanged in the urine, with 80 percent excreted in the form of inactive metabolites, largely N^4-acetylsulfamethoxazole. Both drugs have similar half-lives of 8 to 12 hours in patients with normal renal function. With renal insufficiency, nonrenal metabolism and clearance of both drugs increase. Significant changes in the elimination half-life of trimethoprim do not occur until the GFR falls below about 30 ml/min, whereas the total clearance of SMX shows little change even in patients with advanced renal failure.[70] However, inactive SMX metabolites accumulate in patients with renal failure and may be associated with hypersensitivity reactions or insoluble urinary precipitates. Peritoneal dialysis removes little TMP, SMX, or their metabolites.[71] Although most studies have found efficient hemodialytic removal of TMP and SMX, dialytic clearance of SMX metabolites is poor, leading to some confusion regarding the need for supplemental doses after hemodialysis. Similarly, the more extensive protein binding of TMP and N^4-acetylsulfamethoxazole suggests that less removal of these compounds will occur during continuous hemofiltration techniques (e.g., CAVH, CAVHD) than of the less highly protein-bound SMX.

Dosing guidelines for TMP-SMX in patients with renal failure who are being treated with high doses needed for *P. carinii* infections are not clearly defined (Table 10-5). Monitoring of blood drug levels would be ideal, but is not routinely available, and use of alternative agents should be considered in patients with advanced renal insufficiency.

Sulfadiazine

Sulfadiazine is a relatively short-acting sulfonamide derivative used in combination with pyrimethamine for the treatment of central nervous system (CNS) toxoplasmosis. The major renal toxicity of sulfadiazine is crystalluria, which may occur in 5 percent or more of patients treated with the large doses needed to treat severe cerebral toxoplasmosis (2 to 8 g/d), due to the low solubility of the drug in an acidic urine.[72] Patients usually present with typical features of renal colic, but may also be relatively asymptomatic. Volume depletion due to fever, vomiting, or diarrhea and a low urine pH predispose patients to sulfadiazine crystalluria. "Shocks of wheat" crystals of sulfadiazine or the metabolites N-acetylsulfadiazine or 2-sulfanilamido-pyrimidine may be seen in the urine[73] (Fig. 10-2). The calculi are radiolucent

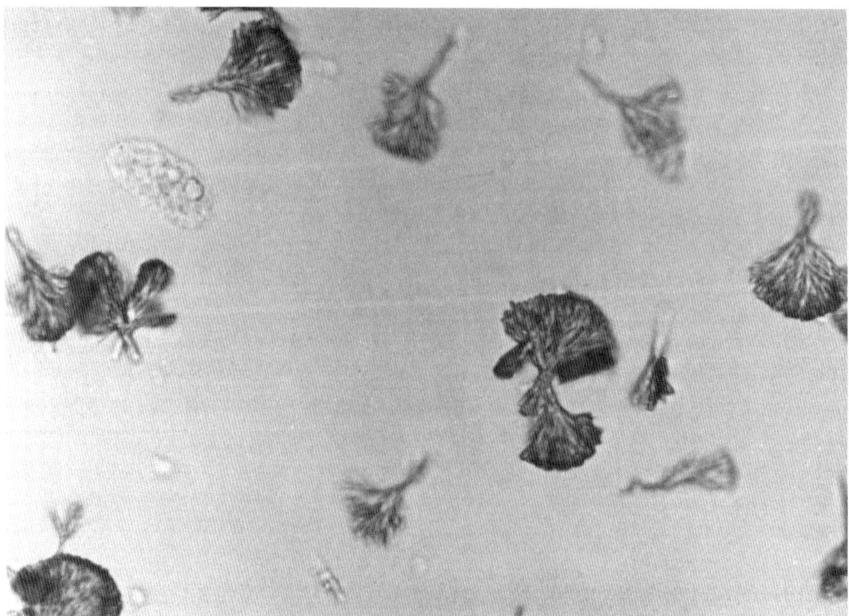

Fig. 10-2. "Shocks of wheat" crystals in urine sediment of a patient with sulfadiazine-induced ARF. (From Oster et al.,[73] with permission.)

by plain radiography. Ultrasonography usually shows multiple echogenic foci or sludge in the collecting system; hydronephrosis may or may not be present. Bilateral urinary tract obstruction may cause oligoanuric ARF requiring temporary dialysis, and placement of ureteral or percutaneous stents may be necessary for the acute management of urinary tract obstruction. Administration of oral or intravenous fluids and alkaline diuresis to achieve a urine pH greater than 7.15 rapidly reverses the renal insufficiency in most cases.[72] Sulfadiazine can be continued in some patients if adequate volume repletion (2 to 3 L/d) and urinary alkalinization with 6 to 12 g of sodium bicarbonate to keep the urine pH greater than 7.15 can be maintained, although the dose may need to be reduced.[73] In most patients, alternative therapies are probably preferred. Severe ARF due to allergic interstitial nephritis has also occurred with sulfadiazine.

Sulfadiazine is excreted into the urine by both glomerular filtration and tubular secretion. Fifteen to 40 percent of the drug is excreted in the acetylated form. Protein binding, normally 30 to 55 percent, is reduced in patients with renal insufficiency. In patients with severe renal failure, the normal half-life of 8 to 17 hours may be prolonged up to 35 hours, with markedly reduced urinary excretion of the active drug and concomitantly elevated plasma levels. Although sulfadiazine is cleared to some extent by hemodialysis, the clinical significance of this is not well defined. Precise dosing guidelines have not been established in patients with renal failure, and avoidance of sulfonamides is generally recommended in those with significant azotemia. The suggested dose adjustments in Table 10-5 may be used if sulfadiazine treatment is necessary.

Pentamidine

Originally developed for treatment of trypanosomiasis and leishmaniasis, pentamidine has become a mainstay of therapy for *P. carinii* infection in patients with AIDS. The incidence of ARF in AIDS patients treated with pentamidine has ranged from 25 percent to as high as 95 percent in different studies. In most cases the renal failure is relatively mild and nonoliguric, although more severe ARF may occur in up to 5 percent of patients. Dialysis is only rarely required, usually in patients who are severely ill and receiving other nephrotoxic agents. The need for dialysis in patients with pentamidine-related ARF is associated with a high mortality. The onset of ARF usually occurs after 7 to 12 days of therapy, with recovery of kidney function beginning within a week of stopping the drug. A return to baseline function is generally seen within several weeks. The urinalysis typically shows mild proteinuria, pyuria, glycosuria, and granular casts. Gross hematuria has also rarely been seen.

Risk factors for pentamidine-induced ARF include use of other nephrotoxic drugs and underlying renal insufficiency. The role of volume depletion as an exacerbating factor has been suggested by studies in experimental animal models as well as a greater incidence of nephrotoxicity in patients who receive pentamidine as outpatients without supplemental intravenous fluids, compared with well-hydrated inpatients. Pentamidine-induced ARF is more likely to occur with a prolonged course of therapy and large cumulative doses. The risk of nephrotoxicity has been correlated with serum levels of the drug by some investigators.[74] Although others have failed to confirm this association, the use of inhaled pentamidine, which produces low serum levels of the drug, has only very rarely been associated with the development of ARF.

Few reports of the renal histopathologic features of pentamidine-associated ARF in humans are available. Degenerative changes in the proximal tubule have been described and, in experimental animals, dose-dependent renal toxicity correlates with swelling and degeneration of renal tubular epithelial cells. Although the kidneys are a major site of tissue accumulation of pentamidine, the mechanism underlying the renal toxicities of this drug are unknown. It has been postulated that pentamidine may precipitate nucleic acids within renal tubular epithelial cells, resulting in depletion of the intracellular nucleotide pool required for energy-dependent cellular functions.

Pentamidine may also cause renal tubular dysfunction and fluid-electrolyte disturbances. Hyperkalemia, often associated with hyperchloremic metabolic acidosis, has been reported in 25 to 95 percent of AIDS patients treated with pentamidine. This usually occurs after more than a week of therapy, in patients who have also developed ARF. Urinary magnesium wasting and hypomagnesemia, which may be associated with cardiac arrhythmias and symptomatic hypocalcemia, may persist for months after cessation of pentamidine therapy.[75] Hypocalcemia, which is seen during 2 to 12 percent of courses of pentamidine therapy, may also complicate pentamidine-induced pancreatitis. Although hyponatremia in patients with pentamidine-induced ARF has been noted, it is not clear to what extent this is directly related to pentamidine, because hyponatremia is such a common complication in patients with HIV infection. Although hypoglycemia is a well-recognized complication of pentamidine treatment,[74] diabetes mellitus with ketoacidosis has also been reported.[76]

Despite significant tissue accumulation of pentamidine in the kidneys, less than 5 percent of a dose is excreted in the urine over 24 hours. Although small amounts may be found in the urine for 6 to 8 weeks after a dose, renal excretion accounts for less than 10 percent of total body clearance. Intermediate and terminal plasma half-lives of 5 to 6 hours and 10 to 15 days, respectively, are not significantly altered in patients with impaired renal function.[77] Pentamidine is extensively tissue and protein bound, with a volume of distribution that exceeds 3 L/kg.

Although these pharmacokinetic characteristics suggest that dosing modification is not necessary in patients with renal insufficiency,[78] some authors do recommend dose reductions for patients with significant renal impairment (Table 10-5), although this may not reduce the incidence of pentamidine-induced ARF. The large volume of distribution and extensive tissue and protein binding suggest that little drug would be removed with dialysis, so dose supplements after hemodialysis are probably unnecessary.

Pyrimethamine

Pyrimethamine, an inhibitor of dihydrofolate reductase used for malaria prophylaxis, acts synergistically with sulfadiazine against *Toxoplasma gondii* and is used to treat cerebral toxoplasmosis. It does not appear to be nephrotoxic. Like TMP, which is chemically similar to pyrimethamine, and cimetidine, pyrimethamine inhibits renal creatinine secretion and reduces creatinine clearance without affecting the inulin clearance or GFR.[79] Therefore, an increase in the serum creatinine concentration may be observed within the first few days after pyrimethamine is started.

Pyrimethamine is highly protein bound, has a volume of distribution of about 2.4 L/kg, and a mean plasma half-life of about 80 to 105 hours. In patients with normal kidney function, only 1 to 4 percent of a single dose is excreted into the urine during each of the first 7 to 10 days, but small amounts of pyrimethamine and its metabolites continue to appear in the urine for up to 30 to 50 days, so that 16 to 32 percent of a single dose may eventually be excreted in the urine.[80] Dose adjustments are probably not necessary in patients with renal failure, although accumulation of pyrimethamine may occur during prolonged therapy with the typical daily maintenance doses of 25 to 75 mg used for treatment of cerebral toxoplasmosis.

Dapsone

A sulfone antibiotic chemically related to the sulfonamides, dapsone has been used for the treatment of leprosy and dermatitis herpetiformis, and for the treatment and prophylaxis of quinine-resistant *Plasmodium falciparum* malaria. Dapsone is now used in patients with HIV infection as an alternative to TMP-SMX and aerosolized pentamidine for PCP prophylaxis, and to a lesser extent for treatment of acute *P. carinii* infection.

Nephrotic syndrome, ARF with hemoglobinuria due to dapsone-induced intravascular hemolysis, and renal papillary necrosis have been rarely reported in patients receiving dapsone. Mild hyperkalemia has been reported to occur more frequently in patients treated with a combination of dapsone and TMP than with TMP-SMX, whereas hyperkalemia has not been found in patients receiving dapsone alone. As discussed earlier, this may be related to a recently observed drug interaction between dapsone and TMP, which results in higher plasma concentrations of both drugs when used together.[66] The elevated TMP levels may be responsible for the observed increase in plasma potassium concentrations, because TMP has recently been shown to inhibit renal potassium excretion and cause reversible hyperkalemia by an amiloridelike action on distal nephron apical sodium channels.[63–65]

Dapsone is primarily metabolized by hepatic N-hydroxylation and acetylation. The mean serum half-life is about 1 to 3 days and the volume of distribution is about 2 L/kg. In patients with normal kidney function, about 10 to 20 percent of an oral dose appears in the urine within the first few days after a dose, although up to 70 percent may eventually be excreted in the urine, mostly as metabolites and glucuronide or sulfate conjugates.[81,82] Because dapsone is extensively bound to plasma proteins, little drug is likely to be removed by dialysis. No specific guidelines for dose adjustments of dapsone in patients with renal insufficiency are available, although some dose reduction may be advisable.

Atovaquone

Atovaquone is a hydroxynaphthoquinone recently approved for oral treatment of mild to moderate PCP in patients who are intolerant of TMP-SMX. The drug also has antimicrobial activity against *P. falciparum* and *T. gondii*. There have been no nephrotoxic reactions or fluid-electrolyte disturbances yet reported with clinical or experimental use of the drug.

Atovaquone is apparently not metabolized, but undergoes biliary secretion with an enterohepatic cycle and ultimate fecal excretion. Little if any atovaquone appears in the urine. The terminal serum elimination half-life is on the order of 2 to 3 days. Circulating drug is virtually completely protein bound (personal communication, Burroughs Wellcome, 1994).[83] No information is yet available on the effects of renal insufficiency or dialysis on atovaquone pharmacokinetics, although it would appear unlikely that either would significantly alter drug metabolism or levels.

Primaquine

The combination of clindamycin and primaquine, an 8-aminoquinolone that has been used in the treatment of malaria, appears to be effective therapy for PCP. Primaquine has several important toxicities, including methemoglobinemia, hemolytic anemia in glucose-6-phosphate dehydrogenase (G6PD) deficient individuals, and granulocytopenia, but does not appear to be directly nephrotoxic or a cause of fluid-electrolyte disturbances.

Primaquine is rapidly, but variably, absorbed from the gastrointestinal tract, then widely distributed into tissues with a variable volume of distribution that may be as much as 150 to 300 L. The drug is rapidly and extensively metabolized, with a terminal elimination half-life of 3 to 8 hours. Less than 4 percent of active drug appears in the urine over 6 days in patients with normal kidney function, although over 60 percent is excreted as various metabolites.[84,85] Although no specific information is available, it is unlikely that renal insufficiency or dialysis has a clinically significant effect on primaquine pharmacokinetics, although metabolites may accumulate. Clindamycin, which is used in conjunction with primaquine, is not nephrotoxic and does not require dose adjustments in patients with renal insufficiency.

Paromomycin

Paromomycin is an aminoglycoside that is usually administered orally in divided doses of 1.5 to 2 g/d to treat intestinal amebiasis and cryptosporidiosis in AIDS patients. Parenteral paromomycin, which is not presently available in the United States, has also been used to treat cryptosporidial cholangiopathy. Very little paromomycin is normally absorbed after oral administration, and therefore it does not cause significant systemic or renal toxicities.[86] As with neomycin, another oral "nonabsorbable" aminoglycoside, caution in patients with ulcerative lesions of the bowel is urged because absorption may occur and lead to nephrotoxicity. Dose adjustments in patients with renal insufficiency should not be needed with oral paromomycin, but will be necessary for parenteral use of the drug.

ANTIMYCOBACTERIAL AGENTS
Isoniazid

No nephrotoxicity or fluid-electrolyte complications have been attributed to isoniazid (INH). INH is only minimally protein bound and distributes in a volume of about 0.6 L/kg. Fifty to 95 percent of a dose is excreted in the urine within 24 hours in patients with normal kidney function, mostly as metabolites. Plasma levels and urinary excretion are dependent on genetically determined rates of hepatic acetylation. The normal serum half-life varies widely from about 1 to 10 hours, in a bimodal distribution based on acetylator phenotype. In the presence of renal failure, the half-life is usually within this normal range, but may be prolonged in some patients.[87]

Dose adjustments for INH are not needed in patients with renal failure, although some have recommended a reduction in the dose from 300 to 200 mg/d in patients with severe renal failure (GFR <10 ml/min) who are not being treated with dialysis. The usual daily dose should be given after a hemodialysis treatment, because as much as 46 to 90 percent of a dose may be removed during the treatment. Significant amounts of INH were removed by hourly exchanges of peritoneal dialysis in a child with INH poisoning and extremely elevated plasma INH levels, but standard doses of 300 mg/ d are usually recommended for patients on CAPD. Pyridoxine supplements of 50 to 100 mg/d are necessary while patients are receiving INH to avoid INH-related neurotoxicities.[88]

Rifampin

ARF is an uncommon but well-described complication of rifampin therapy, particularly with intermittent, interrupted, or otherwise discontinuous drug therapy.[1,89] Fewer cases have been associated with continuous therapy. Patients may present within minutes to hours of a dose with lumbar or abdominal pain, vomiting, rigors, fever, hypotension, malaise, diarrhea, myalgias, rash, and edema, with the abrupt onset of ARF, which is often oliguric. Rarely, patients may be relatively asymptomatic or develop ARF of more insidious onset. Serum complement levels are usually normal. Urinalysis reveals proteinuria, which may be in the nephrotic range; microscopic or macroscopic hematuria; and less commonly, eosinophiluria. Dialysis has been required in many cases. Complete recovery usually occurs over a period of several months, although some patients do not fully recover renal function. A variety of renal tubular abnormalities have also been described in patients treated with rifampin, such as glucosuria, renal potassium wasting, urinary acidification defects, an increase in the fractional excretion of uric acid, and nephrogenic diabetes insipidus. Rifampin increases the hepatic metabolism of cortisol and other glucocorticosteroids. This may precipitate an acute adrenal crisis with hypotension, hyponatremia, and hyperkalemia in patients with adrenal insufficiency, including those on replacement therapy. The dose of steroids in patients with known adrenal insufficiency should therefore be at least doubled when rifampin is being administered.[90]

Antirifampin antibodies have been found in the serum of patients treated with rifampin, particularly those with ARF and acute toxic reactions with hemolysis,[91] suggesting that ARF in these patients may be an immunologically mediated process. Not all patients with rifampin-associated ARF have detectable antirifampin antibodies, however. These antibodies can also be found in some rifampin-treated patients without ARF or other toxicities, so their pathogenetic role remains a bit uncertain. Rechallenge with rifampin after an episode of ARF may be accompanied by recurrence of ARF, particularly in those with antirifampin antibodies, and should be avoided if at all possible.

Histologic changes with rifampin-induced ARF consist primarily of tubulointerstitial nephritis with a mononuclear cellular infiltrate and occasional eosinophils, interstitial edema, and acute tubular necrosis. Glomeruli are usually normal, although mild mesangial proliferation may be seen. Rarely, renal cortical necrosis with glomerular capillary fibrin thrombi has been described. Immunofluorescent studies are usually negative, but have rarely demonstrated immunoglobulin and complement deposition. Electron microscopy is also usually normal, although mesangial, paramesangial, and subendothelial electron-dense deposits have occasionally been seen. Rapidly progressive (crescentic) glomerulonephritis, interstitial nephritis, mesangial proliferative glomerulonephritis, and thrombotic thrombocytopenic purpura (TTP)[92] have also been rarely associated with rifampin therapy.

Immunoglobulin light chains, usually κ alone or both κ and λ, have been reported in the urine of patients receiving rifampin without clinical manifestations of kidney disease, as well as in the urine and renal biopsies of patients with rifampin-related ARF.[93] Histologic findings in the latter group of patients have included dense eosinophilic proteinaceous casts and focal and segmental glomerular sclerosis, which has been noted to be similar to the findings seen in multiple myeloma and light-chain nephropathy.[94]

Between 10 and 25 percent of a dose of rifampin is excreted unchanged in the urine over 24 hours, staining the urine (as well as other body fluids) orange-brown. Up to 40 percent of an administered dose is excreted as metabolites. About 70 to 90 percent of rifampin is bound to plasma proteins. The half-life varies from about 2.5 to 5 hours, and is only minimally prolonged in patients with severe renal failure, although serum levels do tend to be somewhat elevated in these patients compared with normals. Despite this, dose adjustments are not necessary in patients with renal insufficiency. Because neither hemodialysis nor peritoneal dialysis removes significant amounts of rifampin, supplemental doses are not needed in patients with ESRD.[87]

Rifabutin

Rifabutin is a semisynthetic rifamycin antibiotic that is similar to rifampin, with in vitro activity against *Mycobacterium avium-intracellulare* and *M. tuberculosis*. Like rifampin, rifabutin colors urine and other body fluids an orange-brown color. Although mild azotemia has been noted in some patients treated with rifabutin, a specific relationship to the drug has not been established, and no other definite nephrotoxicity of rifabutin has been reported.[95]

Rifabutin is extensively metabolized to over 20 metabolic products. Following a single oral dose, about 5 percent is excreted unchanged in the urine in 24 hours, with a urine concentration greatly exceeding that of plasma. Fifty percent of a dose may be excreted in the urine, largely as metabolites, over several days.[96] The drug is 85 percent protein bound, and is widely distributed in tissues with a volume of distribution about 15 times total body water.[96] The elimination half-life in patients with varying degrees of renal insufficiency has been reported to be between 11 and 26 hours, which is less than that observed in other patients (45 to 67 hours) (data on file, Adria Laboratories). The reasons for this are not clear, although the volume of distribution may be lower in patients with renal insufficiency, and further study of this drug's pharmacokinetics are needed. Dose adjustments, however, are probably not needed for patients with renal insufficiency. No information is available regarding the dialytic clearance of rifabutin, but significant clearance is unlikely given its large volume of distribution and extensive protein and tissue binding.

Ethambutol

Several cases of ARF due to tubulointerstitial nephritis have been attributed to ethambutol, although in each case other antituberculous drugs were also prescribed. Ethambutol reduces renal excretion of uric acid, producing elevations in the serum uric acid level in many patients.

Table 10-6. Dosing Recommendations: Ethambutol, Pyrazinamide, Capreomycin[a]

| | Recommended Dose by GFR (ml/min) | | |
Drug/Usual Dose	50–90	10–50	<10
Ethambutol			
15–25 mg/kg PO qd	15 mg/kg qd	15 mg/kg q24–36h	15 mg/kg q48h
Pyrazinamide			
15–30 mg/kg PO qd	Usual	10–20 mg/kg qd or 40–60 mg/kg 3 times/wk	
Capreomycin			
1 g IM qd	0.5–1 g qd	0.25–0.5 g q24–48h	0.25 g q48–72h

[a] Hemodialysis (HD) and peritoneal dialysis (PD):
Ethambutol: avoid, or use dose recommended for GFR <10 ml/min, give dose post-HD.
Pyrazinamide: avoid, or use 30–60 mg/kg 3 times/week on nondialysis days.
Capreomycin: use dose recommended for GFR <10 ml/min.

Approximately 60 to 80 percent of an orally administered dose of ethambutol appears in the urine in individuals with normal kidney function, mostly as unchanged drug. About 20 to 30 percent is bound to plasma proteins. Renal clearance of ethambutol, about 7 ml/min/kg, greatly exceeds GFR, indicating that tubular secretion contributes to its clearance. Plasma clearance is markedly reduced in patients with renal insufficiency, with the serum half-life increasing from 3 to 4 hours in patients with normal renal function to between 7 and 15 hours in patients with renal failure.[87] Although significant clearance of ethambutol with hemodialysis (mean dialysance approximately 50 ml/min) and peritoneal dialysis has been reported, the total amount of drug removed may actually be rather small. Dosing recommendations are provided in Table 10-6. Given the risk of ocular toxicity even with reduced doses, which may result in inadequate antimycobacterial therapy, it may be best to use alternative agents in patients with renal insufficiency.

Pyrazinamide

Although a high incidence of hepatotoxicity initially limited the widespread use of pyrazinamide, this drug is now used in lower doses in combination with other antimycobacterial agents to treat multidrug-resistant tuberculosis. The most frequent side effect is hyperuricemia, which occurs in up to 40 percent of patients. This is often associated with polyarthralgias, with acute gouty arthritis occurring less commonly. Pyrazinamide and its main metabolite pyrazinoic acid suppress uric acid secretion by the renal proximal tubule, probably by competitive inhibition of peritubular urate anion exchange, an effect used to investigate clinical disorders of urate homeostasis. Pyrazinamide-induced hyperuricemia may be difficult to control with allopurinol because, despite reducing uric acid production, allopurinol also leads to an accumulation of pyrazinoic acid, which further suppresses uric acid excretion. Rifampin appears to increase the urinary excretion of both uric acid and pyrazinoic acid, which may explain the observation that hyperuricemia and arthralgias are less common in patients receiving both drugs than in those receiving pyrazinamide alone.[97] Acute interstitial nephritis has been reported in a patient receiving multiple drugs for treatment of tuberculosis, which resolved only after pyrazinamide was discontinued. A case of pyrazinamide-associated rhabdomyolysis with myoglobinuric ARF has recently been reported.[98] In transplant patients, pyrazinamide may indirectly affect renal function by causing a reduction in cyclosporine levels, which may predispose to development of acute transplant rejection.[99]

Pyrazinamide is rapidly and completely absorbed after oral administration with an elimination half-life of about 8.5 to 9.5 hours.[87] Only a tiny fraction appears in the urine as unchanged drug. The major pathway of metabolism appears to be microsomal deamidation to pyrazinoic acid. The plasma half-life of pyrazinamide is not significantly altered in patients with renal insufficiency, although its metabolite pyrazinoic acid may accumulate. Pyrazinamide and its metabolites are effectively cleared by dialysis, with 15 to 43 percent of a dose removed as pyrazinamide and up to 70 percent of a dose removed as pyrazinamide and metabolites during 3 to 4.5 hours of hemodialysis.[100] Dosing guidelines for patients with renal insufficiency are shown in Table 10-6, although it is often recommended that use of pyrazinamide be avoided in patients with significant renal insufficiency.

Clofazamine

The antileprotic drug clofazamine is used in combination therapy of disseminated *M. avium-intracellulare* infection in patients with AIDS. No renal toxicity has been associated with the use of clofazamine, although the urine, as well as other body fluids and skin, may turn reddish-brown. A recent report implicated clofazamine in the development of proximal renal tubular acidosis, but only limited details were provided.[101]

Clofazamine is slowly and only partially absorbed from the gastrointestinal tract, then accumulates in adipose cells and reticuloendothelial tissues. The elimination half-life is about 70 days. Less than 1 percent of a dose is excreted in the urine. No dosage adjustments are required for renal failure or after dialysis.

Capreomycin

Capreomycin is a polypeptide antibiotic produced by *Streptomyces capreolus* with activity against *M. tuberculosis,* used as a second-line agent for treatment of multidrug-resistant tuberculosis. Capreomycin must be administered parenterally by deep intramuscular injection. The drug is both ototoxic and nephrotoxic. Renal insufficiency, which is usually mild and may be associated with low-grade proteinuria,[102,103] often does not require discontinuation of the drug, although in one case fatal renal failure occurred in a patient treated with capreomycin. The mechanism of capreomycin-related ARF is not known. In some patients, renal insufficiency may be due in part to intravascular volume depletion, as a salt-wasting effect of capreomycin has been described.[104,105] A direct toxic effect is also likely, with findings of acute tubular necrosis being described in several cases. Because eosinophilia is not uncommon in patients receiving capreomycin, a component of allergic interstitial nephritis is perhaps also possible, but has not been yet documented.

Electrolyte abnormalities, including potentially severe hypokalemia and hypocalcemia, hypomagnesemia, hyponatremia, and metabolic alkalosis have also been reported in patients receiving capreomycin.[103–105] These disturbances may occur in the absence of capreomycin-induced renal insufficiency. The electrolyte abnormalities appear to be readily reversible upon discontinuation of the drug, but may recur with drug rechallenge. Urinary studies have revealed an inappropriate natriuresis, kaliuresis, and magnesuria, without glycosuria or phosphaturia. The hypocalcemia has for the most part been attributed to hypomagnesemia. Elevated plasma renin levels have been reported in several cases, and in one instance, urinary and plasma aldosterone levels were thought to be inappropriately elevated.[105] In one report, in which the authors likened the renal effects of capreomycin to aminoglycoside-induced renal tubular abnormalities and Bartter syndrome, high doses of spironolactone, but not indomethacin, corrected the hypokalemia and metabolic alkalosis.[105]

Between 32 and 87 percent of a 1-g dose is excreted unchanged in the urine within 12 hours. Urinary excretion and total clearance are markedly reduced in patients with renal insufficiency, without a change in the volume of distribution. In one study, the terminal elimination half-life of capreomycin was about 5 hours in individuals with normal kidney function, about 17 to 18 hours when the creatinine clearance was between 20 and 51 ml/min, and 58 hours in patients on dialysis.[106] In a limited study in only three patients, the hemodialysis clearance of capreomycin was reported to be between 0.9 and 2.7 L/h, with extraction ratios of 0.08 to 0.57, resulting in the removal of 35 to 144 mg during a 3-hour hemodialysis treatment. Based on these findings, the authors recommended that the dose of capreomycin be administered after a treatment in order to avoid removal by hemodialysis.[106] Dosage adjustments are needed for patients with renal insufficiency (Table 10-6).

Ciprofloxacin and Ofloxacin

These two fluoroquinolone antimicrobials, which have a broad antimicrobial spectrum of activity, are increasingly included in treatment regimens for infection of *M. avium-intracellulare* and multidrug-resistant tuberculosis. Preclinical toxicologic studies with ciprofloxacin revealed an obstructive nephropathy caused by needle-shaped crystals within the renal tubules, accompanied by an interstitial inflammatory infiltrate. These pathologic changes and the associated renal dysfunction were attributed to a foreign body reaction triggered by the intrarenal precipitation of ciprofloxacin and/ or its metabolites, which are insoluble in alkaline urine. Crystal formation and renal inflammation occur only in animals with alkaline urine. In these animal studies, renal dysfunction occurred with doses above those that produced crystalluria alone.[107] Crystalluria can occur in normal humans receiving large doses of ciprofloxacin and when the urine is highly alkaline, although the crystalluria has not been associated with a decline in kidney function, perhaps because of the spherical shape of the crystals.[108,109] However, patients receiving high doses of ciprofloxacin should maintain adequate hydration and, if possible, avoid a highly alkaline urine pH. Crystalluria has not been documented in patients receiving ofloxacin, although ofloxacin crystals can form in alkaline urine left at room temperature for 24 hours.[109]

Mild and transient elevations of blood urea nitrogen or creatinine concentration have been noted rarely in patients receiving ciprofloxacin and ofloxacin. Rare instances of glucosuria, hematuria, pyuria, and proteinuria in patients treated with ofloxacin have been noted in postmarketing surveillance (written communication, McNeil Pharmaceutical, 1993), although these abnormalities may not be directly drug related. Cases of more severe ciprofloxacin-associated ARF have also been reported, usually associated with features suggestive of a hypersensitivity reaction and an acute interstitial nephritis.[110,111] Fever has often been present, along with rash, nausea, vomiting, arthralgias, and myalgias less commonly. Eosinophilia may also be present. The urinalysis may show pyuria, microscopic hematuria, granular casts, and eosinophiluria. In one patient without renal insufficiency, hematuria with red blood cell casts recurred during three separate courses of therapy. In only one instance, after an overdose of ciprofloxacin in a patient with a urine pH of 7, was ARF with transient crystalluria reported. Ciprofloxacin-induced ARF has been oliguric in about 25 percent of reported cases but only one reported patient required temporary dialysis. Renal function generally recovers spontaneously within 2 to 4 weeks (range, 4 days to 8 weeks). A short course of steroids was used in several cases, but there are no controlled data to indicate whether this treatment enhances recovery of renal function. Histopathologic findings have included an acute interstitial nephritis, with a lymphocytic and plasma cell infiltrate and occasional eosinophils and granulomatous changes, with normal glomeruli and blood vessels and negative immunofluorescence studies. In one instance, electron microscopy revealed epithelial vacuolization, thought to be consistent with a toxic, rather than hypersensitivity, injury.

ARF associated with elevated cyclosporine levels has occurred in renal transplant patients receiving both ciprofloxacin and cyclosporine, possibly related to inhibition of hepatic metabolism of cyclosporine by ciprofloxacin. However, no evidence of altered cyclosporine kinetics was noted in transplant patients receiving 750 mg of ciprofloxacin orally twice daily for up to 7 days.[112] Ofloxacin does not appear to interact with cyclosporine.

Ciprofloxacin has an oral bioavailability of 70 to 85 percent, which is dramatically reduced by concurrent administration of divalent cation-containing medications, such as antacids containing aluminum, magnesium, and calcium-salts, antacids, and iron supplements.[113,114] The divalent cations present in formulations of didanosine may also interfere with ciprofloxacin absorption.[115] Ciprofloxacin is about 15 to 40 percent protein bound, with a steady-state volume of distribution of 2.5 to 4.0 L/kg. Approximately 15 to 20 percent of the absorbed drug is hepatically metabolized by cytochrome P-450-mediated oxidation and conjugation reactions. Fifty to 70 percent of a dose is excreted unchanged into the urine over 48 hours, with the rest excreted in the stool via an enterohepatic cycle and urinary excretion of metabolites. The renal clearance of ciprofloxacin is approximately 250 to 450 ml/min in normal volunteers, implying significant tubular secretion of the drug. Consistent with this is the observation that probenecid inhibits the renal excretion of ciprofloxacin and prolongs the terminal elimination half-life, which is normally 3 to 4 hours.[116] In patients with renal insufficiency, the renal clearance of the drug is impaired, with elevated levels of both ciprofloxacin and its metabolites. The serum half-life becomes prolonged to 5 to 10 hours when the GFR falls below 20 ml/min/1.73 m^2.[117,118] Ciprofloxacin hemodialysis extraction coefficients of 0.21 to 0.31 with cuprophane membranes and clearances of 40 to 55 ml/min have been reported, although less than 30 percent of an administered dose is removed.[117,118] Although the total amount of drug removed by peritoneal dialysis is small, therapeutic drug levels are obtained in peritoneal dialysate after oral or intravenous administration of ciprofloxacin.[119,120] Although not all authors recommend dose adjustments for patients with renal insufficiency, some dose reduction may be advisable, especially in patients receiving high doses and in whom there are coexisting illnesses that may impair metabolic (nonrenal) clearance of the drug (Table 10-7).

Table 10-7. Dosing Recommendations: Ciprofloxacin, Ofloxacin, Clarithromycin[a]

	Recommended Dose by GFR (ml/min)		
Drug/Usual Dose	50–90	10–50	<10
Ciprofloxacin			
250–750 mg PO bid	Usual	250–500 mg bid	250–500 mg qd
400 mg IV q12h	Usual	q12–24h	q24–48h
Ofloxacin			
400 mg PO/IV q12h	Usual	200–400 mg qd	100–400 mg q24–48h
Clarithromycin			
250–500 mg PO bid	Usual	Usual	qd

[a] Hemodialysis (HD) and peritoneal dialysis (PD):
Ciprofloxacin: 250 mg PO bid, 400 mg IV q24h.
Ofloxacin: 100 mg bid (HD), use dose recommended for GFR <10 ml/min (PD).
Clarithromycin: use dose recommended for GFR <10 ml/min (no data).

Like ciprofloxacin, oral absorption of ofloxacin is also impaired by concurrent administration of antacids and certain other medications. Between 70 and 90 percent of a dose of ofloxacin is excreted in the urine, mostly as unchanged drug, with less than 5 percent appearing as metabolites. Ten to 30 percent is bound to plasma proteins, and the steady-state volume of distribution is about 1.5 L/kg. Renal clearance, about 195 ml/min, exceeds GFR, indicating a contribution from tubular secretion.[121,122] Recent studies with rat renal brush border membrane vesicles suggest that ofloxacin may be transported by an organic cation transport system.[123] The normal serum half-life of about 5 to 10 hours is prolonged to between 20 and 50 hours in patients with a GFR less than 10 ml/min, with a close correlation between creatinine clearance and urinary elimination and total plasma clearance. The volume of distribution does not change with renal insufficiency.[124-126] Less than 5 to 15 percent of a dose of ofloxacin is removed by CAPD.[126-128] The fractional clearance of ofloxacin with hemodialysis is about 15 to 25 percent, with removal of only about 10 percent of a dose.[124,126,129,130] Dosing recommendations for patients with renal insufficiency are outlined in Table 10-7.

MISCELLANEOUS DRUGS

Clarithromycin and Azithromycin

These two macrolide antibiotics, which are chemically related to erythromycin and are active against a variety of common respiratory, skin, and soft tissue infections, may also have a role in the management of *M. avium-intracellulare* infections, *Toxoplasma* encephalitis, and cryptosporidiosis. Severe acute tubulointerstitial nephritis has been reported in one patient treated with azithromycin, which was irreversible despite treatment with prednisone and resulted in the need for chronic dialysis.[131]

Clarithromycin has a mean terminal elimination half-life of about 2 to 8 hours. As much as 40 percent of a dose may be excreted in the urine, with another 5 to 10 percent excreted as the 14(R)-hydroxy metabolite. Renal clearance of clarithromycin is about 100 to 200 ml/min in a young, healthy population, but is reduced in elderly patients. Clarithromycin is about 70 percent bound to plasma proteins.[132,133]

Only about 5 to 15 percent of orally administered azithromycin is recovered in the urine. This drug has a long terminal elimination half-life, which has been reported to vary from 30 hours to as much as 5 days, with a mean of about 60 hours.[134,135] Although not specifically studied yet, azithromycin probably does not require dose adjustments for renal insufficiency, whereas clarithromycin may in patients with advanced renal insufficiency (Table 10-7). The effects of dialysis on the pharmacokinetics of these two drugs are not known.

CONCLUSIONS

As the pharmaceutical armamentarium used in patients with HIV infection expands, renal toxicities are also likely to become increasingly recognized, particularly given the frequent polypharmacy employed in patients with AIDS and the use of "nontraditional" therapies by some patients.[136–138] The clinician must therefore maintain a high level of suspicion regarding potential drug toxicities and interactions, especially in patients with impaired renal function.

REFERENCES

1. Berns JS, Cohen RM, Stumacher RJ, Rudnick MR: Renal aspects of therapy for human immunodeficiency virus and associated opportunistic infections. J Am Soc Nephrol 1:1061, 1991
2. Bennett WM, Aronoff GR, Golper TA et al: Drug Prescribing in Renal Failure. Dosing Guidelines for Adults. 2nd Ed. American College of Physicians, Philadelphia, 1991
3. Gopinath R, Hutcheon M, Cheema-Dhadli S, Halperin M: Chronic lactic acidosis in a patient with acquired immunodeficiency syndrome and mitochondrial myopathy: biochemical studies. J Am Soc Nephrol 3:1212, 1992
4. Chattha G, Arieff AI, Cummings C, Tierney LM Jr: Lactic acidosis complicating the acquired immunodeficiency syndrome. Ann Intern Med 118:37, 1993
5. Connolly KJ, Allan JD, Fitch H et al: Phase I study of 2'-3'-dideoxyinosine administered orally twice daily to patients with AIDS and AIDS-related complex and hematologic intolerance to zidovudine. Am J Med 91:471, 1991
6. Crowther MA, Callaghan W, Hodsman AB, Mackie ID: Dideoxyinosine-associated nephrotoxicity. AIDS 7:131, 1993
7. Warner WL: Toxicology and pharmacology of adenine in animals and man. Transfusion 17:326, 1977
8. de Miranda P, Good SS, Yarchoan R et al: Alteration of zidovudine pharmacokinetics by probenecid in patients with AIDS or AIDS-related complex. Clin Pharmacol Ther 46:494, 1989
9. Chatton JY, Munafo A, Chave JP et al: Trimethoprim, alone or in combination with sulphamethoxazole, decreases the renal excretion of zidovudine and its glucuronide. J Clin Pharmacol 34:551, 1992
10. Kremer D, Munar MY, Kohlhepp SJ et al: Zidovudine pharmacokinetics in five HIV seronegative patients undergoing continuous ambulatory peritoneal dialysis. Pharmacotherapy 12:56, 1992
11. Gallicano KD, Tobe S, Sahai J et al: Pharmacokinetics of single and chronic dose zidovudine in two HIV positive patients undergoing continuous ambulatory peritoneal dialysis (CAPD). J AIDS 5:242, 1992
12. Singlas E, Taburet AM, Borsa Lebas F et al: Didanosine pharmacokinetics in patients with normal and impaired renal function: influence of hemodialysis. Antimicrob Agents Chemother 36:1519, 1992
12a.Dudley MN, Graham KK, Kaul S et al: Pharmacokinetics of stavudine in patients with AIDS or AIDS-related complex. J Infect Dis 166:480, 1992

13. Yusufi ANK, Szczepanska-Konkel M, Kempson SA et al: Inhibition of human renal epithelial Na$^+$/P$_i$ cotransport by phosphonoformic acid. Biochem Biophys Res Commun 139:679, 1986
14. Loghman-Adham M, Dousa TP: Dual action of phosphonoformic acid on Na$^+$-phosphate cotransport in opossum kidney cells. Am J Physiol 263:F301, 1992
15. Farese RV, Schambelan M, Hollander H et al: Nephrogenic diabetes insipidus associated with foscarnet treatment of cytomegalovirus retinitis. Ann Intern Med 112:955, 1990
16. Jacobson MA, Gambertoglio JG, Aweeka FT et al: Foscarnet-induced hypocalcemia and effects of foscarnet on calcium metabolism. J Clin Endocrinol Metab 72:1130, 1991
17. MacGregor RR, Graziani AL, Weiss R et al: Successful foscarnet therapy for cytomegalovirus retinitis in an AIDS patient undergoing hemodialysis: rationale for empiric dosing and plasma level monitoring. J Infect Dis 164:785, 1991
18. Sawyer MH, Webb DF, Balow JE, Strauss SE: Acyclovir induced renal failure: clinical course and histology. Am J Med 84:1067, 1988
19. Becker BN, Fall P, Hall C et al: Rapidly progressive acute renal failure due to acyclovir: case report and review of the literature. Am J Kidney Dis 22:611, 1993
20. Eck P, Silver SM, Clark EC: Acute renal failure and coma after a high dose of oral acyclovir (letter). N Engl J Med 325:1178, 1991
21. Rashed A, Azadeh B, Abu-Romeh SH: Acyclovir-induced acute tubulo-interstitial nephritis. Nephron 56:436, 1990
22. Davenport A, Goel S, Mackenzie JC: Neurotoxicity of acyclovir in patients with end-stage renal failure treated with continuous ambulatory peritoneal dialysis. Am J Kidney Dis 6:647, 1992
23. MacDiarmaid-Gordon AR, O'Connor M, Beaman M, Ackrill P. Neurotoxicity associated with oral acyclovir in patients undergoing dialysis. Nephron 62:280, 1992
24. Jones T, Alderman C: Acyclovir clearance by CAVHD (letter). Intensive Care Med 17:125, 1991
25. Swan SK, Munar MY, Wigger MA, Bennett WM: Pharmacokinetics of ganciclovir in a patient undergoing hemodialysis. Am J Kidney Dis 17:69, 1991
26. Boulieu R, Bastien O, Bleyzac N: Pharmacokinetics of ganciclovir in heart transplant patients undergoing continuous venovenous hemodialysis. Ther Drug Monit 15:105, 1993
27. Mannering GJ, Deloria LB: The pharmacology and toxicology of the interferons: an overview. Ann Rev Pharmacol Toxicol 26:455, 1986
28. Kurzrock R, Gutterman JU, Talpaz M: Interferons-α, β, γ: basic principles and preclinical studies. p. 246. In DeVita VT, Hellman S, Rosenberg SA (eds): Biological Therapy of Cancer. JB Lippincott, Philadelphia, 1991
29. Lisker-Melman M, Webb D, DiBisceglie AM et al: Glomerulonephritis caused by chronic hepatitis B virus infection: treatment with recombinant human alpha-interferon. Ann Intern Med 111:479, 1989
30. Johnson RJ, Gretch DR, Yamabe H et al: Membranoproliferative glomerulonephritis associated with hepatitis C virus infection. N Engl J Med 328:465, 1993
31. Lane HC: The role of α-interferon in patients with human immunodeficiency virus infection. Sem Oncol, (suppl. 7) 18:46, 1991
32. Quesada JR, Talpaz M, Rios A et al: Clinical toxicity of the interferons in cancer patients: a review. J Clin Oncol 4:234, 1986

33. Gresser I, Maury C, Tovey M et al: Progressive glomerulonephritis in mice treated with interferon at birth. Nature 263:420, 1976
34. Lane HC, Davey V, Kovacs JA et al: Interferon-α in patients with asymptomatic human immunodeficiency virus (HIV) infection. Ann Intern Med 112:805, 1990
35. Averbuch SD, Austin HA, Sherwin SA et al: Acute interstitial nephritis with the nephrotic syndrome following recombinant leukocyte A interferon therapy for mycosis fungoides. N Engl J Med 310:32, 1984
36. Lederer E, Truong L. Unusual glomerular lesion in a patient receiving long-term interferon alpha. Am J Kidney Dis 20:516, 1992
37. Schilling PJ, Kurzrock R, Kantarjian H et al: Development of systemic lupus erythematosus after interferon therapy for chronic myelogenous leukemia. Cancer 68:1536, 1991
38. Kramer P, Bijnen AB, Ten Kate FWJ, Jeekel J: Recombinant leukocyte interferon A induces steroid-resistant acute vascular rejection episodes in renal transplant recipients. Lancet 1:989, 1984
39. Freundlich B, Jimenez SA, Steen VD et al: Treatment of systemic sclerosis with recombinant interferon-gamma: a phase I/II clinical trial. Arthritis Rheum 35:1134, 1992
40. Bocci V, Pacini A, Muscettola M et al: Renal filtration, absorption and catabolism of human alpha interferon. J Interferon Res 1:347, 1981
41. Wills RJ: Clinical pharmacokinetics of interferons. Clin Pharmacokinet 19:390, 1990
42. Hirsch MS, Tolkoff-Rubin NE, Kelly AP, Rubin RH: Pharmacokinetics of human and recombinant leukocyte interferon in patients with chronic renal failure who are undergoing hemodialysis. J Infect Dis 148:335, 1983
43. Tokazewski-Chen SA, Marafino BJ, Stebbing N: Effects of nephrectomy on the pharmacokinetics of various cloned human interferons in the rat. J Pharmacol Exp Ther 227:9, 1983
44. Llanos A, Cieza J, Bernardo J et al: Effect of salt supplementation on amphotericin B nephrotoxicity. Kidney Int 40:302, 1991
45. Bullock NE, Luke RG, Nuttall CE, Bhathena D: Can mannitol reduce amphotericin B nephrotoxicity: double-blind study and description of new vascular lesions in kidneys. Antimicrob Agents Chemother 10:555, 1976
46. Sawaya BP, Weihprecht H, Campbell WR et al: Direct vasoconstriction as a possible cause for amphotericin B-induced nephrotoxicity in rats. J Clin Invest 87:2097, 1991
47. Zager RA, Bredl CR, Schimpf BA: Direct amphotericin B-mediated tubular toxicity: assessments of selected cytoprotective agents. Kidney Int 41:1588, 1992
48. Heyman SN, Stillman IE, Brezis M et al: Chronic amphotericin nephropathy: morphometric, electron microscopic, and functional studies. J Am Soc Nephrol 4:69, 1993
49. Dukes CS, Perfect JR: Amphotericin B-induced malignant hypertension episodes (letter). J Infect Dis 161:588, 1990
50. Lyman CA, Walsh TJ: Systemically administered antifungal agents: a review of their clinical pharmacology and therapeutic applications. Drugs 44:9, 1992
51. Graybill JR, Stevens DA, Galgiani JN et al: Itraconazole treatment of coccidioidomycosis. Am J Med 89:282, 1990
52. Sharkey PK, Rinaldi MG, Lerner CJ et al: High dose itraconazole in the treatment of severe mycoses, abstracted. 28th Interscience Conference on Antimicrobial Agents and Chemotherapy. Abstract no. 575, p.210, 1988

53. Phillips P, Graybill JR, Fetchick R, Dunn JF: Adrenal response to corticotropin during therapy with itraconazole. Antimicrob Agents Chemother 31:647, 1987

54. Debruyne D, Ryckelynck J-P: Clinical pharmacokinetics of fluconazole. Clin Pharmacokinet 24:10, 1993

55. DeMuria D, Forrest A, Rich J et al: Pharmacokinetics and bioavailability of fluconazole in patients with AIDS. Antimicrob Agents Chemother 37:2187, 1993

56. Oono S, Tabei K, Tetsuka T, Asano Y: The pharmacokinetics of fluconazole during haemodialysis in uraemic patients. Eur J Clin Pharmacol 42:667, 1992

57. Berl T, Wilner K, Henrich WL: Pharmacokinetics of fluconazole in renal failure, abstracted. J Am Soc Nephrol 4:245, 1993

58. Grant SM, Clissold SP: Itraconazole: a review of its pharmacodynamic and pharmacokinetic properties, and therapeutic use in superficial and systemic mycoses. Drugs 37:310, 1989

59. Smith D, Van de Velde V, Woestenborghs R, Gazzard BG: The pharmacokinetics of itraconazole in AIDS patients. J Pharm Pharmacol 44:618, 1992

60. Boelaert J, Schurgers M, Matthys E et al: Itraconazole pharmacokinetics in patients with renal dysfunction. Antimicrob Agents Chemother 32:1595, 1988

61. Medina I, Mills J, Leoung G et al: Oral therapy for *Pneumocystis carinii* pneumonia in the acquired immunodeficiency syndrome—a controlled trial of trimethoprim-sulfamethoxazole versus trimethoprim-dapsone. N Engl J Med 323:776, 1990

62. Greenber S, Reiser IW, Chou S-Y, Porush JG: Trimethoprim-sulfamethoxazole induces reversible hyperkalemia. Ann Intern Med 119:291, 1993

63. Velazquez H, Perazella MA, Wright FS, Ellison D: Renal mechanism of trimethoprim-induced hyperkalemia. Ann Intern Med 119:296, 1993

64. Choi MJ, Fernandez PC, Patnaik A et al: Trimethoprim-induced hyperkalemia in a patient with AIDS. N Engl J Med 328:703, 1993

65. Schlanger LE, Kleyman TR, Ling BN: K$^+$-sparing diuretic actions of trimethoprim: inhibition of Na$^+$ channels in A6 distal nephron cells. Kidney Int 45:1070, 1994

66. Lee BL, Medina I, Benowitz NL et al: Dapsone, trimethoprim, and sulfamethoxazole plasma levels during treatment of *Pneumocystis* pneumonia in patients with the acquired immunodeficiency syndrome (AIDS): evidence of drug interactions. Ann Intern Med 110:606, 1989

67. Modest GA, Price B, Mascoli N: Hyperkalemia in elderly patients receiving standard doses of trimethoprim-sulfamethoxazole (letter). Ann Intern Med 120:437, 1994

68. Pennypacker LC, Mintzer J, Pitner J: Hyperkalemia in elderly patients receiving standard doses of trimethoprim-sulfamethoxazole (letter). Ann Intern Med 120:437, 1994

69. Canaday DH, Johnson JR: Hyperkalemia in elderly patients receiving standard doses of trimethoprim-sulfamethoxazole (letter). Ann Intern Med 120:437, 1994

70. Paap CM, Nahata MC: Clinical use of trimethoprim-sulfamethoxazole during renal dysfunction. Drug Intell Clin Pharm 23:646, 1989

71. Halstenson CE, Blevins RB, Salem NG, Matzke GR: Trimethoprim-sulfamethoxazole pharmacokinetics during continuous ambulatory peritoneal dialysis. Clin Nephrol 22:239, 1984

72. Molina J-M, Belenfant X, Doco-Lecompte T et al: Sulfadiazine-induced crystalluria in AIDS patients with toxoplasma encephalitis. AIDS 5:587, 1991

73. Oster S, Hutchison F, McCabe R: Resolution of acute renal failure in toxoplasmic encephalitis despite continuance of sulfadiazine. Rev Infect Dis 12:618, 1990

74. Comtois R, Pouliot J, Vinet B et al: Higher pentamidine levels in AIDS patients with hypoglycemia and azotemia during treatment of *Pneumocystis carinii* pneumonia. Am Rev Respir Dis 146:740, 1992

75. Nielsen H: Hypomagnesaemia associated with pentamidine therapy. AIDS 8:561, 1994

76. Herchline TE, Plouffe JF, Para MF: Diabetes mellitus presenting with ketoacidosis following pentamidine therapy in patients with acquired immunodeficiency syndrome. J Infect 22:41, 1991

77. Conte JE: Pharmacokinetics of intravenous pentamidine in patients with normal renal function or receiving dialysis. J Infect Dis 163:169, 1991

78. Vöhringer H-F, Arasteh K: Pharmacokinetic optimisation in the treatment of *Pneumocystic carinii* pneumonia. Clin Pharmacokinet 24:388, 1993

79. Opravil M, Keusch G, Luthy R: Pyrimethamine inhibits renal secretion of creatinine. Antimicrob Agents Chemother 37:1056, 1993

80. LeLiboux A, Duquesne H, Montay G et al: Pharmacokinetics of pyrimethamine in healthy young volunteers using a new solid phase extraction/HPLC method. Eur J Drug Metab Pharmacokinet 3:284, 1991

81. Zuidema J, Hilbers-Modderman ESM, Merkus FWHM: Clinical pharmacokinetics of dapsone. Clin Pharmacokinet 11:299, 1986

82. May DG, Porter JA, Utrecht JP et al: The contribution of N-hydroxylation and acetylation to dapsone pharmacokinetics in normal subjects. Clin Pharmacol Ther 48:619, 1990

83. Hughes WT, Kennedy W, Shenep JL et al: Safety and pharmacokinetics of 566C80, a hydroxynaphthoquinone with anti-*Pneumocystis carinii* activity: a phase I study in human immunodeficiency syndrome virus (HIV)-infected men. J Infect Dis 163:843, 1991

84. Breckenridge A, Back DJ, Edwards IG et al: The clinical and biochemical pharmacology of primaquine. p. 65. In Wernsdorfer WH, Trigg PI (eds): Primaquine: Pharmacokinetics, Metabolism, Toxicity and Activity. Wiley, Chichester, 1987

85. Fletcher KA, Price Evans DA, Gilles HM et al: Studies of the pharmacokinetics of primaquine. Bull WHO 59:407, 1981

86. Bissuel F, Cotte L, Rabodonirina M et al: Paramomycin: an effective treatment for cryptosporidial diarrhea in patients with AIDS. Clin Infect Dis 18:447, 1994

87. Ellard GA: Chemotherapy of tuberculosis for patients with renal impairment. Nephron 64:169, 1993

88. Siskind MS, Thienemann D, Kirlin L: Isoniazid-induced neurotoxicity in chronic dialysis patients: report of three cases and a review of the literature. Nephron 64:303, 1993

89. Davis CE, Carpenter JL, Ognibene AJ, McAllister K: Rifampin-induced acute renal failure. South Med J 79:1012, 1986

90. Venkatesan K: Pharmacokinetic drug interactions with rifampicin. Clin Pharmacokinet 22:47, 1992

91. Mauri JM, Fort J, Bartolome J et al: Antirifampicin antibodies in acute rifampicin-associated renal failure. Nephron 31:177, 1982

92. Fahal IH, Williams PS, Clark RE, Bell GM: Thrombotic thrombocytopenic purpura due to rifampicin (letter). BMJ 304:882, 1992

93. Graber CD, Jebaily J, Galphin RL, Doering E: Light chain proteinuria and

humoral immunoincompetence in tuberculous patients treated with rifampin. Am Rev Respir Dis 107:713, 1973

94. Soffer O, Nassar VH, Campbell WG, Bourke E: Light chain cast nephropathy and acute renal failure associated with rifampin therapy: renal disease akin to myeloma kidney. Am J Med 82:1052, 1987

95. O'Brien RJ, Lyle MA, Snider DE Jr: Rifabutin (Ansamycin LM 427): a new rifamycin-S derivative for the treatment of mycobacterial diseases. Rev Infect Dis 9:519, 1987

96. Battaglio R, Pianezzola E, Salgarollo G et al: Absorption, disposition and preliminary metabolic pathway of ^{14}C-rifabutin in animals and man. J Antimicrob Chemother 26:813, 1990

97. Sarma GR, Acharyulu GS, Murthy PVK et al: Role of rifampicin in arthralgia induced by pyrazinamide. Tubercle 64:93, 1983

98. Namba S, Igari T, Nishiyama K et al: A case of pyrazinamide-associated myoglobinuric renal failure. Jpn J Med 30:468, 1991

99. delCerro LAJ, Hernandez FR: Effect of pyrazinamide on ciclosporin levels (letter). Nephron 62:113, 1992

100. Lacroix C, Hermelin A, Guiberteau R et al: Haemodialysis of pyrazinamide in uraemic patients. Eur J Clin Pharmacol 37:309, 1989

101. Soriano V, Morenao V, Alba A et al: Kussmaul respiration and abdominal pain secondary to metabolic acidosis in AIDS patients with disseminated *Mycobacterium avium* complex infection receiving clofazamine. AIDS 7:894, 1993

102. Garfield JW, Jones JM, Cohen NL et al: The auditory, vestibular and renal effects of capreomycin in humans. Ann NY Acad Sci 135:1039, 1966

103. Aquinas M, Citron KM: Rifampicin, ethambutol and capreomycin in pulmonary tuberculosis, previously treated with both first and second line drugs: the results of 2 years of chemotherapy. Tubercle 53:153, 1972

104. Holmes AM, Hesling CM, Wilson TM: Capreomycin-induced serum electrolyte abnormalities. Thorax 25:608, 1970

105. Steiner RW, Omachi AS: A Bartter's-like syndrome from capreomycin, and a similar gentamicin tubulopathy. Am J Kidney Dis 7:245, 1986

106. Lehmann CR, Garrett LE, Winn RE et al: Capreomycin kinetics in renal impairment and clearance by hemodialysis. Am Rev Respir Dis 138:1312, 1988

107. Schlüter G: Toxicology of ciprofloxacin. p. 61. In Neu HC, Weuta H (eds): Proceedings of the First International Ciprofloxacin Workshop. Excerpta Medica, Amsterdam, 1986

108. Thorsteinsson SB, Bergan T, Oddsdottir S et al: Crystalluria and ciprofloxacin, influence of urinary pH and hydration. Chemotherapy 32:408, 1986

109. Bergan T, Rohwedder R, Thorsteinsson SB: Significance of crystalluria caused by quinolones. Rev Infect Dis, suppl. 5, 11:S1395, 1989

110. Wolfson JS, Hooper DC: Overview of fluoroquinolone safety. Am J Med, suppl. 6A, 91:153S, 1991

111. Lo WK, Rolston KVI, Rubenstein EB, Bodey GP: Ciprofloxacin-induced nephrotoxicity in patients with cancer. Arch Intern Med 153:1258, 1993

112. Lang T, deVillaine JF, Garraffo R, Touraine J-L: Cyclosporine (cyclosporin A) pharmacokinetics in renal transplant patients receiving ciprofloxacin. Am J Med, suppl. 5A, 87:82S, 1989

113. Bergan T, Dalhoff A, Rohwedder R: Pharmacokinetics of ciprofloxacin. Infection, suppl. 1, 16:S3, 1988

114. Wise R, Griggs D, Andrews JM: Pharmacokinetics of the quinolones in volunteers: a proposed dosing schedule. Rev Infect Dis, suppl. 1, 10:S83, 1988

115. Sahai J, Gallicano K, Oliveras L et al: Cations in the didanosine tablet reduce ciprofloxacin bioavailability. Clin Pharmacol Ther 53:292, 1993

116. Wingender W, Beerman D, Foerster D et al: Mechanism of renal excretion of ciprofloxacin, a new quinolone carboxylic acid derivative, in humans. Chemioterapia, suppl. 2, 4:403, 1985

117. Boelaert J, Valcke Y, Schurgers M et al: The pharmacokinetics of ciprofloxacin in patients with impaired renal function. J Antimicrob Chemother 16:87, 1985

118. Singlas E, Taburet AM, Landru I et al: Pharmacokinetics of ciprofloxacin tablets in renal failure: influence of haemodialysis. Eur J Clin Pharmacol 31:589, 1987

119. Golper TA, Hartstein AI, Morthland VH, Christensen JM: Effects of antacids and dialysate dwell times on multiple-dose pharmacokinetics of oral ciprofloxacin in patients on chronic ambulatory peritoneal dialysis. Antimicrob Agents Chemother 31:1787, 1987

120. Shalit I, Kitzes-Cohen R, Rapaport J et al: Pharmacokinetics of ciprofloxacin in patients receiving peritoneal dialysis and being treated for peritonitis. Rev Infect Dis, suppl. 5, 11:1072, 1989

121. Lamp KC, Bailey EM, Rybak MJ: Ofloxacin clinical pharmacokinetics. Clin Pharmacokinet 22:32, 1992

122. Monk JP, Campoli-Richards DM: Ofloxacin: a review of its antibacterial activity, pharmacokinetic properties and therapeutic use. Drugs 33:346, 1987

123. Okano T, Maegawa H, Inui K-I, Hori R: Interaction of ofloxacin with organic cation transport systems in rat renal brush-border membranes. J Pharmacol Exp Ther 255:1033, 1990

124. Fillastre JP, Leroy A, Humbert G: Ofloxacin pharmacokinetics in renal failure. Antimicrob Agents Chemother 31:156, 1987

125. Höffler D, Koeppe P: Pharmacokinetics of ofloxacin in healthy subjects and patients with impaired renal function. Drugs, suppl. 1, 34:51, 1987

126. Flor S, Guay D, Opsahl et al: Pharmacokinetics of ofloxacin in healthy subjects and patients with varying degrees of renal impairment. Int J Clin Pharmacol Res 11:115, 1991

127. Chan MK, Chau PY, Chan WWN: Ofloxacin pharmacokinetics in patients on continuous ambulatory peritoneal dialysis. Clin Nephrol 28:277, 1987

128. Passlick J, Wonner R, Keller E et al: Single and multiple dose kinetics of ofloxacin in patients on CAPD. Peritoneal Dial Int 9:267, 1989

129. Dörfler A, Schulz W, Burkhardt F, Zichner M: Pharmacokinetics of ofloxacin in patients on haemodialysis treatment. Drugs, suppl. 1, 34:62, 1987

130. Kampf D, Borner K, Pustelnik A: Multiple dose kinetics of ofloxacin and ofloxacin metabolites in haemodialysis patients. Eur J Clin Pharmacol 42:95, 1992

131. Mansoor GA, Panner BJ, Ornt DB: Azithromycin-induced acute interstitial nephritis (letter). Ann Intern Med 119:636, 1993

132. Davey PG: The pharmacokinetics of clarithromycin and its 14-OH metabolite. J Hosp Infect, suppl. A, 19:29, 1991

133. Chu S-Y, Sennello LT, Bunnell ST et al: Pharmacokinetics of clarithromycin, a new macrolide, after single ascending oral doses. Antimicrob Agents Chemother 36:2447, 1992

134. Chave J-P, Munafo A, Chatton J-Y et al: Once-a-week azithromycin in AIDS patients: tolerability, kinetics, and effects on zidovudine disposition. Antimicrob Agents Chemother 36:1013, 1992

135. Foulds G, Shepard RM, Johnson RB: The pharmacokinetics of azithromycin in human serum and tissues. J Antimicrob Chemother, suppl. A, 25:73, 1990
136. Lee BL, Safrin S: Interactions and toxicities of drugs used in patients with AIDS. Clin Infect Dis 14:773, 1992
137. Hess B, Raisin J, Zimmerman A et al: Tubulointerstitial nephropathy persisting 20 months after discontinuation of chronic intake of germanium lactate citrate. Am J Kidney Dis 21:548, 1993
138. Hirschtick RE, Dyrda SE, Peterson LC: Death from an unconventional therapy for AIDS (letter). Ann Intern Med 120:694, 1994

11

Renal Imaging in Patients with HIV Infection

Michael C. Hill
Diane K. Huntington

INTRODUCTION

Patients with human immunodeficiency virus (HIV) infection may develop renal and genitourinary tract diseases that are directly HIV related.[1] They can also be afflicted by renal diseases that affect the general population, such as acute bacterial pyelonephritis or renal stone disease. The coexistence of two diseases in these patients is also not uncommon, so that any renal imaging finding has to be closely correlated with imaging findings from other organs of the body, and also with the patient's clinical history, laboratory findings, and any treatment that the patient is receiving.[2]

Because there are many ways to image the kidneys, any radiographic evaluation has to be tailored based on the patient's specific clinical symptoms and signs.[1,2]

RENAL FAILURE

Ultrasound is the initial study of choice in patients with renal failure as it is noninvasive and does not involve the administration of intravenous contrast necessary for an intravenous urogram (IVU) or computed tomography (CT) scan.[3] The normal kidney is usually less echogenic than the adjacent liver.[4] Using the liver as a comparison in an HIV-infected patient can be misleading, however, because hepatic disease can cause a diffuse increase in liver echogenicity, which may be due to fatty infiltration of the liver.[5] If the kidneys appear sonographically normal, then acute renal failure is perhaps more likely to be reversible, such as when due to volume depletion or use of nephrotoxic drugs.[3,6] On the other hand, the kidney parenchyma may be very echogenic. This sonographic finding, often referred to as "medical renal disease,"[4] may be seen with HIV-associated nephropathy (HIVAN)[3,6–13] (Fig. 11-1). This is, however, a nonspecific finding, as many causes of parenchymal renal disease due to varying pathologies, unassociated with HIV, can give a similar echogenic appearance with ultrasonography.[4] In patients with HIV infection, this sonographic finding may be associated with irreversible renal failure.[3] In patients with HIVAN, this increased renal echogenicity is believed to reflect focal segmental glomerulosclerosis and the associated interstitial and tubular changes seen with HIVAN.[11,14,15] Renal size in HIVAN is usually normal or slightly enlarged and does not decrease much, even with end-stage renal disease.[7,10,14,15]

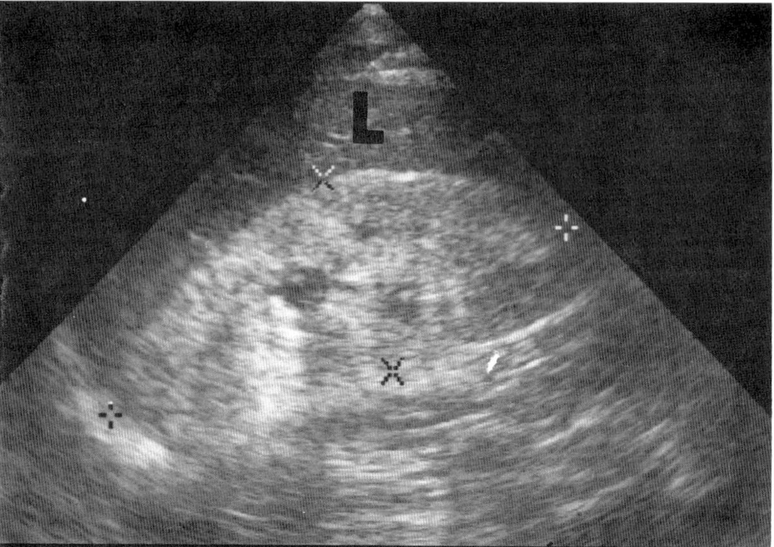

Fig. 11-1. Longitudinal ultrasound image of the right kidney demonstrating diffuse increase in echogenicity throughout the renal parenchyma seen with HIV-associated nephropathy. L, liver.

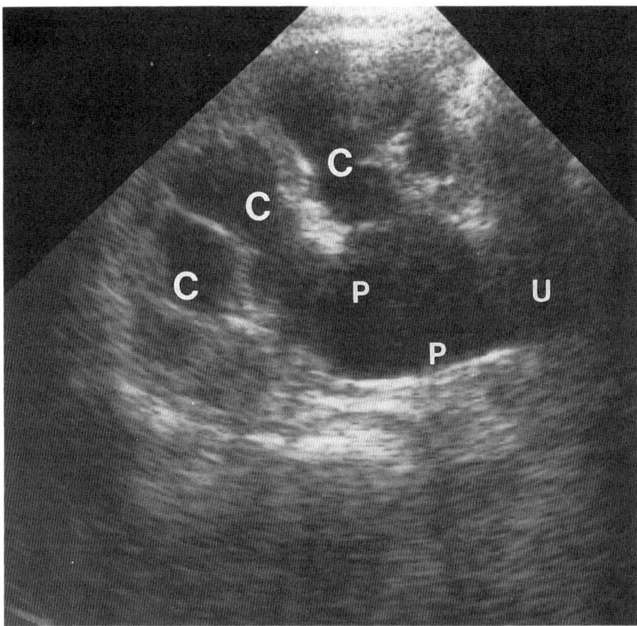

Fig. 11-2. Hydronephrosis due to retroperitoneal lymphadenopathy secondary to AIDS-related lymphoma. Longitudinal sonogram of the right kidney demonstrates moderate to marked dilatation of the calyces (C), pelvis (P), and the proximal right ureter (U). The left kidney was also hydronephrotic.

The presence of bilateral hydronephrosis necessitates examination of the retroperitoneum to rule out obstructing retroperitoneal lymphadenopathy, usually due to acquired immunodeficiency syndrome (AIDS)-related lymphoma (Fig. 11-2). If the cause of obstruction cannot be ascertained by ultrasound, then a CT scan with oral and rectal contrast, but without intravenous contrast, should be performed to more fully evaluate the retroperitoneum and pelvis.[16] In some cases of obstruction, there may be little or no evidence of dilatation of the collecting system.[17,18] If obstruction is clinically suspected, a nuclear medicine study using technetium DTPA (diethylenetriamine-pentaacetic acid) or technetium MAG3, a percutaneous nephrostomy, or retrograde pyelography should be considered for further evaluation.[18,19]

Obstructive uropathy has also been described in AIDS patients with renal failure receiving sulfadiazine for central nervous system (CNS) toxoplasmosis, due to intratubular precipitation of crystals and formation of stones composed of sulfadiazine or its metabolites. These patients present with renal failure and may have typical symptoms of renal colic, or may be relatively asymptomatic. Sonography may show the kidneys to be normal, or reveal echogenic nonshadowing sludge and/or a varying number of echogenic stones in the pelvicalyceal system, with or without hydronephrosis or hydroureter.[20–24] The stones may very rarely be visible on plain abdominal radiographs, but are usually radiolucent. Ureteral obstruction can be detected with intravenous urography, and noncontrast enhanced abdominal-pelvic CT scans may also show stones. Focal areas of echogenicity in the renal pyramids, due to small stones in the renal tubules, may also be seen. They typically disappear over a number of days with volume expansion and alkalinization of the urine, with improvement in the patient's renal function.[20–24]

RENAL INFECTION

The most common cause of hematuria in patients with AIDS is urinary tract infection.[25] Imaging procedures are not necessary in the majority of patients with acute pyelonephritis as the diagnosis is easily made on clinical grounds and by examination of the urine. The patients that require imaging are those who fail appropriate antibiotic therapy and are still symptomatic 48 to 72 hours after the initiation of treatment.[26,27] The initial imaging procedure can be ultrasound. In uncomplicated acute pyelonephritis, the kidney may be enlarged and hypoechoic while an intrarenal or perinephric abscess will be identified as a complex fluid collection in or around the kidney[26] (Fig. 11-3). Such abscesses can, when necessary, be drained using

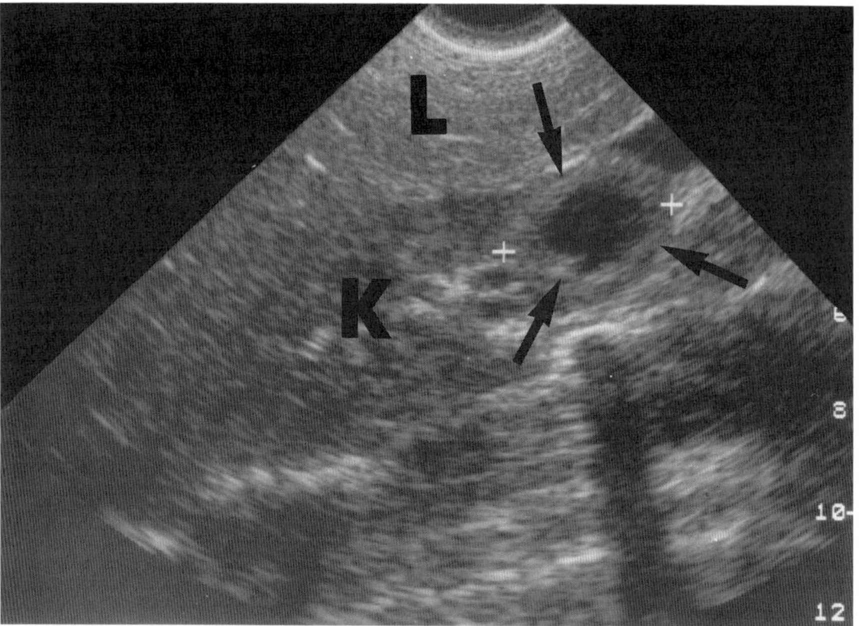

Fig. 11-3. Longitudinal sonogram of the right kidney (K) demonstrating a thick-walled abscess (*arrows*) in the lower pole. L, liver.

either ultrasound or CT guidance.[28] With focal pyelonephritis (lobar neph-
ronia), a focal hypoechoic or hyperechoic area may be seen on ultrasonography, which is not a true abscess but represents focal infection of a renal
pyramid.[26,27] These lesions are often better seen on a contrast-enhanced CT
scan as focal areas of reduced enhancement.[27] Infection related to renal
stone disease and hydronephrosis due to an obstructing stone or unsuspected
ureteropelvic junction obstruction may also be seen sonographically.[29] If the
ultrasound examination is normal, and the patient is still symptomatic, a
CT scan should be performed both without and with intravenous contrast.
Small abscesses missed by ultrasound may be detected in this fashion, as
ill-defined fluid collections in or around the kidney.[27] CT may also detect
air in the renal parenchyma, or in the pelvicalyceal system secondary to
emphysematous pyelonephritis.[26]

AIDS-related opportunistic infections such as *Pneumocystis carinii, Mycobacterium avium-intracellulare* (MAI), and cytomegalovirus (CMV) can involve the kidneys.[30–37] *P. carinii* is the most common opportunistic infection
in AIDS patients and may disseminate from the lungs to visceral organs
including the kidneys. This has been associated with the use of aerosolized
pentamidine.[31,34,35,37] On ultrasound, tiny bright echogenic areas, due to
inflammatory foci, are seen not only in the kidneys, but also in the liver,
spleen, and lymph nodes.[31,34,35,37] In the kidneys, these areas are mainly
located in the cortex and are usually 3 to 4 mm in size, but can be larger,
especially in other organs such as the spleen.[34,37] Initially, these tiny lesions
may not be detectable on a CT scan. These lesions eventually calcify, due
to progression of the disease, at which time they do become apparent on
CT[34,37] (Fig. 11-4). Calcification of these tiny areas does not necessarily
mean that the disease is quiescent.[16]

Punctate calcifications in the kidneys are not specific for *P. carinii,* but
can also be found in disseminated MAI, CMV, and candidiasis.[30,33,36,38] In
MAI, the punctate densities may be in the cortex or medulla and may be
calcified on CT and so can be indistinguishable from the lesions associated
with disseminated *P. carinii.*[30,36] Similar findings have also been reported
in disseminated CMV.[33] Hepatic and renal calcifications have also been
described in patients with treated systemic candidiasis.[38] These calcifications are usually less well defined and much larger than those associated
with disseminated *P. carinii,* MAI, and CMV. Fungus balls can form in the
pelvicalyceal system, appearing sonographically as well-defined round to
oval echogenic areas that do not shadow.[39]

Mycobacterium tuberculosis in patients with AIDS can spread hematoge-
nously from the lungs to other organs, including the kidneys,[16] producing
caseating cavitary lesions in the renal pyramids that spread into the adjacent calyces (ulcerocavernous lesion). These lesions can be identified by ultrasound or CT as irregular thick-walled cavities in the kidney that commu-
nicate with the pelvicalyceal system and are associated with thinning of the
renal cortex.[40] Renal parenchymal calcification may also be present. Fibrosis

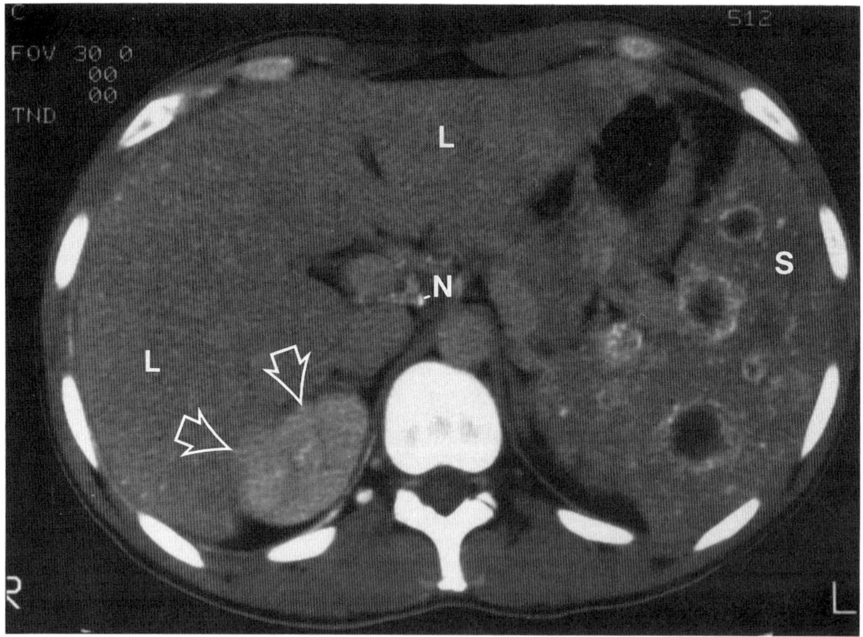

Fig. 11-4. Tiny punctate densities are identified in the upper pole of the right kidney (*arrows*) in a patient with disseminated *P. carinii*. Multiple punctate calcifications are also seen in the liver (L), lymph nodes (N), and spleen (S).

resulting from renal tuberculosis may produce contraction of the renal pelvis, distortion of the ureters, and hydronephrosis.[40]

RENAL STONE DISEASE

In an HIV-infected patient with acute flank pain and hematuria, in whom renal stone disease is suspected, the imaging choices include ultrasonography and intravenous urography.[41] A plain radiograph of the abdomen and pelvis may show a calcified stone in the kidneys, along the pathway of either ureter or in the bladder.[29,41] There may be a delayed nephrogram/pyelogram on the obstructed side on the IVU.[29] Ultrasound is good at visualizing renal and bladder stones, but is of little value in detecting stones in the ureter, except at the ureterovesicle junction.[41] It may be used, however, in conjunction with plain radiographs, if an IVU is contraindicated.

Punctate calcifications can be seen in the renal parenchyma with disseminated infections including *P. carinii,* MAI, and CMV, as discussed above.[30–37] Amphotericin B, which is used intravenously to treat disseminated fungal infections, can also cause renal calcifications. There are also a variety of other causes of renal cortical or medullary calcification (nephro-

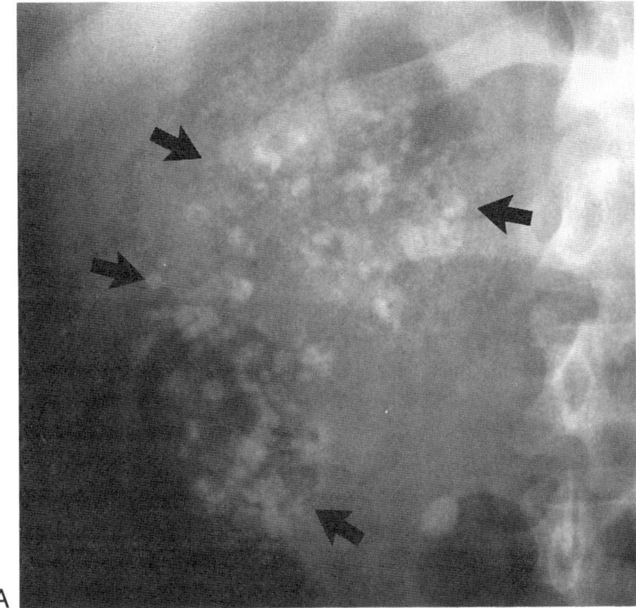

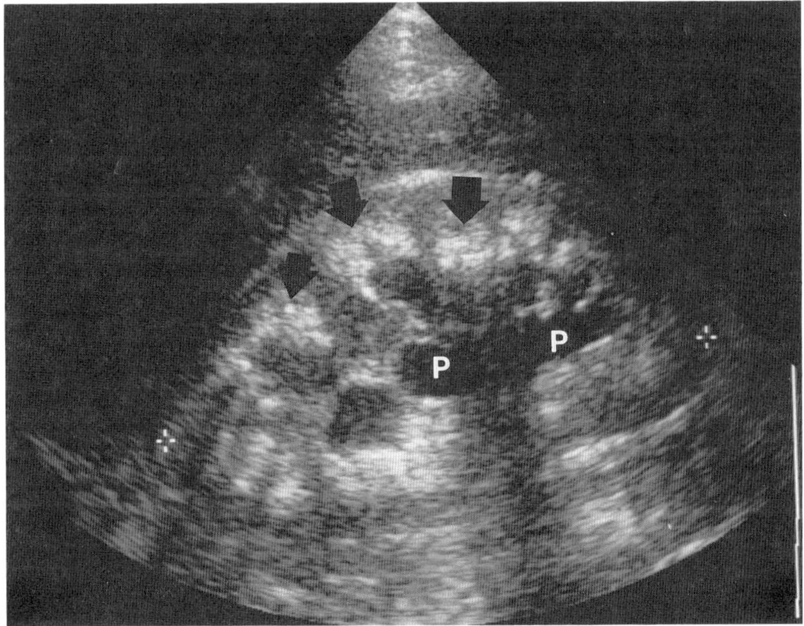

Fig. 11-5. (A) Supine radiograph of the abdomen showing diffuse calcifications (nephrocalcinosis) throughout the right kidney *(arrows)*. A calcified stone is also identified in the proximal right ureter. **(B)** Longitudinal sonogram of the right kidney demonstrating mild dilatation of the pelvicalyceal system (P) with focal areas of calcifications in the area of the renal pyramids *(arrows)*.

Table 11-1. Renal Calcifications in HIV Patients

Infections
    Pneumocystis carinii
    Mycobacterium tuberculosis
    Mycobacterium avium-intracellulare
    Cytomegalovirus
    Candida albicans
Drugs
    Sulfadiazine
    Amphotericin B
    Analgesic nephropathy
Hypercalcemia
    Hyperparathyroidism
    Malignancies
    Vitamin D intoxication
    Milk-alkali syndrome
Miscellaneous
    Medullary sponge kidney
    Hyperuricemia
    Renal tubular acidosis
    Sarcoidosis
    Sickle cell disease
    Oxalosis

calcinosis), not directly related to HIV infection[29] (Table 11-1 and Fig. 11-5).

RENAL MASSES

Renal masses are often detected incidentally on sonograms or CT scans performed to image other organs (Table 11-2). Uncommonly, an AIDS patient with hematuria will have a renal imaging study that reveals a mass.

Table 11-2. Renal Masses in HIV Infection

Benign
    Cystic
        Simple cyst
        Polycystic kidney disease
        Acquired renal cystic disease
        Abscess
    Solid
        Angiomyolipoma
        Adenoma
Malignant
    Solid
        AIDS-related lymphoma
        Renal cell carcinoma
        Metastatic tumors

Cystic Renal Masses

Simple renal cysts are very common and appear as lucent defects during the nephrogram phase of an IVU.[42] They may also cause a mass effect on the adjacent pelvicalyceal system. The sonogram will demonstrate a smooth thin (2 to 3 mm) wall and echofree fluid with good through-transmission.[42] If there is doubt about whether a cyst is benign because of internal echoes or septations within the cyst, focal or diffuse thickening of the wall of the cyst, or calcification of the cyst wall, a CT scan both without and with contrast should be performed.[43] The scan without contrast is used to detect calcification within the kidney or within the wall of the cyst itself, while the administration of contrast will demonstrate the degree of wall enhancement surrounding the fluid-filled center. The density of the fluid within the cyst should never exceed 20 to 25 Hounsfield units (HU).[42,43] If the fluid measures greater than this, hemorrhage into the cyst, possibly from an underlying tumor, has to be considered, so careful evaluation of the cyst wall with contiguous thin CT sections (3 to 5 mm) is necessary. It should be remembered that a thick-walled abscess can mimic a necrotic tumor, and so clinical correlation with the imaging findings is necessary.

If it cannot be determined whether a renal mass is benign or malignant (indeterminate mass), a magnetic resonance imaging (MRI) scan can be performed both without and with gadolinium.[44] If this does not resolve the problem, consideration has to be given to operative resection of the mass. Ultrasound or CT-guided needle biopsy should only be performed if clinical circumstances dictate that the patient is not an operative candidate, or where lymphoma of the kidney is a strong likelihood.

The autosomal dominant or adult type of polycystic kidney disease may be discovered on an ultrasound or CT scan of the patient presenting with high blood pressure or renal failure. The kidneys will be large and contain multiple cysts that range in size from millimeters to centimeters.[42] Internal echoes within the cysts by ultrasonography may be due to hemorrhage. The cysts may also have curvilinear and punctate calcifications in their walls.

Solid Renal Masses

The most common cause of solid renal masses in HIV-infected patients is renal lymphoma.[16,45–48] On ultrasound, these are seen as single or multiple hypoechoic masses in the kidney (Fig. 11-6), which may infiltrate into the renal sinus and diffusely enlarge the kidney.[47] Lymphomas may also grow around the capsule of the kidney to envelop it.[47] Similar findings will be present on CT scan.[45,46] These masses do not enhance with intravenous contrast, as they are hypovascular. It is important to do a contrast-enhanced CT scan to detect these masses, however, as they may not be evident on a non-contrast-enhanced scan. Renal lymphoma is usually associated with disease in the adjacent retroperitoneal lymph nodes and in organs such as

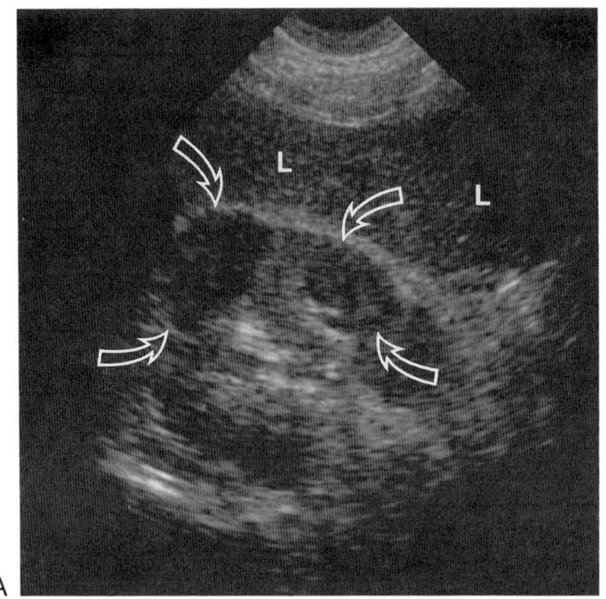

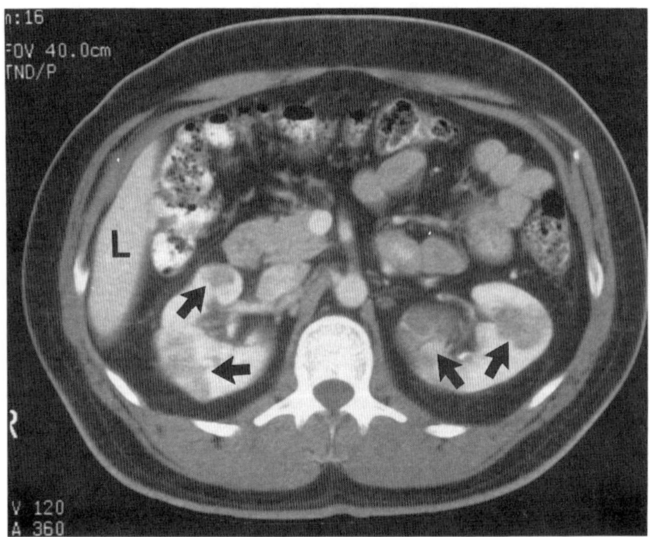

Fig. 11-6. **(A)** Transverse sonogram of the right kidney showing AIDS-related renal lymphoma as two hypoechoic masses *(arrows)* in the right kidney. L, liver. **(B)** Contrast-enhanced CT scan demonstrating multiple low-density masses *(arrows)* in both kidneys in patient with AIDS-related lymphoma. No retroperitoneal lymphadenopathy is seen. L, liver.

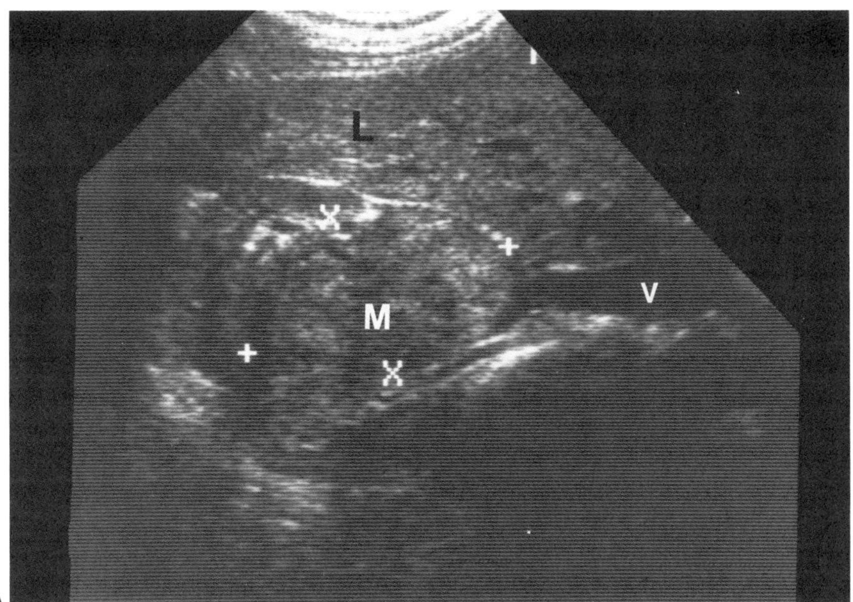

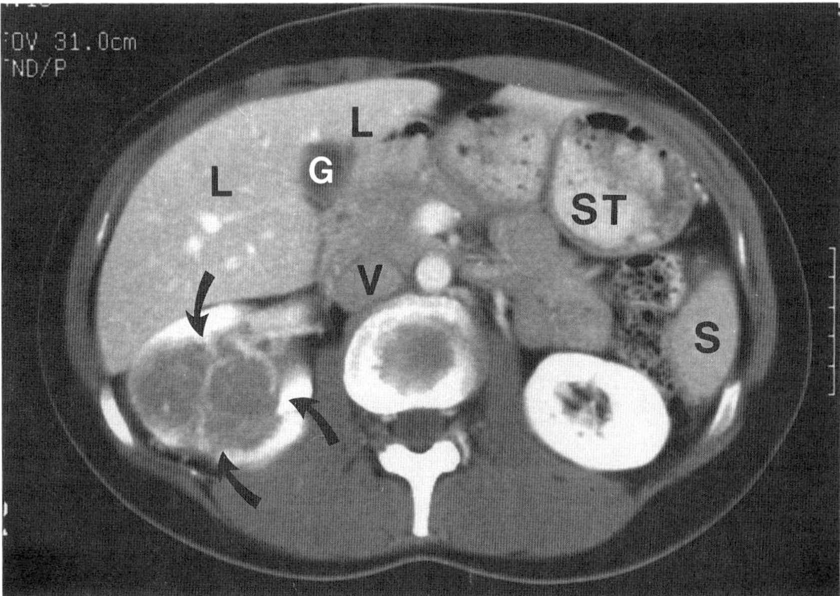

Fig. 11-7. Hypernephroma of the right kidney in an AIDS patient. **(A)** Transverse sonogram of the right kidney demonstrating a solid mass (M). L, liver; V, inferior vena cava. **(B)** Contrast-enhanced CT scan demonstrating a solid vascular mass *(arrows)* in the right kidney. There is no evidence of invasion of the inferior vena cava (V), liver metastasis, or retroperitoneal lymphadenopathy. G, gallbladder; ST, stomach; S, spleen.

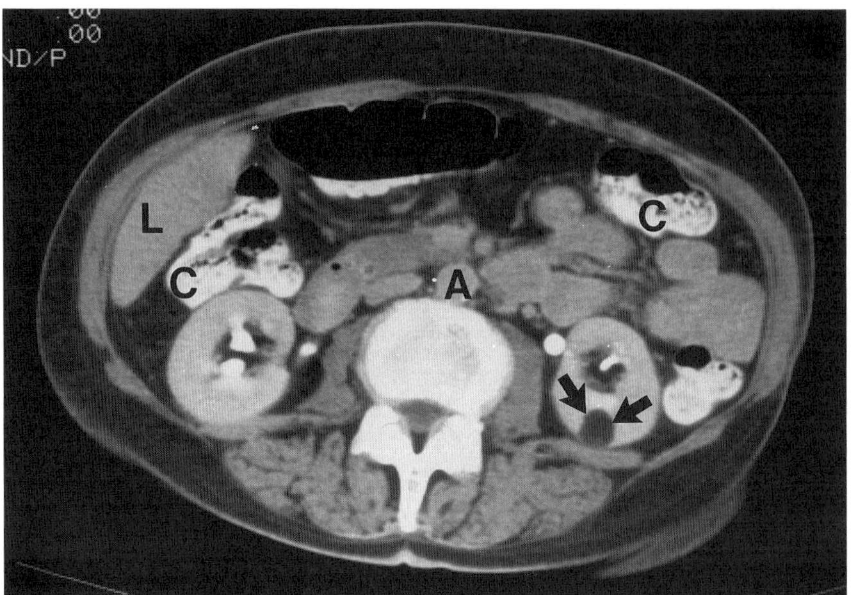

Fig. 11-8. Contrast-enhanced CT scan demonstrates a renal angiomyolipoma as well-defined mass of fat density in the left kidney *(arrows)*. L, liver; C, colon; A, aorta.

the liver, spleen, and adrenal gland. However, the kidneys may be the only site of involvement.[45,46,48] Kaposi sarcoma usually involves the kidney only microscopically, and so cannot usually be seen with imaging techniques.[16]

Other solid mass lesions of the kidney such as renal cell carcinoma may also be found[43,49] (Fig. 11-7), which may be seen on ultrasound or CT to invade the renal vein into the inferior vena cava. There may be adjacent retroperitoneal lymphadenopathy along with liver metastasis. MRI is an alternate imaging technique to CT in staging the extent of renal cell carcinoma and may show venous invasion by the tumor, often better than CT.[44]

Not all solid mass lesions of the kidney in the AIDS patient are malignant. The most common benign renal tumor is an angiomyolipoma. It has a characteristic appearance, being echogenic on ultrasound while the CT scan may show that it contains fat[43](Fig. 11-8).

CONCLUSION

Radiologic imaging of the kidneys and genitourinary tract plays a very important role in the clinical evaluation and management of patients with AIDS, particularly in the setting of acute renal failure, hematuria or possible nephrolithiasis, and in the evaluation of renal masses. Proper use of the various imaging modalities that are available requires close collaboration between clinicians and radiologists.

REFERENCES

1. Jeffrey RB: Abdominal imaging in the immunocompromised patient. Radiol Clin North Am 30:579, 1992
2. Federle MP: A radiologist looks at AIDS: imaging evaluation based on symptom complexes. Radiology 166:553, 1988
3. Nugent PA, Hill MC, Dunwoody WJ et al: Sonography of renal failure in AIDS. J Ultrasound Med 9:S19, 1990
4. Huntington DK, Hill SC, Hill MC: Sonographic manifestations of medical renal disease. Semin Ultrasound CT MR 12:290, 1991
5. Schneiderman DJ, Arenson DM, Cello JP et al: Hepatic disease in patients with the acquired immune deficiency syndrome (AIDS). Hepatology 7:925, 1987
6. Valeri A, Neusy AJ: Acute and chronic renal disease in hospitalized AIDS patients. Clin Nephrol 35:110, 1991
7. Rao TKS: Human immunodeficiency virus (HIV) associated nephropathy. Annu Rev Med 42:391, 1991
8. Soni A, Agarwal A, Chander P et al: Evidence for an HIV-related nephropathy: a clinico-pathological study. Clin Nephrol 31:12, 1989
9. Carbone L, D'Agati V, Cheng JT, Appel GB: Course and prognosis of human immunodeficiency virus-associated nephropathy. Am J Med 87:389, 1989
10. Bourgoignie JJ, Meneses R, Ortiz C et al: The clinical spectrum of renal disease associated with human immunodeficiency virus. Am J Kidney Dis 12:131, 1988
11. Langs C, Gallo GR, Schacht RG et al: Rapid renal failure in AIDS-associated focal glomerulosclerosis. Arch Intern Med 150:287, 1990
12. Yee JM, Raghavendra BN, Horii SC, Ambrosino M: Abdominal sonography in AIDS, a review. J Ultrasound Med 8:705, 1989
13. Townsend RR, Jeffrey RB: Ultrasonography in AIDS. Ultrasound Q 7:293, 1989
14. Hamper UM, Goldblum LE, Hutchins GM et al: Renal involvement in AIDS: sonographic-pathologic correlation. AJR 150:1321, 1988
15. Schaffer RM, Schwartz GE, Becker JA et al: Renal ultrasound in acquired immune deficiency syndrome. Radiology 153:511, 1984
16. Miller FH, Parikh S, Gore RM et al: Renal manifestations of AIDS. Radiographics 13:587, 1993
17. Kamholtz RG, Cronan JJ, Dorfman GS: Obstruction and the minimally dilated renal collecting system: US evaluation. Radiology 170:51, 1989
18. Naidich JB, Rackson ME, Mossey RT, Stein HL: Nondilated obstructive uropathy: percutaneous nephrostomy performed to reverse renal failure. Radiology 160:653, 1986
19. Mettler FA, Guiberteau MJ: Genitourinary system. p. 237. In: Essentials of Nuclear Medicine Imaging. WB Saunders, Philadelphia, 1991
20. Christin S, Baumelou A, Bahri S et al: Acute renal failure due to sulfadiazine in patients with AIDS. Nephron 55:233, 1990
21. Oster S, Hutchison F, McCabe R: Resolution of acute renal failure in toxoplasmic encephalitis despite continuance of sulfadiazine. Rev Infect Dis 12:618, 1990
22. Farinas MC, Echevarria S, Sampedro I et al: Case report: renal failure due to

sulphadiazine in AIDS patients with cerebral toxoplasmosis. J Intern Med 233: 365, 1993

23. Hein R, Brunkhorst R, Thon WF et al: Symptomatic sulfadiazine crystalluria in AIDS patients: a report of two cases. Clin Nephrol 39:254, 1993

24. Simon DI, Brosius FC, Rothstein DM: Sulfadiazine crystalluria revisited: the treatment of toxoplasma encephalitis in patients with acquired immunodeficiency syndrome. Arch Intern Med 150:2379, 1990

25. Miles BJ, Melser M, Farah R et al: The urological manifestations of the acquired immunodeficiency syndrome. J Urol 142:771, 1989

26. Goldman SM, Fishman EK: Upper urinary tract infection: the current role of CT, ultrasound and MRI. Semin Ultrasound CT MR 12:335, 1991

27. Soulen MC, Fishman EK, Goldman SM, Gatewood OMB: Bacterial renal infection: role of CT. Radiology 171:703, 1989

28. Lang EK: Renal, perirenal and pararenal abscesses: percutaneous drainage. Radiology 174:109, 1990

29. Banner MP: Calculous disease. p. 1752. In Pollack HM (ed): Clinical Urography. WB Saunders, Philadelphia, 1990

30. Falkoff GE, Rigsby CM, Rosenfield AT: Partial, combined cortical and medullary nephrocalcinosis: US and CT patterns in AIDS-associated MAI infection. Radiology 162:343, 1987

31. Radin DR, Baker EL, Klatt EC et al: Visceral and nodal calcification in patients with AIDS-related *Pneumocystis carinii* infection. AJR 154:27, 1990

32. Radin DR: Intraabdominal *Mycobacterium tuberculosis* vs *Mycobacterium avium-intracellulare* infections in patients with AIDS: distinction based on CT findings. AJR 156:487, 1991

33. Towers MJ, Withers CE, Hamilton PA et al: Visceral calcification in patients with AIDS may not always be due to *Pneumocystis carinii*. AJR 156:745, 1991

34. Spouge AR, Wilson SR, Gopinath N et al: Extrapulmonary *Pneumocystis carinii* in a patient with AIDS: sonographic findings. AJR 155:76, 1990

35. Lubat E, Megibow AJ, Balthazar EJ et al: Extrapulmonary *Pneumocystis carinii* infection in AIDS: CT findings. Radiology 174:157, 1990

36. Bray HJ, Lail VJ, Cooperberg PL: Tiny echogenic foci in the liver and kidney in patients with AIDS: not always due to disseminated *Pneumocystis carinii*. AJR 158:81, 1992

37. Bargman JM, Wagner C, Cameron R: Renal cortical nephrocalcinosis: a manifestation of extrapulmonary *Pneumocystis carinii* infection in the acquired immunodeficiency syndrome. Am J Kidney Dis 17:712, 1991

38. Shirkhoda A: CT findings in hepatosplenic and renal candidiasis. J Comput Assist Tomogr 11:795, 1987

39. Kintanar C, Cramer BC, Reid WD, Andrews WL: Neonatal renal candidiasis: sonographic diagnosis. AJR 147:801, 1986

40. Goldman SM, Fishman EK, Hartman DS et al: Computed tomography of renal tuberculosis and its pathological correlates. J Comput Assist Tomogr 9:771, 1985

41. Hill MC, Rich JI, Mardiat JG, Finder CA: Sonography vs. excretory urography in acute flank pain. AJR 144:1235, 1985

42. Hayden CK, Swischuk LE: Renal cystic disease. Semin Ultrasound CT MR 12: 361, 1991

43. Bosniak MA: The small (≤3.0 cm) renal parenchymal tumor: detection, diagnosis, and controversies. Radiology 179:307, 1991

44. Semeleka RC, Shoenut JP, Kroeker MA et al: Renal lesions: controlled compari-

son between CT and 1.5 T MR imaging with nonenhanced and gadolinium-enhanced fat-suppressed spin echo and breath-hold FLASH techniques. Radiology 182:425, 1992
45. Radin DR, Esplin JA, Levine AM, Ralls PW: AIDS-related non-Hodgkin's lymphoma: abdominal CT findings in 112 patients. AJR 160:1133, 1993
46. Nyberg DA, Jeffrey RB, Federle MP et al: AIDS-related lymphomas: evaluation by abdominal CT. Radiology 159:59, 1986
47. Townsend RR, Laing FC, Jeffrey RB, Bottles K: Abdominal lymphoma in AIDS: evaluation with US. Radiology 171:719, 1989
48. Mohler JL, Jarow JP, Marshall FF: Unusual urological presentations of acquired immune deficiency syndrome: large cell lymphoma. J Urol 138:627, 1987
49. Smith SJ, Bosniak MA, Megibow AJ et al: Renal cell carcinoma: earlier discovery and increased detection. Radiology 170:699, 1989

Dialysis and Transplantation in Patients with HIV Infection

Rashmi Vijayvargiya
Juan P. Bosch

INTRODUCTION

The growth of the human immunodeficiency virus (HIV) epidemic and the considerable number of HIV-infected patients developing renal failure has resulted in an increasing need for providing renal replacement therapy.

Although renal replacement therapy may maintain life in HIV-infected patients, its impact on survival may be limited compared with the course of the retroviral infection itself. Improved survival may result because of better understanding of the disease and its prevention, and advancements in antiretroviral therapy and the treatment of opportunistic infections.

PREVALENCE OF HIV INFECTION IN DIALYSIS PATIENTS

Hemodialysis

The prevalence of HIV infection among patients with end-stage renal disease (ESRD) treated with hemodialysis varies widely depending on the geographic location of the unit and the demographics of the patient population. The largest of the initial studies was performed by Marcus et al.[1] who surveyed 1,324 patients in 28 dialysis centers in 12 states. HIV seropositivity was assessed by Western blot techniques. The prevalence of HIV seropositivity ranged from 0.3 to 2.6 percent depending on the location of the dialysis unit and the demographics of the individual patient populations. The overall seroprevalence was 0.98 percent. This variability in seroprevalence rates and overall prevalence in the U.S. ESRD population has been observed in several other studies and reviews.[2–7] The seroprevalence was higher in patients tested in eight centers located in areas from which a high cumulative incidence of acquired immunodeficiency syndrome (AIDS) had been reported. However, this study[1] suffered from possible bias because patients volunteered for HIV testing, which may have resulted in either overestimation or underestimation of the true prevalence of HIV infection.

Reiser et al.[8] also documented a high point prevalence of HIV seropositivity in ESRD patients treated with hemodialysis in an area with a high incidence of AIDS. From January 1, 1986 through June 30, 1989, 320 chronic hemodialysis patients at the Brookdale Hospital Medical Center were tested for the presence of antibody to HIV, using enzyme-linked immunosorbent assay (ELISA) as well as Western blot techniques. Thirty-nine patients (12 percent) had serologic evidence of HIV infection. Thirty-four (87 percent) of the 39 HIV-seropositive patients were asymptomatic at the start of the study, whereas 3 had AIDS-related complex (ARC) and two had AIDS.

To assess the epidemiology of HIV infection in a large ESRD population, a collaborative study was conducted in Boston and Baltimore in the early 1980s.[9] Among 435 patients in Baltimore and 90 patients in Boston, 2.8 percent and 3.3 percent of patients, respectively, were HIV seropositive by ELISA and Western blot techniques. Among 100 frozen serum samples obtained from another population of patients treated for ESRD with hemodialysis in Boston in 1980, only one was seropositive. Many repeatedly ELISA positive but Western blot negative specimens were observed in each of the three groups studied. Two important conclusions can be drawn from these data. The point prevalence of patients exposed to HIV in these two hemodialysis populations was well in excess of the seroprevalence noted concurrently in the general population by Red Cross Blood Centers in those two cities. These point prevalences were substantially higher than those reported from dialysis centers in other large cities as well. Because the patients were not evaluated for risk factors, it is possible that some or even all patients had been infected as a result of sexual activity or intravenous drug use. Second, the proportion of specimens that was repeatedly ELISA positive but Western blot negative was striking, especially among the stored serum samples.

The high prevalence of HIV-1 infection in populations at risk in Miami prompted a seroepidemiologic study of both HIV-1 and human T-cell leukemia virus type 1 (HTLV-1, a closely related virus) infection in patients with ESRD treated with chronic hemodialysis.[7] One hundred twenty-nine patients treated with hemodialysis in 1986 and 1987 were tested for antibody against both viral antigens by ELISA. Seroreactive samples for HIV-1 and/or HTLV-1 were confirmed by Western blot and, for HTLV-1, by viral cultures. Thirty patients (23.2 percent) had evidence of retroviral infection (22 for HIV-1 alone, 4 for HTLV-1 alone, and 4 for both HIV-1 and HTLV-1). The most frequent risk factors were intravenous drug use, followed by blood transfusion. Patients exposed to HIV-1 had lower T4/T8 ratios and higher mortality than those with HTLV-1 infection alone. The authors concluded that HTLV-1, as well as HIV-1 infection, is endemic in chronic dialysis centers in Miami. The clinical consequences of HTLV-1 infection in relatively immunocompromised patients treated with chronic hemodialysis remains to be established.

Kimmel et al.[10] studied 392 ESRD patients treated with renal replacement therapy from 1984 to 1992 in Washington, DC. The prevalence of exposure to HIV was 7.9 percent. Twenty-three HIV-infected patients were treated with hemodialysis. The HIV-infected ESRD patients were younger than uninfected patients. The mean age of the HIV-infected patients treated with hemodialysis was 37.5 years, compared with 49.8 years for the uninfected patients ($P < .002$). The majority of patients were black males. In contrast to other studies, most patients had homosexual behavior as the risk factor for HIV infection.

Alter et al.[11] surveyed dialysis centers reporting patients with HIV infection from 1985 to 1989. In 1985 only 244 (0.3 percent) patients reported from 11 centers were HIV infected. No patient had clinical AIDS. In 1989 1,248 patients from 26 dialysis centers (1 percent) were HIV infected. Six hundred sixty-three had clinical AIDS, and 585 were asymptomatic HIV-infected patients. This suggested a threefold increase in the prevalence of HIV seropositivity in the dialysis population over a short period. Ten percent of the centers and 19 percent of the patients were reported from New York City, where HIV infection is known to be highly prevalent. In general, the geographic distribution of dialysis patients with HIV infection was similar to that reported for all cases of AIDS.

In 1990 the Centers for Disease Control and Prevention (CDC), in collaboration with the Health Care Financing Administration, performed a mail survey of chronic hemodialysis centers in the United States. This study determined trends in hemodialysis-associated diseases. Of 1,995 centers surveyed, 1,882 (94 percent) centers responded, representing 140,608 patients and 36,907 staff members. Twenty-six percent of centers reported providing hemodialysis for patients infected with HIV, and 1.1 percent of dialyzed patients had known HIV infection.[12] These data suggest that the prevalence of HIV infection in the U.S. ESRD population has plateaued.

Continuous Ambulatory Peritoneal Dialysis

Little is known about the prevalence of HIV infection among continuous ambulatory peritoneal dialysis (CAPD)-treated ESRD patients. Rubin[13] studied the prevalence of HIV infection in an ESRD population treated with CAPD in Jackson, Mississippi. Eighty-two patients aged from 7 to 72 years were tested for HIV antibody. Seven (9 percent) were positive by both ELISA and Western blot techniques. This high prevalence of HIV seropositivity was attributed to transmission of HIV infection through frequent blood transfusions before routine screening of blood in 1986.

Of 392 ESRD patients who entered a dialysis program in Washington, DC, 31 or 7.9 percent were HIV infected.[10] Eight of the 31 (25.8 percent) patients elected to start CAPD, but the proportion of HIV-infected patients treated with CAPD was similar to that in the entire ESRD population. The high prevalence can be attributed to the geographical location of the unit in an area with a high incidence of AIDS. Table 12-1 summarizes data regarding the prevalence of HIV infection in ESRD patients in selected populations treated with CAPD and hemodialysis.

Table 12-1. Prevalence of HIV-Infected ESRD Patients

Modality	Authors	Year	Population	Prevalence (%)
HD	Marcus et al.[1]	1986–1987	National	0.98
HD	Perez et al.[2]	1986–1987	Miami, FL	23.2
HD	Chirgwin et al.[4]	1981–1987	Brooklyn, NY	39
HD	Reiser et al.[8]	1986–1989	Brooklyn, NY	12
HD	Baltimore		Baltimore, MD	2.8
	Boston Collabotative Study[9]	1980	Boston, MA	3.3
HD	Kimmel et al.[10]	1984–1992	Washington, DC	8.1
HD	Alter et al.[11]	1989	National	1
HD	CDC and HCFA Survey[12]	1990	National	1.1
CAPD	Rubin[13]	1986	Jackson, MS	9
CAPD	Kimmel et al.[10]	1984–1992	Washington, DC	7.5

Abbreviations: HD, hemodialysis; CAPD, continuous ambulatory peritoneal dialysis.

HIV Testing in the ESRD Population

Screening surveys have relied primarily on ELISA to detect antibodies against HIV. However, the sensitivity of this test in patients with chronic renal failure is uncertain. There is a high false-positive rate using standard ELISA testing for HIV infection in the dialysis population. This has been attributed to the development of antibodies to the H-9 cell line, which is derived from HLA class II antigens.[14] Dialysis patients are often exposed to these antigens as a result of multiple blood transfusions. Peterman et al.[15] found 25 (4.8 percent) of 520 patients treated with hemodialysis were seropositive for antibody to HTLV-III by ELISA. Four had high reactivity on ELISA and also had a positive Western blot evaluation. Twenty-one had low ELISA reactivity, negative Western blot tests, and negative cultures. The low ELISA reactivity among the dialysis patients represented false-positive test results rather than impaired ability to produce antibodies. The false-positive ELISA test results in these patients were due to exposure to H-9 cell line antigens during blood transfusions. Frequent blood transfusions induced cross-reacting antibodies against determinants of these cells used to culture HIV. Patients with low ELISA reactivity received more transfusions in the dialysis center than seronegative controls from the same centers. The HTLV-III culture technique is relatively insensitive, as only one patient in the high ELISA reactivity group was culture positive. The authors of this study concluded that frequent blood transfusions place dialysis patients at risk for HIV infection, but more commonly lead to false-positive results using the ELISA.

Arnow et al.[14] tested 83 chronic hemodialysis patients for HIV infection. Five (6 percent) of the patients had positive screening ELISA at low reactivity. Four of these five patients had antibodies to H-9 cellular antigens. Comparison of the five seropositive patients to control subjects matched for age, sex, and duration of dialysis showed no significant differences in the number of lymphocytes or helper/suppressor T-cell ratio between the groups. Specimens with this low level of reactivity are usually culture and Western blot negative, and are typically considered false positives. Six months later, screening ELISA results and Western blot analyses were negative in these five patients, using a newer assay with improved specificity.

Routine Use of HIV Testing in Dialysis
Patients

The most important reasons to conduct HIV testing in patients with ESRD are to diagnose current illness, to identify asymptomatic HIV-infected persons who could benefit from prophylactic and antiretroviral treatments, to minimize the risk of transmission in health care settings, and to implement education in safe sexual practices (Table 12-2).

Reiser et al.[8] found during their $3\frac{1}{2}$ year study that 87 percent (34 of 39)

Table 12-2. Benefits of Routine HIV Testing in ESRD Patients

Possible benefit from antiretroviral prophylaxis and prophylaxis for specific infections leading to improved survival

Institution of behavioral modification techniques to prevent spread of infection to others

Benefit for infection control purposes

Screening prior to transplantation

of HIV-infected patients were asymptomatic at the beginning of the study, and 72 percent (28 of 39) remained asymptomatic for a mean period of 14 months (range 1 to 42 months). In the same study, 25 percent (10 of 39) of HIV-positive patients did not volunteer a risk factor for infection until after the positive HIV serology was obtained. Thus, this study suggested the importance of routine HIV testing in the ESRD population, because a significant number of patients in an area of endemic HIV infection were infected in the absence of obvious risk factors.

SURVIVAL

Hemodialysis

Survival of HIV-infected patients with ESRD is variable and depends on the patient's stage of infection. Early reports were uniformly pessimistic and suggested that survival of patients with AIDS and ESRD was dismal.[16,17] A study by Rao et al.[16] performed between January 1982 and December 1986, among 750 patients with AIDS, showed 43 (5.7 percent) developed irreversible renal failure (AIDS-associated nephropathy). Twelve patients were not dialyzed, and all died of uremia within 1 month. Of the remaining 31 patients who were hemodialyzed, 5 survived more than 3 months and 2 lived 7 and 9 months each. In another group of 18 hemodialysis patients who used intravenous drugs and developed AIDS during maintenance dialysis therapy, all died within 3 months of diagnosis. None of these 18 patients were tested for HIV antibody before initiation of hemodialysis; their renal failure was presumed to be due to heroin nephropathy. The authors suggested that maintenance hemodialysis was not effective in prolonging life, either in patients with AIDS-associated nephropathy and uremia, or in patients with ESRD in whom AIDS developed during the course of maintenance dialysis. They also suggested that hemodialysis may be useful only in the management of potentially reversible acute renal failure in patients with AIDS.

A study by Ortiz et al.[17] considered 51 adults with HIV infection, including 20 chronic hemodialysis patients in whom HIV infection was documented before or concurrently with the development of symptomatic chronic renal failure, and 31 patients with HIV-associated nephropathy requiring chronic maintenance hemodialysis. Patients were followed to evaluate survival on outpatient dialysis in relation to the clinical stage of the HIV infection, regardless of when infection was acquired. The 17 patients who developed AIDS died a mean of 93 days after starting hemodialysis. On the other hand, 12 asymptomatic HIV carriers were alive after a mean follow-up of 488 days on chronic hemodialysis. Five hemodialysis patients with ARC were alive after a mean of 564 days. This study showed that in asymptomatic carriers and in patients with ARC, maintenance hemodialysis can provide meaningful, long-term life support. Clearly more experience is needed to identify which specific complications may carry a worse prognosis and which, if any, may be compatible with meaningful survival on hemodialysis.

Feinfeld et al.[18] reported a mean survival in patients with AIDS and ESRD treated with hemodialysis of 13.2 months, whereas HIV-infected ESRD patients at earlier stages of disease survived, on average, 15.7 months. Survival in patients with AIDS was significantly shorter than for less symptomatic HIV-infected patients. This study suggested that the approach to such patients should be individualized. Despite previous reports that dialysis patients with AIDS do very poorly,[16,17] in this study five patients with AIDS all lived more than 8 months on maintenance dialysis, and three survived over 1 year. The authors concluded that patients with AIDS treated with maintenance hemodialysis do not necessarily have only a 1 to 3 month life expectancy. Survival of 12 months or more is possible, even with recurrent opportunistic infections, probably because of use of antiretroviral therapy and improvements in treating opportunistic infections.

A study by Kimmel et al.[10] assessed the life expectancy of HIV-infected patients treated with hemodialysis and CAPD. Survival time for each individual patient was determined by the number of months between first and last dialysis, or death. Patients were entered into the chronic hemodialysis or CAPD programs according to standard clinical criteria. Approximately 8 percent of both the hemodialysis and CAPD population were HIV infected. Nearly two-thirds of the patients had stage IV infection. Mean survival time in HIV-infected patients treated with hemodialysis was 14.7 months. Age, HIV status, and stage of HIV infection were predictors of survival in hemodialysis patients, whereas sex and race were not. Mean survival time for the entire non-HIV-infected hemodialysis population (n = 361) was 44 months (Fig. 12-1).

Continuous Ambulatory Peritoneal Dialysis

Little has been written regarding the role of CAPD in the treatment of HIV-infected patients with ESRD. A major problem in the care of HIV-infected CAPD patients is the possible development of malnutrition. Several investigators have argued that the serum albumin level in CAPD patients correlates with protein catabolic rate, suggesting that a low serum albumin is the result of insufficient protein intake with resultant protein malnutrition. Many CAPD patients do not ingest the daily amount of protein required

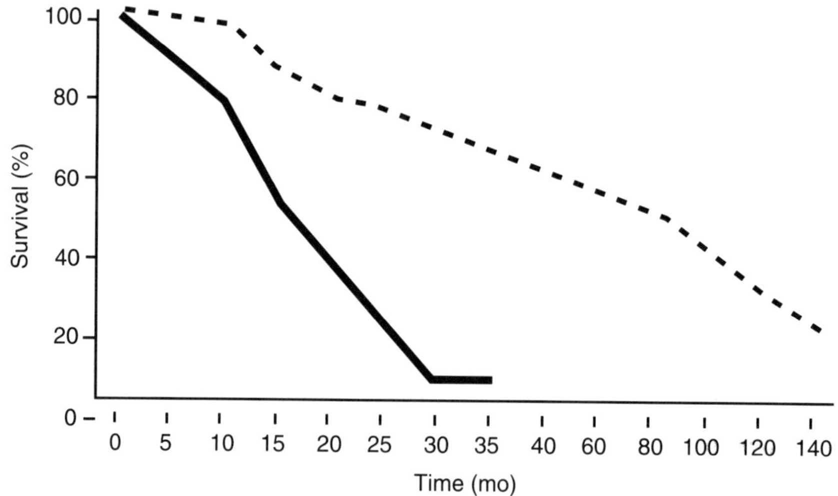

Fig. 12-1. Kaplan-Meier survival curves for HIV-infected patients with ESRD, treated with hemodialysis (*solid line*), and uninfected hemodialysis patients (*broken line*). The curves are significantly different ($P < .001$, log rank test). (Data from Kimmel et al.[10])

to maintain nitrogen balance. Protein losses imposed by the treatment may result in increased morbidity and mortality.

In a study by Kimmel et al.[10] eight HIV-infected patients elected to start CAPD. HIV-infected ESRD patients treated with CAPD had lower mean serum albumin concentration at the time of their first dialysis treatment, compared with the hemodialysis patients. There were no significant differences in mean age or the distribution of patients with regard to racial background or renal or comorbid disease between HIV-infected patients treated with CAPD and hemodialysis. Mean survival of noninfected patients with ESRD treated with CAPD was 41.6 months, significantly longer than the mean 17.9 months survival in HIV-infected ESRD patients treated with CAPD (Fig. 12-2). When HIV-infected ESRD patients were analyzed separately, there was no difference in mean survival time (14.7 versus 17.9 months) between patients treated with hemodialysis and CAPD (Fig. 12-3). Treatment modality, therefore, was not a significant factor in determining survival for HIV-infected patients with ESRD.

It is possible that albumin loss during CAPD might have negatively impacted on survival in patients treated with peritoneal dialysis. This might be a consideration in HIV-infected patients treated with CAPD, because nutrition may be an important factor in the survival of HIV-infected patients. However, HIV-infected CAPD patients in the study had a survival rate that was not significantly different from that of patients treated with hemodialysis, in spite of their lower mean serum albumin level at the time of initiation of CAPD treatment and the protein losses imposed by the treat-

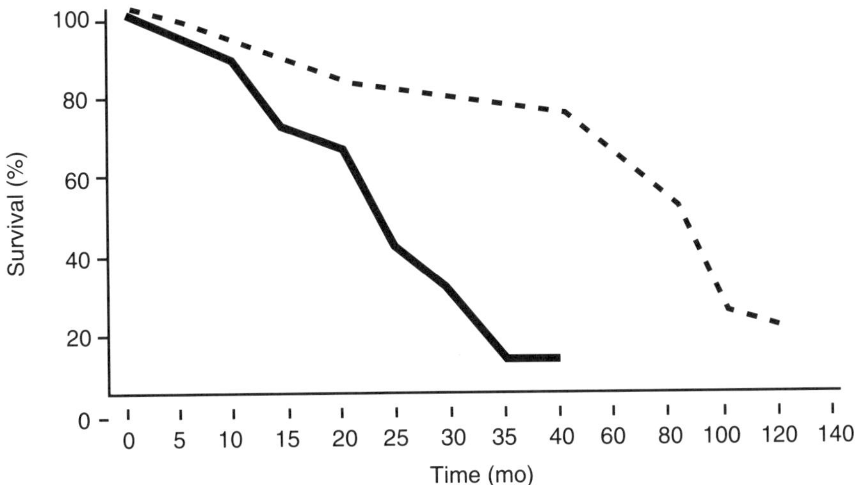

Fig. 12-2. Kaplan-Meier survival curves for HIV-infected patients with ESRD, treated with CAPD (*solid line*), and uninfected CAPD patients (*broken line*). The curves are significantly different ($P < .001$, log rank test). (Data from Kimmel et al.[10])

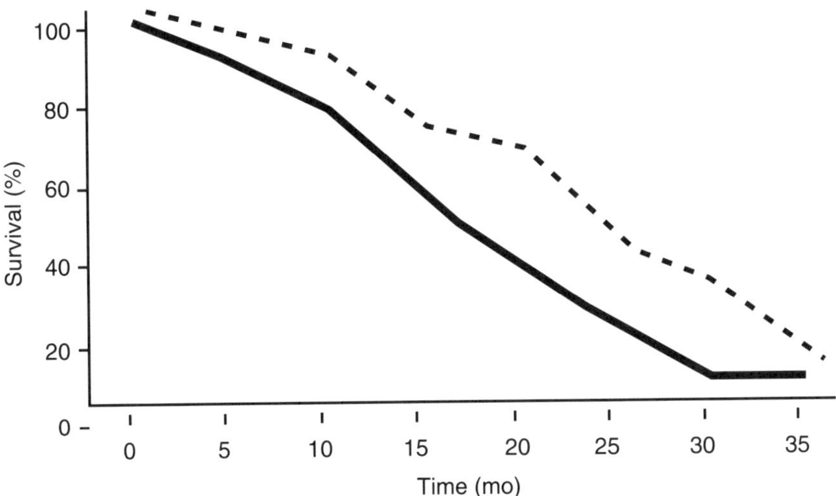

Fig. 12-3. Kaplan-Meier survival curves for HIV-infected patients with ESRD, treated with hemodialysis (*solid line*), and CAPD (*broken line*). There is no significant difference between the curves. (Data from Kimmel et al.[10])

ment. There was no difference in the number of hospitalizations, or the prevalence of dementia between the two groups of HIV-infected patients treated for ESRD.

Tebben et al.[19] studied the outcome of HIV-infected ESRD patients treated with CAPD. These patients were retrospectively studied from 1987 to 1992. Survival was defined as the percentage of patients remaining on CAPD at defined time intervals after initiation of CAPD. Mortality was higher in patients with stage IV compared with asymptomatic HIV infection (CDC classes II and III). Hospitalization rates were higher in patients with advanced infection. One- and 2-year patient survival on CAPD was 58 percent and 54 percent, respectively. The median survival of 12.1 months from the time of diagnosis of AIDS in 14 of 27 patients in this study compared favorably to the survival of patients with AIDS without ESRD. The authors concluded that survival of HIV-infected patients with ESRD maintained on CAPD is correlated with the stage of HIV infection. They also concluded that survival of AIDS patients with ESRD maintained on CAPD is not substantially worse than survival of AIDS patients without ESRD reported in the literature.

The decision to dialyze patients with AIDS with advanced renal failure often involves complex considerations regarding patient outcomes. However, asymptomatic HIV-infected patients and patients with ARC can do well for months or years during dialytic therapy.[10,18] Moreover, patients with AIDS who develop acute renal failure often recover most or all renal function.[16]

Rao et al.[16] and Bourgoignie et al.[20] recommended consideration of each HIV-infected patient's candidacy for renal replacement therapy on an individual basis, obtaining advance directives whenever possible. The presence of progressive neurologic disease and dementia in patients with AIDS makes the benefit of dialysis more difficult to justify and may require early termination of renal replacement therapy. Recent advances in AIDS research have enabled physicians to prolong symptom-free intervals, to improve treatment of opportunistic infections, and to prolong productive life span even after the occurrence of an AIDS-defining illness.

Improved treatments have extended the survival time of persons with AIDS. In the early years of the epidemic the average time from diagnosis of AIDS to death was less than 12 months. More recent estimates suggest that that time interval has increased to up to 20 months.[21,22] Further improvements in antiretroviral therapy have been effective in prolonging the asymptomatic state in patients whose CD4 cell counts declined to $500/mm^3$ or less.[23]

MODALITY SELECTION

As with any patient, consideration should be given to the impact of the renal replacement therapy on the lifestyle of the patient when selecting treatment modality in patients with HIV infection and ESRD. If the patient

Table 12-3. Potential Advantages of Hemodialysis in HIV-Infected ESRD Patients

Improves bleeding diathesis by correcting platelet dysfunction
Modality of choice in patients with early dementia or in patients with wasting disorder
Preferred modality in patients who are noncompliant, or in whom the diagnosis of acute or chronic renal failure is uncertain

has a strong preference for flexibility in diet, active lifestyle, and employment, CAPD may be a preferred treatment modality. However, even mild AIDS-related dementia, which may prevent a patient from performing exchanges, can be considered a great obstacle in choosing CAPD. Asymptomatic HIV-infected patients and patients with ARC may do well treated in center hemodialysis programs, but may also be good candidates for CAPD or home hemodialysis. Patients with AIDS who have frequent opportunistic infections requiring hospitalizations may be better treated with center hemodialysis. The decision to initiate maintenance dialysis for patients with AIDS is not straightforward, particularly because several groups found AIDS patients developing ESRD usually die within weeks to months despite intensive dialysis and nutritional support.[16,17]

Although there are no hard and fast rules regarding choice of modality of renal replacement therapy in HIV-infected patients with ESRD, we review some medical guidelines for selecting dialysis for patients, in order to provide optimal therapy and quality of life. Hemodialysis is the preferred mode of dialysis when treating sick, hospitalized patients, especially if there is uncertainty regarding the diagnosis of acute or chronic renal failure. Center hemodialysis is best recommended in patients who have early dementia or in patients who are noncompliant. CAPD should be avoided in patients with wasting disorders, as protein losses imposed by the treatment may worsen the patient's nutritional status (Table 12-3).

The initiation of hemodialysis partially corrects the defects responsible for platelet dysfunction. However, patients treated with hemodialysis still have a higher risk of hemorrhagic events because of repeated exposure to heparin. Acute bleeding may occur at many sites: gastrointestinal blood loss, subdural and retroperitoneal hematomas, and the vascular access. In addition to acute bleeding episodes, patients treated with hemodialysis are exposed to chronic blood loss with each treatment. Patients with uremic coagulopathy, HIV-mediated thrombocytopenia, and other bleeding diatheses in whom systemic heparinization should be avoided may also benefit from treatment with CAPD (Table 12-4). Peritoneal dialysis may also be beneficial when intravascular insertion of foreign bodies in septic patients is contraindicated. Inability to create an adequate vascular access is always a relative indication for CAPD. Staff who care for HIV-infected patients treated with CAPD may have lower risk of exposure to blood and needle sticks. During hemodialysis, blood membrane interactions may induce cytokine stimulation, which may theoretically enhance viral replication.[24] Gen-

Table 12-4. Potential Advantages of CAPD in HIV-Infected ESRD Patients

Decreased transfusion requirements, facilitating the use of antiretroviral therapy
Decreased occupational exposure of dialysis staff to infection due to lower frequency of venipuncture
Avoid anticoagulation in patients with known bleeding disorders
Avoid vascular access and its complications such as bacteremia and access failure
Less activation of the immune system including cytokine and lymphocyte stimulation with concurrent increased viral replication
Preferred modality in patients with intravenous drug use

erally, cellulosic-based membranes have a greater capacity to activate complement and attenuate granulocyte responses, leading to chronic stimulation of the immune system.[25] In contrast, CAPD utilizes a natural membrane to remove nitrogenous waste products. There is, however, no data that such immune stimulation is deleterious to patients with HIV infection treated with hemodialysis.

ANEMIA AND THE USE OF ERYTHROPOIETIN

Although inadequate production of erythropoietin (EPO) is the most important factor in the pathogenesis of anemia in ESRD, it is not the only factor responsible for anemia in HIV-infected ESRD patients.[26] Other factors such as opportunistic infection and the concurrent use of bone marrow suppressive agents may play an important role in the pathogenesis of anemia. The use of recombinant human EPO in HIV-infected patients has been shown to be of benefit.[27] This therapy is also effective in patients treated with zidovudine.[28] The presence of active infection or liver disease may interfere with the effectiveness of treatment with EPO. The release of lymphokines and tumor necrosis factors during inflammation or infection may inhibit erythropoiesis despite the administration of EPO. Seizures are uncommon in carefully monitored patients, except when hypertension is not controlled or when patients have previous seizure disorders (e.g., associated with primary central nervous system [CNS] pathology such as cryptococcal meningitis, toxoplasmosis, or CNS tuberculosis).

PLACEMENT OF VASCULAR ACCESS

The benefits of early establishment of vascular access should be emphasized. Arteriovenous (A-V) fistula surgery should be performed as early as possible before the initiation of hemodialysis to permit maturation. Delayed surgery, synthetic grafts, and early use of accesses may be associated with increased risk of complications. Indwelling catheters should be avoided, if possible, because of the high rate of infection.[29,30] Early placement of an A-V fistula is preferable to the use of a synthetic graft for vascular access.

THROMBOSIS AND BLEEDING IN HIV-INFECTED ESRD PATIENTS

Patients with HIV infection may have a hypercoagulable state that may lead to recurrent access thrombosis. Several endothelium-dependent physiologic antithrombotic mechanisms have been recently recognized that may be involved in the pathogenesis of HIV-associated hypercoagulability. The major currently known antithrombotic factors are antithrombin III, protein C, protein S, and the fibrinolytic system. Inherited defects in each of these factors can cause serious thrombotic tendencies. Abnormalities such as protein S deficiency, and increased plasminogen activator inhibitor activity have been observed in HIV-infected patients.[31] Whether the HIV infection is associated with endothelial injury, or other inherited factors contribute to such thrombotic tendencies, is unknown. On the other hand, HIV-infected ESRD patients may also have bleeding diatheses. This may not only be secondary to qualitative platelet dysfunction, but also thrombocytopenia, which may be due to medication effects, bone marrow damage or infiltration, or secondary to HIV-immune-mediated mechanisms.[32] Thrombotic thrombocytopenic purpura is another complication of HIV infection that may contribute to bleeding diathesis and renal insufficiency[33] (see Ch. 6).

RISK OF PERITONITIS

HIV infection might be associated with a higher rate of peritonitis, because of immunosuppression, compared with that in uninfected patients with ESRD treated with CAPD. Dressler et al.[34] reported a high incidence of pseudomonal and candidal peritonitis in HIV-infected patients treated with CAPD. They followed 71 patients with ESRD treated with CAPD. Seven were HIV positive and five were considered to be at high risk for HIV infection, but were seronegative. Fifty-nine patients were at low risk for HIV infection. The total peritonitis rate was higher in both the high-risk and HIV-infected groups when compared with that in the low-risk population. Peritonitis usually culminated in catheter removal and in conversion of the patients to hemodialysis. The high-risk patients had similar socioeconomic backgrounds and dialysis exchange techniques compared with patients in the low-risk group. The patients in the high-risk group had more gram-positive infections. These authors suggested that factors related to HIV infection might have influenced the type of pathogens isolated during peritonitis in HIV-infected patients treated with CAPD. This study included patients at high risk for HIV infection, therefore less is known about the natural history of peritonitis in the HIV-infected patients.

Tebben et al.[19] demonstrated a higher risk of peritonitis, as well as a higher percentage of infections attributed to pseudomonas and fungi, in HIV-infected patients treated with CAPD. This was attributed, in part, to a behavioral component, because an increased incidence of peritonitis was observed in the patients who were active parenteral drug users. An element of superimposed immunodeficiency, however, in that population cannot be ruled out. The type of CAPD system (closed versus open) may also affect peritonitis rates.

However, Kimmel et al.[10] reported that peritonitis rates were similar in HIV-infected and uninfected CAPD patients. This group of patients was primarily composed of patients with homosexual behavior as the risk factor for the development of AIDS. Wasser et al.[35] also found no difference in the prevalence of peritonitis in HIV-infected patients compared with uninfected ESRD patients treated with CAPD. Perhaps differences between these populations explain the conflicting results regarding peritonitis in HIV-infected CAPD patients. Clearly we need more information about host defense factors and skin colonization in HIV-infected patients treated with CAPD.

HIV p24 antigen has been detected in a patient's peritoneal dialysis effluent, although no viral isolation studies were performed. Correa-Rotter et al.[36] concluded that the dialysis fluid of HIV-infected patients may contain antigen, and is therefore potentially infective. The authors discussed possible factors such as variability in viral replication or permeability of the peritoneal membrane that could influence the presence of viral antigen in peritoneal fluid. Breyer and Harbison[37] demonstrated that replication competent HIV can be recovered from peritoneal dialysis effluent, despite normal membrane characteristics, the absence of active peritoneal inflammation, and appropriate antiretroviral therapy. They cultured the peritoneal dialysis fluid from two asymptomatic HIV-seropositive patients and one patient with AIDS. HIV was isolated from both the dialysis effluent and blood of two of the three patients tested. The isolation of HIV from peritoneal dialysis effluent suggests that such fluid could be a source of viral transmission. All three patients in this study were receiving zidovudine, which did not abrogate recovery of virus from the peritoneal dialysis effluent. However, this study did not attempt to quantify viral titers present in cell-free dialysate, or to determine the minimum volume of dialysate necessary to obtain a positive culture. Because the majority of recoverable virus resides in the cellular contents of the dialysate effluent, the volume of dialysate needed for positive culture might vary with the cell count of the fluid. It is unknown whether the ability to recover HIV from dialysate correlates with patients' CD4 counts.

As with all issues of exposure to HIV, it is difficult to quantify the risk that exposure to peritoneal dialysis effluent might pose to health care workers or family members of HIV-seropositive individuals. The titers of virus in the dialysate are lower than in blood and serum. The findings, however, suggest that such fluid could potentially be a source of viral transmission. The need for conscientious application of universal precautions both in and outside the hospital is imperative. Various infection control policies for HIV-infected CAPD patients have been suggested (Table 12-5).

Table 12-5. Universal Precautions for Providing CAPD Treatment to HIV-Infected Patients

1. Use universal precautions when obtaining blood and body fluids.
2. Used dialysate bags should be placed in a covered container. At the end of the day, dialysate should be disposed of in a sink or toilet.
3. Gloves, apron, and face shields should be worn while disposing of dialysate.
4. Avoid splashing of dialysate when emptying bags into the toilet; 200 ml of a 1:10 dilution of bleach should be poured into the sink or toilet and left for 30 minutes after the disposal of dialysate.
5. Empty bags, tubing, and cycler sets should be placed into red plastic trash bags labeled "INFECTIOUS" waste. Hands must be washed after these procedures.
6. HIV-infected patients and their families performing CAPD must be educated regarding infection control practices to be followed at home.

(Modified from Centers for Disease Control and Prevention[43] with permission.)

RISK OF NOSOCOMIAL TRANSMISSION IN THE DIALYSIS SETTING

The possibility of transmission of HIV to health care workers has been of concern since the identification of HIV as the cause of AIDS. The cumulative results of several studies of health care workers have shown that they are at an extremely low but finite risk of occupational infection with the virus.[38–41] The predominant occupational risk for infection is through accidental needle stick exposure; however the risk of infection after exposure to HIV-infected blood through a needle stick is less than 0.5 percent.[40]

Alter et al.[11] suggested that the risk of transmission of hepatitis B virus is much greater than that of HIV, and the current established measures for prevention of transmission of hepatitis B virus can be used to minimize the risk of transmission of HIV. Hepatitis B vaccination prevents infection in the general population, but in the ESRD population the response to vaccination remains inadequate.[42] Reactivation of hepatitis B surface antigenemia can occur in patients with HIV infection. Carmen et al.[42] reported a patient who had reactivation of hepatitis B viral infection with reappearance of hepatitis B surface antigenemia in the setting of coinfection with HIV-1. At the initiation of hemodialysis in 1980, this patient, who used intravenous drugs, was found to be anti-hepatitis B surface antibody positive, but hepatitis B surface antigenemia was absent. He had a renal transplant that was subsequently rejected. The antibody titers gradually declined. He was later found to be transiently positive for hepatitis B surface antigen. The authors suggested that infection was probably latent and reactivation may have occurred during the period of immunosuppression. Therefore it seems reasonable to follow antigen levels at frequent intervals in ESRD patients with other viral infections in addition to HIV. Isolated dialysis space or machines are not recommended for treatment of most HIV-infected ESRD patients.[43] Patients who have communicable diseases such as tuberculosis or other mycobacterial infections should be isolated from other patients for 7 to 10 days while

Table 12-6. Universal Precautions for Providing Hemodialysis Treatment to HIV-Infected Patients

1. Dialyzers may be reused but the use of individual dialyzers must be restricted to individual patients.
2. Centers that wish to use high-flux dialysis may consider the use of a separate system for patients with HIV infections.
3. Nondisposable supplies that are not restricted to individual patients must be sterilized between uses.
4. Sodium hypochlorite or formaldehyde, which effectively eradicates HIV, should be used to disinfect dialysate pathways.
5. Gloves must be worn for contact with blood or body fluids, mucous membranes, or nonintact skin of the patient.
6. Hands must be washed immediately before and after patient care.
7. Gowns, masks, and goggles must be worn if aerosolization or splattering of blood or body fluids is likely.
8. Sharp instruments must be handled with great care and discarded immediately in containers designed for this purpose. Used venipuncture needles must not be recapped.
9. Blood spills must be cleaned promptly with disinfectant such as 1:10 dilution of bleach.
10. Refrain from direct patient care if you have exudative lesions.
11. The Employee Health Service should be contacted in cases of accidental needle stick or mucous membrane exposure.

(Modified from Centers for Disease Control and Prevention,[43] with permission.)

drug therapy is initiated. Our policy is to clean and disinfect machines between uses by HIV-infected and other patients. Dialyzers can be reused according to standard procedures for cleaning and testing. Clear labeling of dialyzers and attention to accuracy are required at all times.

The CDC has issued guidelines for providing dialysis treatment to HIV-infected patients.[43] These guidelines cover the use of universal precautions (Table 12-6) to limit nosocomial and occupational spread of HIV infection in the dialysis unit, and policies and procedures that should be used in the care of HIV-infected ESRD patients.

RENAL TRANSPLANTATION AND HIV INFECTION

The HIV epidemic has posed problems for the transplantation community because the use of potent immunosuppressive drugs and the occurrence of intercurrent infections may complicate the already increased potential of HIV infection for morbidity and mortality in transplant patients.

Transmission in the Peritransplant Period

Perioperative blood transfusions or the transplanted organ are the major sources of primary HIV infection in transplant recipients. Most transplant patients receive multiple blood transfusions before or in association with renal transplantation.

A 30-year-old organ donor sustained massive head injuries and required transfusion of 56 units of blood and blood products.[44] This patient died after 2 days. Initial testing of his serum was negative for HIV; however, at the time of transplantation a second evaluation revealed he was HIV seropositive. This suggested that the transfusions had transiently diluted the patient's serum and resulted in a falsely negative HIV antibody test. The recipient of his kidney was seronegative at the time of transplantation but seroconverted by day 51. However, he demonstrated no signs or symptoms of HIV infection 1 year after transplantation. After transplantation, the recipient's blood was periodically assayed for viral p24 antigen and HIV antibody. HIV p24 antigen was detected as early as 1 day after transplantation. p24 titers declined on the fourth day after transplantation, but levels rose until seroconversion.

In potential cadaveric organ donors, HIV antibody testing should be performed on pretransfusion sera or on sera obtained several hours after massive transfusion of blood products. If possible, repeat serum samples for HIV antibody testing should be obtained as close to organ harvesting as possible.

Ward et al.[45] studied two patients in whom HIV antigen was detected within 4 and 16 days after transplantation. In both patients HIV antibody was not detected until 36 days and 27 days, respectively, after the detection of HIV antigen. These findings are consistent with earlier studies that showed that immunosuppressive medications do not delay the humoral immune response to HIV infection in transplant recipients.

In some high-risk geographic areas, 15 to 20 percent of homosexual men who test negative by ELISA may be infected with HIV.[46] Martin et al.[47] reported the case of a renal allograft recipient who developed symptoms suggestive of AIDS. Serologic studies revealed that the donor was HIV infected. Retrospective testing of stored sequential serum samples showed that the recipient was serologically HIV negative before transplantation. p24 antigen was detected in the recipient 21 days after transplantation. The authors suggested that in addition to p24 antigen, elevated β_2-microglobulin levels may be a useful marker for HIV infection before seroconversion in donors.

Simmonds et al.[48] described a case of HIV transmission by transplantation of organs and tissues procured during the "window" period. This study reviewed the processing of all the transplanted organs from the donor, tested stored donor lymphocytes for HIV-1 by viral culture and the polymerase chain reaction, and tested samples for HIV antibody and antigen from four organ recipients (two of whom received a kidney) who seroconverted 26 and 54 days after transplantation. The other two patients who received liver and kidney transplants died. Stored sera from donors that was subsequently tested was positive for HIV p24 antigen and HIV antibody. They concluded that HIV antigen testing may allow earlier detection of infectious donors, thus closing somewhat the "window" of seronegativity.

Thus several case reports have suggested that HIV can be transmitted by solid organs and some forms of tissue transplantation.[44,47,48] The screening tests that are currently used cannot rule out a false-negative test result occurring during the "window" period or because of other factors such as massive blood transfusions. It is widely accepted that a window of seronegativity of 6 to 8 weeks duration may exist after infection with HIV. During this time an antibody response may not be detected.[49,50] Studies using polymerase chain reaction for detection of integrated HIV proviral DNA in peripheral blood mononuclear cell fractions of high-risk individuals suggest that this period of silent infection could last for several months before the appearance of detectable antibody levels by ELISA and Western blot techniques.[51,52] The exclusion of donors whose behavior may place potential recipients at risk for HIV infection may be important, but could negatively impact on organ availability. Careful evaluation of prospective donors' medical histories may help exclude donors recently infected with HIV-1. Special care must be taken to ensure that tissue from intravenous drug user, hemophiliac, and homosexual donors is not HIV infected. The approaches to prevention of transmission of infection via transplantation should include screening of prospective donors for risk factors and laboratory markers of HIV-1 infection, including circulating HIV antigens.

The risk of transmission of HIV infection via kidney transplants appears to be low. It has been lower since December 1985, when routine screening of transplant donors was initiated. The capacity of the transplanted kidney to transmit the virus has been well documented in at least 25 cases[53-55] reporting transmission of HIV infection via this route. In each of these case reports, the donor was a member of a high-risk group. The outcome in the transplanted patients, however, has not been as uniformly poor as has been assumed. Transfusion may play a role in the success rate for kidney transplants. Screening of blood donors has probably been effective in reducing the potential of transfusions to transmit HIV infection. It is not clear if patients who were infected with HIV before transplantation have different outcomes compared with patients who became infected after transplantation.

Milogram et al.[53] reported the case of a 38-year-old woman with no known sexual contacts. In July 1982 she received a cadaver renal allograft. The patient was treated with antilymphocyte globulin, steroids, and azathioprine for a brief period but was later placed on cyclosporine. One month postoperatively the patient was readmitted with cytomegalovirus (CMV) infection. The infection was complicated by massive gastrointestinal bleeding. By this time she had received 75 units of blood before and after transplantation. She developed antibodies to HTLV-III 3 months after renal transplantation. Her course was remarkable for frequent viral infections and a decreasing requirement for immunosuppression. One year after transplantation she received no further immunosuppression. Her renal function remained normal. Kaposi sarcoma was detected in an axillary lymph node biopsy 19 months after transplantation. She died 25 months after transplantation with neurologic deterioration associated with CMV infection.

Feduska et al.[54] reviewed the course of 2,550 kidney transplant recipients treated between 1964 and 1986. A low incidence of AIDS, *Pneumocystis carinii* pneumonia (PCP), Kaposi sarcoma, and lymphoma was observed in these patients. Three recipients developed AIDS. The mode of transmission in one patient was sexual and in two patients was via blood transfusion. One HIV-infected patient died of a perforated appendix and generalized peritonitis 1 month after transplantation. This patient received multiple transfusions. The perioperative course was complicated by PCP and hepatitis C. The second patient died with PCP, Kaposi sarcoma, and staphylococcal septicemia 9 months after transplantation. The third patient died of candida septicemia 34 months after transplantation.

L'age Stehr et al.[55] described four patients who had received cadaveric kidney grafts in 1984 from donors at high risk for the development of AIDS. The three kidney donors had a history of intravenous drug use. Five of the six donated kidneys were transplanted. After transplantation, four recipients were treated with immunosuppressive regimens consisting of steroids and intravenous cyclosporine. All four patients had a similar clinical course. Two to 7 weeks after transplantation, they experienced transient episodes of fever, and pronounced leukopenia and lymphopenia lasting up to 2 months. In all four patients, leukopenia with altered T4/T8 ratios occurred over time. Immunosuppressive medications were continued and the clinical course of HIV infection did not seem to be accelerated. Limited information is available about the fifth recipient who became HIV positive 8 months after transplantation.

In a study by Carbone et al.[56] two patients developed HIV infection after transplantation. Both patients received only low-dose immunosuppressive therapy, had no episodes of rejection for several years, and had excellent renal function at the time they developed opportunistic infections. Both patients died after multiple opportunistic infections that occurred more than 2 years after transplantation. The types of infection were unusual in that toxoplasmosis, disseminated CMV, and aspergillosis usually occur in the early transplant period. In both of these patients, the immunologic profiles were consistent with HIV-related immunodeficiency. The first patient had an inverted T4/T8 ratio of 0.37 with an absolute T4 count of 3/μl. The second patient had a T4/T8 ratio of 1.8 with an absolute T4 cell count of 19/μl. Both patients developed disseminated CMV infection. The profound depletion of T4 cells and loss of B-cell responsiveness was more characteristic of AIDS than of low-dose immunosuppressive therapy. Theoretically the depression of cell-mediated immunity seen in AIDS could prolong allograft survival. This probably occurred in the above cases because these patients maintained allograft survival after 1 year of transplantation despite minimal immunosuppression.

Because either AIDS or immunosuppressive medications can depress cell-mediated immunity, predisposing to the development of opportunistic infections, the appearance of infection alone is insufficient to diagnose AIDS in transplanted HIV-infected patients. During the first 6 months after transplantation, infections are usually bacterial, although other opportunistic infections such as disseminated CMV, aspergillosis, and toxoplasmosis can occur.[56–59] Deaths due to severe infection are unlikely in the later transplant period. However, certain features such as the type of infection, the humoral response to the infection, characteristics of T-cell lymphocyte subsets, the timing of the infection after transplantation, and the amount and type of immunosuppressive therapy used can help distinguish infection related to immunosuppressive therapy alone from that seen in HIV-induced immunodeficiency.[56]

Schwartz et al.[59] reviewed the course of 53 patients in whom HIV infection was caused by liver, kidney, bone, or heart transplantation or blood transfusion. The cumulative incidence of AIDS was significantly lower in 40 transplant patients treated with an immunosuppressive regimen including cyclosporine, compared with 13 transplant patients receiving immunosuppressive therapy without cyclosporine. Cyclosporine cannot prevent the progression of HIV-1 infection, but may have a moderating effect on the progression of disease in HIV-infected persons if it is administered as early as possible after infection.[60] In patients with AIDS, however, toxic effects may be observed secondary to increased immunosuppressive effects leading to increased risk of infections in patients treated with cyclosporine. Further information regarding the outcome of immunomodulation with cyclosporine in HIV-infected transplant patients would be useful.

Post-transplant Course of Previously HIV-Infected Patients

There has been a high incidence of systemic fungal, bacterial, and CMV infection, as well as recurrent localized herpes simplex and candidal infection in HIV-infected patients after their transplantation. Shaffer et al.[61] described rejection episodes in two HIV-infected patients. One patient died of overwhelming gram-negative sepsis 8 weeks after kidney transplantation. The other patient died 9 months after kidney transplantation after sustaining seven major bacterial infections, disseminated CMV infection, and lactobacillus bacteremia.

Oliveira et al.[62] described an HIV-infected patient who had two episodes of allograft rejection within the first 2 months after transplantation. He died 2 years after transplantation with progressive CMV infection and recurrent PCP. Tzakis et al.[63] studied 25 whole organ recipients treated from 1981 through 1988. Eleven patients were infected with HIV before transplantation, although this was not known until later in eight recipients. The other 14 patients were infected perioperatively. The organs transplanted were the liver, heart, and kidney. Six of these patients were alive after a mean of 3.3 years. Survival was not different in the seroconverter (patients who converted after transplantation) and prevalent (patients who were HIV positive before transplant) groups at any point up to 5 years after transplantation. The AIDS-free interval of recipients who seroconverted after transplantation was far less than in control hemophiliac patients who seroconverted after blood transfusions. The reasons for these discrepancies are not known.

Isolated case reports suggest that administration of immunosuppressive therapy after transplantation renders HIV-infected transplant patients more susceptible to opportunistic and other infections.[64] HIV is tropic for T cells, particularly the CD4 helper lymphocytes, which play a central role in the initiation of allograft rejection.[65] In the resting cell, HIV replication is limited until cellular activation develops. After activation, production of mature virus leads to cell death. Asymptomatic individuals who have been seropositive for HIV before transplant had considerable rejection activity after transplantation. Rejection episodes may result in administration of increased immunosuppressive therapy, which may promote viral replication and may be detrimental to the patient.[56] Inhibition of interleukin-2 (IL-2) production, caused by cyclosporine, also decreases the expression of HIV.[66] Prompt et al.[67] suggested that inhibition of IL-2 production by steroids may enhance viral expression and cell death. A major effect of cyclosporine is the inhibition of IL-2-dependent T-lymphocyte proliferation and differentiation of T cells expressing CD4, the primary target cells and receptors for HIV.

Anecdotal observations[60] have suggested that cyclosporine may modify the progression of HIV infection. Erice et al.[64] suggested that use of cyclosporine in a series of HIV-infected patients was not associated either with a better outcome or decreased development of AIDS. Most case reports did not include details regarding the prophylactic regimens used after transplantation to prevent opportunistic infections. Clinical experience with the results of therapy with zidovudine on outcome is needed. The role of immunosuppressive therapy in HIV-infected transplant recipients is uncertain as most of the cases were reported before zidovudine was available. Approximately 50 percent of HIV-infected transplant patients suffer an accelerated course with early deaths from opportunistic infections.[67,68] The contribution of rejection and use of immunosuppressive medications to the outcome of transplant recipients with HIV infection are unknown. Further studies are necessary to evaluate factors that are important in determining the mortality and morbidity of graft and patient survival in HIV-infected transplant patients.

Because of the prognostic implications of infection with HIV, it is reasonable to follow some guidelines for treating HIV-infected recipients of transplanted organs with antiretroviral drugs. Clinical management of patients who are found to be infected with HIV after transplantation should include administration of zidovudine, and perhaps other antiretroviral agents. The efficacy and optimal therapy of such patients, is however, unknown.

Because immunosuppressive agents predispose HIV-infected patients to infectious complications, it seems reasonable to avoid transplantation in HIV-infected patients. Acute rejection is possible in HIV-infected transplant recipients, as the capacity to respond to allogeneic stimulation in such patients remains relatively intact. However, the incidence of opportunistic infections is increased severalfold in such patients. Although the proper therapeutic approach to conventional immunosuppression in HIV-infected transplant patients is unknown, the use of the more potent immunosuppressive medications such as antithymocyte globulin, and OKT3 monoclonal antibodies should probably be avoided. More studies must be performed in this relatively small subset of transplanted patients to evaluate the natural history of the disease and guide proper therapy and management.

REFERENCES

1. Marcus R, Favero MS, Banerjee S et al: Prevalence and incidence of human immune deficiency virus among patients undergoing long term hemodialysis. Am J Med 90:614, 1991
2. Perez G, Ortiz-Interian C, Lee H et al: Human immunodeficiency virus and human T cell leukemia virus type 1 in patients undergoing maintenance hemodialysis in Miami. Am J Kidney Dis 14:39, 1989
3. Villanueva Sy, De Medina M, Perez G et al: Prevalence of human immunodeficiency virus antibodies and hepatitis B markers among patients having hemodialysis (letter). Ann Intern Med 105:968, 1986
4. Chirgwin K, Rao TKS, Landesman SH: HIV infection in a high prevalence hemodialysis unit. AIDS 3:731, 1989
5. Schoenfeld P, Feduska NJ: Acquired immunodeficiency syndrome and renal disease: Report of National Kidney Foundation National Institute of Health Task Force on AIDS and Kidney Disease. Am J Kidney Dis 15:14, 1990
6. Glassock RJ, Cohen AH, Danovitch G et al: Human immunodeficiency virus infection and the kidney. Ann Intern Med 112:35, 1990
7. Perez GO, Ortiz C, De Medina M et al: Lack of transmission of human immunodeficiency virus in chronic hemodialysis patients. Am J Nephrol 8:123, 1988
8. Reiser WI, Shapiro WB, Porush GJ: The incidence and epidemiology of human deficiency virus infection in 320 patients treated in an inner city hemodialysis center. Am J Kidney Dis 16:26, 1990
9. Baltimore-Boston Collaborative Study Group: Human immunodeficiency virus infection in hemodialysis patients. Arch Intern Med 148:617, 1988
10. Kimmel PL, Umana WO, Simmens SJ et al: Continuous ambulatory peritoneal dialysis and survival of HIV infected patients with end-stage renal disease. Kidney Int 44:373, 1993
11. Alter MJ, Favero MS, Tokars JI: National surveillance of dialysis associated disease in United States, 1989. Am Soc Artif Intern Organs J 37:97, 1991
12. Tokars JI, Alter MJ, Favero MS et al: National surveillance of hemodialysis associated disease in the United States, 1990. Am Soc Artif Intern Organs J 39:71, 1993
13. Rubin J: Prevalence of HIV virus among patients undergoing continuous ambulatory peritoneal dialysis. Trans Am Soc Artif Intern Organs 35:144, 1989
14. Arnow PM, Fellner S, Harrington R et al: False positive results of screening for antibodies to human immunodeficiency virus in chronic hemodialysis patients. Am J Kidney Dis 11:383, 1988
15. Peterman TA, Lang GR, Milos NJ et al: HTLV-III/LAV infection in hemodialysis patients. JAMA 255:2324, 1986

16. Rao TKS, Friedman EA, Nicastri AD: The types of renal disease in the acquired immunodeficiency syndrome. N Engl J Med 316:1062, 1987
17. Ortiz C, Meneses R, Jaffe D et al: Outcome of patients with human immunodeficiency virus on maintenance hemodialysis. Kidney Int 34:248, 1988
18. Feinfeld DA, Kaplan R, Dressler R et al: Survival of human immunodeficiency virus-infected patients on maintenance dialysis. Clin Nephrol 32:221, 1989
19. Tebben JA, Rigsby OM, Selwyn AP et al: Outcome of HIV infected patients on continuous ambulatory peritoneal dialysis. Kidney Int 44:191, 1993
20. Bourgoignie JJ, Meneses R, Pardo V: AIDS associated nephropathy. Adv Nephrol 17:113, 1988
21. Hellinger FJ: Updated forecasts of the costs of medical care for persons with AIDS. Public Health Rep 105:1, 1990
22. Barlett JA: Chronic management and counseling for persons with HIV infection. p. 1965. In Wyngaarden JB, Smith LH, Bennett JC (eds): Cecil Textbook of Medicine. 19th Ed. WB Saunders, Philadelphia, 1992
23. Volberding PV, Lagakos SW, Koch MA et al: Zidovudine in asymptomatic human immunodeficiency virus infection. A controlled trial in persons with fewer than 500 CD4-positive cells per cubic millimeter. N Engl J Med 322:941, 1990
24. Bourgoignie JJ, Interian CO: Impact of human immunodeficiency virus on the treatment of uremia. Sem Dialysis 1:187, 1988
25. Schulman G, Hakim RM: Recent advances in the biocompatibility of hemodialysis membranes. Nephrol Dial Transplant 6:10, 1993
26. Eshback JW: The anemia of chronic renal failure: pathology and the effect of recombinant erythropoietin. Kidney Int 35:171, 1989
27. Henry DH, Jembsek JG, Levin AS et al: Recombinant human erythropoietin and the treatment of anemia in patients with AIDS or advanced ARC not receiving zidovudine. J AIDS 5:847, 1992
28. Phair JP, Abeles RI, Mcneill MV et al: Recombinant human erythropoietin treatment: investigational new drug protocol for the anemia of acquired immunodeficiency treatment. Arch Intern Med 153:2669, 1993
29. Brock JS: HIV and HD related vascular access. J Vascular Surg 16:904, 1992
30. Nannery WB, Stoldt HS, Fares LG: Hemodialysis access operation performed upon patients with human immunodeficiency virus. Surg Gynaecol Obstet 173:387, 1991
31. Lafeuillade A, Alessi MC, Poizot M et al: Endothelial cell dysfunction in HIV infection. J AIDS 5:127, 1992
32. Karpatkin S, Nardi M: Auto immune anti-HIV-1 gp 120 antibody with antiidiotype like activity in sera and immune complexes of HIV-1-related immunologic thrombocytopenia. J Clin Invest 89:356, 1992
33. Leaf NA, Laubenstein LJ, Raphael B et al: Thrombotic thrombocytopenic purpura associated with human immunodeficiency virus type 1 infection. Ann Intern Med 109:194, 1988
34. Dressler R, Peters AT, Lynn RI: Pseudomonal and candidal peritonitis as a complication of continuous ambulatory peritoneal dialysis in HIV infected patients. Am J Med 86:787, 1989
35. Wasser WG, Boyle MJ, Brandon S et al: HIV positivity does not predispose peritoneal dialysis patients to peritonitis, abstracted. Am Soc Nephrol 2:369, 1991
36. Correa-Rotter R, Saldivar S, Soto LE et al: Recovery of HIV antigen in peritoneal dialysis fluid. Peritoneal Dial Int 10:67, 1990

37. Breyer JA, Harbison MA: Isolation of human immunodeficiency virus from peritoneal dialysate. Am J Kidney Dis 21:23, 1993
38. Tokars JI, Marcus R, Culver DH et al: Surveillance of HIV infection and zidovudine use among health care workers after occupational exposure to HIV infected blood. Ann Intern Med 118:913, 1993
39. Ippolito G, Puro V, Decarli G et al: The risk of occupational human immunodeficiency virus infection in health care workers. Arch Intern Med 153:1451, 1993
40. Marcus R, and the CDC Cooperative Needle Stick Surveillance Group: Survey of health care workers exposed to blood from patients infected with the human immunodeficiency virus. N Engl J Med 319:1118, 1988
41. Gerberding JL, Bryant-Leblane CE, Nelson K et al: Risk of transmitting the human immunodeficiency virus to health care workers exposed to patients with AIDS and AIDS related conditions. J Infect Dis 156:1, 1987
42. Ortiz-Interian CJ, de Medina MD, Perez GO et al: Recurrence and clearance of hepatitis B surface antigenemia in a dialysis patient infected with the human immunodeficiency virus. Am J Kidney Dis 16:154, 1990
43. Centers for Disease Control and Prevention: Recommendation for providing dialysis treatment to patients infected with human T-lymphotropic virus type III/lymphadenopathy associated virus. MMWR 35:376, 1986
44. Bowen PA II, Lobel SA, Caruana R et al: Transmission of human immunodeficiency virus (HIV) by transplantation: clinical aspects and time course analysis of viral antigenemia and antibody production. Ann Intern Med 108:46, 1988
45. Ward JW, Holmsberg SD, Allen JR et al: Transmission of human immunodeficiency virus by blood transfusion screened as negative for HIV antibody. N Engl J Med 318:473, 1988
46. Mayer KH, Stoddard AM, McCusker J et al: Human T-lymphotropic virus type III in high risk antibody negative homosexual men. Ann Intern Med 104:194, 1986
47. Martin DH, Pearson JE, Kumar P et al: Sequential measurement of B2 microglobulin levels, p24 antigen levels, and antibody titres following transplantation of a HIV virus infected kidney allograft. J AIDS 4:1118, 1991
48. Simmonds RJ, Holmberg SD, Hurwitch R: Transmission of human immunodeficiency virus type 1 from a seronegative organ and tissue donor. N Engl J Med 326:726, 1992
49. Kessler HA, Blaaw B, Spear J et al: Diagnosis of human immunodeficiency virus infection in seronegative homosexuals presenting with an acute viral syndrome. JAMA 258:1196, 1987
50. Ranki A, Valle SL, Krohn M et al: Long latency precedes overt seroconversion in sexually transmitted human immune deficiency virus infection. Lancet 2:589, 1987
51. Imagawa DT, Lee MH, Wolinsky SM et al: HIV type I infection in homosexual men who remain seronegative for prolonged periods. N Engl J Med 320:1459, 1989
52. Wolinsky SA, Rinaldo CR, Kwoe S et al: HIV virus type-I infection in a median of 18 months before a diagnostic western blot: evidence from a cohort of homosexual men. Ann Intern Med 111:961, 1989
53. Milogram M, Esquenazi V, Fuller L et al: Acquired immunodeficiency syndrome in a transplant patient. Transplant Proc, suppl. 2:S17, 1985
54. Feduska NJ, Perkins MA, Meltzer J et al: Observations relating to the incidence of acquired immune deficiency syndrome and other possibly associated condi-

tions in a large population of renal transplant recipients. Transplant Proc 19: 2161, 1987

55. L'age-Stehr J, Schwartz A, Offerman G et al: HTLV-III infection in kidney transplant recipients. Lancet 2:136, 1985

56. Carbone LG, Cohen DJ, Hardy MA et al: Determination of acquired immunodeficiency syndrome (AIDS) after renal transplantation. Am J Kidney Dis 11:387, 1988

57. Rubin RH, Wolfsin JS, Cosin AB: Infection in the renal transplant recipient. Am J Med 70:405, 1981

58. Peterson PK, Rergusin R, Fryd DS et al: Infectious diseases in hospitalized renal transplant recipients: a prospective study of a complex and evolving problem. Medicine 61:360, 1982

59. Schwartz A, Offerman G, Keller F et al: The effect of cyclosporine on the progression of human immunodeficiency virus type 1 infection transmitted by transplantation. Data on 4 cases and review of the literature. Transplantation 55:95, 1993

60. Klatzmann D, Laporte JP, Achour A et al: Cyclosporin A treatment for human immunodeficiency virus infected transplant recipients. Transplant Proc 19:1828, 1987

61. Shaffer D, Pearl RH, Jenkins RL et al: HTLV III/LAV infection in kidney and liver transplantation. Transplant Proc 19:2176, 1987

62. Oliveira DBG, Winearls CG, Cohen J et al: Severe immunosuppression in a renal transplant recipient with HTLV III antibodies. Transplantation 41:260, 1985

63. Tzakis AG, Cooper MH, Dunner JS et al: Transplantation in HIV positive patients. Transplantation 49:354, 1990

64. Erice A, Rhame FS, Heussner RC et al: Human immunodeficiency virus infection in patients with solid organ transplant: report of five cases and review. Rev Infect Dis 13:537, 1991

65. Daligleish AG, Beverly PCL, Claphan PR et al: The CD4 (T4) antigen is an essential component of the receptor for the AIDS retrovirus. Nature 312:763, 1987

66. Andriew JM, Even P, Venet A et al: Effects of cyclosporin A on T cell subsets in human immunodeficiency virus disease. Clin Immunol Immunopathol 46:181, 1988

67. Prompt CA, Reiss MM, Grillo FM et al: Transmission of AIDS virus at renal transplantation. Lancet 2:672, 1985

68. Rubin RH, Jenkins RL, Shaw BW Jr: The acquired immunodeficiency syndrome and transplantation. Transplantation 44:1, 1987

13

HIV and Dialysis: Occupational Risk and Medical Legal Implications

Joel Neugarten
Paul L. Kimmel

DIALYSIS OF HIV-INFECTED PATIENTS

Prevalence and Length of Survival

Surveys of the end-stage renal disease (ESRD) Program in the United States indicate that the prevalence of human immunodeficiency virus (HIV)-infected patients in dialysis programs rose rapidly between 1985 and 1987 followed by a plateauing at approximately 1 percent of the dialysis population.[1] Between 1985 and 1991, the proportion of dialysis centers dialyzing HIV-infected patients increased from 11 to 29 percent, corresponding to an increase in the prevalence of HIV infection from 0.3 to 1.2 percent (1,914 infected patients in a total dialysis population of 155,877).[1] Acquired immunodeficiency syndrome (AIDS) complicating ESRD is most frequently acquired through intravenous drug use or as a complication of multiple blood transfusions for the treatment of anemia in the pre-erythropoietin era.[2–4] HIV infection may also be acquired through renal transplantation or secondary to risk factors in common with the general population.[4] The prevalence of HIV infection in single dialysis centers varies widely from 0 to 39 percent, depending on the geography of the facility and demographics of the patient population.[2–15] The highest reported prevalence rate (39 percent) was seen in an inner city facility located in New York City, the epicenter of the AIDS epidemic.[10] In 1990, 9 percent of the centers dialyzing HIV-infected patients and 20 percent of the infected patients were located in New York City.[16] Centers dialyzing HIV-infected patients were located in 44 states, the District of Columbia, and Puerto Rico.[16] Twenty-one percent of the centers and 41 percent of the infected patients were located in six large metropolitan areas in a geographic distribution similar to that for all cases of AIDS.[16]

Survival of HIV-infected patients with ESRD is variable and depends on the stage of infection. Early reports were uniformly pessimistic and suggested that survival of patients with AIDS and ESRD was dismal.[8,17] More recent data suggest that the survival of HIV-infected patients on dialysis may be prolonged in patients in the early stages of infection.[9,18–20] These data are important because approximately half of HIV-infected dialysis patients are asymptomatic.[16] Several investigators have suggested that ESRD does not adversely influence the survival of AIDS patients and report a median patient survival of approximately 1 year, similar to the median patient survival for all cases of AIDS.[19,20] A recent study reported a mean survival time of 15.5 months for HIV-infected patients with stage III or IV infection at the time of initiation of dialysis, compared with a mean survival of 44 months among non-HIV-infected dialysis patients.[18] Stage of HIV infection is a major factor determining length of survival in most studies.[19,20]

No difference in mean survival time has been observed between HIV-infected patients treated with hemodialysis and those treated with continuous ambulatory peritoneal dialysis (CAPD).[18] A recent large series found that the peritonitis rate and the etiologic agents of peritonitis in HIV-infected patients were similar to non-HIV-infected CAPD patients.[18] In addition, this study found no difference in the number of hospitalizations between HIV-infected patients treated with hemodialysis and CAPD.[18] In contrast, a number of reports suggest an increased rate of peritonitis and in particular, a high incidence of pseudomonal and fungal infections among HIV-infected CAPD patients.[20,21] The increased peritonitis rate in HIV-infected patients was attributed to behavioral factors.[20,21] Arguably then, hemodialysis and CAPD appear to be equally good treatment alternatives for HIV-infected patients with ESRD.

Dialysis Procedures

The Centers for Disease Control and Prevention (CDC) has issued guidelines for providing dialysis treatment to HIV-infected patients.[22] HIV-infected patients need not be isolated from the general dialysis population.[22] In fact, such isolation violates federal and in many cases state and local antidiscrimination laws (discussed below). Dialyzers may be reused, but use of individual dialyzers must be restricted to individual patients.[22] Nondisposable supplies that are not restricted to individual patients must be sterilized between uses.[22] Standard infection control and environmental control procedures including routinely practiced disinfection and sterilization techniques are adequate to prevent transmission of infection by eradicating HIV from dialysis equipment and work surfaces.[22] Sodium hypochlorite or formaldehyde, used to disinfect dialysate pathways of dialysis machines, effectively eradicate HIV.[22] The Association for the Advancement of Medical Instrumentation recommends that written procedures should specify whether and how hemodialyzer reprocessing will be performed.[23] Dialysis facilities must also comply with Occupational Safety and Health Administration (OSHA) regulations designed to prevent transmission of blood-borne infections in the workplace.[24] These regulations encompass universal precautions and are discussed below.

Peritoneal dialysis could potentially decrease the risk of occupational exposure to HIV due to the lower frequency of venipuncture. However, recent studies suggest that spent peritoneal dialysis effluent may also be a potential source of viral transmission.[25,26] Replication-competent HIV has been recovered from cells present in the peritoneal effluent of two of three HIV-infected CAPD patients, notwithstanding zidovudine treatment.[25] In a second study, HIV antigen was detected in the dialysis effluent of two of three other HIV-infected CAPD patients.[26] Health care workers employed by hospital or dialysis facilities must comply with universal precautions and wear gowns, gloves, and facial protection when changing bags or disposing of spent dialysate.[21] Spent dialysate should be disposed of in the sewer. Disposable tubing and empty dialysate bags must be placed in plastic bags properly labeled to indicate they contain biohazardous material prior to disposal as mandated by federal, state, and local regulations.[24] In addition, HIV-infected patients and their families performing CAPD must be educated regarding infection control practices to be followed at home.

OCCUPATIONAL RISK OF HIV TRANSMISSION IN THE DIALYSIS UNIT

Risk to Health Care Workers

Data derived from prospective studies of health care workers with occupational exposure to HIV indicate that the risk of transmission after percutaneous injury by needles or sharp instruments contaminated with HIV-infected blood is approximately 0.25 percent.[27–33] A prospective national surveillance study conducted by the CDC of health care workers exposed to blood or body fluids of HIV-infected patients reported a 0.36 percent rate of seroconversion among those with percutaneous exposure (4 of 1,103).[27] Combining data from 21 reported prospective studies, HIV infection was transmitted to nine health care workers who sustained 3,625 percutaneous injuries exposing them to HIV-infected blood (0.25 percent).[28] One seroconversion was documented after 1,007 mucous membrane exposures.[28] The splash incident resulting in HIV transmission involved a large quantity of blood contaminating a large area of mucous membrane contamination. No seroconversions occurred after exposure of nonintact skin.[28]

Most data on transmissibility of HIV after percutaneous injury are derived from prospective studies that primarily examined percutaneous injuries from needles contaminated with highly infectious blood from patients hospitalized with late stages of HIV infection.[28–33] In addition, many source patients were not receiving antiretroviral therapy and most percutaneous injuries involved hollow bore needles, which tend to transfer a larger inoculum of blood than do solid sharp objects such as scalpels and suture needles.[28–33] In the setting of dialysis, large gauge dialysis cannula would transfer even larger inocula of blood. In fact, the risk of transmission after a percutaneous injury may vary widely and attempts to calculate an overall risk of HIV transmission are complicated by varying infectivity of source patients and varying types and severity of injuries sustained by individual health care workers. The principal determinant of risk is the infectivity of the blood contaminating the wound.[34] Infectivity of blood varies with the stage of HIV infection of the source individual. Viral titers in the blood increase exponentially as HIV infection progresses from the asymptomatic stage to full-blown AIDS.[35] A recent study suggests that HIV-infected patients with chronic renal insufficiency or ESRD treated with dialysis have a higher prevalence of plasma viremia compared with HIV-infected patients without renal disease.[36] Because HIV infectivity may be related to the magnitude of viable virus in the inoculum, this high prevalence has important implications for health care workers treating HIV-infected ESRD patients.

Other determinants of risk include the size of the inoculum of blood, the type and severity of injury (superficial versus deep penetrating injuries), and the use of gloves. In an in vitro needle stick model, it was shown that the volume of blood transferred increased in proportion to needle size and the depth of penetration but was reduced by a glove barrier.[34] Moreover, gloves provided a more effective barrier to blood transmission from hollow bore needles than solid bore needles.[34] The effect of antiretroviral therapy on infectivity has not been ascertained.

There is currently no data to suggest patient to patient, patient to staff, or staff to patient transmission of HIV in the United States ESRD program. One multicenter study performed serial HIV testing in patients from 28 dialysis units.[3] No episode of seroconversion was documented among 254 patients after 1 year. In another multicenter study examining the seroprevalence of HIV antibody among 112 dialysis workers who denied nonoccupational risk factors, no case of infection was detected.[37] However, the low participation rate of 70 percent qualifies interpretation of this study. Single-center studies from dialysis facilities with a high seroprevalence also fail to demonstrate nosocomial transmission.[10,38] Of concern is a report of HIV infection in 12 of 18 patients from one dialysis facility located outside of the United States.[39] Two additional infected patients were detected among 55 dialysis patients in four nearby units. Both these patients were previously dialyzed in the high prevalence dialysis unit. Because the infected patients did not belong to a high-risk group, the possibility was raised that the patients may have been infected through contaminated filters or tubing.[39] However, the blood transfusion histories of infected patients were not reported.[39]

Thirty-three health care workers in the United States are documented to have acquired HIV infection through occupational exposure.[40,41] Seroconversion was documented by a negative baseline serology obtained immediately after injury.[41] These cases include 28 percutaneous injuries, 4 mucocutaneous exposures, and 1 injury causing both percutaneous and mucocutaneous exposure.[41] An additional 69 health care workers infected with HIV who did not have behavioral or transfusion risks were classified as possible cases of occupational transmission.[41] All these individuals reported past percutaneous or mucocutaneous exposures to blood, body fluids, or laboratory specimens, but seroconversion was not documented.[40,41]

Seroprevalence studies among health care workers at high risk of occupational exposure have failed to demonstrate a high prevalence of HIV infection.[42-44] However, voluntary seroprevalence studies may seriously underestimate HIV infection if those health care workers who already knew or suspected they were infected declined to participate in the study.[45] Comparisons between voluntary and blinded seroprevalence studies often indicate that those who decline to participate are more likely to be infected with HIV.[45] In a cross-sectional study of over 1,300 dentists and other dental care professionals, only one dentist not engaged in high-risk behavior was found to be infected.[42] Among 3,420 orthopedic surgeons participating in a seroprevalence study, no surgeon not at increased risk for HIV due to behavioral risk factors was found to be infected.[43] Data derived from combining 13 studies performed between 1985 and 1988 that examine the seroprevalence of HIV among health care workers show a prevalence of 0.32 percent (21 of 6,619).[44] This prevalence is similar to that seen in the general population

(0.12 to 0.80 percent).[44] Even in highly endemic areas of Africa, where infection-control guidelines were not routinely followed, a disproportionate prevalence of HIV infection among health care workers was not observed.[46]

Risk to Dialysis Staff

The risk of patient to staff transmission of HIV in the dialysis unit can be estimated, although not precisely. The risk of injury and exposure varies depending on the type of procedure performed, the technique employed, the degree of adherence to infection-control practices, the medical condition, technical skill and experience of the health care worker, and the prevalence of HIV in the dialysis unit population. The risk of seroconversion after a percutaneous injury involving HIV-infected blood depends on the infectivity of the patient, the severity and type of injury, and the type of needle or instrument causing the injury. Injuries involving solid sharp objects and patients in early stages of HIV infection may be associated with a lesser risk of transmission than the 0.25 percent figure suggested by prospective studies that primarily evaluated hollow bore needle stick injuries from highly infectious source patients in late stages of HIV infection. On the other hand, the large bore needles used to cannulate arteriovenous fistulas are more likely to introduce a large inoculum of blood than standard needles. In addition, the high prevalence of viremia in dialysis patients may enhance infectivity.[36] The risk from a single procedure can be calculated as the product of (1) the risk of seroconversion after a single contaminated needle stick, (2) the proportion of HIV-positive persons in the dialysis patient population, and (3) the incidence of percutaneous injuries.[47] Cumulative risk is determined by the equation $1 - [1 - w]^{xyz}$, where w represents the probability of seroconversion after a single needle stick, x represents the time period measured in years, y represents the number of needle sticks per year, and z represents the proportion of HIV-infected patients in the patient population.[48–50]

In order to calculate risk, one must estimate the prevalence of HIV-infected persons in the patient population. Seroprevalence among patient populations varies widely depending on the geography of the dialysis facility and the demography of the patient population. In addition, one must also ascertain the incidence of percutaneous injuries among dialysis workers. The incidence of needle stick injuries among dialysis workers employed by a large provider of dialysis services was 1 in 2,000 dialyses performed in 1990.[4] Using a seroconversion rate of 0.25 percent and an HIV seroprevalence of 1.0 percent among dialysis patients, the risk of transmission of HIV infection from patient to staff is 1 in 80 million dialyses. Assuming 200,000 dialysis patients nationwide undergo three dialysis treatments per week, our model predicts that one dialysis worker will be infected with HIV as a result of occupational transmission each 2.6 years. In an individual dialysis unit with 100 patients and a 10 percent seroprevalence of HIV, the risk of HIV transmission is 1 per 8 million dialyses. In such a unit, one dialysis worker will be infected with HIV as a result of occupational transmission each 513 years. Assuming a dialysis worker initiates seven dialyses per day, the annual risk for individual employees in this unit is 0.02 percent and the cumulative 10-year risk is 0.21 percent. These risks may be compared with those faced in other occupations. The annual risk of death among police and firefighters is on the order of 0.2 percent.[51]

Risk to the Patient

Five patients were infected with HIV transmitted during invasive dental procedures performed by a Florida dentist with AIDS.[52] Epidemiologic data support direct dentist to patient transmission.[52] The five patients were infected with HIV strains with nucleotide sequences and amino acid signature patterns closely related to the strain infecting the dentist.[52] The dentist did not consistently comply with recommended infection control guidelines.[52] Barrier precautions were not always properly implemented, gloves were occasionally reused after washing, and sterilization techniques did not comply with recommended guidelines.[52] Nevertheless, transmission could not be explained by these breaches and the precise mode of transmission has not been determined.[52] Aside from this cluster in Florida, no other cases of transmission of HIV infection from health care provider to patient has been documented.[52] "Look-back" studies that have identified and tested more than 20,000 patients who underwent invasive procedures performed by HIV-infected physicians or dentists have failed to detect additional cases of HIV transmission.[53] Although inadequate scientific data are currently available to assess the precise risk of HIV transmission from infected health care workers to patients, that risk appears to be extremely small.[54]

The risk that a cluster of cases might arise due to transmission from a single infected practitioner to multiple patients defies quantitation. However, one can calculate the risk of sporadic HIV transmission to patients undergoing procedures performed by an HIV-infected health care worker. The risk of sporadic transmission in the dialysis unit may be calculated from the product of the probability of percutaneous injury to the HIV-infected health care worker; the probability that the health care worker's blood will contact the patient's blood, mucous membranes, or nonintact skin after an injury; and the probability of seroconversion after exposure to the worker's blood. However, in the context of arteriovenous fistula cannulation, no data are available to estimate how often the blood of an injured worker will contact the patient's blood, mucous membranes, or nonintact skin. Because such contact is highly unlikely to occur, the prospect of worker to patient transmission also appears to be extremely unlikely.

UNIVERSAL PRECAUTIONS

The CDC has developed infection-control guidelines to prevent transmission of HIV, hepatitis, and other blood-borne infections in the health care setting.[55] Recently promulgated OSHA regulations give legal authority to these guidelines.[24] Universal precautions entail the use of these infection-control precautions for all patients where there exists a risk of exposure to blood or body fluids capable of transmitting HIV, irrespective of the perceived risk that a given patient carries the virus.[55] Because clinical assessment of HIV status is unreliable, the blood and certain potentially infectious body fluids (including peritoneal fluid and all body fluids visibly contaminated by blood) of all patients are considered infectious and appropriate protective measures must be used.[55] Gloves must be worn when contacting blood, body fluids, mucous membranes, or contaminated surfaces and when performing phlebotomies, starting intravenous devices, or performing invasive procedures.[55] Masks and eye protection must be worn in situations where blood or body fluids may contact mucous membranes and gowns must be worn where splashing may occur.[55] These guidelines also provide procedures for the safe handling and disposal of needles and sharp objects and set forth recommendations concerning the use of resuscitative devices and the exclusion from patient care of health care workers with exuding lesions or weeping dermatitis.[55] In addition, universal precautions encompass standard infection control practices such as appropriate handwashing and require that instruments and other reusable equipment be disinfected and sterilized between uses.[55]

Compliance with universal precautions by physicians and other health care workers has been poor.[56–60] Several studies indicate that 50 percent or more of health care workers fail to comply with universal precautions and that 25 percent of needles are recapped contrary to CDC guidelines.[56–60] The reasons given by health care workers for failing to comply with universal precautions include lack of knowledge and the presence of emergency circumstances.[58] Rubin and Lief[61] surveyed 89 satellite dialysis units in 1990 and found that infection control precautions were inconsistently followed. Whereas barrier precautions were properly used in over 75 percent of facilities known to treat HIV-infected patients, these precautions were used in less than one-half of the units in which HIV-infected patients were not known to be dialyzed.[61]

Educational efforts alone are often ineffective in increasing compliance with universal precautions.[62] An intensive educational program to foster compliance with universal precautions was associated with only a modest increase in compliance,[62] while one-time educational programs were ineffective in increasing compliance.[63,64] In one study, more than 50 percent of all procedures and more than three-fourths of surgical procedures were not in compliance with recommended guidelines both before and after an educational program.[63] In other studies, educational programs to reduce the frequency of needle recapping were totally ineffective.[64,65] In contrast, a policy of mandatory compliance and employee accountability may prove effective in increasing compliance with universal precautions.[66] Monitoring and employee accountability significantly increased compliance with universal precautions more than threefold during the performance of major procedures and by 66 percent overall.[66] In an earlier study at the same institution, educational efforts that did not include monitoring and accountability were judged ineffective.[57] Another successful program to increase compliance with handwashing similarly relied on conspicuous observation and immediate feedback.[67]

Universal precautions have been shown to be effective in reducing cutaneous and mucous membrane exposure of health care workers to blood and body fluids.[68–70] It has been estimated that two-thirds of nonparenteral occupational exposures could be prevented by adherence to universal precautions.[71] In a study examining self-reported exposures to blood and body fluids, it was found that the incidence of cutaneous exposures decreased nearly 50 percent after training in universal precautions.[68] In another study, implementation of universal precautions and a mandatory educational program led to a nearly 50 percent increase in barrier use and a nearly 50 percent reduction in the number of nonparenteral exposures.[69]

Whether or not universal precautions can reduce percutaneous injuries in health care workers is unclear.[28,29,33,56,65,70–77] It has been estimated by some investigators that 20 to 40 percent of needle stick injuries to health care workers could be prevented by adherence to universal precautions.[56,71,72] Preventable exposures included injuries due to needle recapping and improper disposal.[29] However, a reduction in the frequency of percutaneous injuries as a result of implementing universal precautions has not been consistently demonstrated.[70] In two surveillance studies of occupational exposure to HIV, only 5 and 14 percent of needle stick injuries were judged to be avoidable.[28,33] Notwithstanding a decrease in disposal-related needle stick injuries, several studies have found that the introduction of needle disposal systems and educational programs failed to reduce total needle stick injuries.[65,73] No reduction in the frequency of needle stick injuries was documented after implementation of universal precautions nor were such injuries reduced in those health care workers who complied with universal precautions as compared with those who did not.[65,73–77]

OSHA REGULATIONS

The Occupational Safety Health Act imposes two broad duties on employers.[78] The general duty clause requires all employers to provide a workplace that is "free from recognized hazards that are causing or are likely to cause death or serious physical harm to employees."[78] Employers also have a duty to comply with all regulations promulgated by OSHA.[78] The Department of Labor has recently promulgated regulations that implement OSHA standards to prevent blood-borne disease.[24] These standards mandate that health care employers prepare an Exposure Control Plan.[24] This plan must include an exposure determination that identifies all work-related tasks and procedures in which percutaneous or mucocutaneous exposure to blood or potentially infectious materials may occur and identifies all job classifications that involve these tasks and procedures.[24] The plan must also include a schedule and method of implementation of specific standards designed to minimize or eliminate occupational exposure to blood-borne pathogens.[24] These standards relate to universal precautions, engineering and work practice controls, personal protective equipment, housekeeping, hepatitis B vaccination, postexposure evaluation and follow-up, hazard communication, employee training, and recordkeeping.[24] The plan must also include procedures for evaluating the circumstances surrounding work-related exposure incidents.[24] Mandated engineering controls, designed to isolate or remove blood-borne hazards from the work environment, include the provision of appropriate personal protective equipment and properly labeled puncture-resistant containers for disposal of sharps.[24] Mandated work practice controls, designed to reduce the likelihood of exposure by changing the way a task is performed, include prohibiting needle recapping, requiring handwashing after glove removal, and requiring removal of personal protective equipment after employees leave work areas.[24] In addition, employers must provide training for employees identified in the exposure determination and ensure that employees comply with safe work practices and properly use personal protective equipment.[24] OSHA regulations are enforced through inspections and imposition of fines and may result in imprisonment where violations result in death.

OSHA regulations relating to post-HIV-exposure evaluation and counseling are discussed in detail below.

CDC GUIDELINES FOR PREVENTING HIV TRANSMISSION IN THE HEALTH CARE SETTING

The CDC has issued recommendations for preventing transmission of HIV and hepatitis B virus infection in health care settings.[54] The CDC defined the term invasive procedure to include "surgical entry into tissue, cavities or organs or repair of major traumatic injuries," cardiac catheterization, angiography, invasive obstetric procedures, and major dental procedures.[79] Exposure-prone procedures were defined as those procedures associated with the transmission of hepatitis B virus despite adherence to universal precautions.[54] These procedures involved "digital palpation of a needle tip in a body cavity or simultaneous presence of a [surgeon's] . . . fingers and a needle or other sharp instrument or object in a poorly visualized or highly confined anatomic site."[54] Certain oral, cardiothoracic, colorectal, and obstetric/gynecologic procedures were identified as exposure-prone because they carry a risk that the surgeon will suffer a percutaneous injury and that his blood will contact the patient's wound, body cavity, or mucous membranes.[54] The CDC guidelines state that health care workers who do not perform invasive procedures and who adhere to universal precautions pose no risk of transmission of HIV to patients.[54] Invasive procedures that lack the characteristics of exposure-prone procedures pose a "substantially lower risk if any" of transmission of HIV.[54] The CDC concluded that current scientific knowledge does not support the imposition of practice restrictions on HIV-infected health care workers who perform invasive procedures not identified as exposure-prone if they practice recommended techniques, adhere to universal precautions, and follow recommended sterilization and disinfection procedures.[54]

Because dialysis does not involve any invasive or exposure-prone procedures, CDC guidelines would not support imposition of worksite restrictions on HIV-infected workers who adhere to universal precautions and follow recommended techniques and infection control procedures. Nor do the CDC guidelines support mandatory HIV testing of dialysis employees insofar as the guidelines conclude that health care workers who do not perform invasive procedures and who adhere to universal precautions pose no risk of transmission of HIV to patients.[54] Although CDC guidelines are not legally binding unless incorporated into governmental regulations, they do establish scientific principles and standards of conduct used by courts to determine negligence in tort actions and to evaluate alleged discriminatory practices under a "significant risk" standard (see below).[80] Many states are currently in the process of developing such guidelines for HIV-infected health care workers.

HIV TESTING
False-Positive Rate

There is a high false-positive rate with standard enzyme-linked immunosorbent assay (ELISA) testing for HIV antibody among dialysis patients.[4,22] A positive ELISA has a relatively low predictive value for HIV infection in the dialysis population.[4,22] This has been attributed to the development of antibodies to a H9 cell line derived HLA class II antigen. Dialysis patients are often repeatedly exposed to this antigen as a result of multiple blood transfusions.[4,22] Of 2,806 dialysis patients who underwent testing, 200 showed a positive ELISA for HIV antibody; however, only 77 were positive by Western blotting.[4] The 4 to 5 percent false-positive rate among dialysis patients is severalfold higher than the 0.17 percent false-positive rate seen among blood donors.[22]

Discriminatory Practices Involving HIV Test Results

Although state and local laws generally govern the informed consent and confidentiality requirements for HIV testing, the recently enacted Americans with Disabilities Act limits the discretion of dialysis facilities to require that patients be tested.[81] A practice of requiring transient dialysis patients to submit to HIV testing for the purpose of excluding admission of infected patients clearly violates the Act and subjects a dialysis facility to the possibility of reimbursement sanctions by the Department of Health and Human Services (HHS) and actions by the Justice Department for civil monetary damages and injunctive relief.[80] The facility may also be subject to private actions for monetary damages, injunctive relief, and attorney's fees and costs.[80] Such practices may also violate state statutes or local law. In 1990, the Council of Nephrology Social Workers surveyed the transient dialysis acceptance practices of 100 randomly selected dialysis units.[82] Nearly two-thirds of units required HIV testing.[82] Nearly one-quarter of the units would not accept HIV-infected transient patients and in an additional one-quarter the facility's acceptance policy was unclear.[82] Prompted by 92 complaints from the HIV Legal Clinic of the District of Columbia School of Law, the Office of Civil Rights of HHS investigated the acceptance policies and procedures of dialysis units in eight states.[83] The complaints alleged that the units refused to accept HIV-infected patients or isolated infected patients in violation of antidiscrimination statutes.[83] Nearly two-thirds of the complaints have been resolved, in some cases with the Office of Civil Rights requiring corrective measures (Mauro Montoya, personal communication, 1993).

The question of whether a dialysis facility may require mandatory pre-admission HIV testing or whether it may require routine testing of all its patients entails assessment of several factors. At issue is an interpretation of the Americans with Disabilities Act and applicable state and local antidiscrimination laws and an assessment of how test results will be used, including the consequences to patients who decline testing or who test positive. The Americans with Disabilities Act extends to disabled individuals comprehensive rights, protections, and remedies aimed at eliminating discrimination against individuals with disabilities in the private as well as public sectors.[81] Persons with AIDS, as well as asymptomatic individuals infected with the HIV virus, are disabled within the meaning of the Americans with Disabilities Act and are thus entitled to all the protections it affords to the disabled.[80] Title III of the Act prohibits discrimination based on disability "in the full and equal enjoyment of . . . services [and] facilities . . . of any place of public accommodation."[81] Title III also provides that no individual shall be denied, on the basis of disability, the opportunity to participate in or benefit from a covered entity, nor shall he be afforded a service or accommodation that is unequal, different, or separate.[81] Thus, the provisions of Title III unequivocally prohibit the denial of services by a dialysis provider to an individual solely on the basis of HIV infection. Title III, however, does not prohibit exclusion of disabled individuals who pose a "significant risk" in the form of a "direct threat to the health and safety of others" where the risk cannot be eliminated by reasonable modifications in policies, practices, or procedures.[81] However, as discussed earlier, the risk of transmission of HIV from dialysis patient to caregiver arguably does not constitute a "significant risk" nor pose a direct threat to the health and safety of the staff or other patients.

The Americans with Disabilities Act also limits the discretion of dialysis facilities to establish eligibility requirements.[81] Eligibility criteria may not screen out individuals with disabilities, "unless such criteria can be shown to be necessary for the provision of the . . . services . . . being offered."[81] This provision prevents a dialysis provider from requiring that a prospective patient undergo HIV testing as a means of screening out infected individuals, unless knowledge of test results was required to safely provide dialysis to that patient or to other patients. In the case of hepatitis B, serologic testing is required to safely provide dialysis to the facility's patient population. The results of hepatitis B testing will result in modifications in practices and procedures to protect staff and other patients from infection, most notably isolation of the infected patient and use of dedicated equipment.[84] This is not the case for HIV infection, where no modifications or accommodations in practices and procedures are required to dialyze HIV-infected patients.[22]

Theoretically, knowledge of a patient's HIV status might reduce the exposure of health care workers to blood and body fluids of the patient by motivating strict compliance with universal precautions and encouraging changes in dialysis procedures or techniques that reduce exposure but are not practical for all patients. However, modifications in practice that unduly burden the patient may themselves be discriminatory. Moreover, scientific data do not demonstrate benefits from routine HIV testing to identify patients for infection control purposes.[28,70,85–89] Observational studies have shown that knowledge of a patient's HIV status does not increase compliance with recommended precautions, decrease exposure frequency, or decrease the risk of infection for health care workers.[28,70,85–89] Intraoperative exposure of surgical personnel to blood and body fluids is not influenced by the knowledge or perception that a patient is seropositive.[70,85,86] The CDC has concluded that routine testing of all patients is not recommended to prevent transmission of HIV in the workplace and that testing is unlikely to supplement universal precautions in further reducing the already low risk of occupational transmission of HIV.[87–89] The CDC has recently issued additional guidelines that recommend that health care providers offer voluntary and confidential HIV counseling and testing under certain circumstances discussed below.[90] The purpose of such testing is not to supplement universal precautions or to protect the health care provider, but to obtain for the patient the health benefits that result from early diagnosis and treatment.[90] Thus, mandatory serologic screening is prohibited as a means of denying dialysis services to infected patients seeking admission to a dialysis facility or seeking transient dialysis.

The Americans with Disabilities Act also requires that a dialysis provider make reasonable modifications in policies, practices, or procedures to accommodate an HIV- or hepatitis-B-infected patient where such modifications are necessary to enable the patient to undergo dialysis.[81] Furthermore, failure to make these modifications constitutes discrimination unless the modifications would "fundamentally alter the nature of . . . [the] services [offered]. . . ."[81] These provisions would prohibit exclusion of hepatitis-B-infected patients and require dialysis units to provide isolation areas and dedicated equipment only if courts held that these accommodations are reasonable. In the case of HIV, dialysis of infected patients does not necessitate any modifications whatsoever on the part of the dialysis facility.[22] CDC guidelines mandate universal precautions for all patients and do not require dialysis facilities to institute any additional precautions or procedures or modify waste disposal practices in caring for HIV-infected patients.[22] Moreover, dialysis units are prohibited from offering dialysis-related services that are unequal, different, or separate unless required to eliminate a significant risk to the safety of patients and staff. In the case of hepatitis B, isolation is clearly required to prevent spread of infection within the facility.[84] In the case of HIV, however, the CDC has concluded that isolation is not necessary for infection control.[22] Thus, isolation of HIV-infected patients is discriminatory behavior that violates the Americans with Disabilities Act.

Routine Testing of Dialysis Patients

HIV testing of individual dialysis patients is clearly indicated in certain specific circumstances. HIV testing is indicated, after informed consent is obtained in accordance with state and local law, before renal transplantation, to confirm a suspected medical diagnosis of AIDS, and to ascertain the serologic status of the source patient after a significant staff exposure to blood or other potentially infectious materials. In addition, we suggest that voluntary and confidential HIV counseling and testing be offered to all dialysis patients with a diagnosis of focal glomerulosclerosis, a history of intravenous drug use, or other high-risk behavior and to those who received blood transfusions between 1978 and 1985. On the other hand, attempts to *compel* selected patients to submit to HIV testing based solely on their sexual preference, history of drug use, or other high-risk behavior is discriminatory under the Americans with Disabilities Act (discussed below).

Early detection of HIV infection through routine testing of dialysis patients in accordance with state and local law may be associated with benefits to both the patient and the community at large.[90] Infected patients will receive early therapeutic intervention as a result of early diagnosis. In addition, counseling of infected individuals to avoid high-risk behavior may reduce the spread of HIV in the community. However, routine HIV testing must not to be adopted as a substitute for universal precautions. Patients may be infected with other blood-borne pathogens and HIV testing will not detect a newly infected patient before seroconversion. Moreover, infected patients detected by routine screening and those who decline HIV testing may not be denied medical care, provided suboptimal care, or offered a different class of care (i.e., isolation of infected patients).[81]

The CDC recommends voluntary and confidential HIV counseling and testing of patients at risk in acute care hospitals and associated clinics.[90] It recommends that these facilities encourage health care providers to question their patients about risk factors and offer voluntary and confidential HIV counseling and testing to those at risk.[90] Hospitals with a seroprevalence exceeding 1 percent or an AIDS prevalence exceeding 1 per 1,000 discharges, are encouraged to offer HIV counseling and testing routinely to patients aged 15 to 54 years.[90] Informed consent for testing should be obtained as required by state and local law and confidentiality of test results must be maintained.[90] The CDC also encourages other health care facilities to offer counseling and voluntary HIV testing based on the seroprevalence of HIV in their patient population, which may be determined by anonymous testing of a sample group.[90]

Thus, the CDC recommends that dialysis facilities associated with acute care hospitals and those with a high seroprevalence offer voluntary and confidential HIV counseling and testing after informed consent is obtained in accordance with state and local law. In 1991, 30 percent of dialysis units routinely tested all new admissions for HIV and 19 percent routinely tested their patients after admissions.[1] The merits of routine HIV testing in free-standing dialysis units with a low seroprevalence are not directly addressed by the CDC recommendations. Moreover, many states do not require informed consent for HIV testing and dialysis facilities are able to sample patients' blood without their knowledge. Thus, dialysis facilities in some states may adopt testing policies and procedures that do not conform with the voluntary and informed testing procedure envisioned by the CDC recommendation. Nevertheless, the same arguments used to support voluntary testing in acute care facilities and those with a high seroprevalence—early diagnosis and preventing community spread of HIV—are applicable to the general dialysis population with a seroprevalence of approximately 1 percent nationwide.

We suggest that elements in an HIV surveillance program should include procedures for obtaining and documenting informed consent, providing pre- and post-test counseling, limiting access to test results, and safeguarding confidentiality as required by state and local law. In light of CDC guidelines that conclude that no special precautions are required to dialyze HIV-infected patients, we suggest that a positive test result not be disseminated to the general staff. Moreover, as discussed earlier, knowledge of patients' serologic status does not contribute to staff safety where adherence to universal precautions is the rule. Access to test results may safely be limited to the facility's medical director, the head nurse, and the treating nephrologist. The treating nephrologist or the medical director, with the consent of the treating nephrologist, may be assigned the responsibility of informing the patient of test results and providing counseling. A specially trained social worker, knowledgeable in CDC recommendations for preventing transmission of HIV, may help provide counseling.[87,88] Restricting access to test results will protect against unauthorized dissemination and possible tort liability for failing to take reasonable precautions to protect the confidentiality of the test results and will also assure that a positive test will not decrease the level of care provided to the infected patient.

Testing of Dialysis Staff

The Americans with Disabilities Act affords HIV-infected health care workers protection against employment discrimination based on serologic status.[81] Its provisions may preclude compulsory pre-employment HIV screening or compulsory employee surveillance for HIV. The Act permits the use of eligibility criteria to screen out HIV-infected health care workers only if the criteria are "necessary for the provision of the . . . services . . . being offered."[81] If infected health care workers pose a significant risk of transmitting HIV to patients that cannot be eliminated by reasonable accommodations, then compulsory testing of staff would be permissible. However, the CDC has concluded that health care workers who do not perform invasive procedures and adhere to universal precautions pose no risk of HIV transmission to patients.[54] Because dialysis unit staff do not perform invasive procedures, infected workers do not pose a significant risk of HIV transmission. Thus, staff may not be subjected to compulsory testing. Moreover, management may not single out an employee and require them to submit to testing solely because the employee is perceived to be at high risk for infection due to sexual preference or other high-risk behavior. Individuals engaged in high-risk behavioral activities, if perceived to be infected with HIV, are disabled within the meaning of the Act, whether or not they are actually infected, and thus entitled to its protections.[80,81] Dialysis units may, however, offer voluntary and confidential HIV testing to staff as long as the facility does not impose sanctions for failure to participate or change work assignments in the event of a positive test.

The situation may arise where the management of a dialysis unit has knowledge that an employee is infected with HIV. Clearly, dismissal or a change in work assignment based solely on serologic status is discriminatory behavior under the Americans with Disability Act. Moreover, a facility may not modify an infected employee's work assignment or require an employee to disclose their serologic status or submit to HIV testing unless the employee poses a significant risk of HIV transmission to patients that cannot be eliminated by reasonable accommodations. Thus, even where the employee poses a significant risk of contagion, the dialysis facility is required to reasonably accommodate the employee's physical and mental limitations. The unit must modify the employee's duties and responsibilities to permit the employee to engage in as many of their job duties as they can competently perform.[80] Because dialysis staff do not perform invasive procedures, they do not pose a significant risk to patients merely because they are infected with HIV. However, exceptions can be envisioned. For example, a history of noncompliance with universal precautions in an employee with exposed weeping, exudative lesions might pose such a risk. In addition, HIV-related physical or mental limitations may impair an employee's ability to provide quality care. On the other hand, remote or speculative risks are not cognizable. The HIV-infected health care worker must be evaluated on an individual basis with respect to the types of procedures performed, mental and physical capabilities, record of adherence to infection control practices, technical skill and expertise, and the possibility that reasonable modifications in procedural techniques may accommodate their disability.[80]

A related question is whether HIV-infected dialysis nurses or technicians pose a cognizable risk under the doctrine of informed consent. The informed consent doctrine does not require disclosure to the patient of all risks of proposed procedures, such as access cannulation.[91] The duty to inform patients of a potential risk is "a function not only of the severity of the injury, but also of the likelihood the injury will occur. Regardless of the severity [of injury], if the probability [of injury] is so small as to be practically nonexistent, then the possibility of that injury occurring cannot be considered a material factor in a rational assessment of whether to engage in the activity. . . ."[91] The CDC has concluded that HIV-infected health care workers who do not perform invasive procedures and who adhere to universal precautions do not pose a risk.[22] Arguably, it then follows that dialysis-related procedures performed by HIV-infected staff do not fall within the doctrine of informed consent.

POSTEXPOSURE EVALUATION, COUNSELING, AND PROPHYLAXIS

Postexposure Evaluation and Counseling

CDC guidelines recommend that after an injury that exposes a health care worker to the blood of an HIV-infected patient, the worker undergo periodic HIV testing over at least a 1-year period (a baseline determination followed by repeat testing at 6 weeks and at 3, 6, and 12 months).[87,88] Counseling must include a discussion of the modes of HIV transmission and recommendations to prevent transmission pending a final determination of whether seroconversion has occurred.[87,88] These recommendations involve major lifestyle changes that impact on childbearing decisions and include use of barrier contraception.

An effective exposure assessment protocol must ensure that employees immediately bring exposure incidents to the attention of the management of the dialysis facility. Mandated procedures for postexposure evaluation and follow-up are set forth in detail in OSHA regulations.[24] The facility management is required to provide immediate and confidential medical evaluation, counseling, and follow-up.[24] The route of exposure and the attendant circumstances must be documented.[24] We suggest that documentation be performed even if the exposure is not deemed "significant." We also suggest that the dialysis facility designate its medical director to perform the postexposure medical evaluation, provide postexposure counseling that strictly conforms to CDC guidelines, manage issues relating to antiretroviral prophylaxis, and provide follow-up care. Where feasible and not prohibited by state and local law, the source patient must be identified and his or her identity documented.[24] When state and local law require consent for HIV testing and the source patient's refusal precludes testing, documentation is required.[24] When consent is not required by law or after legally required consent is obtained, the source patient's blood must immediately be tested for HIV and hepatitis viral serology if the patient is not already known to be infected.[24] The results of these tests must be documented.[24] OSHA regulations also require that the source patient's test results be made available to the exposed employee.[24] The employer must also inform the exposed employee of applicable laws and regulations that protect the confidentiality of the identity and serologic status of the source patient.[24] In the event of unauthorized dissemination of the source patient's test results by the exposed employee, failure to document these instructions may subject the facility to tort liability for failing to take reasonable precautions to protect the confidentiality of the test result. Where informed consent was obtained from the source patient, we suggest that the medical director or the treating nephrologist inform the patient of test results and provide post-test counseling in strict accordance with CDC guidelines.[87,88] Where informed consent is not legally required and was not in fact obtained, OSHA regulations provide no guidance as to whether or not to inform the source patient of test results; however, state and local law may require that the source patient be apprised of test results. Blood from the exposed staff member must be collected immediately after consent is obtained and tested to document baseline serologic status.[24] If the employee consents to blood collection but refuses HIV testing, the blood specimen must be preserved for at least 90 days from the exposure incident.[24] Testing of baseline serology must be promptly performed if the employee changes their mind within 90 days of the exposure and elects to have their blood tested.[24]

The physician responsible for postexposure evaluation and follow-up must be given a copy of the applicable OSHA regulations, documentation of the route of exposure and attendant circumstances, a description of the employee's duties that relate to the exposure incident, relevant employee medical records, and results of the source patient's HIV testing and hepatitis serologies.[24] We suggest that the evaluating physician document and explain the decision-making process as it relates to antiretroviral prophylaxis and document that counseling has been provided that strictly conforms to CDC guidelines.

The evaluating physician must prepare a written opinion.[24] The employer must obtain a copy of the written opinion and provide a copy to the exposed employee within 15 days of completion of the evaluation.[24] The written opinion must document that the employee has been informed of the results of the evaluation and has been told about diseases that may result from exposure to blood or body fluids and require further follow-up or treatment.[24] OSHA regulations require that all other findings and diagnoses made by the examining physician must remain confidential and may not be included in the written opinion.[24] The dialysis facility must maintain confidential records of employees with occupational exposures for at least the duration of employment plus 30 years.[24] These records must include results of postexposure medical examinations, testing, and follow-up, and a copy of the evaluating physician's written opinion.[24] The record must also include a copy of the information the employer is required to provide to the evaluating physician pursuant to OSHA regulations, including a description of the exposed employee's duties related to the exposure incident, documentation of the route of exposure and attendant circumstances, and results of the source patient's blood testing if available.[24]

Antiretroviral Prophylaxis

A recent study suggests that HIV-infected patients with chronic renal insufficiency or ESRD treated with dialysis have a higher prevalence of plasma viremia compared with HIV-infected patients without renal disease.[36] This relationship is independent of infection-related parameters such as stage of disease, CD4 count, and antiretroviral therapy.[36] Because HIV infectivity may be related to the magnitude of viable virus in the inoculum, the high prevalence of plasma viremia in hemodialysis patients has important implications for dialysis unit staff providing care to HIV-infected ESRD patients. The high prevalence of viremia in infected dialysis patients may be an important consideration for medical directors, occupational health officers, and dialysis health care workers in deciding whether to start antiretroviral therapy after percutaneous exposure to infected blood.

The role, if any, for postexposure zidovudine prophylaxis is controversial. A statement issued by the Public Health Service in 1990 concluded that data derived from animal studies were inadequate to assess the efficacy of zidovudine as prophylaxis for health care workers with occupational exposure to HIV.[92] In animal models, administration of zidovudine simultaneously with or immediately after retroviral exposure suppressed viral replication and altered the course of retroviral infection but did not prevent infection.[27,93-95] Also, efficacy of prophylaxis diminished as the time from infection until institution of drug therapy increased.[27,93-95] Moreover, the natural history of retroviral infection in animal models differs from that in man, limiting extrapolation of data to humans.[27,93-95]

The CDC is conducting a prospective surveillance study of the risk of infection and patterns of use and toxicity of zidovudine in health care workers after occupational exposure to HIV.[27] Thirty-one percent of 848 subjects with percutaneous exposures elected to take zidovudine. That proportion increased from 5 percent in 1988 to over 40 percent in 1992.[27] Despite zidovudine prophylaxis, one of these individuals became infected with HIV.[27] Seventy-five percent of those electing to take zidovudine reported side effects including, in descending order of frequency, nausea, malaise, fatigue, headache, vomiting, and other gastrointestinal complaints.[27] Thirty-one percent did not complete the course of treatment. No seroconversions occurred among 224 HIV-exposed Italian health care and public safety workers receiving zidovudine prophylaxis in a dose of 1,000 to 1,250 mg/d.[96] The proportion of subjects accepting prophylaxis in this study increased between 1988 and 1990 and reached a level of 20 percent.[96] Anemia, neutropenia, and hepatotoxicity were encountered infrequently but did not require discontinuation of therapy.[96] However, constitutional symptoms occurred in 50 percent and led to discontinuation of prophylaxis in 29 subjects.[96] In reported studies, the proportion of subjects discontinuing treatment prematurely ranged from 13 to 50 percent.

Failure of postexposure zidovudine prophylaxis has been documented in eight health care workers who suffered percutaneous exposures.[27] The time from exposure to the first dose of zidovudine ranged from ½ to 12 hours and the duration of treatment ranged from 8 to 54 days.[27] Five of the source individuals were receiving zidovudine.[27] The time to documentation of seroconversion ranged from 24 to 121 days.[27] Failure of postexposure zidovudine prophylaxis has been described in five additional cases with massive nonoccupational exposure to HIV.[27] From these data it can be concluded that any protection afforded by zidovudine prophylaxis is not absolute. Because zidovudine suppresses viral replication in animal models but fails to prevent infection, postexposure zidovudine prophylaxis may theoretically delay seroconversion and require extended postexposure serologic follow-up. However, delayed seroconversion has not been observed in animal studies or after failed prophylaxis in humans.[97] Nevertheless, because of the potential for delayed seroconversion, extended follow-up is indicated.[93]

The proportion of health care workers electing postexposure zidovudine prophylaxis at University of California at San Francisco—San Francisco General Hospital (UCSF-SFGH) and at the National Institutes of Health (NIH) Clinical Center is approximately 75 percent.[94] At the NIH, zidovudine prophylaxis is offered to nonpregnant health care workers presenting within 24 hours after percutaneous or mucous membrane exposure to blood or blood-containing body fluid known to be infected with HIV.[94] Renal or hepatic disease is a relative contraindication to administration of zidovudine.[94] A dose of 1,200 mg of zidovudine is administered daily for 6 weeks.[94] At UCSF-SFGH, zidovudine prophylaxis is recommended to nonpregnant health care workers who have incurred a massive exposure to HIV (injection or transfusion of infected blood). This group "endorses" prophylaxis after serious parenteral exposure (deep needle sticks).[94] Zidovudine prophylaxis is also available, but not encouraged for employees with less severe exposures.[94] A dose of 1,000 mg of zidovudine is administered daily for 4 weeks.[94] It has been suggested that stratification to identify high-risk exposures might help clarify the indications for zidovudine prophylaxis.[94] Factors to be considered include (1) the nature of the exposure, including the route and severity of exposure, the type of body fluid involved, and the age of the specimen, (2) characteristics of the source patient, including stage of HIV infection, presence of viremia, and treatment status, and (3) the interval between exposure and presentation.[94] Counseling of exposed health care workers must include a discussion of the risk of acquiring HIV infection, the limited nature of the animal data suggesting efficacy of zidovudine, potential short- and long-term toxicities, evidence of teratogenicity in experimental animals, the lack of adequate data to evaluate carcinogenicity, the diversity of opinion among medical experts, the need for extended follow-up, and the need to use barrier techniques to prevent contraception and to prevent sexual transmission of HIV.[21] If zidovudine is to be administered, the physician must obtain informed consent that clearly documents the aforementioned discussion and that indicates that use of zidovudine as a postexposure prophylactic agent is not an approved indication for the drug. Clinical and laboratory monitoring of treatment requires, at a minimum, fortnightly complete blood counts, platelet counts, and blood chemistries including liver function tests and muscle enzymes.[94,95] The legal liability of the physician for use of zidovudine for an unapproved indication has not been established.

Often the HIV status of the source patient will not be known immediately. If the patient is perceived to be at high risk for HIV infection, the exposed health care worker may elect to begin zidovudine prophylaxis and discontinue treatment if the source patient is later found not to be infected.[94]

TORT LIABILITY

In most states, worker's compensation statutes govern compensation for transmission of HIV infection to salaried employees such as nurses, technicians, and custodial workers, arising from or in the course of employment.[98,99] Pursuant to exclusivity clauses contained in the worker's compensation statutes of most states, tort actions are barred except for intentional torts by the employer.[98,99] However, in one large state an employer may be subject to third party liability in a products liability action.[80]

Recently promulgated OSHA regulations give legal authority to universal precautions. Although other CDC guidelines may not be legally binding, they establish a professional standard of care to which defendants may be held in actions for negligence where defendants failed to adhere to recommended practices.[80] Although the failure of a dialysis facility to adhere to OSHA regulations may or may not conclusively establish negligence, such failure is, at a minimum, evidence of negligence. In a negligence action based on the fear of contracting AIDS brought by a nonemployee exposed to the blood or body fluids of a patient, some states require proof by the plaintiff that the exposure involved HIV-infected blood or body fluids.[80] State case law governing liability in actions based on the fear of contracting AIDS is reviewed elsewhere[80] and tort liability for failing to take reasonable precautions to protect the confidentiality of HIV test results has been discussed earlier.

CONCLUSION

HIV infection has had a major impact on the practice of nephrology in large metropolitan areas. It has changed the policies and practices governing the way dialysis is performed and has introduced new occupational risks and new forms of governmental intervention into the dialysis unit.

REFERENCES

1. Tokars JI, Alter MJ, Favero MS et al: National surveillance of hemodialysis associated diseases in the United States, 1991. ASAIO J 39:966, 1993
2. Perez G, Ortiz-Interian C, Lee H et al: Human immunodeficiency virus and human T-cell leukemia virus type 1 in patients undergoing maintenance hemodialysis in Miami. Am J Kidney Dis 14:39, 1989
3. Marcus R, Favero MS, Banerjee S et al: Prevalence and incidence of human immunodeficiency virus among patients undergoing long-term hemodialysis. Am J Med 90:614, 1991
4. Glassock RJ: Human immunodeficiency virus (HIV) infection and the kidney. Ann Intern Med 112:35, 1990
5. Villanueva SY, De Medina M, Perez G et al: Prevalence of human immunodeficiency virus antibodies and hepatitis B markers among patients having hemodialysis (letter). Ann Intern Med 105:968, 1986
6. Peterman TA, Lang GR, Milos NJ et al: HTLV-III/LAV infection in hemodialysis patients. JAMA 255:2324, 1986
7. Morrison AJ Jr, Frer CV, Poole CL: Prevalence of human T-lymphotropic virus type III antibodies among patients in dialysis programs at a university hospital. Ann Intern Med 104:805, 1986
8. Rao TKS, Friedman EA, Nicastri AD: The types of renal disease in the acquired immunodeficiency syndrome. N Engl J Med 316:1062, 1987
9. Ortiz C, Meneses R, Jaffe D et al: Outcome of patients with human immunodeficiency virus on maintenance hemodialysis. Kidney Int 34:248, 1988
10. Chirgwin K, Rao TKS, Landesman SH: HIV infection in a high prevalence hemodialysis unit. AIDS 3:731, 1989
11. Rubin J: Prevalence of HIV virus among patients undergoing continuous ambulatory peritoneal dialysis. ASAIO J 35:144, 1989
12. Salahuddin SZ, Groopman JE, Markham PD et al: HTLV-III in symptom-free seronegative persons. Lancet 2:1418, 1984
13. Arnow PM, Fellner S, Harrington R et al: False-positive results of screening for antibodies to human immunodeficiency virus in chronic hemodialysis patients. Am J Kidney Dis 11:383, 1988
14. Baltimore-Boston Collaborative Study Group: Human immunodeficiency virus infection in hemodialysis patients. Arch Intern Med 148:617, 1988
15. Johnston BL, Pode CL, Zito DR et al: Cohort study of human immunodeficiency virus (HIV) antibody testing among patients receiving long-term dialysis at a university hospital. Am J Infect Control 16:235, 1988
16. Tokars JI, Alter MJ, Favero MS et al: National surveillance of dialysis associated diseases in the United States, 1990. ASAIO J 39:71, 1993

17. Bourgoignie JJ, Meseses R, Pardo V: AIDS-associated nephropathy. Adv Nephrol 17:113, 1988
18. Kimmel PL, Umana WO, Simmens SJ et al: Continuous ambulatory peritoneal dialysis and survival of HIV infected patients with end-stage renal disease. Kidney Int 44:373, 1993
19. Feinfeld DA, Kaplan R, Dressler R, Lynn RI: Survival of human immunodeficiency virus-infected patients on maintenance hemodialysis. Clin Nephrol 32:221, 1989
20. Tebben JA, Rigsby MO, Selwyn PA et al: Outcome of HIV infected patients on continuous ambulatory peritoneal dialysis. Kidney Int 44:191, 1993
21. Dressler R, Peters AT, Lynn RI: Pseudomonal and candidal peritonitis as a complication of continuous ambulatory peritoneal dialysis in human immunodeficiency virus-infected patients. Am J Med 86:787, 1989
22. Centers for Disease Control and Prevention: Recommendations for providing dialysis treatment to patients infected with human T-lymphotropic virus type III/lymphadenopathy-associated virus. MMWR 35:376, 1986
23. Recommended Practice for Reuse of Hemodialyzers. Association for the Advancement of Medical Instrumentation. July 28, 1986, p. 2
24. 29 C.F.R. § 1910. 1030, 1991
25. Breyer JA, Harbison MA: Isolation of human immunodeficiency virus from peritoneal dialysate. Am J Kidney Dis 21:23, 1993
26. Correa-Rotter R, Saldivar S, Soto LE et al: Recovery of HIV antigen in peritoneal dialysis fluid. Peritoneal Dial Int 10:67, 1990
27. Tokars JI, Marcus R, Culver DH et al. for the CDC Cooperative Needlestick Surveillance Group: Surveillance of HIV infection and zidovudine use among health care workers after occupational exposure to HIV-infected blood. Ann Intern Med 118:913, 1993
28. Ippolito G, Puro V, De Carli G, and the Italian Study Group on Occupational Risk of HIV Infection: The risk of occupational human immunodeficiency virus infection in health care workers. Arch Intern Med 153:1451, 1993
29. Marcus R, and the CDC Cooperative Needlestick Surveillance Group: Survey of health care workers exposed to blood from patients infected with the human immunodeficiency virus. N Engl J Med 319:1118, 1988
30. Gerberding JL, Bryant-Leblanc CE, Nelson K et al: Risk of transmitting the human immunodeficiency virus, cytomegalovirus, and hepatitis B virus to health care workers exposed to patients with AIDS and AIDS-related conditions. J Infect Dis 156:1, 1987
31. Henderson DK, Fahey BJ, Willy M et al: Risk for occupational transmission of human immunodeficiency virus type 1 (HIV-1) associated with clinical exposure: a prospective evaluation. Ann Intern Med 113:740, 1990
32. McEvoy M, Porter K, Mortimer P et al: Prospective study of clinical, laboratory, and ancillary staff with occupational exposure to blood or body fluids from patients infected with HIV. BMJ 294:1595, 1987
33. Anonymous: Occupational exposure to the human immunodeficiency virus among health care workers in Canada. Can Med J 140:503, 1989
34. Mast ST, Gerberding JL: Factors predicting infectivity following needlestick exposure to HIV: an in vitro model, abstracted. Clin Res 39:381A, 1991
35. Ho DD, Moudgil T, Alam M: Quantitation of human immunodeficiency virus type 1 in the blood of infected persons. N Engl J Med 321:1621, 1989
36. Kimmel PL, VedBrat SS, Pierce PF et al: HIV viral burden in patients with renal disease, abstracted. Am Soc Nephrol 3:313, 1992

37. Berlyne G, Kaczmarek RG, Hamburger S et al: Seroprevalence of antibodies to the human immunodeficiency virus in dialysis workers: results of a multi-center study. Nephron 62:441, 1992
38. Perez GO, Ortiz C, De Medina M et al: Lack of transmission of human immunodeficiency virus in chronic hemodialysis patients. Am J Nephrol 8:123, 1988
39. Buchovsky G, Levin C, Corrales J et al: Epidemic by HIV at a hemodialysis center, abstracted. Programs and Abstracts, IVth International Conference on AIDS, Stockholm, Sweden, June 12–16, 1988, p. 7751
40. Chamberland ME, Conley LJ, Bush TJ et al: Health care workers with AIDS. National surveillance up-date. JAMA 266:3459, 1991
41. Centers for Disease Control and Prevention: Surveillance for occupationally acquired HIV infection—United States, 1981–1992. MMWR 41:823, 1992
42. Klein RS, Phelan JA, Freeman K et al: Low occupational risk of human immunodeficiency virus infection among dental professionals. N Engl J Med 318:86, 1988
43. Centers for Disease Control and Prevention: Preliminary analysis: HIV seroprevalence of orthopedic surgeons, 1991. MMWR 40:309, 1991
44. Gerberding JL: Reducing occupational risk of HIV infection. Hosp Pract 61:63, 1991
45. Schwarcz SK, Bolan GA, Kellogg TA et al: Comparison of voluntary and blinded human immunodeficiency virus type 1 (HIV-1) seroprevalence surveys in a high prevalence sexually transmitted disease clinic population. Am J Epidemiol 137:600, 1993
46. N'galy GB, Ryder R, Quinn TC: Human immunodeficiency virus infection among employees in an African hospital (letter). N Engl J Med 320:1625, 1988
47. Barnet RN: Clinical Laboratory Statistics. 2nd Ed. p. 13, Little, Brown and Company, Boston, 1979
48. Leentvaar-Kuijpers A, Dekker MM, Coutinho RA, Dekker EE: Needlestick injuries, surgeons, and HIV risks. Lancet 335:546, 1990
49. Lowenfils AB, Wormser GP, Jain R: Frequency of puncture injuries in surgery and estimated risk of HIV infection. Arch Surg 124:1284, 1989
50. Hagen MD, Meyer KB, Kopelman RI, Pauker SG: Human immunodeficiency virus infection in health care workers. A method for estimating occupational risk. Arch Intern Med 149:1541, 1989
51. Emanuel EJ: Do physicians have an obligation to treat patients with AIDS? N Engl J Med 318:1686, 1988
52. Ciesielski C, Marianos D, Ou CY et al: Transmission of human immunodeficiency virus in a dental practice. Ann Intern Med 116:798, 1992
53. Mishu B: HIV-infected surgeons and dentists. Looking back and looking forward. JAMA 269:1843, 1993
54. Centers for Disease Control and Prevention: Recommendations for preventing transmission of human immunodeficiency virus and hepatitis B virus to patients during exposure-prone procedures. MMWR 40(RR8):1, 1991
55. Centers for Disease Control and Prevention: Update: universal precautions for prevention of transmission of human immunodeficiency virus, hepatitis B virus, and other bloodborne pathogens in health-care settings. MMWR 37:377, 1988
56. Mangione CM, Gerberding JL, Cummings SR: Occupational exposure to HIV: frequency and rates of underreporting of percutaneous and mucocutaneous exposures by medical housestaff. Am J Med 90:85, 1991
57. Kelen GD, DiGiovanna TA, Celentano DD: Adherence to universal (barrier)

precautions during interventions on critically ill and injured emergency department patients. J AIDS 3:987, 1990
58. Hammond JS, Eckes JM, Gerardo GA, Cunningham DN: HIV, trauma, and infection control: universal precautions are universally ignored. J Trauma 30:555, 1990
59. Goldsmith MF: CDC ponders new HIV guidelines. JAMA 264:1079, 1990
60. Singh V, Raad I, Hamadeh R: AIDS and residency training (letter). Ann Intern Med 114:605, 1991
61. Rubin R, Lief P: Human immunodeficiency virus (HIV) influences the policy and practice of dialysis, abstracted. J Am Soc Nephrol 1:375, 1990
62. Talan DA, Baraff LJ: Effect of education on the use of universal precautions in a university hospital emergency department. Ann Emerg Med 19:1322, 1990
63. Courington KR, Patterson SL, Howard EJ: Universal precautions are not universally followed. Arch Surg 126:93, 1991
64. Edmond M, Khakoo R, McTaggart B, Solomon R: Effect of bedside needle disposal units on needle recapping frequency and needlestick injury. Infect Control Hosp Epidemiol 9:114, 1988
65. Krasinski K, LaCouture R, Holzman RS: Effect of changing needle disposal systems on needle puncture injuries. Infect Control 8:59, 1987
66. Kelen GD, Green GB, Hexter DA et al: Substantial improvement in compliance with universal precautions in an emergency department following institution of policy. Arch Intern Med 151:2051, 1991
67. Leclair JM, Freeman J, Sullivan BF: Prevention of nosocomial respiratory syncytial virus infections through compliance with glove and gown isolation practices. N Engl J Med 317:329, 1987
68. Fahey BJ, Koziol DE, Banks SM, Henderson DK: Frequency of nonparenteral occupational exposures to blood and body fluids before and after universal precautions training. Am J Med 90:145, 1991
69. Wong ES, Stotka JL, Chinchilli VM et al: Are universal precautions effective in reducing the number of occupational exposures among health care workers? A prospective study of physicians on a medical service. JAMA 265:1123, 1991
70. Gerberding JL: Does knowledge of human immunodeficiency virus infection decrease the frequency of occupational exposure to blood? Am J Med 91(3B):3B-308S, 1991
71. Friedland GH, Klein RS: Transmission of the human immunodeficiency virus. N Engl J Med 317:1125, 1987
72. Jagger J, Hun EH, Brand-Elnagger J, Pearson RD: Rates of needle-stick injuries caused by various devices in a university hospital. N Engl J Med 319:284, 1988
73. Ribner BS, Landry MN, Gholson GL et al: Impact of a rigid, puncture resistant container system upon needlestick injuries. Infect Control 8:63, 1987
74. McCormick RD, Meisch MG, Ircink FG, Maki DG: Epidemiology of hospital sharp injuries: a 14-year prospective study in the pre-AIDS and AIDS eras. Am J Med 91(3B):3B-301S, 1991
75. Willy ME, Dhillon GL, Loewen NL et al: Adverse exposures and universal precautions practices among a group of highly exposed health care professionals. Infect Control Hosp Epidemiol 11:351, 1990
76. Franciolo P, Saghafi L, Raselli P: Exposure of health care workers to blood during various procedures: results of two surveys before and after the implementation of universal precautions. Abstract Th.C.602, Program and Abstracts, VIth International Conference on AIDS, San Francisco, June 20–23, 1990, p. 275

77. Linnemann CC, Cannon C, Deronde M, Lanphear B: Failure of educational program, needle disposal containers and universal precautions to decrease needlestick injuries in health care workers. Abstract C8, Third Decennial International Conference on Nosocomial Infections, Atlanta, Georgia, July 31–August 3, 1990, p. 61
78. 29 U.S.C. § 654, 1991
79. Centers for Disease Control and Prevention: Recommendations for prevention of HIV transmission in health-care settings. MMWR 36(2S):1S, 1987
80. Neugarten J: The Americans with Disabilities Act: magic bullet or band-aid for patients and health care workers infected with the human immunodeficiency virus. Brooklyn Law Rev 57:1277, 1992
81. 42 U.S.C. § 12182, 1991
82. Chaney R: HIV testing and transient dialysis. Nephrol News Issues 4:18, 1990
83. Neumann ME: Dialysis units charged with denying transient dialysis care to HIV+ patients. Nephrol News Issues 6:9, 1992
84. Centers for Disease Control and Prevention: Hepatitis-control measures for hepatitis B in dialysis centers. In Viral Hepatitis. Centers for Disease Control and Prevention, Atlanta, Georgia, 1977
85. Gerberding JL, Littell C, Tarkington A, Brown A: Risk of exposure of surgical personnel to patients blood during surgery at San Francisco General Hospital. N Engl J Med 322:1788, 1990
86. Tokars JI, Bell DM, Culver DH et al: Percutaneous injuries during surgical procedures. JAMA 267:2899, 1992
87. Centers for Disease Control and Prevention: Recommendations for preventing transmission of infection with human T lymphotrophic virus type III/lymphadenopathy-associated virus during invasive procedures. MMWR 35:221, 1986
88. Centers for Disease Control and Prevention: Recommendations for preventing transmission of infection with human T-lymphotrophic virus type III/lymphadenopathy-associated virus in the workplace. MMWR 34:681, 1985
89. Centers for Disease Control and Prevention: Update: human immunodeficiency virus infections in health-care workers exposed to blood of infected patients. MMWR 36:285, 1987
90. Centers for Disease Control and Prevention: Recommendations for HIV testing services for inpatients and outpatients in acute-care hospital settings. MMWR 42(RR2):1, 1993
91. Precourt v. Frederick, 481 N.E. 2nd 114 (Mass. 1985)
92. Centers for Disease Control and Prevention: Public Health Service statement on management of occupational exposure to human immunodeficiency virus, including considerations regarding zidovudine postexposure use. MMWR 39(RR-1):1, 1990
93. Henderson DK: Postexposure chemoprophylaxis for occupational exposure to human immunodeficiency virus type 1: current status and prospects for the future. Am J Med 91:3B-312S, 1991
94. Henderson DK, Gerberding JL: Prophylactic zidovudine after occupational exposure to the human immunodeficiency virus: an interim analysis. J Infect Dis 160:321, 1989
95. Gerberding J: Is antiretroviral treatment after percutaneous HIV exposure justified? Ann Intern Med 118:979, 1993
96. Puro V, Ippolito G, Guzzanti E et al: Zidovudine prophylaxis after accidental exposure to HIV: the Italian experience. The Italian Study Group on Occupational Risk of HIV Infection. AIDS 6:963, 1992

97. Gerberding JL, Henderson DK: Use of zidovudine following occupational exposure to human immunodeficiency virus. Clin Infect Dis 15:885, 1992
98. Becker CE, Cone JE, Gerberding JL: Occupational infection with human immunodeficiency virus (HIV). Risks and risk reduction. Ann Intern Med 110:653, 1989
99. Brennan TA: The acquired immune deficiency syndrome (AIDS) as an occupational disease. Ann Intern Med 107:581, 1987

14

Testicular Disease and the Biology of HIV Infection in the Male

Abraham L. Kierszenbaum

INTRODUCTION

Based on its nucleotide sequence homology, structure, and life cycle, the human immunodeficiency virus (HIV) is regarded as a member of the lentivirus family of animal retroviruses. Lentiviruses cause a long-term latent infection in cells and produce slowly progressive, fatal diseases. Two closely related types of HIV, designated HIV-1 and HIV-2, have been identified.

Although these viruses have distinct differences in their genomic structure and antigenicity, they can cause similar clinical syndromes. However, acquired immunodeficiency syndrome (AIDS) is the final stage of a disease caused by HIV-1 infection. AIDS is characterized by significant immunosuppression, including clinical features such as opportunistic infections, malignancies, and degeneration of the central nervous system. HIV-1 primarily infects cells expressing CD4 surface proteins,[1] including helper T cells and macrophages. Studies of HIV-1 pathogenesis have been focused on the progression of infection, in particular the complexities of virus–host interactions preceding the terminal phase of the illness. Strategies are being implemented for preventing sexual transmission of HIV-1 infection as well as for promoting antiviral host responses in HIV-infected patients. In addition, drugs against specific viral targets are under development to either decrease the number of HIV-infected cells or disrupt the HIV life cycle.[2,3]

How Does Semen Transmit HIV-1? What Causes Spermatogenesis Arrest in AIDS Patients?

HIV-1 is principally transmitted through sexual contact. Earlier studies have shown that direct contact with semen is the major mechanism of sexual transmission of HIV-1.[4–8] In addition, spermatogenesis arrest and testicular atrophy are consistent findings in patients with AIDS.[9–12] However, little is known about the initial stages of testicular HIV-1 infection leading to azoospermia and the infective pathway of HIV in the male reproductive tract. Several questions regarding HIV-1 sexual transmission have attracted attention: What is the primary cell host for HIV in semen? What is the pathway followed by HIV-1 to reach semen? Why is spermatogenesis invariably arrested in AIDS patients? As yet, answers to these questions are lacking.

Two components of the cellular fraction of semen have been implicated as the primary host for HIV-1 sexual transmission: sperm and leukocytes. In asymptomatic and symptomatic HIV-seropositive men, HIV-1 appears in semen[4,5] either free in the seminal plasma fraction[6] or in the cellular fraction, associated with sperm[6,8,13] and leukocytes.[14,15] The sperm population in semen decreases in correlation with an arrest of spermatogenesis, whereas leukocytes containing HIV-1, including CD4+ T cells and macrophages, are consistently detected in testes of AIDS patients.[16] The possibility that sperm may be an HIV-1 carrier or vector was suggested by two observations: the presence of CD4-like surface antigens on human sperm surfaces,[8,17] and the identification by transmission electron microscopy of HIV-like particles in sperm of patients with AIDS.[13] In addition, HIV-1 binding in vitro to normal sperm was also determined by electron microscopy and verified by the presence of immunoreactive HIV-1 core protein p24.[8] These observations suggest that normal sperm present in semen can bind HIV-1 and transmit AIDS. At a later stage, when spermatogenesis is disrupted, lymphocytes and macrophages infected with HIV-1 in semen can become the primary source of infection.

However, puzzling questions still remain: How does HIV-1 reach sperm? How effective is the blood-testis barrier and other biologic barriers in preventing HIV-1 access to developing spermatogenic cells and sperm? What is the impact of HIV-1-induced cellular and humoral immune responses on spermatogenesis and sperm transport?

It was widely believed for some time that spermatogenesis and sperm transport along the testicular seminiferous tubules (the site of sperm formation or spermatogenesis) toward the epididymal duct (the site of sperm maturation and storage) take place within a "protected" or "immune privileged" surrounding[18,19] provided by the blood–testis barrier.[20,21] Testicular immune privilege was largely considered to be a passive process, the result of the inability of components of the immune system to interact with spermatogenic cell antigens restricted to privileged or sequestered sites by an effective seminiferous epithelial enclosure. However, recent studies on the pathogenesis of testicular autoimmune disease have shown that downstream regions of the seminiferous tubular epithelial barrier are readily permeable[22] and testicular immune privilege may be an active process resulting from products of the Sertoli cell (the somatic cell component of the seminiferous epithelium). Sertoli cells can suppress interleukin-2 (IL-2) production and T-cell proliferation in vitro.[23]

Our interest in the early stages of HIV-associated testicular alterations and mechanisms of HIV transmission was generated by studies in our laboratory on the characterization of cell–cell and cell–extracellular matrix adhesive molecules expressed during spermatogenesis in rodents and man.[24,25] Cell adhesive molecules include two major classes: Ca^{2+}-dependent cadherins and selectins and Ca^{2+}-independent integrins and cell adhesion molecules (CAMs); the latter are members of the immunoglobulin superfamily.[26] A CD4-like surface antigen, a member of the immunoglobulin superfamily of CAMs, was previously detected in human sperm and reported to be related to the HIV receptor expressed by CD4+ T cells.[8,17] In addition, a human seminal plasma CD4-binding glycoprotein acts as a CD4-masking factor, a property that may play a role in the control of HIV-1 sexual transmission by blocking viral receptor sites.[27] Although these two observations emphasize the relevance assigned to CD4 as an essential receptor for the gp120 coat protein of HIV,[1,28] a CD4-independent mechanism may also account for productive HIV-1 cell infection in vitro.[29,30]

This chapter reviews structural and functional aspects of spermatogenesis, sperm transport, and sperm storage, with particular emphasis on the potential role of local tissue barriers and cell adhesive molecules, including CD4, during the early stages of HIV infection.

SPERMATOGENESIS AND SPERM MATURATION

Structurally, the male reproductive tract can be considered as a long duct with defined segments (Fig. 14-1). These segments are involved in spermatogenesis and sperm transport (testis), and sperm maturation and sperm storage (epididymis) until ejaculation through the vas deferens and urethra. Sperm are produced in the seminiferous epithelium and released into the lumen by a Sertoli-cell-dependent process known as spermiation. Each tangled seminiferous tubule is encircled by testosterone-producing Leydig cells and a network of lymphatic and blood vessels. After their discharge into the fluid environment of the seminiferous tubular lumen, sperm leave the seminiferous tubule through narrow straight tubules called tubuli recti. From straight tubules, the luminal content converges into the rete testis, an intricate labyrinth embedded in the testicular mediastinal stroma surrounded by broad lymph spaces and blood vessels. In the rete testis, the composition of the fluid collected from all seminiferous tubules is then modi-

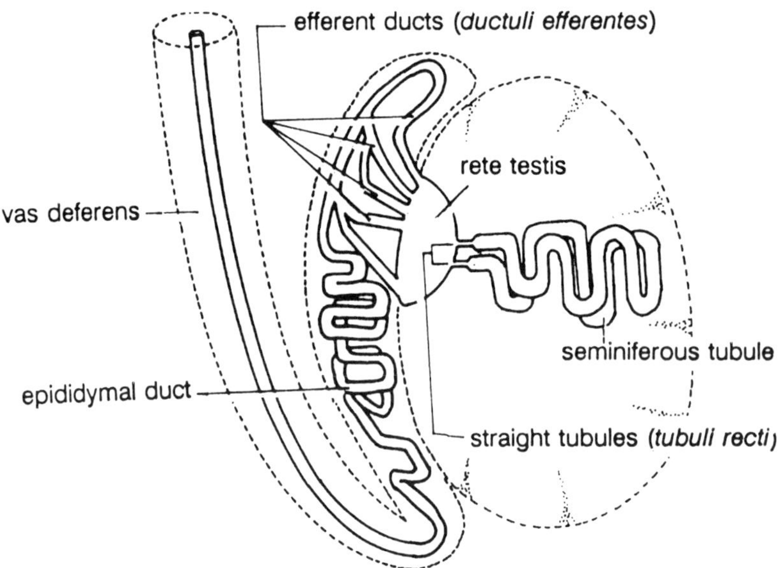

Fig. 14-1. Schematic representation of the interconnected testicular and adjacent extratesticular tubular system. A single highly convoluted seminiferous tubule (located within a lobule, containing one to four seminiferous tubules, not shown), is represented as a closed loop system with two thin and short end arms (straight tubules or tubuli recti). Each arm empties into a network of channels, the rete testis, located in the mediastinal space or hilus of the testis. Five to six efferent ducts (or ductuli efferentes) in the human drain the rete testis, join with each other, and converge into the coiled epididymal duct. The vas or ductus deferens is represented as a tubular structure arising from the caudal portion of the epididymis. Diagram not to scale.

fied, and both sperm and fluid are drained by five to six ductuli efferentes connected to one to two endings of the epididymal duct (Fig. 14-1). Sperm gradually mature as they move along the distal segments of the highly convoluted epididymal duct. The epididymal duct is lined by an absorptive-secretory epithelium, surrounded by a smooth muscle cell wall increasing in thickness distally to the testis. After acquiring fertilizing ability, defined in part by a forward motility pattern, sperm are stored within a complex fluid environment at the distal segment or epididymal tail until ejaculation. Ejaculation starts as an accelerated sperm transit through the vas deferens and concludes in the penile urethra after receiving the product of two secretory glands, the prostate and seminal vesicles, that contribute the bulk of the seminal fluid.

The Seminiferous Tubule and Its Adjacent Vasculature Provide a Protective Biologic Barrier for Sperm Development

Each seminiferous tubule, consisting of a seminiferous epithelium and a centrally located lumen, is surrounded by a continuous wall of contractile myoid cells segregated from the seminiferous epithelium by a basal lamina. Each seminiferous tubule is separated by an intertubular compartment or interstitium containing blood and lymphatic vessels, surrounded by loose connective tissue and androgen-secreting Leydig cells (Fig. 14-2). In rodents, longitudinally oriented intertubular arterioles and intertubular venules running along the seminiferous tubule are linked by a rope-ladder-like peritubular capillary network[31] lined by a continuous, nonfenestrated endothelium. In the human testis, the peritubular capillary plexus is irregular and intertubular arterioles and venules are randomly arranged.[31] Intertubular arterioles and venules supply nutrients and systemic bioregulatory signals to Leydig cells; peritubular capillaries, in turn, supply but do not penetrate the seminiferous epithelium. When compared with brain capillaries, testicular capillaries are more permeable; however, this permeability is significantly lower than in most systemic microvessels. A highly permeable lymphatic system drains fluid and solutes from the interstitium, in particular testosterone secreted by Leydig cells at concentrations 50 to 100 times higher than in peripheral blood.[21,32]

The mammalian seminiferous epithelium contains two cell lineages: the somatic Sertoli cell lineage and the spermatogenic cell lineage. Spermatogenesis results from the interworkings of these two cell lineages. Sertoli cells are the permanent component of the seminiferous epithelium with two significant characteristics: a protracted interphase due to a lack of mitotic cell division after puberty and the display of functional cycles during spermatogenesis, under direct regulation by follicle-stimulating hormone (FSH), androgens, as well as by products generated in adjacent spermatogenic cells. Spermatogenic cells are members of a cell lineage developing from a stem

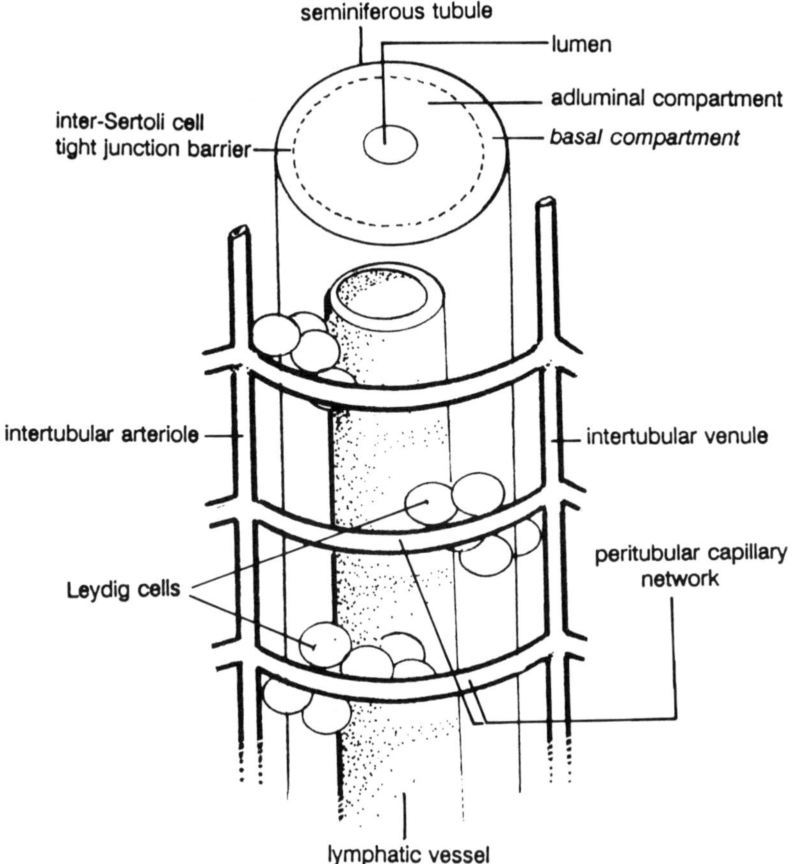

Fig. 14-2. Diagram representing a seminiferous tubule and adjacent components of the intertubular or interstitial space. The seminiferous tubule is lined by the seminiferous epithelium and contains a central lumen. The epithelium is divided by the inter-Sertoli-cell tight junction barrier into two compartments: an adluminal compartment adjacent to the lumen and a basal compartment facing the intertubular space. The intertubular space contains longitudinally oriented intertubular arterioles and intertubular venules. These two types of blood vessels are interconnected by a peritubular capillary network. Clusters of Leydig cells are positioned between the blood vessels and the lymphatic vessel. Diagram not to scale.

cell derived from the primordial germinal cell ancestor. After leaving the stem cell self-renewal cycle, a daughter stem cell initiates a spermatogenic cell lineage consisting sequentially of mitotically dividing spermatogonia, meiotically dividing spermatocytes, and haploid spermatids. Spermatids are involved in a cell differentiation process known as spermiogenesis or sperm formation. Three characteristic events define spermiogenesis: the formation of the acrosome, the development of the flagellum, and the condensation and genetic inactivation of the nucleus.

Spermatogenic cell lineages are replenished continuously after puberty and throughout adulthood and coexist with preceding and subsequent lineages along the seminiferous epithelium.[26,33] A blood-testis barrier monitors the exchange of solutes that originated in components of the intertubular space (including blood vessels), across the seminiferous epithelium. Unlike the blood-brain barrier, where a biologic restriction resides in the endothelium of brain capillaries, it is usually considered that the blood-testis barrier is primarily determined by tight junctions linking adjacent Sertoli cells,[21] with a probable contribution from peritubular myoid cells of the seminiferous tubular wall (Fig. 14-3). Tight or occluding junctions between the basal portions of adjacent columnar Sertoli cells divide the seminiferous epithelium into two compartments: a basal compartment, containing interconnected spermatogonia directly associated with the seminiferous tubular basal lamina, and an adluminal compartment, holding one or more layers of spermatocytes and spermatids insulated from direct access to the vascular environment but contiguous to the intraluminal compartment (Figs. 14-2 and 14-3A). This arrangement places mitotically dividing spermatogonia outside the anatomic barrier, while meiosis and spermiogenesis benefit from the immune privilege provided by the adluminal compartment, protected from autoimmune phenomena.[18,19]

TESTICULAR CAPILLARY ENDOTHELIAL CELLS AS A POSSIBLE TARGET FOR HIV INFECTION AND TRANSMISSION

A major obstacle to understanding the functional relevance of tight junctions between adjacent Sertoli cells as the primary component of a barrier derives from the extensive and orderly distribution of blood and lymphatic vessels around each seminiferous tubule. A recent study on the barrier properties of testicular microvessels has proposed that junctional cleft expansions between capillary endothelial cells form permeability channels.[34] These channels, acting in concert with inter-Sertoli-cell tight junctions, provide supportive and protective functions required for spermatogenesis.[34] Analogous to the blood-brain barrier, where astrocytes maintain blood-brain barrier properties, Leydig cells are closely associated with the blood-lymphatic space (Fig. 14-3A). Leydig cells, which exhibit astrocyte markers,[34] may also have a role in the regulation of the barrier characteristics of testicular capillaries. In the kidney, the glomerular mesangiocapillary network mimics functional characteristics of the blood-testis and blood-brain barriers by its susceptibility to immune-mediated damage. The glomerular capillary loops are lined by a fenestrated layer of endothelial cell cytoplasm, a complex basal lamina, and podocyte-derived slit pores. These structures, responsible for a filtration barrier inserted between the vascular compartment and the Bowman space, can be disrupted by the accumulation of inflammatory cells (monocytes, macrophages, and T cells) and chemical mediators (activation

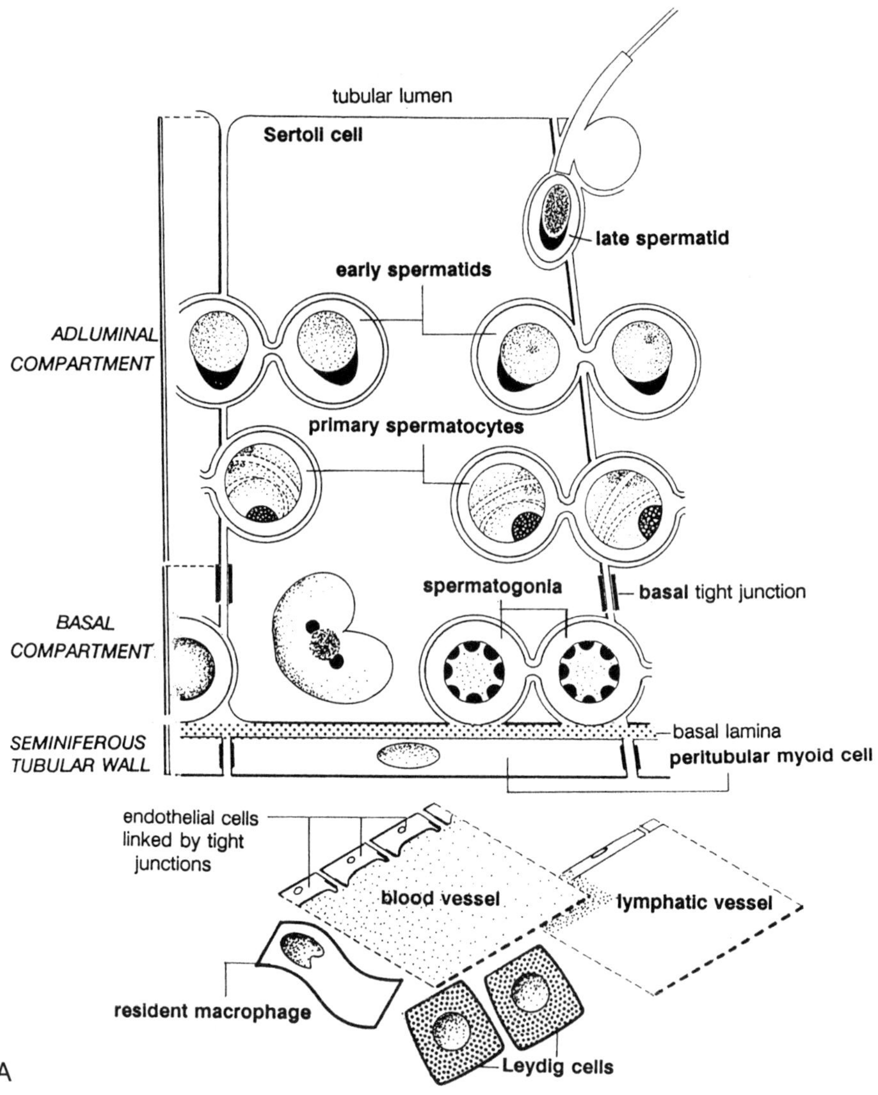

Fig. 14-3. (A) General organization of the seminiferous tubule and intertubular space. A columnar Sertoli cell is linked to adjacent Sertoli cells by basal tight junctions. Basal cell surfaces of Sertoli cells and of spermatogonia are directly associated with the basal lamina and indirectly with peritubular myoid cells (linked by tight junctions represented by vertical black bars). Basal lamina and peritubular myoid cells form the seminiferous tubular wall. Basal tight junctions divide the seminiferous epithelium into two compartments: the adluminal compartment (adjacent to the tubular lumen) and the basal compartment, facing the intertubular space and its components. Spermatocytes (primary and secondary) and spermatids (early and late) are found in the adluminal compartment; spermatogonia occupy the basal compartment. Blood and lymphatic vessels are found in the intertubular compartment, together with Leydig cells and resident macrophages. Blood vessels are lined by endothelial cells joined by tight junctions forming permeability channels acting in concert with Sertoli cell tight junctions to constitute the blood–testis barrier.[34] Diagram not to scale. (*Figure continues.*)

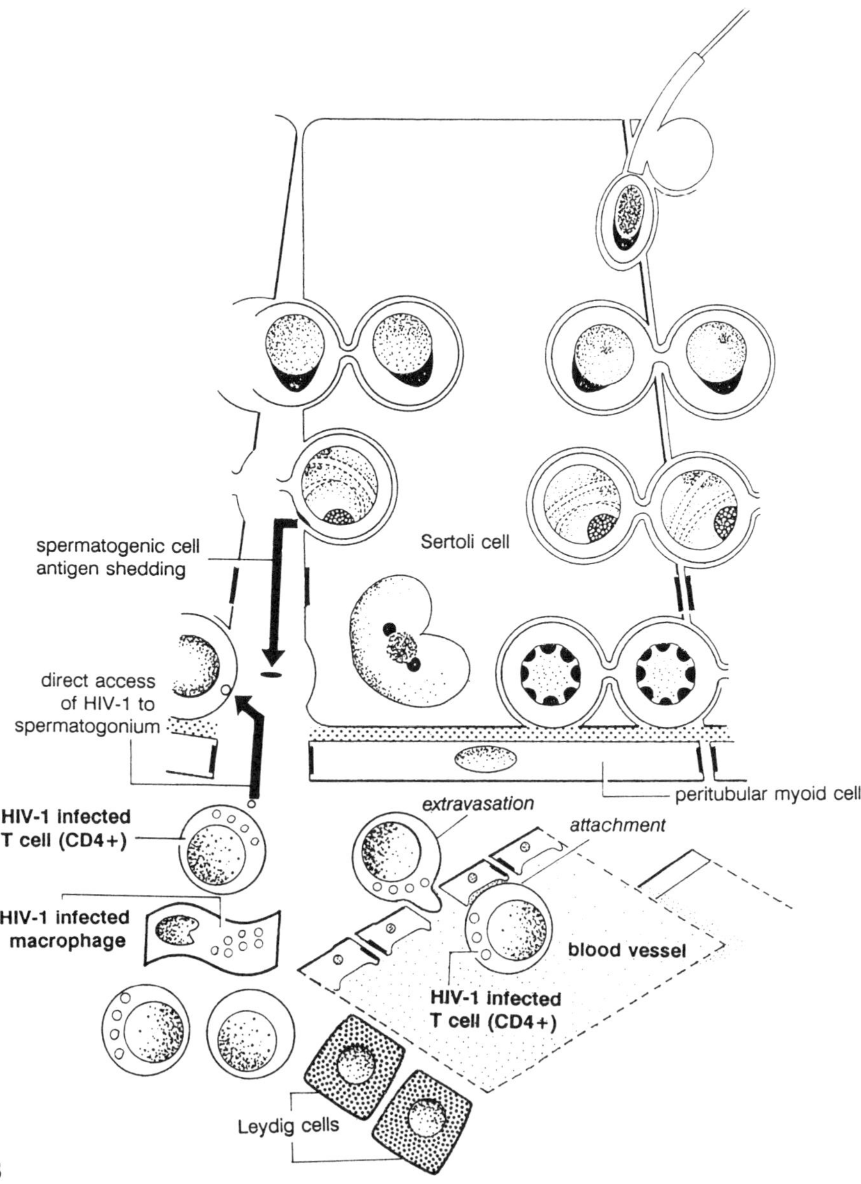

Fig. 14-3 (*Continued*). (**B**) Representation of possible events associated with the presence of CD4+ T cells infected with HIV-1 in the intertubular space after leaving the blood vascular compartment (extravasation) by attaching to endothelial cells and permeating interendothelial cell tight junctions. Disruption of tight junctions linking adjacent Sertoli cells can facilitate the shedding of spermatogenic cell antigens that, in turn, may elicit a response leading to autoimmune orchitis and aspermatogenesis. Macrophages infected with HIV-1 in the intertubular space can contribute to the inflammatory cell infiltrate as well as serve as a source of HIV-1 with possible direct access to a spermatogonium by disrupted inter-Sertoli-cell tight junctions. Diagram not to scale.

of the complement and coagulation system) leading to nephropathy (for a discussion on glomerulonephritis induced by HIV-1, see Ch. 5).

How can we integrate knowledge about the blood-testis, blood-brain, and glomerular mesangiocapillary barriers in HIV-1 infection? Immunohistochemistry, in situ hybridization, and electron microscopy of brain tissue from AIDS patients have shown that viral proteins and nucleic acids are localized in endothelial cells of brain capillaries and less frequently in astrocytes.[35,36] An immunohistochemical analysis of reproductive tissue specimens obtained from AIDS patients at autopsy has shown the presence of CD4 + T-helper lymphocytes (CD4 + T cells), macrophages, and HIV-1 antigens in the intertubular space, in particular surrounding blood vessels and hyalinized seminiferous tubules with absent or incomplete spermatogenesis. Some CD4 +/HIV-1 + cells were detected within the seminiferous epithelium and lumen.[16] Although there is no direct indication of HIV-1 infection of human testicular endothelial cells and macrophages, the uncommon perivascular accumulation of CD4 +/HIV-1 + cells and their cytokine products in the intertubular space suggests a potential threat to the integrity of the blood-testis barrier by disrupting supportive and protective functions of spermatogenesis, including Leydig cell function, favoring access of HIV-1 to developing spermatogenic cells, and providing conditions for leakage of spermatogenic cell antigens capable of precipitating an autoimmune response (Fig. 14-3B). Two observations are relevant to the latter two possibilities: recent in situ hybridization studies have shown the presence of amplified HIV-1 nucleic acids in spermatogonia and their progeny in testicular samples of 11 of 12 men with HIV-1 infection[37] (Fig. 14-4). The presence of specific antibodies against spermatogenic cell antigens in AIDS patients has been reported.[38] In an attempt to place these two observations in a temporal sequence, it may be speculated that during the early phase of HIV-1 testicular infection, HIV-1 can trigger aspermatogenesis by at least three mechanisms. First, a cytopathic effect can result from the disruption of the blood-testis barrier. A disrupted blood-testis barrier can provide HIV-1 direct access to developing spermatogenic cells and enable active viral expression and gradual destruction of spermatogenic cell lineages (Figs. 14-3B and 14-4). Second, a cytotoxic effect leading to cell death can be determined by orchitotoxic viral or viral-induced signaling mediated by cytokines, possibly originating from Sertoli cells or CD4 + T cells and macrophages. Third, an autoimmune destruction of spermatogenic cells can occur in response to specific spermatogenic cell antigens previously secluded from access to the immune system by an intact blood-testis barrier (Fig. 14-3B).

AUTOIMMUNE ORCHITIS AND ORCHITIS INDUCED BY HIV-1

An interesting parallel can be established between AIDS and a model of murine experimental autoimmune orchitis (EAO) by T-cell transfer.[22,39] EAO can be induced by intraperitoneal inoculation of CD4 + T cells obtained

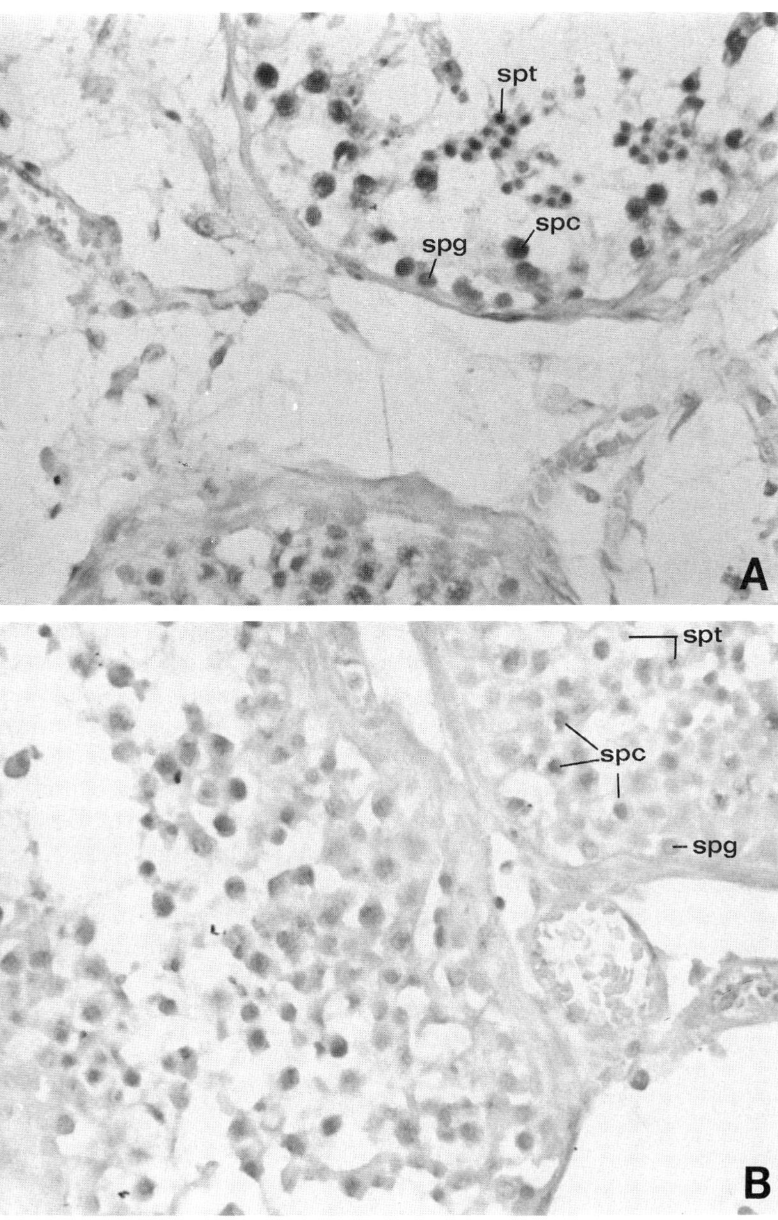

Fig. 14-4. Localization of HIV-1 cDNA in human spermatogenic cells. **(A)** Digoxigenin-11-dUTP was incorporated into polymerase chain reaction amplified HIV-1 DNA using reverse transcription in situ polymerase chain reaction. HIV-1 cDNA was detected by standard in situ hybridization in spermatogonia (spg), spermatocytes (spc), and round spermatids (spt) using an anti-digoxigenin-alkaline phosphatase conjugate. **(B)** The positive signal was lost when nonsense primers were used or the reverse transcription step was omitted. (Photographs courtesy of Dr. Gerard J. Nuovo, Department of Pathology, State University of New York at Stony Brook.) (For additional discussion, see Nuovo G et al.[37])

from mice immunized with spermatogenic cells and previously activated by exposure to testicular antigen or concanavalin A. CD8+ T cells are not required for the transfer of EAO. Testes of EAO mice display characteristic lymphocytic intertubular infiltrates and aspermatogenesis, as do the testes of patients with AIDS.[9–12,16] An antigen-independent disruption of inter-Sertoli-cell junctions (e.g., induced by HIV-1 infection, Fig. 14-3A) can result in the seepage of testicular autoantigens from the adluminal compartment into the intertubular space to provoke immune responses leading to aspermatogenesis.[39]

The pathogenesis of aspermatogenesis induced by either HIV-1 orchitis or EAO as outlined above cannot be placed into the scheme of a disrupted blood-testis barrier without brief consideration of the mechanism by which lymphocytes bind to endothelial cell surfaces and extravasate by a process known as lymphocyte homing. In lymphoid organs, endothelial cell surfaces of venules (known as high endothelial venules) express adhesive molecules (such as tissue-specific addressins and CAMs) involved in lymphocyte homing.[40] Selectins and integrins on lymphocyte cell surfaces (homing receptors) bind to endothelial cell addressins and CAMs (adhesion receptors), allowing lymphocytes to attach and extravasate into a lymphoid organ (lymphocyte homing). Recirculation and homing of lymphocytes are regulated by the immune system, in particular by cytokines (such as IL-1, interferon-γ, and tumor necrosis factor-α) secreted by activated macrophages. Cytokines may increase the expression of endothelial adhesive molecules. Although IL-1 is produced by resident testicular macrophages[39,41] and Sertoli and Leydig cells,[42–44] lymphocyte homing is hardly observed under normal conditions. Whether the expression of endothelial cell addressins and CAMs in testicular endothelial cells is suppressed under basal conditions, or whether testicular immunosuppressive agents prevent lymphocyte homing in the intertubular space to abolish a possible immune response, are both important issues that require further study. It is possible that HIV orchitis and subsequent aspermatogenesis are triggered by a two-step event: first, an initial disruption induced by HIV-1 of the endothelial cell selective functions responsible for the maintenance of an effective blood–testis barrier, facilitating access of CD4+ T cell and macrophages infected with HIV-1 to the intertubular space, and second, HIV-1 infection of spermatogonia and their progeny (Figs. 14-3B and 14-4). The second step needs to be validated by the demonstration of HIV-1 cell surface ligands on spermatogenic cells.

THE STRAIGHT TUBULE–RETE TESTIS REGION AS A VULNERABLE SITE FOR HIV TRANSMISSION

Cuboidal cells fully replace the columnar Sertoli cells when a narrow straight tubule links each end of a seminiferous tubule to the rete testis. The rete testis region is surrounded by an extensive vascular network consisting largely of lymphatic spaces, segments of spiral-shaped arteries, veins, and microvessels.[31] Functionally, the rete testis can be regarded as a collecting, mixing, and modifying station for the contents of all seminiferous tubules, transported by approximately 1,500 converging straight tubules. In addition, the rete testis provides a pressure gradient between seminiferous tubules and the epididymis. Both straight tubules and rete testis are linked by cuboidal-shaped cells linked by less elaborate apical tight junctions (Fig. 14-5), contrasting with the columnar-shaped Sertoli cells of the seminiferous epithelium, connected by impenetrable basal tight junctions (Fig. 14-3A).

Insights concerning the access of inflammatory cells to the straight tubule–rete testis region derive from experimental studies on the pathogenesis of murine EAO by transfer of activated CD4+ T cells, but not by CD8+ T cells.[22,39] Both the adaptive transfer of EAO and HIV-1 orchitis share a common element: CD4+ T cells are pathogenic in both conditions but by different mechanisms. A fundamental notion is that CD4+ T cells recognize exogenous denatured antigenic peptides (such as viral and bacterial components) displayed by specialized presenting cells containing the class II major histocompatibility complex (MHC, also designated human leukocyte antigen, HLA-DR/DQ/DP in human and H-2 in mouse) of cell surface molecules. Class II MHC is primarily expressed by B cells and monocytes/macrophages. CD8+ T cells respond to antigen-presenting cells with class I MHC (HLA-A/B/C/E/F/G classes in humans), which displays peptides from endogenous proteins. Differences in the population of specialized antigen-presenting cells bearing class I or II MHC will influence the host response to antigens of infectious organisms and, therefore, susceptibility to disease.

Macrophages are natural residents of the seminiferous intertubular space, sometimes closely associated with Leydig cell clusters.[41,42] At this location, resident macrophages are class II MHC− in contrast to the preferential distribution of class II MHC+ macrophages in the straight tubule–rete testis region, in particular around the epithelial lining.[45] In human testis, the epithelial lining of rete testis but not luminal sperm are class II MHC+ (HLA-DR+[46]) and transepithelial lymphocytes can be visualized.[47] There is evidence that under normal conditions, spermatogenic cells and sperm do not express HLA antigens.[48]

To place these findings within a working hypothesis, it is possible that the less rigorous epithelial barrier of the straight tubule–rete testis region may be penetrable during early stages of HIV-1 infection by CD4+ T cells infected with HIV-1 trapped by class II MHC-bearing rete testis epithelial cells and antigen-presenting cells, the latter being particularly abundant in this region (Fig. 14-5). Additional histopathologic and immunohistochemical studies of testes from AIDS patients are required to determine whether CD4+, HLA-DR+, and HIV-1+ antigenic sites are detected in the vicinity and inside the straight tubular–rete testis region.

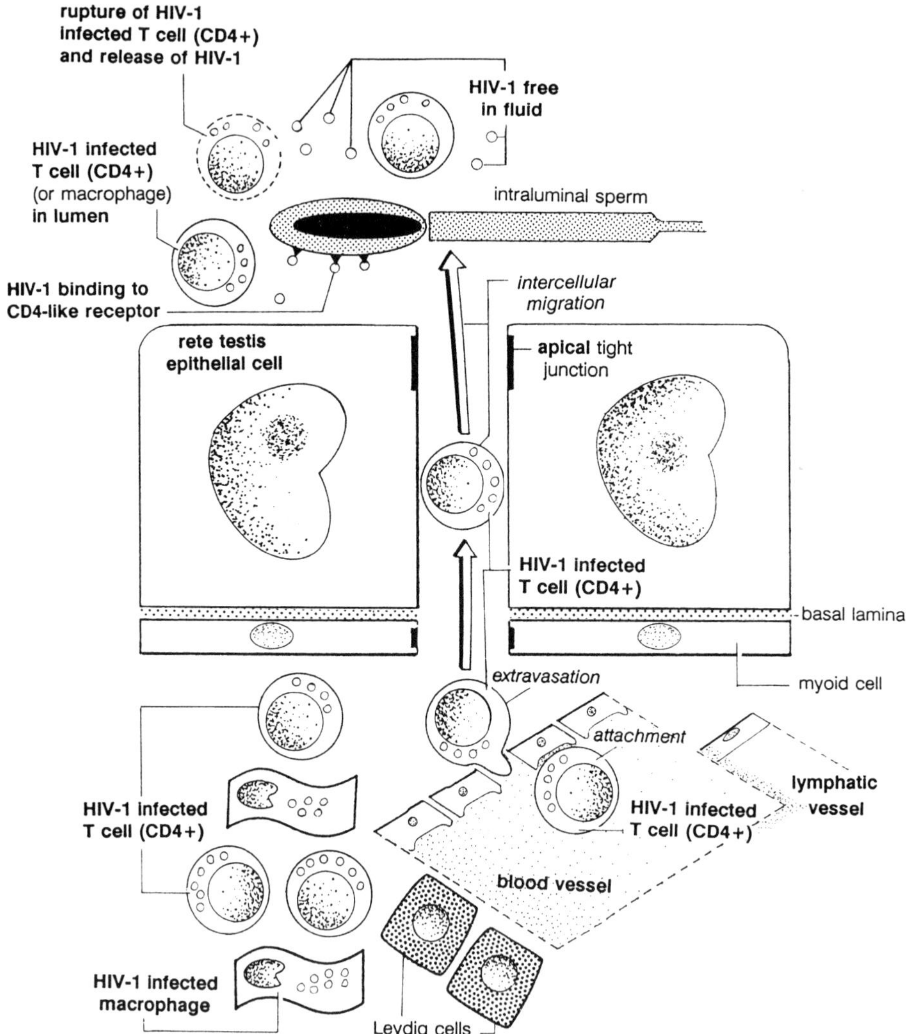

Fig. 14-5. Representation of possible events associated with the presence of HIV-1-infected CD4+ T cells and class II MHC/HLA-DR-containing macrophages in the peri-rete-testis space. The rete testis is lined by a cuboidal epithelium joined by apical tight junctions (contrasting with the basal location of inter-Sertoli cell junctions). Basal surfaces of the rete testis epithelium are associated with a basal lamina and myoid cells. Because of its location in the testicular hilus, the rete testis is surrounded by an extensive network of blood and lymphatic vessels. Resident macrophages (containing class II MHC/HLA-DR antigens) and clusters of Leydig cells are also present. A sperm in transit from the seminiferous tubule to the epididymis is shown in the luminal space. CD4+ T cells are represented leaving a blood vessel by a "hominglike" process after attachment to endothelial cells and extravasation through interendothelial spaces. After transepithelial migration, CD4+ T cells or macrophages infected with HIV-1 can remain intact in the rete testis fluid or become

DOES HIV-1 BIND TO SPERM? DOES HIV-1 BINDING REQUIRE CD4 ANTIGEN?

No matter what the site of entry of HIV-1-infected or bearing cells into the male reproductive tract is, the controversy remains concerning the role of sperm as an HIV-1 carrier or vector during sexual transmission.[8,49] Two major points of discrepancy are: (1) Do human sperm express CD4-like antigens required for HIV-1 binding,[1] and (2) Can active viral replication proceed in sperm known to include an inactivated genome and compact chromatin packaging?[26] Immunofluorescence[8,24,25] and biochemical data[17] support the presence of CD4-like antigens in sperm (rat, Fig. 14-6); however, other studies failed to detect CD4 on sperm.[15,49] Electron microscopic studies have shown HIV-1-like particles attached to the surface of human sperm as well as within sperm, in particular in the mitochondrial region of the tail.[8] These structural observations have been challenged because other investigators failed to detect HIV-1 attachment to sperm, and because genome inactivation in sperm precludes HIV-1 production.[15] In addition, positive viral identification was not confirmed with specific antibodies or DNA probes to HIV-1 components. The proposal that HIV-1 nucleic acid can be integrated within sperm mitochondrial DNA and become infective has been ardently questioned.[50] Although two alternatives to HIV-1 transmission by semen have been considered (for example, by HIV-1-infected CD4 + T cells and macrophages present in semen,[15,49] or by HIV-1 bound to sperm surfaces[8]), a third possibility, resulting from HIV-1 nucleic acid integrated into the sperm genome after infection of a member of the spermatogenic cell progeny,[37] should also be contemplated.

Although it is generally accepted that HIV-1 infection of T cells and macrophages is mediated by CD4 antigens, Fc and complement receptors may be also involved in macrophage infection by opsonized HIV-1. In addition, the glycolipid galactosylceramide can act in vitro as an HIV-1 receptor in astrocytes and neuroblastoma and glioblastoma cell lines by a CD4-independent pathway, contrasting with the infection of brain macrophages and microglia that is CD4-mediated.[29] Furthermore, capillary endothelial cells of human brain in vitro can be infected with HIV-1 by both CD4 − and galactosylceramide-independent mechanisms causing an infection that is productive but noncytopathic.[30] Although it remains to be determined whether infection of these cell types can occur in vivo, the potential HIV-1 binding to sperm by a CD4-independent mechanism needs to be explored.

---

disrupted by local proteases. After disruption, released HIV-1 particles may remain free in the fluid or bind to a CD4-like receptor on intraluminal sperm. Sexual HIV-1 transmission can take place by one or more of the following three possible routes: (1) by CD4 + T cells infected with HIV-1, (2) by HIV-1-sperm "piggyback" transmission, and (3) by free HIV-1 in the seminal plasma. Although not shown, the intraluminal sperm genome may contain HIV-1 nucleic acids derived from the spermatogenic cell progeny infected with HIV-1. Diagram not to scale.

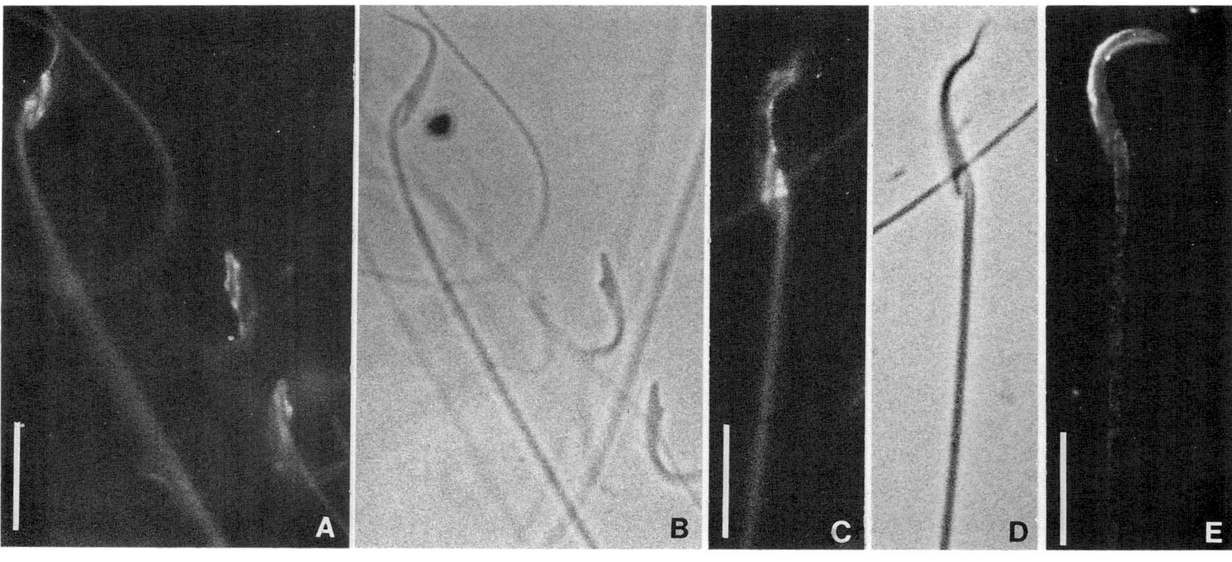

Fig. 14-6. Indirect immunofluorescence of **(A–D)** CD4-like antigen and **(E)** galactosyl receptor in epididymal rat sperm. Sperm were collected from the epididymal tail, washed three times with phosphate-buffered saline (PBS), placed on a microscope glass slide, allowed to attach for 5 minutes, and fixed with 2 percent paraformaldehyde in PBS for 15 minutes. Samples were immunoreacted with mouse anti-rat CD4 (mouse IGg-1)-biotin (MR5115, lot #0303 from Caltag Laboratories, South San Francisco, CA; working dilution of first antibody: 1:50; working dilution of steptavidin-fluorescein: 1:50) and polyclonal antibody to rat hepatic lectin 2/3 (RHL-2/3), an antigen purified from rat liver[54] (working dilution of first antibody: 1:100; second antibody, goat anti-rabbit IgG-fluorescein, working dilution: 1:100). CD4-like immunoreactivity was localized on the ventral surfaces of sperm head (Figs. A–D); RHL-2/3 (designated testis galactosyl receptor[54]) was preferentially detected on the dorsal surfaces of sperm head (Fig. E). RHL-2/3 immunolocalization was used as a control for site location. Bars in Figs. A–E = 20 μm.

An hypothesis has been proposed to bridge the existing controversy regarding the mechanism of HIV-1 transmission by semen. It has been suggested that one or more sperm surface proteins with partial structural homology to CD4 may act as a binding site for gp120 surface protein of HIV-1, allowing HIV-1 to "piggyback" on sperm.[51] This hypothesis regards sperm as a nonproductive HIV-1 vector capable of AIDS transmission to individuals exposed to semen during sexual activity, but in particular by receptive anal intercourse.

The Epididymal Duct, a Potential Site for HIV-1 Infection

The testis may offer two possible entry sites for HIV-infected cells: the seminiferous tubular region and the straight tubule–rete testis region. However, the epididymal duct can be considered as a third alternative. The epididymal duct is lined by columnar principal cells with prominent apical stereocilia, a type of long and branching microvillus-like structure (Fig. 14-7). In addition to principal cells, the epididymal epithelium contains basal cells as well as regionally located apical cells and clear cells. As a whole, the epididymal epithelium provides the necessary environment for sperm maturation and storage, enacted by a balance of absorptive and secretory functions. In addition, a multilayered epididymal periductal sheath of smooth muscle cells contributes to the propulsion of fluid and maturing sperm toward the terminal portion of the duct for storage. Intraepithelial leukocytes, in particular monocytes and lymphocytes, are frequently seen migrating through the epididymal epithelium.[52,53] In situ polymerase chain reaction amplified HIV-1 nucleic acids were not detected in the epididymal epithelium.[37] Therefore, it is conceivable that CD4+ T cells and macrophages infected with HIV-1 can reach the luminal compartment of the epididymal duct and contribute directly (as infecting free HIV-1 particles or CD4+ T cells or macrophages infected with HIV-1) or indirectly through sperm, to sexual transmission of HIV-1 infection (Fig. 14-7).

CONCLUSION

An outline of several possible pathways of HIV-1 transmission has been presented in this chapter within the context of the structure and function of the male reproductive tract (excluding seminal vesicles and prostate). The foregoing discussion has been focused on the mechanism of HIV-1 sexual transmission and causes of aspermatogenesis. The postulated pathways as contributors to HIV-1 transmission in the male have been linked to our current knowledge on the pathogenesis of EAO. Three assumptions have been made in discussing the causes of orchitis induced by HIV-1. First, it has been assumed that viral infection disrupts natural biologic barriers

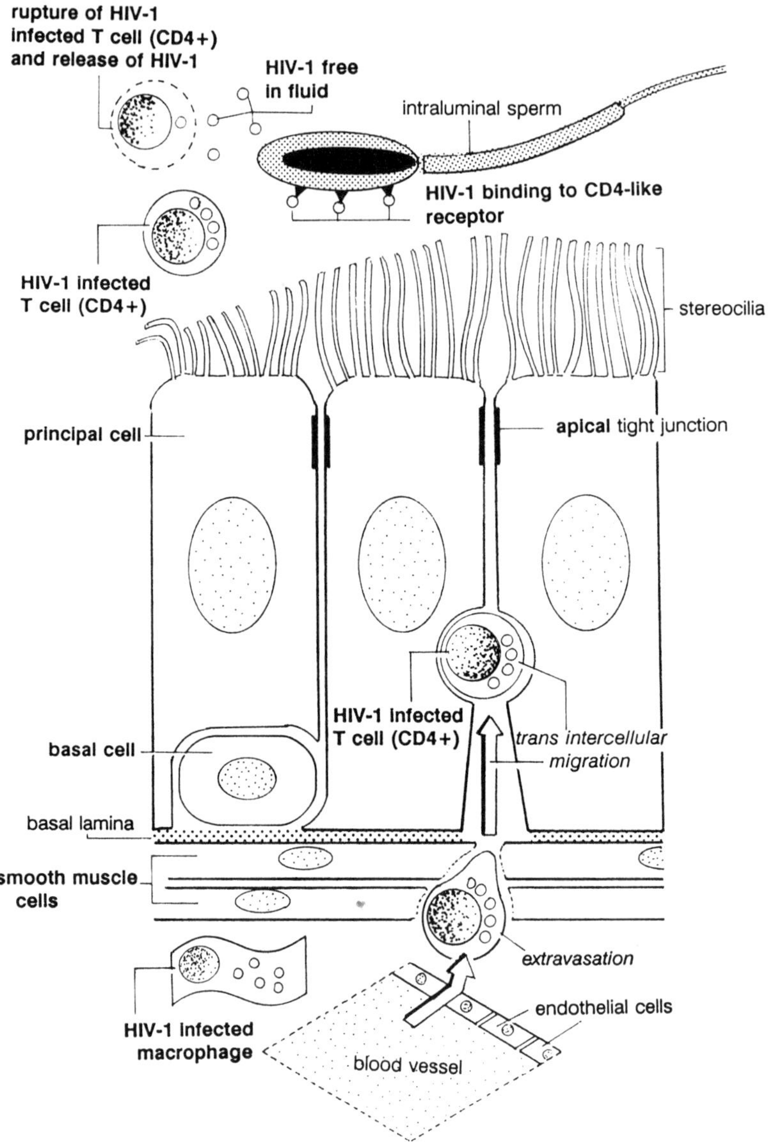

Fig. 14-7. Schematic rendition of the possible pathway of HIV-1 transmission in the epididymal duct. The epididymal epithelium consists of two major cell types: the columnar principal cells and the polygonal basal cells. The apical surfaces of principal cells contain stereocilia (structurally analogous to microvilli but longer); the basal surfaces of both principal and basal cells are related to a basal lamina. The epididymal epithelium is encircled by a multilayer of smooth muscle cells. A CD4+ T cell (or macrophage) infected with HIV-1 is shown leaving a blood vessel between adjacent endothelial cells (extravasation) and permeating the epididymal epithelium. After following an intercellular route, the HIV-infected CD4+ T cell reaches

(blood-testis barrier and intercellular junctions) by introducing cytokine-producing inflammatory cells and CD4+ T cells infected with HIV-1 in the intertubular space by a hominglike mechanism. Second, CD4-like molecules on spermatogenic cell surfaces can facilitate the internalization of HIV-1. Third, amplified HIV-1 DNA localized in members of the spermatogenic cell lineage, suggests the possibility of an HIV-1 infection cycle leading to aspermatogenesis. It needs to be determined whether aspermatogenesis results from direct targeting of spermatogenic cell progenies by HIV-1 nucleic acids, in addition to deficient or modified Leydig cell or Sertoli cell functions or a breakdown of the blood-testis barrier.

ACKNOWLEDGMENTS

I thank Dr. Gregory E. Dean (Department of Urology, Columbia-Presbyterian Medical Center, New York) and Drs. Laura L. Tres and James R. Mertz (Department of Cell Biology and Anatomical Sciences, CUNY Medical School, New York) for their participation in the ongoing study of testicular and sperm cell adhesive molecules, including CD4 and galactosyl receptor. Preliminary results and fruitful discussions led to the development of working hypotheses presented in this chapter. I thank Dr. Gerard J. Nuovo (Department of Pathology, SUNY at Stony Brook) for photographs of HIV-1 nucleic acid localization studies in human testes by polymerase chain reaction in situ hybridization. This work was supported by USPHS Grants HD11884 and HD27685.

REFERENCES

1. Dalgeish AG, Beverley PCL, Clapham PR et al: The CD4 (T4) antigen is an essential component of the receptor for the AIDS retrovirus. Nature 312:763, 1984
2. Haynes BF: Scientific and social issues of human immunodeficiency virus vaccine development. Science 260:1279, 1993
3. Johnston MI, Hoth DF: Present status and future prospects for HIV therapies. Science 260:1286, 1993
4. Ho DD: HTLV-III in the semen and blood of a healthy homosexual man. Science 226:451, 1984

---

the lumen after disrupting apical tight junctions connecting adjacent principal cells. In the luminal space, cells infected with HIV-1 can remain intact in seminal plasma, or break down and release HIV-1 particles. Free HIV-1 particles can then bind to sperm CD4-like receptors. Although not shown, the intraluminal sperm genome may contain integrated HIV-1 nucleic acids derived from a spermatogenic cell progeny infected with HIV-1. Diagram not to scale.

5. Zagury D: HTLV-III in cells cultured from semen of two patients with AIDS. Science 226:449, 1984
6. Borzy MS, Connell RS, Kiessling AA: Detection of human immunodeficiency virus in cell-free seminal fluid. J AIDS 1:419, 1988
7. Bagasura O, Freund M, Weidman J, Harley G: Interaction of immunodeficiency virus with human sperm in vitro. J AIDS 1:431, 1988
8. Scofield VL: Sperm as vectors and cofactors for HIV-transmission. J NIH Res 4:105, 1992
9. De Paepe ME, Waxman M: Testicular atrophy in AIDS: a study of 57 autopsy cases. Hum Pathol 20:210, 1989
10. De Paepe ME, Vuletin JC, Lee MH et al: Testicular atrophy in homosexual AIDS patients: an immune-mediated phenomenon? Hum Pathol 20:572, 1989
11. Yoshikawa Y, Truong LD, Fraire AE, Kim H-S: The spectrum of histopathology of the testis in acquired immunodeficiency syndrome. Modern Pathol 2:233, 1989
12. Dalton ADA, Harcourt-Webster JN: The histopathology of the testis and epididymis in AIDS—a post-mortem study. J Pathol 163:47, 1991
13. Baccetti B, Benedetto A, Burrini AG et al: HIV particles detected in spermatozoa of patients with AIDS. J Submicroscop Cytol Pathol 23:339, 1991
14. Mermin JH, Holodniy M, Katzenstein DA, Merigan TC: Detection of immunodeficiency virus DNA and RNA in semen by the polymerase chain reaction. J Infect Dis 164:769, 1991
15. Anderson DJ, Wolff H, Pudney J et al: Presence of HIV in semen, p. 167. In Alexander NJ, Gabelnick HJ, Spieler JM (eds): Heterosexual Transmission of AIDS. Wiley-Liss, New York, 1990
16. Pudney J, Anderson D: Orchitis and human immunodeficiency virus type 1 infected cells in reproductive tissues from men with the acquired immune deficiency syndrome. Am J Pathol 1:149, 1991
17. Gobert B, Amiel C, Tang J et al: CD4-like molecules in human sperm. FEBS Lett 261:338, 1990
18. Barker CF, Billingham RE: Immunologically privileged sites. Adv Immunol 25:1, 1977
19. Head JR, Billingham RE: Immune privilege in the testis. I. Evaluation of potential local factors. Transplantation 40:423, 1985
20. Setchell BP, Voglmayr JK, Waites GMH: A blood-testis barrier restricting passage from blood into rete testis but not into lymph. J Physiol 200:73, 1969
21. Hinton BT, Turner TT: The seminiferous tubular microenvironment. p. 238. In Desjardins C, Ewing LL (eds): Cell and Molecular Biology of the Testis. Oxford University Press, New York, 1993
22. Tung KSK: Regulation of testicular autoimmune disease. p. 474. In Desjardins C, Ewing LL (eds): Cell and Molecular Biology of the Testis. Oxford University Press, New York, 1993
23. Selawry HP, Kotb M, Herrod HG, Ly Z-N: Production of a factor or factors, suppressing IL-2 production and T cell proliferation by Sertoli cell-enriched preparations. Transplantation 52:846, 1991
24. Dean GE, Mertz JR, Krebs I et al: Expression of cell adhesion molecules during human spermatogenesis in vivo and in vitro, abstracted. J Cell Biol 115:50, 1991
25. Dean GE, Mertz JR, Hensle TW et al: Expression and localization of CD4 in human spermatogenic cells: immunocytochemical and biochemical analysis, abstracted. J Urol 147:380A, 1992
26. Kierszenbaum AL: Mammalian spermatogenesis in vivo and in vitro: a partnership of spermatogenic and somatic cell lineages. Endocrine Rev 15:116, 1994

27. Autiero M, Abrescia P, Guardiola J: Interaction of seminal plasma proteins with cell surface antigens: presence of a CD4-binding glycoprotein in human seminal plasma. Exp Cell Res 197:268, 1991
28. Sweet RW, Truneh A, Hendrickson WA: CD4: its structure, role in immune function and AIDS pathogenesis, and potential as a pharmacological target. Curr Opin Biotechnol 2:622, 1991
29. Harouse JM, Bhat S, Spitalnik SL et al: Inhibition of entry of HIV-1 in neural cell lines by antibodies against galactosyl ceramide. Science 253:320, 1991
30. Moses AV, Bloom FE, Pauza CD, Nelson JA: Human immunodeficiency virus infection of human brain capillary endothelial cells occurs via a CD4/galactosylceramide-independent mechanism. Proc Natl Acad Sci USA 90:10474, 1993
31. Suzuki F, Nagano T: Microvasculature of the human testis and excurrent duct system. Cell Tissue Res 243:79, 1986
32. Bergh A, Damber J-E: Vascular controls in testicular physiology. p. 439. In De Kretser D (ed): Molecular Biology of the Male Reproductive System. Academic Press, New York, 1993
33. Clermont Y: Kinetics of spermatogenesis in mammals. Seminiferous epithelium cycle and spermatogonial renewal. Physiol Rev 52:198, 1972
34. Holash JA, Harik SI, Perry G, Stewart PA: Barrier properties of testis microvessels. Proc Natl Acad Sci USA 90:11069, 1993
35. Wiley CA, Schrier RD, Denaro FJ et al: Cellular localization of human immunodeficiency virus infection within the brains of acquired immune deficiency syndrome patients. Proc Natl Acad Sci USA 83:7089, 1986
36. Stoler MH, Eskin TA, Benn S et al: Human T-cell lymphatic virus type III infection of the central nervous system. A preliminary in situ analysis. JAMA 256:2360, 1986
37. Nuovo G, Becker J, Simsir A et al: HIV-1 nucleic acids localize to the spermatogonia and their progeny: a study by PCR in situ hybridization. Am J Pathol 144:1142, 1994
38. Morrow WJW, Isenberg DA, Sobol RE et al: AIDS virus infection and autoimmunity: a perspective of the clinical, immunological and molecular origins of the autoallergic pathologies associated with HIV disease. Clin Immunol Immunopathol 58:163, 1991
39. Itoh M, Hiramine C, Mukasa A et al: Establishment of an experimental model of autoimmune epididymo-orchitis induced by the transfer of a T-cell line in mice. Int J Androl 15:170, 1992
40. McEver R: Leukocyte-endothelial cell interactions. Curr Opin Cell Biol 4:840, 1992
41. Niemi M, Sharpe RM, Brown WRA: Macrophages in the interstitial tissue of the rat testis. Cell Tissue Res 243:337, 1986
42. Hutson JC: Changes in the concentration and size of testicular macrophages during development. Biol Reprod 43:885, 1990
43. Wang D, Nagpal ML, Calkins JH et al: Interleukin-1β induced interleukin-1α messenger ribonucleic acid expression in primary cultures of Leydig cells. Endocrinology 129:2862, 1991
44. Söder O, Syed V, Callard GV et al: Production and secretion of an interleukin-1-like factor is stage-dependent and correlates with spermatogonial DNA synthesis in the rat seminiferous epithelium. Int J Androl 14:223, 1991
45. Tung KSK, Mahi-Brown CA, Listrom MB: Distribution of histopathology and Ia positive cells in actively induced and passively transferred experimental autoimmune orchitis. J Immunol 138:752, 1987

46. El-Demiry M, James K: Lymphocyte subsets and macrophages in the male genital tract in health and disease. Eur Urol 14:226, 1988
47. Hees H, Wrobel K-H, Elmagd AA, Hees I: The mediastinum of the bovine testis. Cell Tissue Res 255:29, 1989
48. Desoye G, Dohr GA, Ziegler A: Expression of human major histocompatibility antigens on germ cells and early preimplantation embryos. Lab Invest 64:306, 1991
49. Anderson DJ: Mechanisms of HIV-1 transmission via semen. J NIH Res 4:104, 1992
50. Pudney J: Caveats associated with identifying HIV using transmission electron microscopy. p. 197. In Alexander NJ, Gabelnick HJ, Spieler JM (eds): Heterosexual Transmission of AIDS. Wiley-Liss, New York, 1990
51. Root-Bernstein RS, Hobbs SH: Does HIV "piggyback" on CD4-like surface protein of sperm, viruses and bacteria? Implications for co-transmission, cellular tropism and the induction of autoimmunity in AIDS. J Theor Biol 160:249, 1993
52. Reid BL, Cleland KW: The structure and function of the epididymis. I. The histology of the rat epididymis. Aust J Zool 5:223, 1957
53. Hoffer AP, Hamilton DW, Fawcett DW: The ultrastructure of the principal cells and intraepithelial leucocytes in the initial segment of the rat epididymis. Anat Rec 175:169, 1973
54. Abdullah M, Kierszenbaum AL: Identification of rat testis galactosyl receptor using antibodies to liver asialoglycoprotein receptor: purification and localization on surfaces of spermatogenic cells and sperm. J Cell Biol 108:367, 1989

15

Molecular Biology of HIV-1 and Kidney Disease

Ram R. Shukla

Paul L. Kimmel

Ajit Kumar

INTRODUCTION

Human immunodeficiency virus type 1 (HIV-1) is the etiologic agent of the acquired immunodeficiency syndrome (AIDS).[1–3] AIDS is primarily characterized by a continuous depletion of circulating T lymphocytes, especially the helper/inducer type (CD4). The decrease in the CD4 cell population impairs the immune response of the infected individual, resulting in susceptibility to opportunistic secondary infections and tumors.[4–6]

Although AIDS is primarily associated with dysfunctional immune surveillance of the infected individual, other organs such as brain, skin, and kidney are also affected. The nephropathologic complications observed in patients infected with HIV-1 include proteinuria and focal glomerulosclerosis (FGS), and immune complex nephropathy.[7–12] A certain population of patients infected with HIV-1 develop a nephropathy characteristic of HIV-1 infection, termed HIV-associated nephropathy (HIVAN).[7,8,11,12] However, the molecular mechanisms underlying the pathogenesis of HIVAN are unknown.

A number of recent reviews have covered details of the various aspects of HIV-1 pathogenesis, including its molecular structure, mechanisms of infection, and regulation.[4–6,13–18] In this chapter, we focus on the review of information relevant to the regulation of expression of HIV-1 genes by HIV-1 regulatory gene products and host gene products, and the molecular characteristics of the infection of renal tissue by HIV-1. In addition, we present a hypothesis to explain the pathogenic mechanisms involved in the development of HIV-1-associated FGS.

MOLECULAR BIOLOGY OF HIV-1

HIV-1 Virion

HIV-1 is a prototypical retrovirus belonging to the lentivirus subfamily of *Retroviridae*. As observed under the electron microscope, the HIV-1 viral particle is an icosahedron, with a diameter of 110 μm (Fig. 15-1). It contains a cylindrical core or nucleocapsid surrounded by an outer lipid bilayer. The

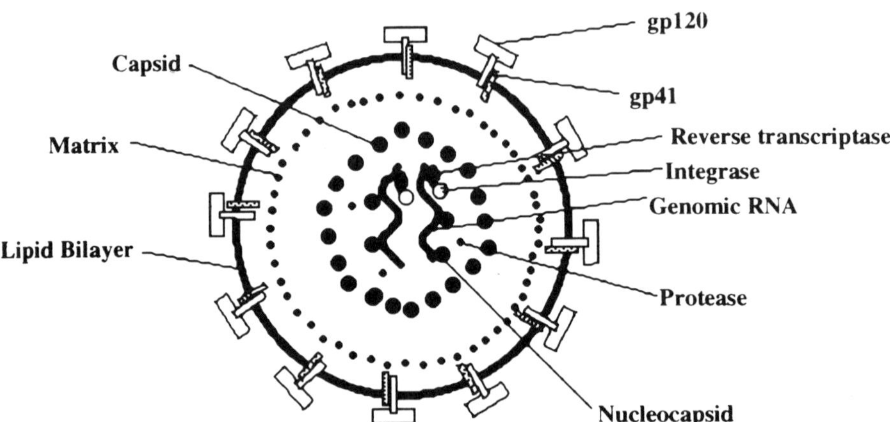

Fig. 15-1. Structure of HIV. The virion contains an outer coat, consisting of a lipid bilayer and a matrix, which surrounds the nucleocapsid core. The nucleocapsid contains the genomic RNA and associated viral proteins.

nuclear core houses two copies of a single-stranded RNA genome in association with the *gag*-derived viral proteins p24, p17, p9, and p7. p24 is the major protein of the core whereas p17 is myristylated and associates with the inner surface of the lipid bilayer. The other viral proteins associated with the genomic RNA are reverse transcriptase (RT) (p55/p63, an RNA-dependent DNA polymerase), protease (p12), and integrase (p11), all derived from the *pol* gene. The surface of the virion contains spikes formed by the *env*-derived glycoproteins gp120 (the external surface envelope protein) and gp41 (a transmembrane protein). gp120 is associated with the central region of gp41 by hydrophobic interactions. The region of gp120, exposed on the surface of the virion, contains the binding site for cellular receptor(s) and the major antibody neutralizing domain.[13,14,16,18]

The major mode of infection of cells by HIV-1 involves the interaction of gp120 present on the viral particle surface with the cellular CD4 receptor. During the process of virus binding the V1 region of CD4 interacts with a conserved domain near the C-terminal end of gp120. Because changes in the conformation of gp120 molecules disrupt this interaction, it would appear that other regions of gp120, in addition to the conserved region, play a role during CD4 receptor binding. In addition, cells that lack CD4 receptors can also be infected by HIV-1, suggesting that there are other pathways of HIV-1 entry into cells. Human skin fibroblasts, brain-derived glial cells, brain capillary endothelial cells, fetal adrenal cells, and certain other human cells lacking CD4 receptors can all be infected by HIV-1.[16,18] The mechanism of CD4-independent viral entry in these cells is not clear. However, the presence of other cellular receptors for HIV-1 has been reported in certain cell types. Parts of HIV-1 gp120, other than the CD4 binding domain, may play a role in HIV-1 entry in CD4 negative cells. Certain brain-derived cells contain a potential HIV-1 fusion receptor called galactosyl ceramide (Gal C), which binds to the V3 domain of CD4.[19] The same receptors may be important in the infection of bowel-derived cells.[20] Not all brain cells, however, express this receptor. It is possible that these receptors do not provide the most common pathway of viral entry in CD4 − cells. Other potential receptors that provide an attachment site for gp120 or gp41 may be involved in CD4 independent entry of virus. For example, membrane-associated mannose-binding factor on placental cells may be another HIV receptor for CD4 − cells.[21] In addition, a 180-kd receptor may be involved in the infection of glioma cells.[22] This protein's interaction with gp120 results in the induction of tyrosine kinase activity in these cells. Yet another mechanism for viral entry may involve lymphocyte-function-associated antigen 1 (LFA-1) adhesion molecules, which are important for cell–cell fusion.[23] In addition to receptor-mediated virus entry, there is evidence for the transfer of entire virus particles by cell–cell contact. Such transfers have been shown to occur in macrophage to lymphocyte, and lymphocyte to epithelial cell contacts.[24,25] Such cell to cell virus transfer is not prevented by neutralizing antibodies.[25]

Life Cycle of HIV-1

The first step in HIV-1 infection involves the binding of virus to a target cell as described above. This event is followed by the fusion of the virus with the cell membrane via the transmembrane viral protein gp41 and the internalization of the viral core. In the cytoplasm, proviral DNA is synthesized from the genomic RNA. This reaction is catalyzed by the viral RT enzyme, which uses the host cell tRNA as a primer to reverse transcribe the RNA genome.[26] RNase H, an RNA degrading enzyme associated with RT, digests the genomic RNA from the newly synthesized cDNA/RNA hybrid, and the second strand of the proviral DNA is synthesized. This reaction also duplicates the regulatory sequences, the long terminal repeats (LTRs), at both the 5' and 3' ends of the proviral DNA. Recently, it has been shown that in resting T cells the reverse transcription reaction is inefficient and an accumulation of incomplete and relatively labile DNA results.[27] Activation of T cells by mitogens, antigens, and/or cytokines is required for completion of reverse transcription and integration.[27,28] In the cytoplasm the proviral DNA exists as a nucleoprotein complex. The 3' end of each DNA strand is cleaved to expose 3'-OH groups before the proviral DNA moves to the nucleus. During the integration process, the host chromosomal DNA undergoes a staggered cut and the recessed ends of the viral and host DNA are joined. This is followed by repair of the gap between the host and viral DNA. A ligation step completes the integration process. This integration reaction is mediated by the viral integrase enzyme.[29] Once the virus incorporates itself in the host genome, its genes are expressed just like any other host gene.[13,14,16,30] Figure 15-2 shows a diagrammatic representation of the HIV-1 life cycle.

The primary infection of an individual by HIV-1 is characterized by an initial burst of viremia and a significant decrease in the number of CD4+ T cells within the first 3 to 6 weeks. Afterwards, plasma virus levels decrease while the level of CD4+ T cells rises. This period is followed by a long period of clinical latency. In late stages of HIV-1 infection, the viral load in the plasma increases again, the CD4+ count falls sharply, and full-blown AIDS ensues.[4,5] T cells, the primary target of HIV-1 infection, are generally present in the G_0 (nonreplicative) cell cycle state. Although the T cells can be infected by HIV-1, they do not produce mature infectious virions unless activated.[31,32] Activation of T cells by antigens, mitogens, cytokines, and/ or interleukins and viral proteins of other heterologous viruses provides a permissive environment for HIV-1 replication.[17,30–32]

However, reports have demonstrated that a true microbiologic latency may not exist as believed earlier, because the virus replicates in lymphoid tissue at a very high rate in patients at every stage of HIV-1 infection.[33] Likewise, high levels of HIV-1 in plasma during all stages of infection have been found using competitive polymerase chain reaction (PCR), a highly sensitive technique to determine viral RNA levels.[34] These observations therefore suggest that in some tissues virus is efficiently replicating at all

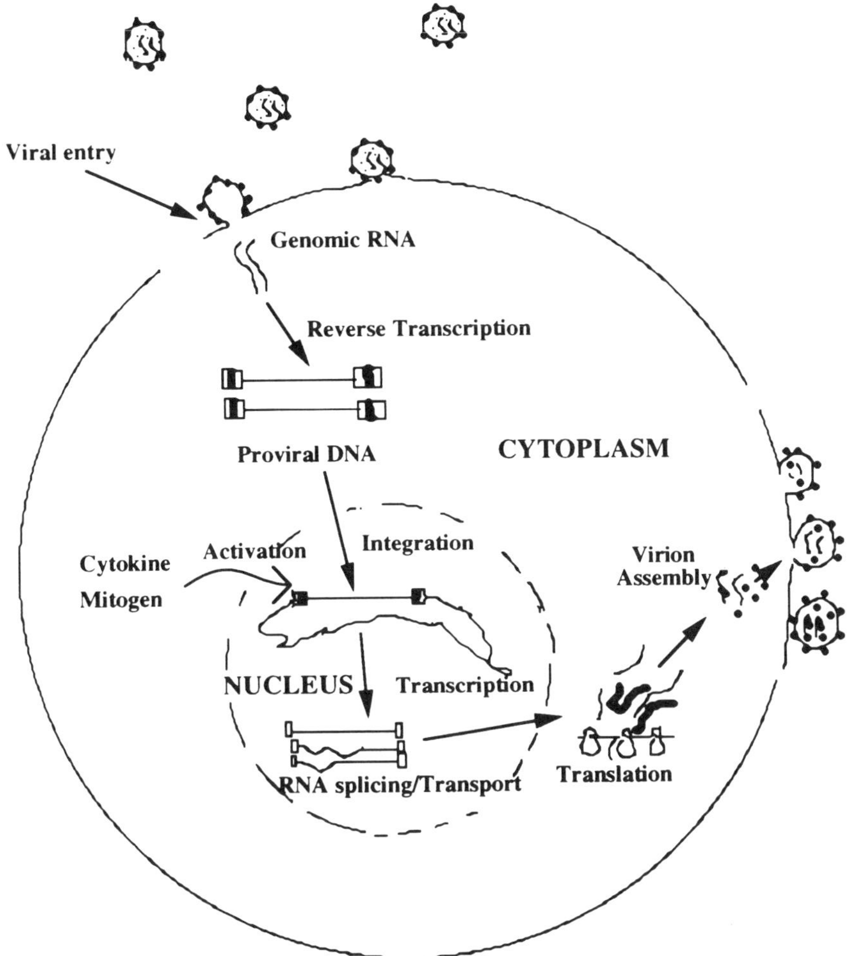

Fig. 15-2. The life cycle of HIV-1. Entry of the virus, in a cell, is followed by synthesis of proviral DNA by reverse transcription. Proviral DNA migrates to the nucleus where it integrates in the genome of the infected cell. Afterwards, viral genes are expressed like host genes. Following the production of various viral proteins and genomic RNA, new virion particles are assembled that bud from the cell membrane.

stages of infection whereas in other tissues virus remains latent until activated by mitogenic signals.

Structure of the HIV-1 Genome

Like a typical retrovirus, the HIV-1 genome contains a noncoding region of a regulatory sequence element and genes encoding the structural proteins, Gag, Pol, and Env.[35,36] The genome of HIV-1 is a 9.7-kilobase (kb) single-

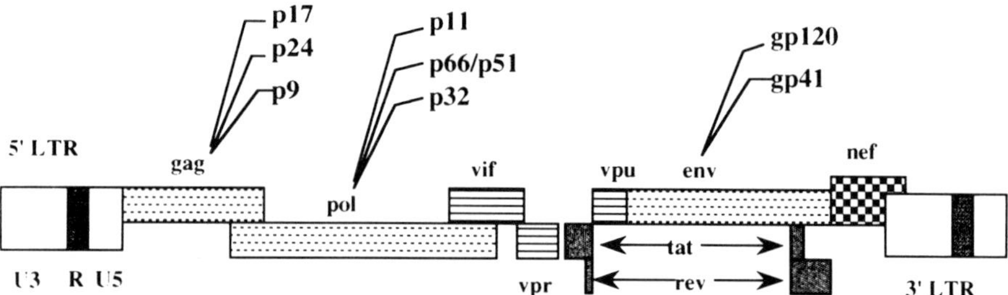

Fig. 15-3. Organization of genes in the HIV-1 genome. The protein encoding region for various genes is depicted with boxes. The peptide products of structural genes are also shown.

stranded RNA. It is more complex than a conventional retroviral genome (Fig. 15-3). In addition, the HIV-1 genome also contains six regulatory genes, namely *nef, rev, tat, vif, vpu,* and *vpr.* The products of these regulatory genes play critical role(s) at various stages of the HIV-1 life cycle. In addition to the regulatory genes, the complexity of the HIV-1 genome is compounded by the presence of at least four splice donor and six splice acceptor sites. These sites generate over 20 distinct transcripts that have almost every viral gene as the first open reading frame (ORF).[18] The HIV-1 mRNA transcripts can be separated into three major size categories (Fig. 15-4). The first category is the unspliced, 9.0-kb genomic RNA that encodes the *gag* and *pol* gene products. The second is the singly spliced, 4-kb set of transcripts that encode the *env, vif, vpr,* and *vpu* gene products.[37] This intermediate class is heterogeneous, containing at least 12 members. The last category is the doubly spliced, 2-kb transcripts that code for Tat, Rev, and Nef.[38,39]

The transcripts encoding Tat and Rev are polycistronic, but the *tat* mRNAs produce mostly Tat, while the *rev* transcripts produce large amounts of both Rev and Nef. The *nef* mRNAs are the most abundant of the three early HIV-1 transcripts.[38,39] The *rev* transcripts are present in moderate amounts, whereas the *tat* mRNAs are only present in low amounts.[38,39] All the multiple spliced mRNAs lack rev responsive element (RRE), making their expression Rev independent.[18]

Regulatory Element

The regulatory sequence element, corresponding to the promoter of a eukaryotic gene, is located within the LTR. A copy of the LTR is present at both the 5' and 3' ends of the proviral DNA of HIV-1. The HIV-1 LTR is composed of 634 nucleotides (nts). It can be divided into three regions: (1) a core region having sequences necessary for the initiation of transcription; (2) an enhancer region to which host-cell-specific factors or viral transcription factors bind; and (3) a negative regulatory element (NRE), which is required for the repression of viral transcription. The LTRs also contain sequences crucial for viral integration into the host chromosome. Although LTRs are present at

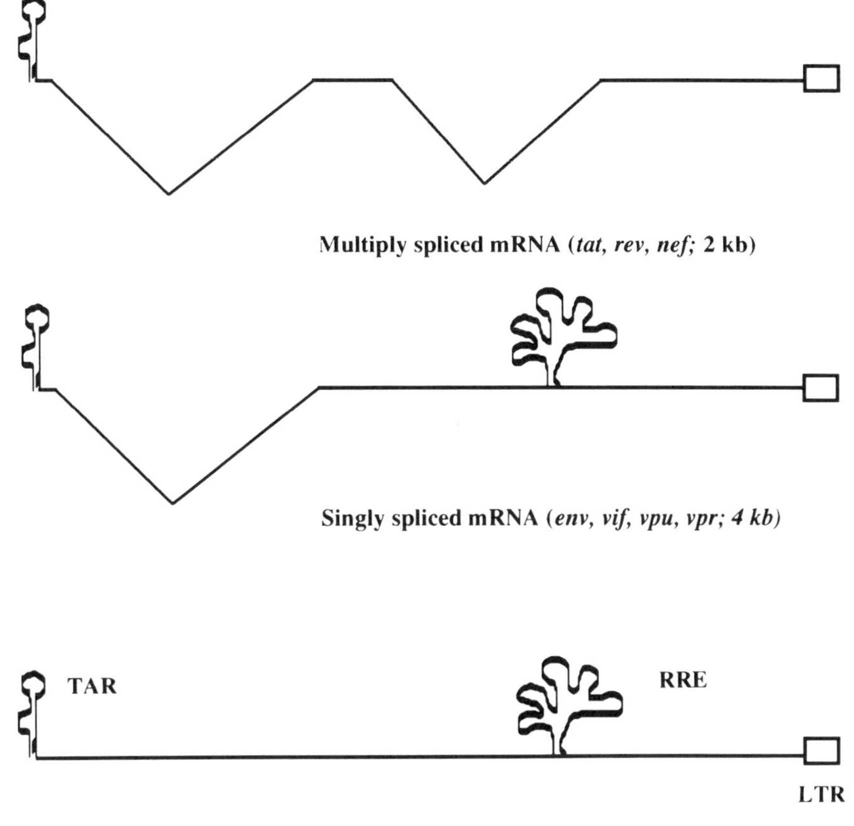

Fig. 15-4. HIV-1 mRNA transcripts. The pattern of splicing and protein products derived from each transcript are indicated.

both ends of the provirus, the 5′ LTR is used as the promoter for transcription whereas the 3′ LTR is used for polyadenylation.[13,15,18]

Structural Genes

HIV-1 contains genes for the three conventional structural proteins Gag, Env, and Pol, characteristic of all the lentiviruses.[35] Both Gag and Pol are translated from the full-length viral mRNA as polyprotein precursors, p55 for Gag and p160 for Pol. The *gag* and *pol* genes overlap by 241 nts and *pol* is in the − 1 reading frame relative to the *gag* reading frame. A ribosomal frame shift mechanism is responsible for the expression of the *pol* gene, due to a homopolymeric sequence or slippage sequence at the *gag-pol* overlap region followed by a hairpin loop structure.[40] The low frequency of this frame shift occurrence results in a predominant production of *gag*-derived proteins compared with *pol*-derived proteins.[18]

The 55-kd *gag* precursor polyprotein, p55, is cleaved by the viral protease, producing the p24, p17, p9, and p7 proteins.[41] These proteins make up the nucleocapsid core of the HIV-1 virion. The 160-kd *pol* precursor polyprotein, pr 160$^{gag\ pol}$, contains 1,003 amino acids and produces p10 (protease), p66 (RT/RNase H), and p32 (integrase), by the action of viral protease. The p66 protein undergoes cleavage to release a C-terminal 14-kd protein that forms a heterodimer with the N-terminal protein, p51, and is believed to have RNase H activity.[14,18]

RT is an RNA-dependent DNA polymerase that synthesizes proviral DNA using tRNA as a primer. During the reverse transcription reaction, RNase H carries out both endo- as well as exo-nucleolytic degradation of RNA from the DNA:RNA hybrids, except for a short stretch of purine residues. This polypurine tract serves as the primer for the synthesis of the plus strand of proviral DNA. HIV-1 RT, due to the lack of proofreading function, causes a high frequency of misincorporations (1:1,700 to 1:4,000), resulting in a high rate of mutation in the newly synthesized viral particles.[26] The HIV-1 integrase, required for the integration of the proviral DNA into the host cell genome, contains an endonucleolytic activity that removes two nts from the 3' ends of the proviral DNA.[29]

The *env* gene mRNA is a singly spliced polycistronic transcript that codes for a 160-kd env precursor protein, called gp160.[36,37] The Env precursor protein is folded and dimerized in the rough endoplasmic reticulum (RER), and cleaved into the N-terminal gp120 and C-terminal gp41.[42] These peptides remain attached to each other even after cleavage.[18] In the golgi apparatus they are glycosylated and sulfated. The Env protein contains at least 20 epitopes that are distinguished in antibody and cellular recognition. The V3 hypervariable region of gp120, consisting of a loop between two cysteine residues, is the primary immunodominant domain of the Env proteins.[43–45] The gp120 and gp41 peptides also allow binding of the virus to the CD4 receptor on the host cell and eventual membrane to virus fusion.[16]

Regulatory Genes

The HIV-1 regulatory protein Tat (transactivator) is a 15-kd, 86 amino acid protein.[46] The Tat protein is a trans-activator protein, and is required for productive viral replication.[47,48] Tat binds to a trans-activation response element, TAR RNA, present at the 5' end of the viral transcript (+1 to +57). In the absence of Tat, the majority of viral transcripts are prematurely terminated, but when Tat binds to TAR RNA, the production of full-length viral transcripts is significantly increased. Tat-mediated trans-activation is cell type specific and requires host cell proteins.[49,50] A number of TAR binding cellular proteins have been identified; however, the mechanism of their effect on Tat function is not understood.[51,52] In addition to its role in viral gene transcription, Tat also has cytotoxic effects.[53–55] Tat increases the expression of tumor necrosis factor (TNF) in acutely and chronically infected T cells by activating the TNF gene promoter.[55]

Rev (regulator of virion expression) is another important viral protein required for the expression of HIV-1 structural proteins.[49,50] It is a 19-kd protein, generated from a doubly spliced mRNA transcript.[56] Rev binds to a complex stem loop RNA structure called RRE, present in the *env* gene.[57-60] The precise mechanism of Rev function is not known; however it has been hypothesized that alterations in nucleocytoplasmic transport and mRNA splicing may play crucial roles in this process.[61-66]

Nef (negative factor) is another HIV-1 regulatory protein of 206 amino acids, encoded by a multiply spliced mRNA.[56,67] Like Tat and Rev, Nef is an early viral protein and its ORF is conserved in HIV-1, HIV-2, and simian immunodeficiency virus (SIV)-2, suggesting an important function of Nef during the viral life cycle.[68,69] The Nef protein is myristylated and phosphorylated, and is associated with phosphorylated structures in the cytoplasm.[70] In addition, it binds to GTP and has GTPase activity. Nef also has protein kinase activity and can undergo autophosphorylation.[70] Another effect of Nef includes inhibition of the transcription factor nuclear factor of the Kappa light-chain enhancer in B cells (NF-κB) binding activity in T cells activated by mitogens.[71] Initially proposed as an inhibitor of HIV-1 replication, the precise function of Nef remains unclear.[72]

The Vif gene product can be translated from a 5.0-kb singly spliced[67] or a 2.5-kb doubly spliced transcript.[73] Vif, a 23-kd cytoplasmic protein, has been labeled the virion infectivity factor.[74-76] Vif is not necessary for viral replication but is necessary for newly synthesized virions to have full infectivity. The mechanism of Vif function is not known.[75,77,78]

Vpu is a unique product of HIV-1, with no parallel protein in other primate lentiviruses. The *vpu* gene product, encoded by a polycistronic mRNA, is an 81 amino acid 15- to 20-kd protein.[79-81] Vpu, a phosphorylated protein, is associated with the cytoplasmic membrane of infected cells where it is involved in the efficient release of newly formed virions from the cell surface.[80-83]

The vpr gene product is encoded by a 2.5-kb doubly spliced transcript, producing either a 77 or 96 amino acid, 15-kd protein.[84-86] Vpr increases the rate of viral replication and cytopathic effects in T cells. The vpr protein is packaged within the viral particle with each particle containing about 100 copies.[84,87] vpr increases the rate of viral replication and cytopathic effects in T cells. Vpr also activates, in trans, a number of viral and cellular promoters and may produce the initial Tat-independent transcription.[84,87]

Mechanism of HIV-1 Gene Expression

The expression of a eukaryotic gene and the function of its protein product may be regulated at several levels. These include (1) transcription of the gene in response to a specific mitogenic signal or cell-type-specific gene expression due to the presence of a specific transcription factor; (2) the processing of the precursor mRNA by alternative splicing; (3) selective restric-

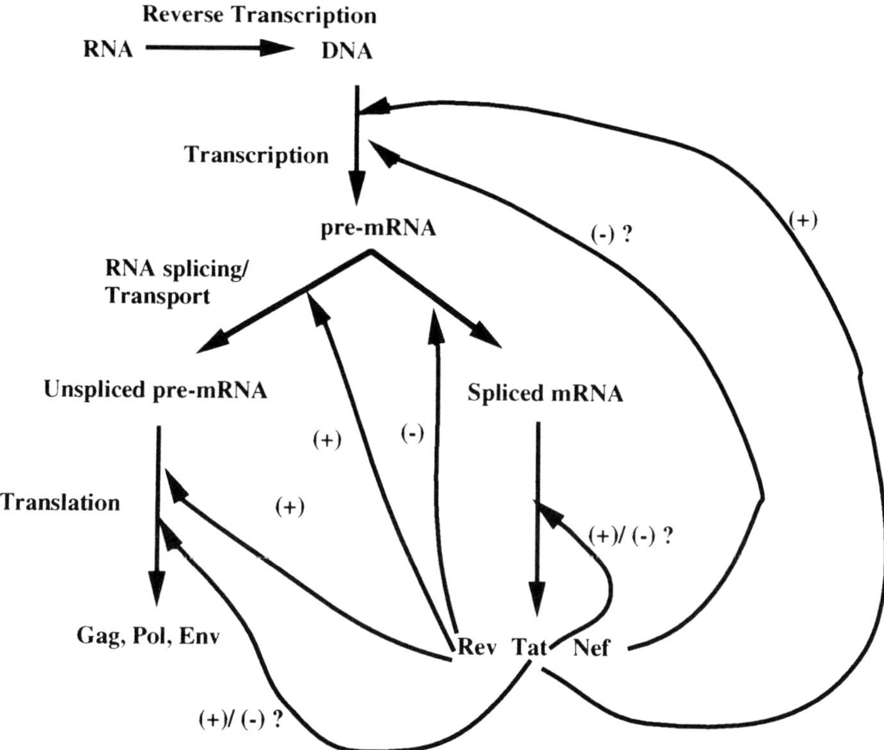

Fig. 15-5. Complexity of the regulation of HIV-1 gene expression. The major steps in the regulation of HIV-1 gene expression are reverse transcription, transcription, mRNA splicing, and nucleocytoplasmic export of spliced/unspliced mRNA and translation. Steps at which viral proteins play regulatory roles are indicated. (+) or (−) represent positive or negative modes of regulation by viral proteins.

tion of mRNA transcripts to the cytoplasm or the nucleus; and (4) regulation at the level of translation by frame shifting or the use of multiple initiation signals. Additionally, the activity of a protein may be regulated by post-translational modifications. The genes of HIV-1 contain sequences recognized by the host cell gene expression machinery. Therefore, the expression of HIV-1 genes is regulated in a manner similar to other eukaryotic genes, for example, at the level of transcription and alternative splicing. However, the expression of HIV-1 genes is more complex due to its cell-specific expression, and the presence of unique viral regulatory sequences and viral proteins such as Tat and Rev, which alter the host cell metabolism for the advantage of the virus (Fig. 15-5). The viral proteins Tat and Rev play crucial roles in the regulation of viral gene expression at the transcriptional and post-transcriptional levels.

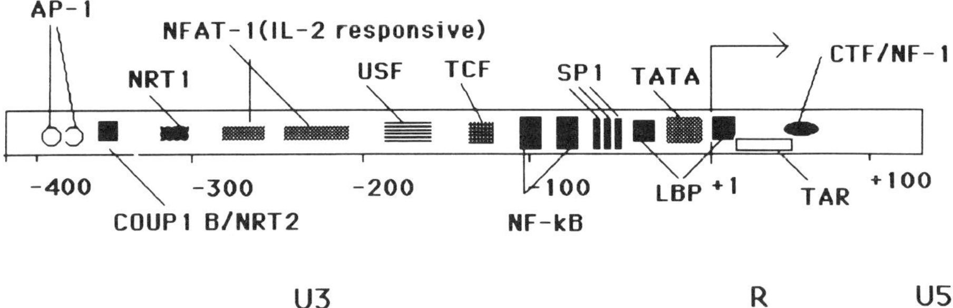

Fig. 15-6. Organization of the HIV-1 LTR. The binding site for each transcription factor is indicated.

Transcriptional Regulation

Regulation by transcription factors. As stated previously, the 5′ LTR acts as the promoter for HIV-1 gene expression, whereas the 3′ LTR is used as the polyadenylation site. The LTRs are composed of 634 nts of noncoding sequences and contain three regions in the order 5′-U3, R, and U5-3′ (Fig. 15-6). The U3 region consists of 453 to 456 nts, the R region is 98 nts, and the U5 region is 83 to 85 nts long.[88,89] The U3 region contains the binding site for host and viral transcription factors and extends up to the transcription start site. The R region starts at the transcriptional initiation site and contains the Tat responsive element, the TAR RNA.[14,15,18,51,73] The U5 region is downstream of the transcription unit and contains G-T rich clusters, necessary for efficient polyadenylation.[90] In most cell types, HIV-1 LTR is a weak promoter due to the presence of specific negative regulatory sequences within the 5′ LTR or a lack of a cell-type-specific factor(s) necessary for transcription.[13,18,51,91,92] The presence of the TAR stem loop structure at the mRNA start site and the low efficiency of the RNA polymerase, which usually falls off the transcript before completion of transcription, also decreases the efficiency of transcription.[93–97]

The regulation and transcriptional efficiency of the HIV-1 LTR has been primarily studied by using chloramphenicol acetyl transferase (CAT) reporter systems, DNase footprinting, and cell infection studies using proviral DNA. In the reporter system, LTR sequences are cloned upstream of the CAT gene. The CAT gene encodes a bacterial enzyme that catalyzes the acetylation of chloramphenicol. The HIV-1 LTR directs the transcription of the CAT mRNA using the transcription factors of the transfected cell. The efficiency of the transcription is proportional to the transcriptional efficiency of the LTR sequences in transfected cells[98] (Fig. 15-7). DNase I footprinting is used to define the binding sites of transcription factors and other regulatory factors to LTR. DNase footprinting involves the incubation of LTR DNA with nuclear extract or purified transcription factors, followed by treatment

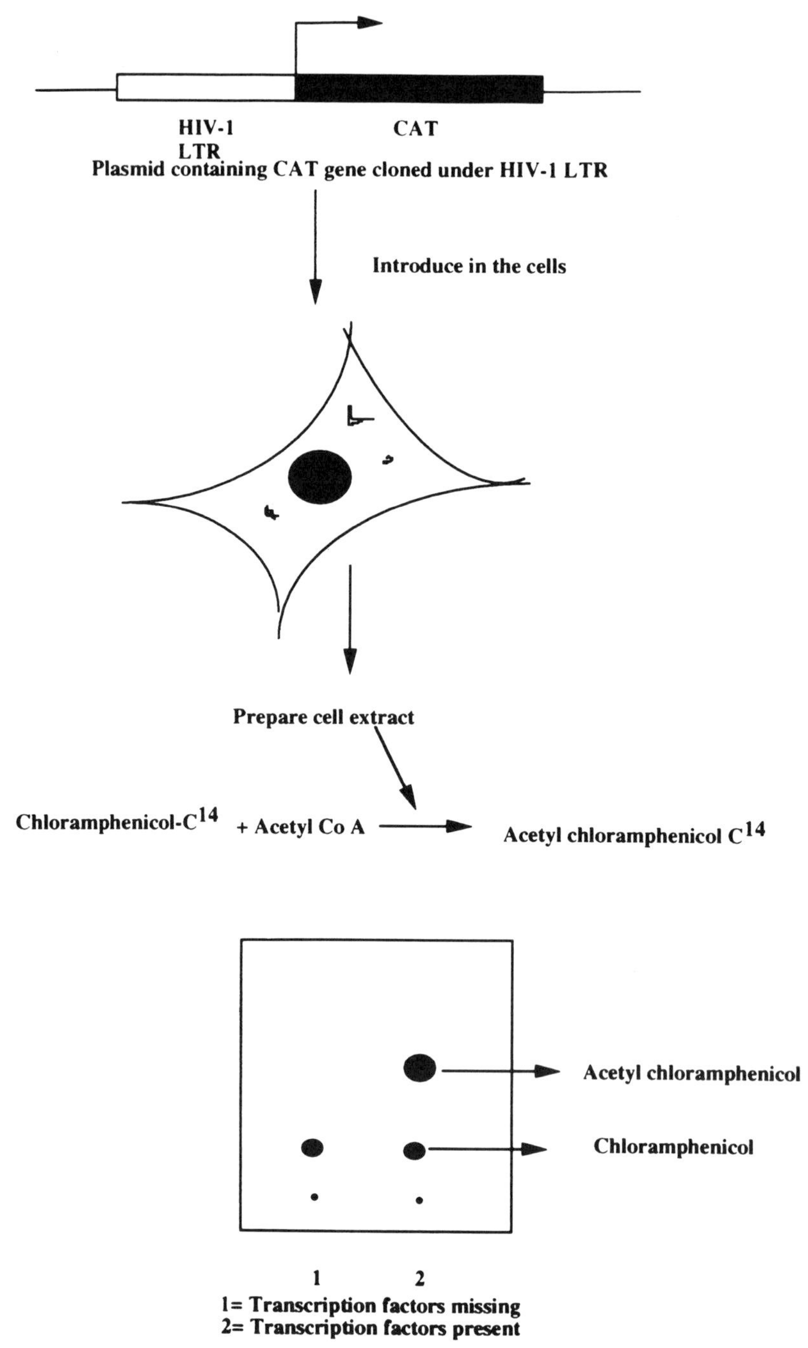

Fig. 15-7. The CAT reporter system for studying the function of HIV-1 LTR. Major steps involved in the assay are construction of the reporter plasmid by cloning the LTR sequences in a eukaryotic expression vector, cloning of the gene encoding CAT enzyme downstream of the LTR, transfection of the reporter plasmid in the desired cells, preparation of cell lysate, and assaying the enzyme activity.

of the reaction mixture with DNase I. Regions of DNA, to which proteins bind, are protected from digestion whereas unbound DNA is degraded. In a separate reaction, DNA alone is incubated with DNase. Analysis of the digestion products from the two reactions on a polyacrylamide gel results in the formation of a DNA ladder. By comparing the band pattern with and without protein, the sequence(s) required for a factor's binding can be deduced. In the following section we will review information regarding those transcription factors that play regulatory roles in the expression of HIV-1 LTRs.

An extremely low level of LTR-driven HIV-1 transcription, referred to as basal transcription, occurs in the absence of cell activation signals such as cytokines, growth factors, or viral trans-activator proteins. Basal transcription is regulated by constitutively expressed transcription factors such as TF-IID and SP1, due to their binding to respective binding motifs in LTR.[51] Mutations in both the SP1 and TF-IID binding sites result in a large decrease in HIV-1 gene expression.[99] Binding of TF-IID to TATA BOX nt -22 to -27 at the site of transcriptional initiation through its component TATA binding protein or TBP mediates the formation of an initiation complex by the interaction between TF-IID, TF-IIA, TF-IIB, TF-IIE, TF-IIF, TF-IIH, and RNA polymerase II.[100,101] In addition, TF-IID is also required for the function of other transcription factors such as SP1 and NF-κB.[102] An inhibitor of TF-IID-mediated transcription, a 123-kd TATA binding protein, has also been identified; however, the functional significance of this protein is unknown.[103] In addition to its role during basal transcription, the TATA box is required for Tat-mediated trans-activation because mutations in the TATA box impair transcriptional activation by Tat.[104,105]

SP1 is a constitutive transcription factor and contains three zinc finger domains that bind to DNA, and two glutamine-rich transcriptional activation domains. There are three functional SP1 binding sites, I (nt -46 to -55), II (nt -57 to -66), and III (nt -68 to -77) in the U3 region of HIV-1 LTR.[99,106] Mutations in two of the three sites cause minimal effects on basal and Tat-mediated transcription.[99] However, simultaneous mutations in all three sites result in a drastic decrease in basal transcription as well as Tat-mediated trans-activation, demonstrating an absolute requirement of at least one SP1 binding site for HIV-1 transcription.[99,107,108]

The interdependence of TF-IID and SP1 function has been shown by the observation that defects in replication of a proviral construct containing mutated SP1 binding sites could be corrected by compensatory mutations in the TATA box.[108] A cellular protein USA (upstream stimulatory activity), is required for the basal LTR expression by TF-IID and SP1 or NF-κB.[109]

Role of NF-κB. A small region of LTR upstream of the 5′ core region contains sequences that comprise the enhancer region. The binding of the cell-specific factor, NF-κB, to this element results in increased HIV-1 LTR expression. NF-κB regulates immunoglobulin gene expression and plays a crucial role in the activation of immune cells as a result of mitogen stimulation.[110] The analysis of the cDNA encoding NF-κB has revealed that it is related to the v-*rel* oncogene, c-*rel* proto-oncogene families, and to the *dorsal* gene of *Drosophila*.[111,112] These proteins share extensive sequence homology at the N-terminal domain, termed the *rel*-homology region. The DNA binding activity of these proteins is present in this region whereas the C-terminal variable region contains the activation domain. A number of related proteins such as p85, p76, p65, and p50 bind to the NF-κB domain of the target DNA.[111] The predominant active form of NF-κB is a heterotetramer of two molecules each of p65 and p50-kd subunits.[13,51,110–112] In uninduced cells NF-κB is localized in the cytoplasm in association with IκB, a 37-kd protein (p37).[113,114] The p50 polypeptide contains the DNA-binding activity, while the p65 subunit allows the complex to be inhibited by IκB.[115] The protein–protein interaction occurs through amino acid repeats called aneurin repeats, present in both p65 and p37. The 50-kd subunit generated by proteolytic cleavage of a precursor polypeptide, p100, is inactive in the absence of the 65-kd polypeptide.[13,51,110–112]

HIV-1 contains two copies of the NF-κB sequence binding motif (GGGACTTTCC) in the U3 region of the LTR.[116–118] The sequences are highly conserved among different HIV-1 isolates, indicating a crucial role for these elements in HIV-1 gene expression. NF-κB is induced through the activation of T lymphocytes by cytokines such as TNF-α or interleukin-1 (IL-1), mitogens such as phorbol myristyl acetate (PMA), or by other viral proteins such as the Tax protein of human T-cell leukemia virus-I (HTLV-1).[116,119–121] This activation results in the induction of second messenger signaling pathways leading to the phosphorylation of IκB. Phosphorylated IκB dissociates from the NF-κB-IκB complex causing the release of the p50-p65 heterodimer of 50- and 65-kd NF-κB subunits. These two polypeptides then migrate to the nucleus where they bind the HIV-1-LTR enhancer region[110–112] (Fig. 15-8). Recently it has been demonstrated that the binding of NF-κB to target sequences alone is not sufficient to induce HIV-1 gene expression. Rather, a protein–protein interaction must occur between NF-κB and SP1 for transcriptional activation.[122]

In addition, the HIV-1 LTR contains binding sites for other transcription factors including upstream stimulatory factor (USF-1), nuclear factor of activated T cells (NFAT-1), cellular factor activator protein (AP-1), chicken ovalbumin upstream promoter-transcription factor (COUP-TF), T-cell factor (site B), c-*myb,* and NRT-1 and NRT-2.[13,51] The binding sites for some of these factors including USF-1, NFAT-1, AP-1, COUP-TF, NRT-1, and NRT-2 are collectively referred to as the negative regulatory element (NRE).[90,123,124] Precise roles for these transcription factors in the regulation of HIV-1 gene expression are not well defined. Deletion studies have yielded conflicting results regarding their roles as negative or positive regulatory factors. For example, in one study, mutations in the USF-1 binding site resulted in a considerable decrease in the expression of LTR[125,126] whereas higher levels of expression were observed in another study.[90] Likewise in one investigation, deletion of the NFAT-1 site resulted in enhanced viral

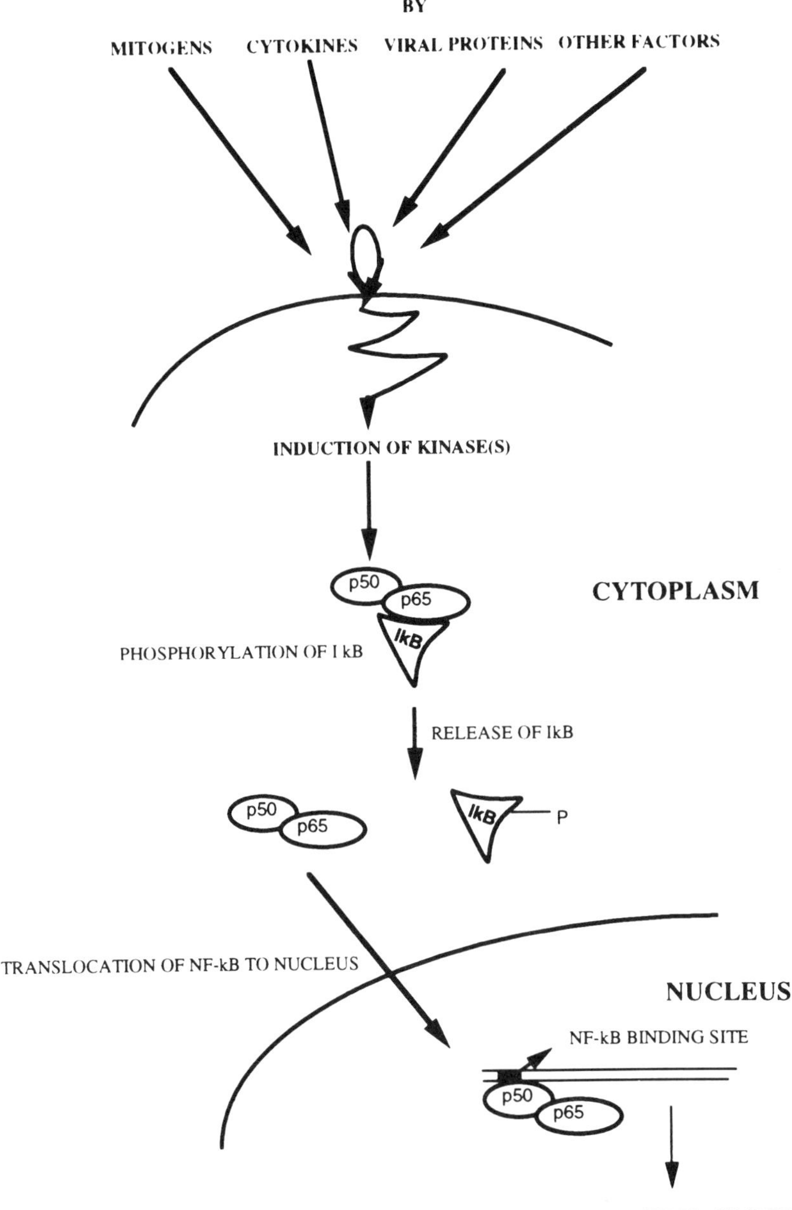

Fig. 15-8. Mechanism of NF-κB mediated activation of HIV-1 transcription. In association with IκB, NF-κB (shown as subunits p50 and p65) remains as an inactive complex in the cytoplasm. Induction of the signal transduction pathways, by external stimuli, causes phosphorylation of the I-κB, which results in the release of NF-κB. NF-κB migrates to the nucleus of the cell where it binds to the DNA sequences of the target gene, leading to an increase in transcription of the gene.

replication,[90] yet other studies did not demonstrate any significant changes in LTR activity due to mutations in this site.[125]

The HIV-1 promoter also contains several protein binding sites downstream of the transcriptional start site. A 63-kd protein, the leader binding protein-1 (LBP-1) or upstream binding protein-1 (UBP-1), binds to nts -16 to $+27$ of the LTR, in the region of transcriptional initiation.[127] LBP-1 also binds the TATA region. The function of LPB-1 binding is not well defined; however, it may affect basal transcription.[127,128]

Cytokine and growth factor mediated regulation. Cytokines can affect the expression of the HIV-1 LTR in a positive or negative fashion.[17,129] Cytokine-mediated changes in the expression of LTR could result from either a direct binding of the cytokine to a response element such as IL-2 or through the activation of a second messenger signaling pathway, as seen with TNF-α or IL-1. Other cytokines and growth factors that activate HIV-1 LTR expression include IL-6, granulocyte-macrophage colony stimulating factor (GM-CSF), and interferon-γ (IFN-γ).[13,18,30,51,129] During viral infection, the interaction of gp120 with CD4 may induce IL-1 and TNF-α expression.[130–132] TNF-α can increase HIV-1 expression in various cell lines.[133–135] IL-1 induces HIV-1 LTR expression in lymphoid[135] and astrocytic cells.[136] IL-6 and GM-CSF, however, increase HIV-1 expression only in monocytic cell lines.[137,138] Both TNF-α and IL-1 induce HIV-1 expression at the level of transcription by inducing NF-κB activation.[119,134,135] TNF-α can work synergistically with either IL-6 or GM-CSF, at the transcriptional or post-transcriptional level.[137] IL-6 and GM-CSF themselves appear to induce HIV-1 expression by post-transcriptional mechanisms.[137]

Treatment of primary monocyte/macrophages with GM-CSF, macrophage colony stimulating factor (M-CSF), IL-3, or IFN-α results in a large increase in HIV-1 production.[137–139] However, prior treatment with IFN-α is necessary for activation by GM-CSF, M-CSF, or IL-3 effects. The upregulation of gene expression is not the only effect of cytokines on HIV-1 gene expression. Some cytokines can decrease HIV-1 gene expression, whereas others have both inductive and inhibitory effects. IFN-γ can decrease HIV-1 expression from acutely and chronically infected cells at the post-translational level by interfering with the budding process.[140] Transforming growth factor-β (TGF-β) is another cytokine that can block the expression of HIV-1 after activation by IL-6, GM-CSF, or a combination of the two. In addition, TGF-β can block the synergistic induction produced by the combination of TNF-α and IL-6.[141] The effect of TGF-β on HIV-1 gene expression may be positive or negative depending on the amount of TGF-β used and the cell type studied.[141–144] Recently we reported the TGF-β-mediated induction of HIV-1 LTR expression in cultured primary human mesangial cells (HMC).[144]

Regulation of HIV-1 gene expression by oncogene products and other agents. HIV-1 LTR expression can also be induced by several oncogene products, protein products of heterologous viruses, hormones, and vitamins. These effects can be mediated by a direct interaction of these agents with LTR sequences or by second messenger signaling and NF-κB induction. The products of *ras, myb,* or *rel* genes have been reported to activate HIV-1 LTR expression.[13] As discussed above, NF-κB is a member of the *rel* oncogene family and can induce HIV-1 replication via the enhancer element. The *ras* proto-oncogene, which encodes GTP binding proteins and can activate protein kinase c or other proto-oncogenes such as c-*fos* or c-*jun,* activates HIV-1 gene expression.[145,146] NF-κB may mediate *ras* activation of HIV-1 LTR.[145,146] Additionally, *ras* activation may be mediated through the AP-1 site in the LTR to which *fos* and *jun* products bind.[13] The c-*myb* product, a cell-type-specific transcription factor highly expressed in immature hematopoietic cells, may also play a role in HIV-1 replication.[147]

Gene products from heterologous viruses can also bind to sequence elements in the HIV-1 LTR, such as the SP1 binding sites, the TATA box, and the NF-κB site, and activate its expression. The viruses that have been shown to increase HIV-1 replication include various herpes viruses (such as herpes simplex virus 1 [HSV-1], cytomegalovirus [CMV], and human herpes virus type 6 [HHV-6], Epstein Barr virus [EBV]), hepatitis B virus (HBV), and HTLV-I.[13] One mechanism by which CMV or HSV may induce HIV-1 gene expression is by the interaction of their immediate early gene products with the USF, LBP, SP1, or NF-κB sites within the LTR.[13] Likewise, different immediate early gene products of EBV also activate HIV-1 LTR expression. For example, LMP-1 and EBNA-1 activate the HIV-1 LTR through the NF-κB site.[13] Two immediate early gene products of adenovirus, E1A and E1B, also activate LTR expression. One possible mechanism for E1A-mediated activation may be its interaction with TF-IID or the TATA region.[148] Finally a 19-kd protein, encoded by the X gene of HBV, can activate LTR expression in transfection experiments.[149] These heterologous viruses may, therefore, act as cofactors in HIV-1 infection by directly influencing HIV-1 replication, HIV-1 cytopathogenicity, or both. These observations are important because patients with AIDS may be infected with these viruses as well. HSV infection, for example, is highly prevalent not only among AIDS patients but also among non-HIV-infected individuals.[150] HSV may remain latent and can be activated by stimuli such as the immunosuppression caused by HIV-1 infection. Activation of HSV will result in the production of HSV gene products that in turn may induce HIV-1 replication. Cases of AIDS patients with HBV infection and EBV infection have also been reported.[150]

Another mechanism by which heterologous viruses can affect HIV-1 infection involves the Fc receptor. This receptor is thought to be the mode of viral entry in the antibody-mediated uptake of HIV-1.[16] HSV coinfection could induce HIV-1 entry by this mechanism.[151] Gene products from heterologous viruses can also act as antigens, resulting in an increase in HIV-1 replication. In addition, uninfected cells become more sensitive to HIV-1 infection after antigen-induced activation.[16]

Lastly, retinoic acid (RA) and vitamin D have also been shown to affect HIV-1 LTR expression. The effect of RA has been found to be cell type specific. In some cases, it inhibits LTR expression induced by PMA or IL-6, but cannot inhibit TNF-induced HIV-1 gene expression.[152] 1,25 dihydroxycholecaliciferol, the most active vitamin D metabolite, also augments the replication of HIV-1 in monocytes.[153]

Tat-mediated TRANS-activation. The Tat protein contains three distinct structural domains: a proline-rich acidic N-terminus, a cysteine-rich central portion, and a positively charged C-terminal basic domain rich in arginine and lysine residues.[154–157] The acidic proline-rich region of Tat has been proposed to serve as an activation domain due to the presence of acidic, polar, and hydrophobic amino acid residues that could form an amphipathic α-helix.[155,158] The cysteine-rich central region, on the other hand, appears to be involved in a metal ion-linked dimerization of Tat.[159] Two other characteristics of Tat, RNA binding[156,159] and nuclear-nucleolar localization, have been attributed to the basic domain.[156,159,160] Tat mutants, lacking the cysteine residues and the TAR binding basic domain, fail to bind TAR and transactivate transcription.[160,161] Tat protein also interacts with several cellular proteins. A 45-kd HeLa nuclear protein, cloned by screening an expression library using Tat as a probe, blocks Tat-mediated trans-activation.[162]

TAR RNA, The Trans-activation Responsive Element

As mentioned earlier, TAR is the cis-acting Tat-responsive element, located at nts +1 to +57 in the R region of the HIV-1 LTR.[91,163,164] The effect of TAR in *trans*-activation is position and orientation dependent.[91,165,166] The TAR RNA sequence folds into a stable secondary stem-loop structure (Fig. 15-9). The structural integrity of the stem region, as well as the six nt loop and the three nt pyrimidine bulge, are crucial for Tat function.[112,165,167–169] The Tat protein binds to TAR RNA at the bulge and mutations in this region cause a loss of trans-activation as well as Tat binding.[170–172]

Mechanisms of TAT Function

In transfection experiments, Tat functions as a potent trans-activator of viral gene expression.[173,174] Tat increases the steady-state level of HIV-1 mRNAs by increasing the rate of transcription, presumably at the transcrip-

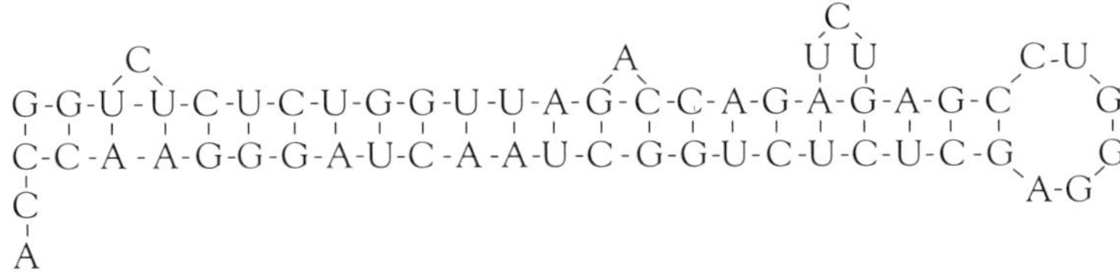

Fig. 15-9. The predicted secondary structure of HIV-1 TAR RNA. The secondary structure was analyzed by McDNAsis v3.2 sequence analysis software.

tional initiation and elongation steps.[93–97] TAR RNA may act as an RNA "enhancer," because its binding by Tat may facilitate the assembly of transcription complexes at the HIV-1 initiation site. It has been postulated that the TAR RNA structure brings Tat to the HIV-1 promoter so it can interact with the transcriptional factors bound to the NF-κB/Sp1 binding sites.[175,176]

In addition, several studies have suggested that Tat may increase the efficiency of the RNA polymerases by helping them stay on the viral transcripts longer.[93,177] Post-transcriptional effects of Tat, such as increasing viral translation, have also been postulated, because the level of viral proteins increases proportionally more than viral mRNA levels during Tat trans-activation.[178]

Involvement of TAR RNA and Cellular Factors in Tat Function

Two lines of evidence suggest host-cell-specific factors are important in Tat-mediated trans-activation. First, mutations in TAR, outside the Tat binding region, result in the loss of the trans-activation response, suggesting that auxiliary factors which interact with TAR RNA play a role in this process. Second, the efficiency of Tat-mediated trans-activation is dependent on cell type. Transient transfection assays have shown that cell types differ in their response to Tat trans-activation by 1,000-fold.[179] Tat trans-activation is very poor in rodent and other nonhuman cell lines.[181] Interestingly, human and mouse or hamster microcell hybrids containing human chromosome 12 are able to support Tat trans-activation.[180,181] These data demonstrate a role of host specific factors, presumably encoded by human chromosome 12, in Tat trans-activation.[180,181] A protein factor(s) from human chromosome 6 may also be important, because it too enhances Tat transactivation in murine cells.[180] These data further suggest the involvement of cell-specific host proteins in Tat trans-activation.

Several groups have demonstrated the binding of cellular factors to TAR RNA.[13,51,182] A number of these proteins have been identified by an RNase protection gel mobility shift assay (Fig. 15-10) and/or ultraviolet (UV) cross-linking of the RNA protein complexes followed by analysis on SDS polyacrylamide gels. In this assay, the target RNA (e.g., TAR RNA) is transcribed in vitro in the presence of a radioactive precursor nucleotide. This uniformly labeled RNA probe is then incubated with nuclear proteins and the formation of RNA-protein complexes takes place. Next, the reaction is treated with ribonuclease (RNase). RNA bound by proteins is protected while unprotected RNA is degraded by RNase. The reaction mixture is then analyzed on a native polyacrylamide gel to resolve the ribonucleoprotein (RNP) complexes. To identify the proteins that bind to RNA, the RNP complexes are exposed to short-wave UV light, causing the covalent attachment of proteins to labeled RNA. These complexes can then be resolved on SDS containing polyacrylamide gel and individual proteins bound to the radioactive RNA can be identified after exposure to x-ray film.

Host cell proteins, p68 (68 kDa) and p185/TRP-1 (185 kDa), two TAR RNA

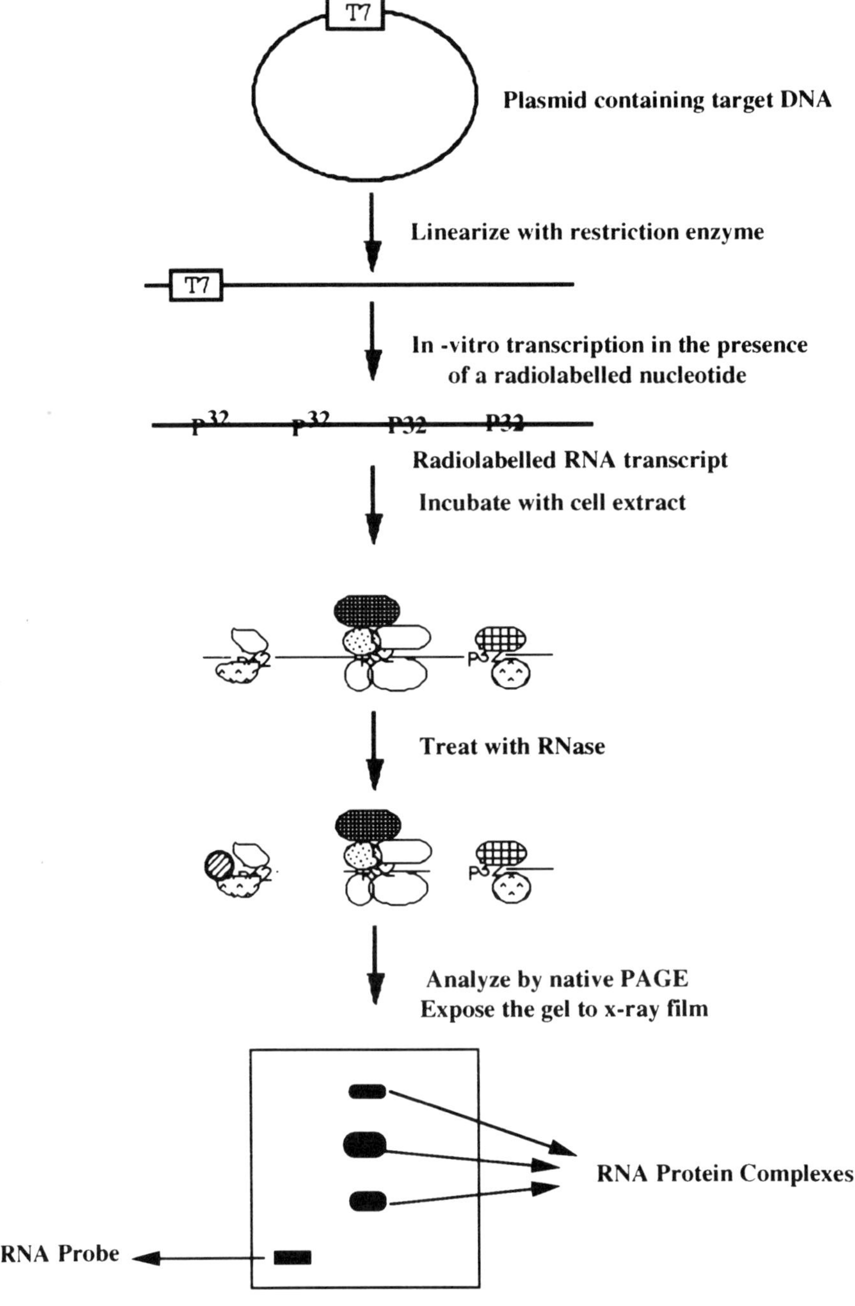

Fig. 15-10. RNase protection gel shift analysis. The steps involved in studying the formation of RNA protein complexes are preparation of a radiolabeled RNA probe in an in vitro transcription reaction, incubation of the RNA probe with proteins, digestion of the unbound RNA with RNase, and analysis of the RNA protein complexes on a native polyacrylamide gel.

loop-binding proteins, a stem binding protein (p140 [140 kd]), and a bulge binding protein (TRP-2), have been identified by this approach.[183–185] The precise function of these proteins in Tat trans-activation is not known; however, induction of Tat-mediated in vitro trans-activation by p68 and p185/TRP-1 has been reported.[183–185] TRP-2 is a family of proteins (70 to 110 kd) that competes with Tat for binding to the bulge region. In the presence of TRP-1, it can enhance in vitro Tat trans-activation.[184]

Another method for isolating RNA binding proteins involves the screening of a cDNA expression library using target RNA as a radioactive probe. This approach also depends on the interaction of RNA with protein and the formation of an RNP complex. Because the RNA is radiolabeled, the cDNA clones expressing the RNA binding protein(s) can be isolated after autoradiography. Using this approach, a cDNA clone encoding a 44-kd TAR RNA binding protein (TRBP) has been isolated from a human cDNA expression library.[186] TRBP binds to the TAR RNA stem region between the bulge and the loop. It *trans*-activates the expression of HIV-1 LTR and other promoters in a nonspecific manner.[186] Recent observations suggest that TRBP belongs to a family of protein kinases, dsI kinase(s), which become activated when bound to double-stranded RNA structures.[187]

Using a similar approach, we have isolated the cDNA for a cytoplasmic protein, clathrin light chain, which binds to TAR RNA in the lower stem region. The function of the clathrin TAR interaction is unknown, but it may play a role during virion maturation (Tatro et al., unpublished results). The interferon-induced, double-stranded-RNA-activated protein kinase, p68, also binds to the TAR RNA stem region and results in a trans-inhibition of translation.[188]

Post-Transcriptional Regulation

Rev-mediated regulation of mRNA splicing and transport. In normal eukaryotic cells, unspliced precursor mRNA transcripts are restricted to the nucleus and only spliced mRNA transcripts are transported to the cytoplasm. However, during HIV-1 replication, structural proteins (Gag, Pol, and Env) are synthesized in the cytoplasm from full-length unspliced or singly spliced pre-mRNA. This necessitates the transport of unspliced/singly spliced viral mRNA to the cytoplasm. The HIV-1 regulatory protein, Rev, mediates the transport of mRNA encoding structural proteins.[49,50,62]

In the initial phase of the viral replication, the viral mRNA consists of a multiple spliced, 2-kb RNA species that encodes the viral regulatory proteins Tat, Rev, and Nef. During the entire course of infection, Tat functions as a trans-activator of viral transcription and thus maintains a positive feedback of viral mRNA for viral replication. In a cell culture model of latency, Pomerantz et al.[189] showed that the transport of mRNA encoding viral structural proteins depends on critical intracellular levels of Rev. As the threshold level of Rev protein in the nucleus is reached, there is a change in the type of transcripts transported to the cytoplasm. The level of multiple spliced 2-

kb species falls considerably, whereas that of unspliced (9-kb) or singly spliced (4-kb) transcripts increases dramatically. The unspliced 9-kb mRNA codes for the structural proteins Gag and Pol whereas the singly spliced 4-kb mRNA codes for viral proteins Env, Vif, Vpu, and Vpr. The transition in the type of mRNA species accumulating in the cytoplasm is regulated by Rev.

Rev is a 19-kd phosphoprotein, primarily localized in the nucleolus and nucleus.[190] We reported an association of Rev with lamin c in the nuclear scaffold of cells constitutively expressing *rev*.[63] Rev has three functional domains, a nuclear localization signal, RRE binding site, and an activation domain. Of the 116 amino acid residues, 8 to 67 are essential for Rev binding to RRE and contain the signals for nucleolar localization and multimerization.[190,191] Multimerization of Rev has been proposed to be essential for the transport of viral RNA and for efficient RRE-rev RNP complex formation.[59,192–194] A role for Rev multimerization in the activation of latent HIV-1 has also been suggested.[194] Although the c-terminal activation domain, composed of amino acid residues 67 to 83, has been shown to be essential for Rev function, the mechanism of its involvement is unknown. Specific mutations in this domain have resulted in the production of *trans*-dominant phenotypes that inhibit the function of rev.[192,195]

Rev function is mediated through its binding to a cis-acting RNA element, RRE, present in the *env* region of viral mRNA.[59,191,194,196] RRE can be mobilized anywhere in the *env* region and is equally functional. Essential minimal RRE sequences have been mapped to 220 nts. RRE contains a complex secondary structure comprising five hairpin loop structures. The secondary structure of RRE is shown in Fig. 15-11. Deletion mutations indicate that only the hairpin loops 1 and 2 are essential both for rev binding and RNA transport. Point mutations that destabilize the RRE RNA hairpin loop 1 also cause the loss of Rev binding and rev function in vivo.[197–199] Therefore, the secondary structure of hairpin loop 1, and not the primary sequence, is required for optimal binding and function. Rev binds to RRE as multimers as shown in in vitro binding reactions.[59,95,193,197]

Several hypotheses have been proposed to explain the mechanism of the function of Rev in RNA transport. According to one theory, the binding of Rev to RRE results in the disruption of spliceosomes. In vitro studies have shown that specific Rev peptides can inhibit mRNA splicing.[65,66] In an alternative proposed mechanism, the binding of Rev to RRE results in the facilitated transport of unspliced mRNA.[60] We showed efficient transport of RRE containing RNA in the presence of Rev in an in vitro RNA transport assay.[63] Conversely, in the presence of Rev, transport of RRE lacking RNA was very inefficient. This experiment further showed that Rev inhibited nuclear scaffold nucleoside triphosphatase, an enzyme thought to be involved in the nucleocytoplasmic transport process.[63] In addition, association of Rev with polysomes and the requirement of Rev for efficient translation of RRE-containing RNA has also been reported.[200,201] None of these hypotheses can entirely explain the mechanism of Rev function. It is therefore probable that

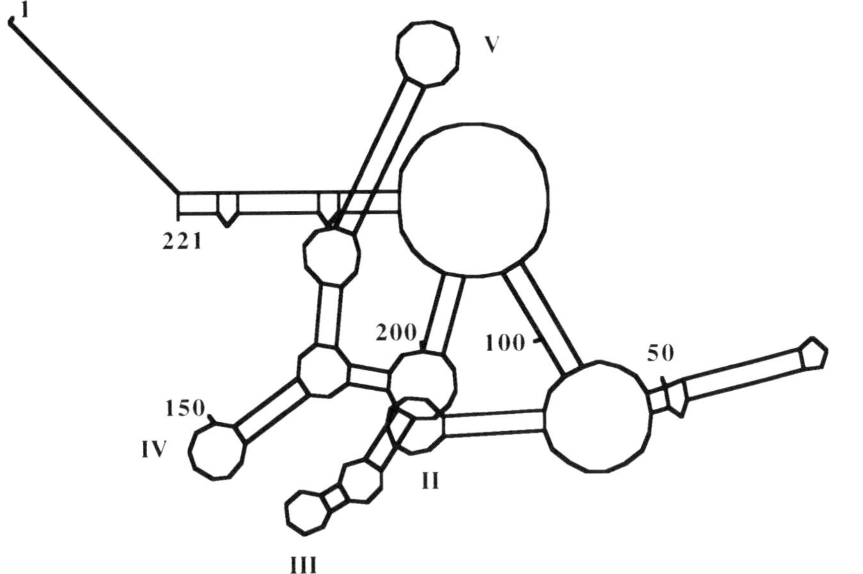

Fig. 15-11. The predicted secondary structure of HIV-1 RRE RNA. The secondary structure was analyzed by McDNAsis v3.2 sequence analysis software. Roman numerals indicate the stem loops of RRE.

a disrupted splicing mechanism concomitant with facilitated transport and translation may be responsible for Rev function.

In addition, because both the splicing and transport of mRNA occur in association with cellular proteins, a role of host proteins in Rev function is possible.[49,50,62] This is further supported by the observation that rev-mediated mRNA transport is host specific[202] (Shukla et al., unpublished results, 1994). Nonhuman cells such as CHO and NIH3T3 fail to become productively infected by HIV-1.[202] Fusion of these cells with human cells, however, results in productive infection. We have recently reported the binding of specific cellular proteins to RRE RNA in vitro in a host-specific manner.[203] Other RRE and Rev-binding proteins have been reported; however, their roles and mechanisms of action are unknown.[204–206] Because both human and murine cells use the same mechanisms of RNA splicing and transport, the existence of a unique mechanism independent of these two processes cannot be excluded.

We have identified two HeLa cell nuclear proteins with molecular weights of 120 and 62 kd that specifically bind to RRE RNA in a host-specific manner. We also observed host-cell-specific formation of RRE nuclear protein complexes because rodent cell nuclear extracts did not form these characteristic complexes, whereas the presence of chromosome 6 in human mouse microcell hybrids supports their formation.[203] Our recent preliminary experiments suggest that factors encoded by human chromosome 6 or 11 are required for Rev-mediated RNA transport (Shukla et al., unpublished results, 1994).

Regulation of HIV-1 Gene Expression at the Level of Translation

In addition to the regulation of HIV-1 gene expression at the level of transcription, splicing, and nucleocytoplasmic transport of the viral RNA, regulation at the level of translation has also been demonstrated. One example of translational regulation is the "leaky scanning" model in which multiple initiation codons are used for translation.[207] For example, Schwartz et al.[208] demonstrated that the *tat* AUG is a stronger initiation signal compared with downstream AUG signals of *rev* or *vpu*. A weak initiation codon of Vpu helps in a predominant expression of upstream initiation codon of *env*. A role of *vpu* in the expression of *env* has been suggested because the removal of the *vpu* initiation codon results in increased expression of *env*.[208,209]

Another mechanism by which HIV-1 gene expression can be regulated at the level of translation is the translation of *gag*- and *pol*-encoded polyproteins from the same precursor mRNA by frame shifting within the *gag* ORF.[40,210] Other mechanisms involving translational regulation of HIV-1 gene expression are mediated by the regulatory proteins Tat and Rev and their respective RNA binding elements TAR and RRE. In addition to its function in the transport of unspliced or singly spliced RNA, Rev is also required for the efficient translation of RRE-containing viral mRNAs.[200,201] Likewise, the presence of Tat alters the translation of TAR-containing RNAs, in both a positive and negative fashion. In in vitro translation experiments, TAR RNA, due to its stem loop secondary structure, inhibited the translation of HIV-1 mRNA, probably by interfering with ribosomal scanning and initiation.[211–213] Addition of Tat to the reaction counteracted the inhibitory effect of TAR, presumably by altering its secondary structure upon binding.[211] Drysdale and Pavlakis,[214] however, reported the downregulation of translation even in the presence of Tat. A possible role for cellular factor(s) in Tat-mediated inhibition of translation was proposed, because inhibition of protein synthesis by cycloheximide abolished the observed inhibitory effects of Tat on HIV-1 mRNA translation.

Yet another mechanism by which TAR modifies HIV-1 mRNA translation may involve the dsI kinase, a kinase activated by interferons, and produced by cells in response to viral infections.[215–220] Activated dsI kinase phosphorylates the α subunit of the eukaryotic initiation factor-2 (eIF-2), which results in the inhibition of translation.[221,222] The inhibition of protein synthesis by interferons through the dsI kinase represents a cellular mechanism for blocking viral infection.[220,223] However, in response to dsI kinase activation, viruses produce small RNA molecules that block dsI kinase activation.[220] The virus-associated (VA) RNA of adenovirus, EBER RNA of the EBV, and TAR RNA of HIV-1 are examples of such double-stranded (ds) small RNAs that inhibit dsI kinase.[224,225] Both inhibitory and stimulatory effects of TAR RNA on the double-stranded kinase have been reported. Gunnery et al.[226] demonstrated the inhibition of dsI kinase activation by TAR RNA.[226] This inhibition was dependent on both the sequence and the secondary structure of the stem and terminal loop of TAR RNA.[226,227] Conversely, a stimulatory effect of TAR RNA on the activation of dsI kinase has been shown in the absence of Tat.[216–218]

MOLECULAR MECHANISMS INVOLVED IN THE PATHOGENESIS OF HIVAN

AIDS may be complicated by HIVAN in approximately 10 percent of patients.[7] The cause of the renal disease itself is unknown but genetic factors or socioeconomic status may be important in its pathogenesis.[7,228,229] In a striking fashion, the disease almost uniformly affects, for unexplained reasons, men rather than women. Preliminary evidence also suggests an association with racial background.[7,228,229] In the United States, renal complications seem to affect specific subsets of patients, primarily blacks.[7,229] Such data suggest that a host response or genetic component may be associated with the incidence of the renal disease.

The common renal syndromes in HIV-1-infected patients include renal insufficiency and nephrotic range proteinuria associated with FGS, and various proliferative glomerulonephritides. HIVAN has characteristic glomerular (collapsing glomerulosclerosis and glomerular epithelial cell changes), tubular (cell simplification and microcystic dilatation), and interstitial (immune cell infiltrate) changes and is marked by the presence of tubular reticular structures (TRS) in endothelial cells.[7,230] Idiopathic FGS is characterized by expansion of the glomerular mesangium (which decreases the glomerular filtration surface) and increased production of mesangial matrix components.[231,232] Decreased matrix degradation in part due to increased expression of tissue inhibitors of metalloproteinases may also play a role in the pathogenesis of glomerulosclerosis.[233,234] Renal function in patients with HIVAN may progress from relatively normal to end-stage renal disease (ESRD), necessitating dialysis, over a period of several days to weeks.[7,235] Such a rapid progression of disease is typically not apparent in gomerulosclerosis of other etiologies, such as diabetic and heroin-associated nephropathy and idiopathic FGS.

The mechanisms involved in the development of HIVAN are unknown. Key issues that must be addressed are (1) is renal tissue productively infected with HIV-1?; (2) does renal disease develop because of the direct effects of HIV-1 gene expression in renal cells?; and (3) do other factors contribute to the development of HIVAN? It is possible that productive infection, associated with the synthesis of viral mRNA and HIV-1 peptides may be important in the pathogenesis of HIVAN. Alternatively, nephropathy may be an indirect result of the presence of HIV-1 in renal tissue. A change in the microenvironment of renal cells, whether a result of renal infection, or due to the presence of infiltrating immune cells, might affect renal cellular growth, proliferation, and function, leading to the development of nephropathy. Finally, circulating HIV-1 peptides might affect the growth and function of renal cells. In the following sections we review in vivo and in vitro data regarding infection of renal cells by HIV-1 and the direct and indirect effects of HIV-1 infection in renal and other cell types, in order to develop a hypothetic scheme to explain the pathogenesis of HIV-associated FGS.

Renal Infection by HIV-1

Cohen and co-workers[236] demonstrated proviral DNA in both the tubular and glomerular epithelium in renal biopsies and autopsy tissue of 10 of 11 patients with HIVAN, by an in-situ hybridization technique. Likewise, renal biopsy tissue of patients infected with HIV-1 with focal glomerulonephritis also contained HIV-1 cDNA in glomerular as well as tubular epithelium. However, when stained for the presence of p24, a *gag*-derived HIV-1 peptide, tubular epithelium showed the presence of p24 in the majority of the patient samples, whereas only one sample showed the presence of p24 in glomerular epithelium. Renal tissue from patients with heroin-associated nephropathy did not reveal the presence of HIV-1 DNA in renal tissue. However, in patients infected with HIV-1 without clinically apparent renal disease, one of the five biopsies showed the presence of HIV-1 cDNA in tubular tissue. Kimmel et al.,[9] using PCR amplification, reported the presence of HIV-1 DNA in glomeruli isolated from renal tissue of patients infected with HIV-1, in both the presence and absence of clinical renal disease. Positive controls included five patients infected with HIV-1 without clinical evidence of renal disease, such as proteinuria premortem, and no light microscopic evidence of nephropathy.

The presence of both HIV-1 DNA and proteins in renal biopsies from patients with HIVAN in the studies of Cohen and co-workers[236] suggests that HIV-1 virus in kidney tissue may be directly responsible for the development of renal disease. However, the presence of HIV-1 DNA in patients infected with HIV-1 without renal disease, reported in both studies,[9,236] indicates that HIV-1 genome in kidney tissue is not sufficient to cause nephropathic changes. Rather, an interplay of specific conditions in different patients may result in the development of renal disease. Although both these reports demonstrate the presence of HIV-1 DNA in renal tissue, it is not known whether HIV-1 genome is actively expressed.

Transgenic animal models of HIV-1 have produced conflicting data regarding the role of HIV-1 gene expression in HIVAN. Leonard et al.[237] used an entire proviral HIV-1 construct for the development of transgenic mice. They failed, however to observe any pathologic changes in the kidney of these animals. Dickie et al.,[238] on the other hand, used a mutant proviral construct, lacking *gag* and *pol* genes, to produce transgenic mice. Three out of eight animals developed FGS similar to that observed in patients infected with HIV-1 with HIVAN. The presence of unspliced, singly spliced, or multiply spliced HIV-1 mRNA was detected in the skin and muscle of these animals. However, the expression of these HIV-1 RNA was modest in relation to the total renal RNA. Total kidney lysates from these animals showed the presence of a 40-kd peptide recognized by HIV-1 antisera specific for gp160. In these transgenic animals, Kopp et al.[239] showed progressive glomerulosclerosis and enhanced renal accumulation of basement membrane components. Immunohistology of kidneys from these animals demonstrated the presence of Rev protein in the sclerotic glomeruli. Interestingly, other HIV-1 peptides such as gp120, gp41, Tat, and Nef were not detected using similar methods. Furthermore, they also observed only two mRNA species, a 2 kb and a 4 kb (corresponding to multiple spliced and singly spliced mRNA) in the kidneys of these animals. Caution must be exercised in interpreting the results from transgenic murine models, because both Tat-mediated *trans*-activation as well as Rev-mediated RNA transport have been shown to require human, cell-type-specific protein[180,181,202] (Shukla et al., unpublished results). As noted previously, in vitro experiments using murine and other rodent cells demonstrated that murine cells do not support[202] HIV-1 gene expression, and that this deficiency can be overcome by fusion of mouse cells with human cells. The presence of only two mRNA species and the absence of *env*-related peptides in the glomeruli of the transgenic mice may suggest a lack of Rev-dependent *env* gene expression in the renal tissue of these animals. Furthermore, because total kidney homogenate was used for protein or RNA analysis, it is possible that the HIV-1 proteins or RNA species were derived from infiltrating cells or circulating blood.

In Vitro Infection of Renal Cells

The mechanism(s) involved in infection of renal cells by HIV-1 is not known. Although infectivity of renal cells has been reported both in vitro and in vivo,[9,240,241] the presence of CD4 or other receptors for HIV-1 on various types of renal cells has not been examined in detail. In a single study, Karlsson-Parra and co-workers[242] demonstrated the presence of CD4 receptors on normal human glomerular cells. This would suggest infection of mesangial cells by the usual route of virus entry (i.e., entry mediated by CD4 receptors). Glomeruli also contain infiltrating macrophages that may be infected with HIV-1. Due to the presence of infiltrating immune cells in the kidneys of patients infected with HIV-1, transfer of virus to renal cells by cell to cell contact is also possible.

In vitro studies have demonstrated differential expression of HIV-1 in various renal cell types. Green et al.,[240] using two different viral strains and transfection conditions, showed that glomerular endothelial cells can support gene expression from both the HIV-1 IIb and HIV-1 MB strains of HIV-1, as demonstrated by the presence of p24 in cell culture supernatants. Mesangial cells, however, could only support gene expression from the HIV-1 MB strain, and their production of p24 was significantly reduced compared with that of endothelial cells. Coculture of mesangial cells with peripheral blood monocytes resulted in considerably increased p24 production. These studies may reflect the lack of a specific factor(s) in mesangial cells that may be required for the efficient replication of both the MB and IIB strains of HIV-1. In contrast to endothelial and mesangial cells, epithelial cells could not support the expression of either of the two HIV-1 strains used. These experiments do not represent natural infection because normal receptor-virus interaction does not occur during transfection. The expression of p24, however, is indicative of the ability of HIV-1 to replicate in mesangial and endothelial cells. The data obtained from in vitro experiments and those obtained from renal tissue of patients infected with HIV-1[9,236,240] may indicate lack of a cell-specific factor(s) required for HIV-1 gene expression in epithelial cells.

Molecular Mechanisms of Disease Progression

The results discussed above do not clearly establish if renal tissue is productively infected by HIV-1. However, in our studies the overwhelming majority (>95 percent) of HIV-infected patients with renal disease showed the presence of HIV-1 genome in the kidney.[9] In addition, we demonstrated the ubiquitous presence of HIV-1 genome in autopsy tissue of patients without the presence of renal lesions,[9] suggesting that the presence of the genomic material in the kidney is not sufficient to induce nephropathy. Triggering and facilitating mechanisms seem likely, therefore, to be associated with nephropathogenesis. Understanding the pathogenesis of such renal disease and nature of such mechanisms might lead to preventive or ameliorative strategies.

Role of HIV-1 Proteins in Renal Disease

Several HIV-1 proteins have cytopathic effects on cells in vitro. gp120 can be cytotoxic to a number of cell types including peripheral blood mononuclear cells, glial cells, neuronal cells, and astrocytes grown in cell culture.[243–248] Exposure of astrocytes to gp120 may cause increased synthesis of cytokines such as IFN-α and -γ, TNF-α, IgG, IL-1, and IL-6.[245,246] Interaction of gp120 with CD4 is essential for this process because soluble CD4 or antibodies to the OKT4 A epitope of CD4 can inhibit induction of IFN.[246] On the other hand, treatment of CD4− brain cells, such as glioma cell lines, with gp120 causes activation of tyrosine kinase activity.[22] HIV-1 gp120 also suppresses lymphocyte proliferation and induces the production of IL-1 β and arachidonic acid products in human monocytes.[249] Other HIV-1 peptides also affect cell metabolism in vitro. The *gag*-derived p24 peptide was shown to inhibit IFN-γ-induced changes in a human monocyte cell line.[250] These *env*- and *gag*-derived peptides could be potentially nephropathogenic because they are present in the HIV-1 virion coat, which interacts with the membranes of target cells.[251] Additionally, gp120 and p24 are shed in the blood, resulting in exposure of renal cells, particularly in the glomerulus, to these viral proteins. The presence of these peptides in renal cells may cause a change in their cytokine levels, which ultimately may alter cellular metabolism leading to increased production of basement membrane components. Alternatively, these viral products can also function to trap immune complexes, which may also alter cell metabolism. Such concepts are clinically meaningful because gp120 and p24 have been demonstrated in renal biopsy material in the form of immune complexes as well as free species.[10,236]

The Tat protein may also act as a viral growth factor because it can be taken up by cells and affect cell growth and proliferation.[252] Recombinant Tat can be a positive or negative regulator of cell growth depending on the cell type and concentration studied.[53,54,253–255] For example, Tat protein stimulates production of TGF-β1 in macrophages.[254] In a transgenic mouse model, animals transgenic for *tat* gene showed the development of skin lesions closely resembling Kaposi sarcoma.[255] Furthermore, Tat may affect the metabolism of renal cells, in that it reportedly affects cell proliferation in a paracrine fashion. The HIV-1 regulatory protein, Rev, inhibits RNA transport in isolated nuclei in vitro.[63] Kopp et al.,[239] in their transgenic animals that developed FGS similar to HIVAN, detected the presence of Rev protein in sclerotic glomeruli. Because other viral proteins were not detected in the affected glomeruli of these animals, a role for rev in the development of nephropathy is possible.

Cellular Mediators of HIVAN

Immune cell infiltration in renal tissue. Both HIV-related FGS and immune complex disease (ICD) are characterized by a dense interstitial infiltrate and tubulopathy[7,8,12,230,256,257] (the latter composed of tubular cell degeneration and microcystic dilatation), which aid in the identification of its HIV-associated nature.[230] The tubular microcystic dilatation in HIVAN shows a striking resemblance to the tubulopathy seen in animal models of spontaneous T-cell-mediated interstitial nephritis.[258] Numerous studies have suggested a role of the interstitial cellular infiltrate in the pathogenesis of nephropathies unassociated with HIV-1 infection.[258–260] The association of progression of several renal diseases, including glomerulonephritis, with interstitial inflammation and fibrosis, rather than glomerular parameters, has been documented in clinicopathologic studies.[261–263] The cellular infiltrate in various interstitial nephritides is composed largely of mononuclear cells, most often T cells, specifically CD4+ or helper T cells.[260] Similarly, T-helper cells constitute a substantial but variable proportion of the lymphocytes in the interstitial infiltrate in HIV nephropathy[256,267] as seen in many renal diseases with interstitial or glomerular inflammation.[260,265] T cells, particularly those characterized by specific T-cell receptors, have been observed in human autoimmune and animal models of diseases, not associated with peripheral T-cell depletion, suggesting specific antigen selection at the site of tissue injury. T-cell dysfunction has also been associated with abnormal glomerular permeability,[268] and abnormal interstitial T cells are found in renal tissue in idiopathic FGS.[269] Macrophages, which may harbor HIV-

1,[264] may also act as effector cells in the pathogenesis of renal diseases of various etiologies.[260,265] Changes in renal structure/functional relationships may result from the modulatory action of cytokines, produced by macrophages, on the metabolism of immune and nonimmune cells and their antigen-presenting function.[260,265,266]

We assessed the cellular infiltrate and measured tissue levels of TGF-β1 and other chemokines, in patients with HIV-1 infection and FGS and HIV-ICD, compared with tissue from patients not infected with HIV-1 with similar nephropathies.[257] The overwhelming majority of HIV-infected patients with renal disease had a prominent interstitial infiltrate of macrophages and lymphocytes,[256] composed primarily of T cells. T cells were present in all the specimens, although the intensity was variable. The total number of interstitial immune cells was significantly greater in tissue from HIVAN compared with tissue from patients with idiopathic FGS.[256] We also demonstrated an increased proportion of interstitial macrophages in HIV-associated renal disease compared with idiopathic FGS.[256]

The presence of T cells in the HIVAN interstitial infiltrate is, however, surprising in a viral infection characterized by marked and progressive peripheral CD4 + T-cell depletion. Why do T cells sequester in renal tissue, associated with nephropathy? Recent reports demonstrate the sequestration of HIV-1 in lymphoid tissue during "clinically latent" phases of infection. Is it possible that renal tissue may serve as another reservoir for the sequestration of T cells infected with HIV-1?[33,264] What mediates T-cell infiltration into renal tissue in HIVANs is unknown. Specific immune cells may elicit a renal tissue response facilitating antigen presentation. A specific population of T cells, capable of mediating nephropathy, has been shown to respond to a "nephritogenic" domain of a renal antigen in an animal model of spontaneous, genetic interstitial nephritis.[270,271] Such mechanisms might be important in the pathogenesis of HIV-associated renal diseases.

Recent data suggest that the functional profile of peripheral T-helper cells[273] differs: a T_{H1} cell, producing primarily IFN-γ and IL-2, a key cell in effecting cell-mediated immune responses, and a T_{H2} cell, producing IL-4 and IL-10, which amplifies B-cell antibody synthesis. A "switch" in T-cell populations has been postulated in the progressive pathogenesis of immune dysregulation in patients infected with HIV-1. T-cell IFN-γ and IL-2 responses decrease, but IL-4 and IL-10 responses increase, as the stage of HIV-1 infection progresses.[272,273] Similar findings have been noted in tissues in subjects with tuberculoid leprosy (high IL-2 and IFN-γ levels) characterized by a good cell-mediated immune response, compared with lepromatous leprosy (high IL-10, IL-4, and perhaps IL-13 levels) with poor cell-mediated immunity.[274] Strutz and Neilson[275] have detailed how specific lymphocytes, secreting IL-2, IL-4, and IFN-γ, may affect macrophage, fibroblast, and tubular epithelial cell function, resulting in the increased synthesis of fibronectin and collagen types I and III, culminating in the development of interstitial fibrosis.

Role of cytokines and growth factors. The role played by cytokines and growth factors in the progression of HIVAN could be protean. If renal cells become infected by HIV-1 through their interaction with CD4 receptors, binding of virus to the CD4 molecule, via gp120, may alter the cellular production of cytokines and growth factors. As discussed above, this has been found to be the case in other cell types. Additionally, gp120 shed in the plasma of infected patients can also bind to CD4 receptors (only poorly described in mesangial cells) on renal cells and alter their cytokine metabolism. Altered cytokine levels could result in altered metabolism of the infected renal cell as well as neighboring uninfected cells. Additionally, the altered cytokine levels of infected cells could increase replication of latent virus in these and other cells. Furthermore, cytokines produced by infiltrating macrophages in renal tissue also may affect the metabolism of renal cells and replication of latent virus. Altered circulating and tissue cytokine and growth factor levels have been reported in patients with AIDS[273,276-278] (reviewed in Refs. 129 and 152). Increased circulating TNF-α and IL-1 β levels have been shown in individuals infected with HIV-1. Increased circulating levels of TGF-β have also been reported in patients infected with HIV-1.[143,278] In addition, IFN-α has been proposed to be a marker of progression of HIV-1 infection.[279] IFN-α and -β can be induced in a variety of cell types by viral infection, and have antiviral activity.[277,280]

Several cytokines and growth factors can modulate the growth of human mesangial cells in culture.[281-283] These include platelet-derived growth factor (PDGF), epidermal growth factor, IL-1, TNF, and TGF-α and -β. These factors may be derived from infiltrating immune cells and may also be secreted by mesangial cells themselves.[281-283] TGF-β has a biphasic effect on the growth and proliferation of mesangial cells. At lower concentrations, it induces proliferation, but at higher concentrations it causes hypertrophic growth of mesangial cells.[281] Studies of experimental animal model systems have suggested a role for TGF-β in the development of glomerulonephritis, because treatment with anti-TGF-β antibodies abrogates the development of disease in these animals.[284] IFN-γ, a product of T lymphocytes, has antiproliferative and protein synthetic effects on mesangial cells[285] and induces the expression of MHC class II antigens in these cells.[286] IFN-α induces the tubular reticular structures that are characteristic of HIV-FGS in lymphoid tissue in vitro.[287]

Cytokines and growth factors could conceivably facilitate the progression of HIVAN in different ways. They can cause the activation of transcription factors whose increased binding to HIV-1 LTR sequences may result in increased transcription of the HIV genome (see section above). We recently demonstrated increased expression of HIV-1 LTR in response to exposure to TGF-β in human mesangial cells in culture.[144] All renal tissue that we evaluated from patients infected with HIV-1 with renal disease stained for TGF-β, in sclerotic areas of glomeruli, in obsolescent glomeruli, and in the interstitium of patients with FGS.[257] Similar findings were documented by us in biopsy tissue from uninfected patients with various renal diseases such as FGS, lupus nephritis, IgA nephropathy, and membranoproliferative glomerulonephritis.[257] TGF-β is therefore nonspecifically associated with sclerotic reactions in human renal tissue, although tissue levels may determine pathologic outcome. Another group has presented similar data.[288]

Cytokines and growth factors may also induce proliferation and matrix synthesis by mesangial cells.[281–283] Recently Mattana et al.[289] reported an increase in the proliferation of human mesangial cells in culture exposed to sera from individuals infected with HIV-1 or supernatants from macrophages infected with HIV-1. This study demonstrates that sera from individuals infected with HIV-1 contain factors, presumably cytokines, that affect the proliferation of mesangial cells.

Recent studies have also demonstrated an alteration in chemotactic cytokine (chemokine) levels in the glomerular tissue of patients infected with HIV-1 who developed HIVAN. Chemokines are low-molecular-weight, pro-inflammatory cytokines that chemotactically attract immune cells into the site of tissue injury.[290] The α-chemokine group acts mainly on neutrophils, although IL-8 has chemotactic properties for CD4+ and CD8+ subsets of human T cells[291] and is produced by activated T cells, fibroblasts, endothelial cells, and human renal cells.[292,293] The β chemokine group, which includes monocyte chemotactic protein-1 (MCP-1) and regulated upon activation, normal t cell expressed and presumably secreted (RANTES), act upon T cells, eosinophils, and basophils. RANTES can activate unstimulated CD4+/CD45RO+ memory T cells as well as both naive and memory phenotypes of stimulated CD4+ and CD8+ cells.[294] Circulating memory T cells produce cytokines upon antigenic restimulation, and can, therefore, function as potent effector cells. Their distribution in tissues may play a critical role in the development of T-cell-mediated autoimmune disorders.[294] In T cells, RANTES expression can be induced after interaction with specific antigens, and can be modulated by growth factors.[295] Additionally, RANTES can be expressed by renal tubular epithelium, nephritogenic antigen-specific CD4+ helper and CD8+ effector T cells, and mesangial cells.[294–296] In the pathogenesis of murine spontaneous interstitial nephritis, a role for RANTES has been suggested.[296] Inflammatory byproducts stimulate the production of MCP-1 by monocytes, macrophages, fibroblasts, endothelial cells, and smooth muscle cells.[297,298] MCP-1 is a chemotactic factor for mononuclear cells and eosinophils into areas of localized tissue injury, but can also activate eosinophils and basophils.[299] Additionally, MCP-1 regulates adhesion molecule expression and cytokine production in human monocytes,[300] and histamine release by basophils.[300] In renal tissue, mesangial cell MCP-1 synthesis can be upregulated by TNF-α, IFN-γ, and aggregates of IgG.[301]

Kimmel and co-workers[302] demonstrated that tissue levels of RANTES, MCP-1, and IL-8 were elevated in renal biopsies from patients with HIV infection and HIV-associated renal disease, compared with idiopathic FGS. This elevation was not simply a consequence of the number of infiltrating immune cells, because no difference in the levels of the cytokines between interstitium and glomeruli was observed.[302] Such data suggest there may be autocrine production of cytokines by glomerular cells in HIVAN, which may be involved in the progression of disease. Therefore, chemokines may play a role in mediating renal tissue damage caused by infiltrating lymphocytes and mononuclear cells. Additionally, specific immune cells, such as infected lymphocytes or monocytes, which produce certain cytokines, might be important in the development of the rapid matrix synthesis characteristic of HIV-related FGS.

Antigen Presentation and Renal Disease

Major histocompatibility complex (MHC) class II protein expression is critical in the presentation of antigen, and in T-cell recognition and activation. Transgenic animal studies have suggested a relationship between increased renal expression of MHC class II protein and murine lupus nephritis, and renal allograft rejection. However, the elevated expression of MHC class II protein alone may not be sufficient for the development of nephropathy.[303] Anti-IFN-γ antibodies blocked kidney-specific, autoreactive T-cell-mediated induction of MHC class II and ICAM-1 expression in cultured tubular epithelial cells derived from the transgenic animals.[304] Clones of these cells secreted a heterogeneous set of cytokines. Recent studies have demonstrated the requirement of "costimulatory" cell–peptide–cell interactions in the interaction of T-helper cells and antigen-presenting cells.[305]

The CD4 molecule, however, serves as both the recognition element for MHC molecules and is the receptor for HIV-1 envelope proteins gp120 and gp41.[306] MHC proteins variably bind HIV-1 peptides.[307,308] Soluble gp120 may also inhibit the binding of MHC class II proteins to CD4.[306] Variability in binding, and in cell signaling in the interaction of HIV peptides, the T-cell receptor, and MHC proteins might lead to anergy by interfering with costimulatory signals[309–312] or HIV-1 peptides might conceivably increase stimulation by functioning as superantigens.[312] Homologs have been detected between regions of HIV-1 viral peptides and HLA molecules.[306,309,313–315] HIV-1 peptides, because of homology with MHC proteins, or as superantigens[316–319] might function as "costimulators" in the interaction of interstitial T cells with antigen-presenting cells, leading to an amplification of the immune response, inflammation, and the generation of a particular set of cytokines that leads to fibrotic responses. HIV-1 gp120 has recently been shown to function as a "costimulator" in the T-cell response.[320] The presence of *env*- and *gag*-coded circulating peptides such as gp41, gp120, and p24 in the renal tissue of HIV-infected patients[109,321] with immune complex nephropathy demonstrates that these HIV-1 peptides could participate in a tissue immune response. These results are generalizable beyond the circulating immune complex disease mechanism because gp120 and gp120–anti-gp120 antigen–antibody complexes are immunomodulatory.[316]

CONCLUSION

All the mechanisms outlined above may potentially be involved in the rapidly progressive renal failure, characterized pathologically by FGS (classic HIVAN) seen in patients with HIV-1 infection. Theoretically, high circulating and local cytokine levels, found in patients with HIV-1 infection or AIDS, might induce increased mesangial cell growth and matrix production, leading to renal insufficiency. Additionally, circulating viral proteins may

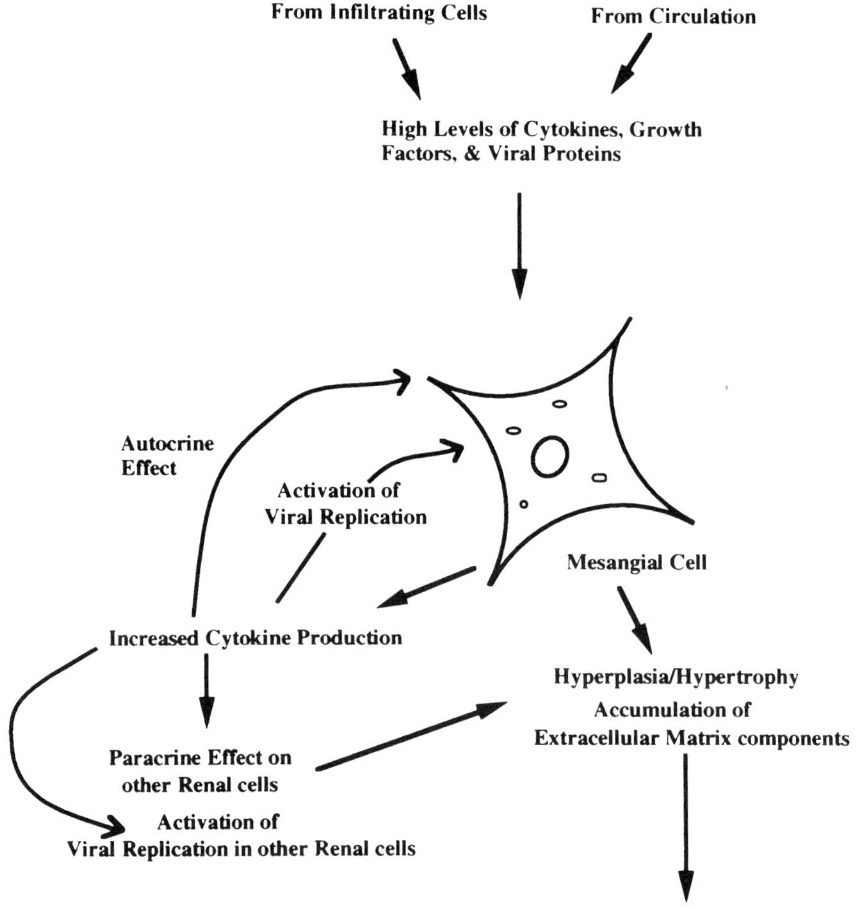

Fig. 15-12. Hypothetical mechanisms of HIVAN development. Various cytokines and viral proteins, present in the circulation or produced in infiltrating cells, may initiate a cycle of events in mesangial cells, such as accumulation of extracellular matrix components, autocrine production of cytokines, activation of viral replication, or paracrine effects in other renal cells. All these events may lead to the development of HIVAN in AIDS patients.

also play a role in the development of renal disease due to their direct effect on the metabolism of renal cells. However, it is possible that multiple mechanisms may be responsible for the disease development and progression in a particular patient. Figure 15-12 shows a schematic hypothetic mechanism by which HIVAN might develop.

Further studies are necessary to elucidate mechanisms whereby the HIV-1 life cycle and productive renal infection with HIV-1 may affect the balance of renal matrix synthesis and catabolism, and interactions between renal and immune cells in specialized microenvironments in different subsets of patients at risk for the development of HIVAN. Carefully controlled experiments and the development of in vitro renal cell culture models, and more detailed immunochemical analysis of human tissue from patients infected with HIV-1 with renal disease will be required to delineate the pathogenic mechanisms underlying the development of HIVAN.

REFERENCES

1. Barre-Sinoussi, F, Chermann JC, Rey F et al: Isolation of a T-lymphotropic retrovirus from a patient at risk for acquired immune deficiency syndrome (AIDS). Science 220:868, 1983
2. Gallo RC, Salahuddin SZ, Popovic M et al: Frequent detection and isolation of cytopathic retroviruses (HTLV-III) from patients with AIDS and at risk for AIDS. Science 224:500, 1984
3. Levy JA, Hoffman AD, Kramer SM et al: Isolation of lymphocytopathic retroviruses from San Francisco patients with AIDS. Science 225:840, 1984
4. Fauci AS: Immunopathogenesis of HIV infection. J AIDS 6:655, 1993
5. Fauci AS: Multifactorial nature of human immunodeficiency virus disease: implications for therapy. Science 262:1011, 1993
6. Weiss RA: How does HIV cause AIDS? Science 260:1273, 1993
7. Bourgoignie JJ: Renal complications of human immunodeficiency virus type I. Kidney Int 37:1571, 1990
8. Glassock RJ, Cohen AH, Danovitch G, Parsa P: HIV infection and the kidney. Ann Intern Med 112:35, 1990
9. Kimmel PL, Ferreira-Centeno A, Farkas-Szallasi T et al: Viral DNA in microdissected renal biopsies of HIV infected patients with nephrotic syndrome. Kidney Int 43:1347, 1993
10. Kimmel PL, Phillips TM, Ferreira-Centeno A et al: HIV-associated immune mediated renal disease. Kidney Int 44:1022, 1993
11. Rao TKS: Human immunodeficiency virus (HIV) associated nephropathy. Ann Rev Med 42:392, 1991
12. Seney FD Jr, Burns DK, Silva FG: AIDS and the kidney. Am J Kidney Dis 16:1, 1990
13. Antoni BA, Stein SB, Rabson AB: Regulation of human immunodeficiency virus infection: implications for pathogenesis. Adv Virus Res 43:53, 1993
14. Greene WC: The molecular biology of human immunodeficiency virus type 1 infection. N Engl J Med 324:308, 1990
15. Haseltine WA: Molecular biology of human immunodeficiency virus (type 1). FASEB J 5:2349, 1991

16. Levy JA: Pathogenesis of human immunodeficiency virus infection. Microbiol Rev 57:183, 1993
17. Pavlakis GN: Structure and function of the human immunodeficiency virus type 1. Sem Liver Dis 12:103, 1992
18. Vaishnav YN, Wong-Staal F: The biochemistry of AIDS. Ann Rev Biochem 60: 577, 1991
19. Bhat S, Spitalnik SL, Gonzalez-Scarano F et al: Galactosyl ceramide or a derivative is an essential component of the neural receptor for human immunodeficiency virus type 1 envelope glycoprotein gp120. Proc Natl Acad Sci USA 8: 7131, 1991
20. Yahi N, Baghdiguian S, Moreau H et al: Galactosyl ceramide (or a closely realted molecule) is the receptor for human immunodeficiency virus type 1 on human colon epithelial HT29 cells. J Virol 66:4848, 1992
21. Curtis BM, Scharnowske S, Watson AJ: Sequence and expression of a membrane associated C-type lectin that exhibits CD4-independent binding of human immunodeficiency virus envelop glycoprotein gp120. Proc Natl Acad Sci USA 89:8356, 1992
22. Schneider-Schaulies J, Schneider-Schaulies S, Brinkman R et al: HIV gp120 receptor on CD4-negative brain cells activates a tyrosine kinase. Virology 191: 765, 1992
23. Hansen JES, Nielsen C, Mathiesen LR et al: Involvement of lymphocyte function associated antigen-1 (LFA-1) in HIV infection: inhibition by monoclonal antibody. Scand J Infect Dis 23:31, 1991
24. Phillips DM, Bourinbaiar AS: Mechanism of HIV spread from lymphocyte to epithelia. Virology 186:261, 1992
25. Gupta P, Balachandran R, Ho M et al: Cell-to-cell transmission of human immunodeficiency virus type 1 in the presence of azidothymidine and neutralizing antibody. J Virol 63:2361, 1989
26. Goff S: Retroviral reverse transcriptase: synthesis, structure, function. J AIDS 3:817, 1990
27. Zack JA, Arrigo SJ, Weitsman SR et al: HIV-1 entry into quiescent primary lymphocytes. Molecular analysis reveals a labile viral structure. Cell 61:212, 1990
28. Zack JA, Cann AJ, Lugo JP et al: HIV-1 production from infected peripheral blood T cells after HTLV-1 induced mitogenic stimulation. Science 240:1026, 1988
29. Brown PO: Integration of retroviral DNA. p. 19. In Swanstron R, Vogt PK (eds): Retroviruses, Strategies of Replication. Springer, New York, 1990
30. Bednarik DP, Folks TM: Mechanism of HIV-1 latency. AIDS 6:3, 1992
31. McDougal JS, Mawle A, Cort SP et al: Cellular tropism of the human retrovirus HTLV-III/LAV I role of T cell activation and expression of the T4 antigen. J Immunol 135:3151, 1985
32. Zagury D, Bernard J, Leonard R et al: Long-term cultures of HTLV-III-infected T cells: a model of cytopathology of T-cell depletion in AIDS. Science 231:850, 1986
33. Pantaleo G, Graziosi C, Demarest JF et al: HIV infection is active and progressive in lymphoid tissue during latent disease. Nature 362:355, 1993
34. Piatak M Jr, Saag MS, Yang LC et al: High levels of HIV-1 in plasma during all stages of infection determined by competitive PCR. Science 259:1749, 1993
35. Varmus H: Retroviruses. Science 240:1427, 1988

36. Muesing MA, Smith DH, Cabradilla CD et al: Nucleic acid structure and expression of the human AIDS/lymphadenopathy retrovirus. Nature 313:450, 1985

37. Schwartz S, Felber BK, Fenyo EM et al: Env and vpu proteins of human immunodeficiency virus type 1 are produced from multiple bicistronic mRNAs. J Virol 64:5448, 1990

38. Robert-Guroff M, Popovic M, Gartner S et al: Structure and expression of tat-, rev-, and nef-specific transcripts of human immunodeficiency virus type 1 in infected lymphocytes and macrophages. J Virol 64:3391, 1990

39. Schwartz S, Felber BK, Benko DM et al: Cloning and functional analysis of multiply spliced mRNA species of human immunodeficiency virus type 1. J Virol 64:2519, 1990

40. Jacks T, Power MD, Masiarz FR et al: Characterization of ribosomal frameshifting in HIV-1 gag-pol expression. Nature 331:280, 1987

41. Marvis RJ, Ahmad N, Lillehoj E et al: The gag gene products of human immunodeficiency virus type 1: alignment within the gag operon reading frame, identification of postranslational modifications, and evidence for alternative gag precursor. J Virol 62:3993, 1988

42. Earl PL, Moss B, Doms, RW: Folding, interaction with GRP78- BiP, assembly, and transport of the human immunodeficiency virus type 1 envelope protein. J Virol 65:2047, 1991

43. Palker TJ, Clark ME, Langlois AJ et al: Type-specific neutralization of the human immunodeficiency virus with antibodies to env-encoded synthetic peptides. Proc Natl Acad Sci USA 85:1932, 1988

44. Rusche JR, Javaherian K, McDanal C et al: Antibodies that inhibit fusion of human immunodeficiency virus-infected cells bind a 24-amino acid sequence of the viral envelope, gp120. Proc Natl Acad Sci USA 85:3198, 1988

45. Capon DJ, Ward RJ: The CD4-gp120 interaction and AIDS pathogenesis. Ann Rev Immunol 9:649, 1991

46. Arya SK, Guo C, Josephs SF, Wong-Staal F: Trans-activator gene of human t-lymphotrophic virus type III (HTLV-III). Science 229:69, 1985

47. Dayton AI, Sodroski JG, Rosen CA et al: The trans-activator gene of the human T cell lymphotrophic virus type iii is required for replication. Cell 44:941, 1986

48. Fisher AG, Feinberg MB, Josephs SF et al: The trans-activator gene of HTLV-III is essential for virus replication. Nature 320:367, 1986

49. Cullen BR: Mechanism of action of regulatory proteins encoded by complex retroviruses. Microbiol Rev 56:375, 1992

50. Rosen CA, Pavlakis GN: Tat and rev: positive regulators of HIV gene expression. AIDS 4:499, 1990

51. Gaynor R: Cellular transcription factors involved in the regulation of HIV-1 gene expression. AIDS 6:347, 1992

52. Rounseville MP, Kumar A: Binding of a host cell nuclear protein to the stem region of human immunodeficiency virus type 1 trans-activation responsive RNA. J Virol 66:1688, 1992

53. Ensoli B, Barillari G, Zaki RC, Wong-Stall F: Tat protein of HIV-1 stimulates growth of cells derived from Kaposi sarcoma lesions of AIDS patients. Nature 345:84, 1990

54. Viscidi RP, Mayur K, Lederman HM et al: Inhibition of antigen-induced lymphocyte proliferation by tat protein from HIV-1. Science 246:1606, 1989

55. Buonaguro L, Brillari G, Chang HK et al: Effects of the human immunodefi-

ciency virus type 1 tat protein on the expression of inflammatory cytokines. J Virol 66:7159, 1992

56. Arya SK, Gallo RC: Three novel genes of human T-lymphotrophic virus type III: immune reactivity of their products with sera from acquired immune deficiency syndrome patients. Proc Natl Acad Sci USA 83:2209, 1986

57. Emerman M, Vazeux R, Paden K: The rev gene product of the human immunodeficiency virus affects envelope-specific RNA localization. Cell 57:1155, 1989

58. Felber BK, Hadzopoulou-Cladaras M, Cladaras C et al: Rev protein of human immunodeficiency virus type 1 affects the stability and transport of the viral mRNA. Proc Natl Acad Sci USA 86:1495, 1989

59. Heaphy S, Dingwall C, Ernberg I et al: HIV-1 regulator of virion expression (rev) protein biding to an RNA stem-loop structure located within the rev response element region. Cell 60:685, 1990

60. Malim MH, Hauber J, Le SY et al: The HIV-1 rev transactivator acts through a structured target sequence to activate nuclear export of unspliced viral mRNA. Nature 338:254, 1989

61. Chang DD, Sharp PA: Regulation of HIV rev depends upon recognition of splice sites. Cell 59:789, 1989

62. Chang DD, Sharp PA: Messenger RNA transport and HIV rev regulation. Science 249:614, 1990

63. Clawson GA, Song YL, Schwartz AM et al: Interaction of human immunodeficiency virus type 1 rev protein with nuclear scaffold nucleoside triphosphate activity. Cell Growth Differ 2:575, 1991

64. Frankhauser C, Izaurralde E, Adachi Y et al: Specific complex of human immunodeficiency virus type 1 rev and nucleolar B23 proteins: dissociation by the rev response element. Mol Cell Biol 11:2567, 1991

65. Kjems J, Frankel AD, Sharp PA: Specific regulation of mRNA splicing in-vitro by a peptide from HIV-1 rev. Cell 67:169, 1991

66. Kjems J, Sharp PA: The basic domain of rev from human immunodeficiency virus type 1 specifically blocks the entry of U4/U5/U6 small nuclear ribonucleoprotein in spliceosome assembly. J Virol 67:4769, 1993

67. Rabson AB, Daugherty DF, Venkatesan S et al: Transcription of novel open reading frames of AIDS retrovirus during infection of lymphocytes. Science 229:1388, 1985

68. Luciw PA, Cheng-Mayer C, Levy JA: Mutational analysis of the human immunodeficiency virus: the orf-b region down-regulates virus replication. Proc Natl Acad Sci USA 84:1434, 1987

69. Terwilliger E, Sodroski JG, Rosen CA et al: Effects of mutations within the 3' orf open reading frame region of human T-cell lymphotropic virus type III (HTLV-III/LAV) on replication and cytopathogenicity. Virology 60:754, 1986

70. Guy B, Kieny MP, Riviere Y et al: HIV F/3' orf encodes a phosphorylated GTP-binding protein resembling an oncogene product. Nature 330:266, 1987

71. Niederman TM, Garcia JV, Hastings WR et al: Human immunodeficiency virus type 1 nef protein inhibits NF-κB induction in human T cells. J Virol 66:6213, 1992

72. Hammes SR, Dixon EP, Malim MH et al: Nef protein of the human immunodeficiency virus type 1: evidence against its role as a transcriptional inhibitor. Proc Natl Acad Sci USA 86:9549, 1989

73. Klotman ME, Wong-Staal F: Human immunodeficiency virus (HIV) gene structure and genetic diversity. In Gallo RC, Jay G (eds): The Human Retroviruses. Academic Press, San Diego, 1991

74. Kan NC, Franchini G, Wong-Staal F et al: Identification of HTLV-III/LAV sor gene product and detection of antibodies in human sera. Science 231:1553, 1986

75. Sodroski J, Goh WC, Rosen C et al: Replication and cytopathic potential of HTLV-III/LAV with sor gene deletions. Science 231:1549, 1986

76. Lee TH, Coligan JE, Allan JS et al: A new HTLV-III/LAV protein encoded by a gene found in cytopathic retroviruses. Science 231:1546, 1986

77. Fisher AG, Ensoli B, Ivanoff L et al: The sor gene of HIV-1 is required for efficient virus transmission in vitro. Science 237:888, 1987

78. Strebel K, Daughtery D, Clouse K et al: The HIV 'A' (sor) gene product is essential for virus infectivity. Nature 328:728, 1987

79. Cohen EA, Terwilliger EF, Sodroski JG et al: Identification of a protein encoded by the vpu gene of HIV-1. Nature 344:532, 1988

80. Strebel K, Klimkait T, Maldarelli F et al: Molecular and biochemical analyses of human immunodeficiency virus type 1 vpu protein. J Virol 63:3784, 1989

81. Strebel K, Klimkat T, Martin MA: A novel gene of HIV-1, vpu, and its 16-kilodalton product. Science 241:1221, 1988

82. Terwilliger EF, Cohen EA, Lu Y et al: Functional role of HIV-1 vpu. Proc Natl Acad Sci USA 86:5163, 1989

83. Klimkait T, Strebel K, Hoggan MD et al: The human immunodeficiency virus type 1-specific protein vpu is required for efficient virus maturation and release. J Virol 64:621, 1990

84. Cohen EA, Terwilliger EF, Jalinoos Y et al: Identification of HIV-1 vpr product and function. J AIDS 3:11, 1990

85. Wong-Staal F, Chandra PK, Ghrayeb J: Human immunodeficiency virus: the eighth gene. AIDS Res Hum Retroviruses 3:33, 1987

86. Cohen EA, Dehni G, Sodroski JG et al: Human immunodeficiency virus vpr product is a virion-associated regulatory protein. J Virol 64:3097, 1990

87. Yuan X, Matsuda Z, Matsuda M et al: Human immunodeficiency virus vpr gene encodes a virion-associated protein. AIDS Res Hum Retroviruses 6:1265, 1990

88. Ratner L, Haseltine W, Patarca R et al: Complete nucleotide sequence of the AIDS virus, HTLV-III. Nature 313:277, 1985

89. Sanchez-Pescador R, Power MD, Barr PJ et al: Nucleotide sequence and expression of an AIDS-associated retrovirus (ARV-2). Science 227:484, 1985

90. Bohnlein S, Hauber J, Cullen BR: Identification of a U5-specific sequence required for efficient polyadenylation within the human immunodeficiency virus long terminal repeat. J Virol 63:421, 1989

91. Lu Y, Touzjian N, Stenzel M et al: Identification of cis-acting repressive sequences within the negative regulatory element of human immunodeficiency virus type 1. J Virol 64:5226, 1990

92. Rosen CA, Sodroski JG, Haseltine WA: The location of cis-acting regulatory sequences in the human T cell lymphotrophic virus type III (HTLV-III/LAV) long terminal repeat. Cell 41:813, 1985

93. Laspia MF, Rice AP, Mathews MB: HIV-1 tat protein increases transcriptional initiation and stabilizes elongation. Cell 59:283, 1989

94. Laspia MF, Rice AP, Mathews MB: Synergy between HIV-1 tat and adenovirus e1a is principally due to stabilization of transcriptional elongation. Genes Dev 4:2397, 1990

95. Marciniak RA, Calnan BJ, Frankel AD et al: HIV tat protein trans-activates transcription in vitro. Cell 63:791, 1990

96. Cullen BR: The HIV-1 tat protein: an RNA sequence-specific processivity factor? Cell 63:655, 1990

97. Cullen BR: Does tat induce a change in viral initiation rights? Cell 73:417, 1993

98. Gorman CM, Moffat LF, Howard BH: Recombinant genomes which express chloramphenicol acetyl transferase in mammalian cells. Mol Cell Biol 2:1044, 1982

99. Harrich D, Garcia J, Wu F et al: Role of SP1-binding domains in in vivo transcriptional regulation of the human immunodeficiency virus type 1 long terminal repeat. J Virol 63:2585, 1989

100. Ptashne M: How eukaryotic transcriptional activators work. Nature 335:683, 1988

101. Buratowski S: The basics of basal transcription by RNA polymerase II. Cell 77:1, 1994

102. Li YC, Ross J, Scheppler JA et al: An in vitro transcription analysis of early responses of the human immunodeficiency virus type 1 long terminal repeat to different transcriptional activators. Mol Cell Biol 11:1883, 1991

103. Garcia JA, Ou S, Lusis AJ et al: Cloning and chromosomal mapping of a human immunodeficiency virus 1 "TATA" element modulatory factor. Proc Natl Acad Sci USA 89:9372, 1992

104. Berkhout B, Jeang KT: Functional roles for the TATA promoter and enhancers in basal and tat-induced expression of the human immunodeficiency virus type 1 long terminal repeat. J Virol 66:139, 1992

105. Olsen HS, Rosen CA: Contribution of the TATA motif to tat-mediated transcriptional activation of human immunodeficiency virus gene expression. J Virol 66:5594, 1992

106. Jones KA, Kadonaga JT, Luciew PA et al: Activation of the AIDS retrovirus promoter by the cellular transcription factor, Sp1. Science 232:755, 1986

107. Leonard J, Parrott C, Buckler-White AJ et al: Variable role of the long-terminal repeat SP1-binding sites in human immunodeficiency virus replication in T lymphocytes. J Virol 63:4919, 1989

108. Ross EK, Buckler-White AJ, Rabson AB et al: Contribution of NF-kappa B and SP1 binding motifs to the replicative capacity of human immunodeficiency virus type 1: distinct patterns of viral growth are determined by T-cell types. J Virol 65:4350, 1991

109. Kretzschmar M, Meisterernst M, Scheidereit C et al: Transcriptional regulation of the HIV-1 promoter by NF-kappa B in vitro. Genes Dev 6:761, 1992

110. Lenardo MJ, Baltimore D: NF-κB: a pleiotropic mediator of inducible and tissue-specific gene control. Cell 58:227, 1989

111. Blank V, Kourilsky P, Israel A: NF-kappa B and related proteins: rel/dorsal homologies meet ankyrin-like repeats. Trends Biochem Sci 17:135, 1992

112. Gilmore TD: NF-kappa B, KBF1, dorsal and related matters. Cell 62:841, 1990

113. Ghosh S, Baltimore D: Activation in vitro of NF-κb by phosphorylation of its inhibitor IκB. Nature 344:678, 1990

114. Zabel U, Baeuerle PA: Purified human κb can rapidly dissociate the complex of the nf-κb transcription factor with its cognate DNA. Cell 61:255, 1990

115. Baeuerle PA, Baltimore D: A 65-kD subunit of active NF-κB is required for inhibition of NF-κB by IκB. Genes Dev 3:1689, 1989

116. Kaufman JD, Valandra G, Roderiquez G et al: Phorbol ester enhances human immunodeficiency virus-promoted gene expression and acts on a repeated 10-base-pair functional enhancer element. Mol Cell Biol 7:3759, 1987

117. Nabel G, Baltimore D: An inducible transcription factor activates expression of human immunodeficiency virus in T cells. Nature 326:711, 1987

118. Wu F, Garcia J, Mitsuyasu R et al: Alterations in binding characteristics of the human immunodeficiency virus enhancer factor. J Virol 62:218, 1988

119. Duh EJ, Maury WJ, Folks TM et al: Tumor necrosis factor α activates human immunodeficiency virus type 1 through induction of nuclear factor binding to the NF-β sites in the long terminal repeat. Proc Natl Acad Sci USA 86:5974, 1989

120. Siekevitz M, Josephs SF, Dukovich M et al: Activation of the HIV-1 LTR by T cell mitogens and the trans-activator protein of HTLV-1. Science 238:1575, 1987

121. Bohnlein E, Siekevitz M, Ballard DW et al: Stimulation of the human immunodeficiency virus type 1 enhancer by the human T-cell leukemia virus type I tax gene product involves the action of inducible cellular proteins. J Virol 63:1578, 1989

122. Perkins ND, Edwards NL, Duckett CS et al: A cooperative interaction between NF-kappa B and SP1 is required for HIV-1 enhancer activation. Embo J 12:3551, 1993

123. Franza BR, Rauscher FJ, Josephs SF et al: The fos complex and fos-related antigens recognize sequence elements that contain AP-1 binding sites. Science 239:1150, 1988

124. Lu Y, Stenzel M, Sodroski JG et al: Effects of long terminal repeat mutations on human immunodeficiency virus type 1 replication. J Virol 63:4115, 1989

125. Zeichner SL, Kim JY, Alwine JC: Linker-scanning mutational analysis of the transcriptional activity of the human immunodeficiency virus type 1 long terminal repeat. J Virol 65:2436, 1991

126. Zeichner SL, Hirka G, Andrews RW et al: Differentiation-dependent human immunodeficiency virus long terminal repeat regulatory elements active in human teratocarcinoma cells. J Virol 66:2268, 1992

127. Jones KA, Luciw PA, Duchange N: Structural arrangements of transcription control domains within the 5'-untranslated leader regions of the HIV-1 and HIV-2 promoters. Genes Dev 2:1101, 1988

128. Boris-Lawrie KA, Brady JN, Kumar A: Sequences within the R region of the long terminal repeat activate basal transcription from the HIV-1 promoter. Gene Express 2:215, 1992

129. Matsuyama T, Kobayashi N, Yammamoto N: Cytokines and HIV infection: is AIDS a tumor necrosis factor disease? AIDS 5:1405, 1991

130. Vyakarnam A, McKeating J, Meager A et al: Tumor necrosis factors (α, β) induced by HIV-1 in peripheral blood mononuclear cells potentiate virus replication. AIDS 4:21, 1990

131. Wahl LM, Corcoran ML, Pyle SW et al: Human immunodeficiency virus glycoprotein (gp120) induction of monocyte arachidonic acid metabolites and interleukin 1. Proc Natl Acad Sci USA 86:621, 1989

132. Merrill JE, Koyanagi Y, Chen ISY: Interleukin 1 and tumor necrosis factor α can be induced from mononuclear phagocytes by human immunodeficiency virus type 1 binding to the CD4 receptor. J Virol 63:4404, 1989

133. Clouse KA, Powell D, Washington I et al: Monokine regulation of human immunodeficiency virus-1 expression in a chronically infected human T cell clone. Immunology 142:431, 1989

134. Israel N, Hazan U, Alcami J et al: Tumor necrosis factor stimulates transcrip-

tion of HIV-1 in human T lymphocytes, independently and synergistically with mitogens. J Immunol 143:3956, 1989

135. Osborn L, Kunkel S, Nabel GJ et al: Tumor necrosis factor α and interleukin 1 stimulate the human immunodeficiency virus enhancer by activation of the nuclear factor κB. Proc Natl Acad Sci USA 86:2336, 1989

136. Swingler S, Easton A, Morris A: Cytokine augmentation of HIV-1 LTR driven gene expression in neural cells. AIDS Res Hum Retroviruses 8:487, 1992

137. Poli G, Bressler P, Kinter A et al: Interleukin 6 induces human immunodeficiency virus expression in monocytic cells alone and in synergy with tumor necrosis factor α by transcriptional and post-transcriptional mechanisms. J Exp Med 172:151, 1990

138. Koyanagi Y, O'Brien WA, Zhao JQ et al: Cytokines alter production of HIV-1 from primary mononuclear phagocytes. Science 241:1673, 1988

139. Poli G, Kinter A, Justement JS et al: Tumor necrosis factor alpha functions in an autocrine manner in the induction of human immunodeficiency virus expression. Proc Natl Acad Sci USA 89:2689, 1992

140. Poli G, Orenstein JM, Kinter A et al: Interferon-γ but not AZT suppresses HIV expression in chronically infected cell lines. Science 244:575, 1989

141. Poli G, Kinter AL, Justement JS et al: TGF-β suppresses HIV expression and replication in infected monocyte/macrophage lineage cells. J Exp Med 173:589, 1991

142. Peterson PK, Gekker G, Chao CC et al: Cocaine potentiates HIV-1 replication in human peripheral blood mononuclear cell cocultures. J Immunol 146:81, 1991

143. Kekow J, Wachsman W, McCutchan A et al: TGF-β and noncytopathic mechanisms of immunodeficiency in HIV infection. Proc Natl Acad Sci 87:8321, 1990

144. Shukla R, Kumar A, Kimmel PL: TGF-β increases the expression of HIV gene in transfected human mesangial cells. Kidney Int 44:1022, 1993

145. Arenzana-Seisdedos F, Israel N, Bachelerie F et al: C-Ha-ras transfection induced human immunodeficiency virus (HIV) transcription through the HIV enhanced in human fibroblast and astrocytes. Oncogene 4:1359, 1989

146. Baldari CT, Macchia G, Massone A et al: P^{21} ras contributes to HIV-1 activation in T cells. FEBS Letter 304:261, 1992

147. Dasgupta P, Saikumar P, Reddy CD et al: Myb protein binds to human immunodeficiency virus 1 long terminal repeat (LTR) sequences and transactivates LTR mediated transcription. Proc Natl Acad Sci USA 87:8090, 1990

148. Horikoshi N, Maguire K, Kralli A et al: Direct interaction between adenovirus E1A protein and the TATA box binding transcription factor IID. Proc Natl Acad Sci USA 88:5124, 1991

149. Seto E, Yen TSB, Peterlin BM et al: Trans-activation of the HIV long terminal repeat by the hepatitis B virus X protein. Proc Natl Acad Sci 85:8286, 1988

150. Nelson JA, Ghazal P, Wiley CA: Role of opportunistic viral-infection in AIDS. AIDS 4:1, 1990

151. Laurence J: Molecular interactions among herpesviruses and human immunodeficiency virus. J Infect Dis 162:338, 1990

152. Poli G, Fauci AS: The effect of cytokines and pharmacologic agents on chronic HIV infection. AIDS Res Hum Retroviruses 8:191, 1992

153. Skolnik PR, Jahn B, Wang MZ et al: Enhancement of HIV replication in monocytes by 1,25 dihydroxycholecalciferol. Proc Natl Acad Sci 88:6632, 1991

154. Garcia JA, Harrich D, Pearson L et al: Functional domains required for tat-

induced transcriptional activation of the HIV-1 long terminal repeat. EMBO J 7:3143, 1988

155. Green M, Loewenstein PM: Autonomous functional domains of chemically synthesized human immunodeficiency virus tat trans-activator protein. Cell 55: 1179, 1988

156. Kuppuswamy M, Subramanian T, Srinivasan A et al: Multiple functional domains of tat, the trans-activator of HIV-1, defined by mutational analysis. Nucl Acid Res 17:3551, 1989

157. Ruben S, Perkins A, Purcell R et al: Structural and functional characterization of human immunodeficiency virus tat protein. J Virol 63:1, 1989

158. Rappaport J, Lee SJ, Khalili K et al: The acidic amino-terminal region of the HIV-1 tat protein constitutes an essential activating domain. New Biologist 1: 101, 1989

159. Frankel AD, Bredt DS, Pabo CO: Tat protein from human immunodeficiency virus forms a metal-linked dimer. Science 240:70, 1988

160. Kamine J, Loewenstein P, Green M: Mapping of HIV-1 tat protein sequences required for binding to TAR RNA. Virology 182:570, 1991

161. Hauber J, Malim M, Cullen BR: Mutational analysis of the conserved basic domain of human immunodeficiency virus tat protein. J Virol 63:1181, 1989

162. Nelbock P, Dillon PJ, Perkins A et al: A cDNA for a protein that interacts with the human immunodeficiency virus tat trans-activator. Science 248:1650, 1990

163. Jakobovits A, Smith DH, Jakobovits EB et al: A discrete element 3' of human immunodeficiency virus 1 (HIV-1) and HIV-2 mRNA initiation sites mediates transcriptional activation by an HIV trans activator. Mol Cell Biol 8:2555, 1988

164. Hauber J, Cullen BR: Mutational analysis of the trans-activation-responsive region of the human immunodeficiency virus type 1 long terminal repeat. J Virol 62:673, 1988

165. Selby MJ, Bain ES, Luciw PA et al: Structure, sequence, and position of the stem-loop in TAR determine transcriptional elongation by tat through the HIV-1 long terminal repeat. Genes Dev 3:547, 1989

166. Sodroski J, Patarca R, Rosen CA et al: Location of the trans-activating region on the genome of human T-cell lymphotrophic virus type III. Science 229:74, 1985

167. Berkhout B, Jeang K-T: Trans-activation of human immunodeficiency virus type 1 is sequence specific for both the single-stranded bulge and loop of the trans-acting-responsive hairpin: a quantitative analysis. J Virol 63:5501, 1989

168. Feng S, Holland EC: HIV-1 tat trans-activation requires the loop sequence within TAR. Nature 334:165, 1988

169. Roy S, Parkin NT, Rosen C et al: Structural requirements for trans activation of human immunodeficiency virus type 1 long terminal repeat-directed gene expression by tat: importance of base pairing, loop sequence, and bulges in the tat-responsive sequence. J Virol 64:1402, 1990

170. Cordingly MG, La Femina RL, Callahan PL et al: Sequence-specific interaction of tat protein and tat peptides with the trans-activation-responsive sequence element of human immunodeficiency virus type 1 in vitro. Proc Natl Acad Sci USA 87:8985, 1990

171. Dingwall C, Ernberg I, Gait MJ et al: Human immunodeficiency virus 1 tat protein binds trans-activation-responsive-region (TAR) RNA in vitro. Proc Natl Acad Sci USA 86:6925, 1989

172. Roy S, Delling U, Chen CH et al: A bulge structure in HIV-1 TAR RNA is required for tat binding and tat-mediated trans-activation. Genes Dev 4:1365, 1990
173. Muesing MA, Smith, DH, Capon DJ: Regulation of mRNA accumulation by a human immunodeficiency virus trans-activator protein. Cell 48:691, 1987
174. Jeang KT, Shank PR, Rabson AB, Kumar A: Synthesis of functional human immunodeficiency virus tat protein in baculovirus as determined by a cell-cell fusion assay. J Virol 62:3874, 1988
175. Berkhout B, Gatgnol A, Rabson AB et al: TAR independent activation of the HIV-1 LTR: evidence that tat requires specific regions of promoters. Cell 62: 757, 1990
176. Southgate CD, Green MR: The HIV-1 tat protein activates transcription from an upstream DNA-binding site: implications for tat function. Genes Dev 5: 2496, 1991
177. Feinberg MB, Baltimore D, Frankel, AD: The role of tat in the human immunodeficiency virus life cycle indicates a primary effect on transcriptional elongation. Proc Natl Acad Sci USA 88:4045, 1991
178. Braddock M, Chambers A, Wilson W et al: HIV-1 tat 'activates' presynthesized RNA in the nucleus. Cell 58:269, 1989
179. Barry PA, Pratt-Lowe E, Unger RE et al: Cellular factors regulate trans-activation of human immunodeficiency virus type 1. J Virol 65:1392, 1991
180. Newstein M, Stanbridge EJ, Casey G et al: Human chromosome 12 encodes a species-specific factor which increases human immunodeficiency virus type 1 tat-mediated trans activation in rodent cells. J Virol 64:4565, 1990
181. Hart CE, Ou CY, Galphin JC et al: Human chromosome 12 is required for elevated HIV-1 expression in human-hamster hybrid cells. Science 246:488, 1989
182. Kumar A, Gatignol A, Jeang K-T et al: Role of cellular factors in tat mediated HIV-1 gene trans-activation. p. 161 In Papas T (ed): Oncogenesis and AIDS. Applied Biotechnology Series. Vol. 7. Gulf Publishing Company, Houston, 1990
183. Marciniak RA, Garcia-Bianco MA, Sharp PA: Identification and characterization of the HeLa nuclear protein that specifically binds to the trans-activation-response (TAR) element of human immunodeficiency virus. Proc Natl Acad Sci USA 87:3624, 1990
184. Sheline CT, Milocco LH, Jones KA: Two distinct nuclear transcription factors recognize loop and bulge residues of the HIV-1 TAR RNA hairpin. Genes Dev 5:2508, 1991
185. Wu F, Garcia J, Sigman D et al: Tat regulates binding of the human immunodeficiency virus trans-activating region RNA loop-binding protein TRP-185. Genes Dev 5:2128, 1991
186. Gatignol A, Buckler-White A, Berkhout B et al: Characterization of a human TAR RNA-binding protein that activates the HIV-1 LTR. Science 251:1597, 1991
187. Gatignol A, Buckler-White A, Jeang KT: Relatedness of an RNA binding motif in human immunodeficiency virus type 1 TAR RNA-binding protein TRBP to human P1/dsI kinase and drosophila staufen. Mol Cell Biol 13:2139, 1993
188. Roy S, Agy M, Hovanessian AG et al: The integrity of the stem structure of human immunodeficiency virus type 1 tat-responsive sequence RNA is required for interaction with the interferon-induced 68,000-M_r protein kinase. J Virol 65:632, 1991

189. Pomerantz RJ, Trono D, Feinberg MB et al: Cells non productively infected with HIV-1 exhibit an aberrant pattern of viral RNA expression: a molecular model for latency. Cell 61:1271, 1990

190. Perkins A, Cochrane AW, Ruben SM et al: Structural and functional characterization of human immunodeficiency virus rev protein. J AIDS 2:256, 1989

191. Cook KS, Fisk GJ, Hauber J et al: Characterization of HIV-1 rev protein: Binding stoichiometry and minimal RNA substrate. Nucl Acid Res 19:1577, 1991

192. Hope TJ, Klein NP, Elder ME et al: Transdominant inhibition of human immunodeficiency virus type 1 rev occurs through formation of inactive protein complexes. J Virol 66:1849, 1992

193. Olsen HS, Cochran AW, Dillon PJ et al: Interaction of the human immunodeficiency virus type 1 rev protein with a structural region in *env* mRNA is dependent on multimer formation mediated through a basic stretch of amino acids. Genes Dev 4:1357, 1990

194. Malim MH, Cullen BR: HIV-1 structural gene expression requires binding of multiple monomers to the viral RRE: implications for HIV-1 latency. Cell 65:241, 1991

195. Benko DM, Robinson R, Solomin L et al: Binding of trans-dominant mutant rev protein of human immunodeficiency virus type 1 to the cis-acting rev-response element does not affect the fate of viral mRNA. New Biol 2:1, 1990

196. Zapp ML, Green MR: Sequence specific RNA binding by the HIV-1 rev protein. Nature 342:714, 1989

197. Daly TJ, Rusche JR, Maione RE et al: Circular dichroism studies of the HIV-1 rev protein and its specific RNA binding site. Biochemistry 29:2971, 1990

198. Olson HS, Nelbock, Cochran AW: Secondary structure is the major determinant for the interaction of HIV rev proteins with RNA. Science 247:845, 1990

199. Dayton ET, Konings DAM, Powell DM et al: Extensive sequence specific information throught the CAR/RRE, the target sequence of the human immunodeficiency virus type 1 rev protein. J Virol 66:1139, 1992

200. D'Agostino DM, Felber BK, Harrison JE et al: The rev protein of human immunodeficiency virus type 1 promotes polysomal association and translation of gag/pol and vpu/env mRNAs. Mol Cell Biol 12:1375, 1992

201. Arrigo SJ, Chen ISY: Rev is necessary for translation but not cytoplasmic accumulation of HIV-1 vif, vpr, and env/vpu 2 RNAs. Genes Dev 5:808, 1991

202. Torono D, Baltimore D: A human cell factor is essential for HIV-1 rev action. EMBO J 9:4155, 1990

203. Shukla R, Kimmel PL, Kumar A: Human immunodeficiency virus type 1 rev-responsive element RNA binds to host cell specific protein. J Virol 68:2224, 1994

204. Vaishnav YN, Vaishnav M, Wong-Staal F: Identification and characterization of a nuclear factor that specifically binds to the rev responsive element (RRE) of human deficiency virus type 1 (HIV-1). New Biol 3:142, 1991

205. Luo Y, Yu H, Peterlin BM: Cellular protein modulates effects of human immunodeficiency virus type 1 rev. J Virol 68:3850, 1994

206. Ruhl M, Mimmelspach M, Bahr GM: Eukaryotic initiation factor 5A is a cellular target of the human immunodeficiency virus type rev activation domain mediating transactivation. J Cell Biol 123:1309, 1993

207. Kozak M: The scanning model for translation: an update. J Cell Biol 108:229, 1989

208. Schwartz S, Felber BK, Pavlakis GN: Mechanism of translation of monocis-

tronic and multicistronic human immunodeficiency virus type 1 mRNAs. Mol Cell Biol 12:207, 1992

209. Willey RL, Maldarelli F, Martin MA et al: Human immunodeficiency virus type 1 vpu protein regulates the formation of intracellular gp160-CD4 complexes. J Virol 66:226, 1992

210. Wilson W, Braddok M, Adams S et al: HIV expression strategies: ribosomal frameshifting is directed by a short sequence in both mammalian and yeast systems. Cell 55:1159, 1988

211. Geballe AP, Gray MK: Variable inhibition of cell free translation by HIV-1 transcripts leader sequences. Nucl Acid Res 20:4291, 1992

212. Parkin NT, Cohen EA, Darveau A et al: Mutational analysis of the 5'noncoding region of human immunodeficiency virus type 1: effects of secondary structure on translation. EMBO J 7:2831, 1988

213. Sengupta DN, Berkhout B, Gatignol A et al: Direct evidence of translational regulation by leader RNA and tat protein of human immunodeficiency virus type 1. Proc Natl Acad Sci USA 87:7492, 1990

214. Drysdale CM, Pavlakis GN: Rapid activation and subsequent down regulation of the human immunodeficiency virus type 1 promoter in the presence of tat: possible mechanism contributing to latency. J Virol 65:3044, 1991

215. Hovanessian AG: The double stranded RNA activated protein kinase induced by interferon: dsRNA-PK. J Interferon Res 6:641, 1990

216. Edery I, Petryshyn R, Sonenberg N: Activation of double-stranded RNA-dependent kinase (dSI) by the TAR region of HIV-1 mRNA: a novel translational control mechanism. Cell 56:303, 1989

217. Sengupta DN, Silverman RH: Activation of interferon-regulated, dsRNA-dependent enzymes by human immunodeficiency virus-1 leader RNA. Nucl Acid Res 17:969, 1989

218. Roy S, Katz MG, Perkin NT et al: Control of interferon-induced p68 kilodalton protein kinase by the HIV-1 tat gene product. Science 247:1216, 1990

219. Szebeni J, Diffenbach C, Wahl SM et al: Induction of alpha interferon by human immunodeficiency virus type 1 in human monocyte-macrophage cultures. J Virol 65:6362, 1991

220. Mathews MB, Shenk T: Adenovirus virus-associated RNA and translation control. J Virol 65:5657, 1991

221. Leroux A, London IM: Regulation of protein synthesis by phosphorylation of eukaryotic initiation factor 2 in intact reticulocytes and reticulocyte lysates. Proc Natl Acad Sci USA 79:2147, 1982

222. Rowland AG, Panniers R, Henshaw EC: The catalytic mechanism of GEF action and competitive inhibition by phosphorylated eIF-2. J Biol Chem 263:5526, 1988

223. Samuel CE: Antiviral actions of interferon, interferon-regulated cellular proteins and their surprisingly selective antiviral activities. Virology 183:1, 1991

224. Bhat RA, Thimmappaya B: Two small RNAs encoded by Epstein Barr virus can functionally substitute for the virus-associated RNAs in the lytic growth of adenovirus 5. Proc Natl Acad Sci USA 80:4789, 1983

225. Bhat RA, Thimmappaya B: Construction and analysis of additional adenovirus substitution mutation confirm the complementation of VAI RNA function by two small RNAs encoded by Epstein-Barr virus. J Virol 56:750, 1985

226. Gunnery S, Rice AP, Robertson HD et al: Tat-responsive RNA of human immunodeficiency virus type 1 can prevent activation of the double-stranded-RNA-activated protein kinase. Proc Natl Acad Sci USA 87:8687, 1990

227. Gunnery S, Green SR, Mathews MB: Tat-responsive region RNA of human immunodeficiency virus type 1 stimulates protein synthesis in vivo and in vitro: relationship between structure and function. Proc Natl Acad Sci USA 89:11557, 1992

228. Bourgoignie JJ, Ortiz-Interiano C, Green DF et al: Race, a co-factor in HIV-1 associated nephropathy. Transplant Proc 21:3899, 1989

229. Cantor ES, Kimmel PL, Bosch JP: Effect of race on the expression of AIDS associated nephropathy. Arch Intern Med 151:125, 1991

230. Cohen AH, Nast CC: HIV-associated nephropathy. A unique combined glomerular, tubular and interstitial lesion. Mod Pathol 1:87, 1988

231. Rennke HG, Klein PS: Pathogenesis and significance of non-primary focal and segmental glomerulosclerosis. Am J Kidney Dis 13:443, 1989

232. Schwartz MM, Korbet SM: Primary focal segmental glomerulosclerosis. Am J Kidney Dis 22:874, 1993

233. Carome MA, Striker LJ, Peten EP et al: Human glomeruli express TIMP-1 mRNA and TIMP-2 protein and mRNA. Am J Physiol 264:F923, 1993

234. Wolthius A, van Goor H, Weening JJ et al: Pathobiology of focal sclerosis. Curr Opin Nephrol Hypertens 2:458, 1993

235. Langs C, Gallo GR, Schacht RG et al: Rapid renal failure in AIDS associated focal glomerulosclerosis. Arch Intern Med 150:287, 1990

236. Cohen AH, Sun NCJ, Shapshak P et al: Demonstration of human immunodeficiency virus in renal epithelium in HIV-associated nephropathy. Mod Pathol 2:125, 1989

237. Leonard JM, Abramczuk JW, Pezen DS et al: Development of disease and virus recovery in transgenic mice containing HIV proviral DNA. Science 242:1665, 1988

238. Dickie P, Felser J, Eckhaus M et al: HIV-associated nephropathy in transgenic mice expressing HIV-1 genes. Virology 185:109, 1991

239. Kopp JB, Klotman ME, Eckhaus M et al: Progressive glomerulosclerosis and enhanced renal accumulation of basement membrane components in mice transgenic for HIV type 1 genes. Proc Natl Acad Sci 89:1577, 1992

240. Green DF, Resnick L, Bourgoignie JJ: HIV infects glomerular endothelial and mesangial, but not epithelial cells in vitro. Kidney Int 41:956, 1992

241. Erice A, Kim Y: In-vitro infection of human renal cells by human immunodeficiency virus: pathogenic implications for HIV-associated nephropathy, abstracted. Clin Res 39:219 1991

242. Karlsson-Parra A, Dimeny E, Fellstron B et al: HIV receptors (CD4 antigen) in normal human glomerular cells. N Engl J Med 320:741, 1989

243. Ameglio F, Capobianchi MR, Castilletti C et al: Recombinant gp120 induces IL-10 in resting peripheral blood mononuclear cells; correlation with the induction of other cytokines. Clin Exp Immunol 95:455, 1994

244. Brenneman DE, Westerbrook GL, Fitzgerald SP et al: Neuronal cell killing by the envelope protein of HIV and its prevention by vasoactive peptide. Nature 335:639, 1988

245. Capobianchi MR, Ameglio F, Fei PC et al: Coordinate induction of INF α and γ by recombinant HIV-1 glycoprotein 120. AIDS Res Hum Retroviruses 9:957, 1993

246. Capobianchi MR, Ankel H, Ameglio F et al: Recombinant gp120 of HIV is a potent interferon inducer. AIDS Res Hum Retroviruses 8:575, 1992

247. Pullium L, West D, Haigword N, Swanson NRA: HIV-1 envelope gp120 alters astrocytes in human brain cultures. AIDS Res Hum Retroviruses 9:439, 1993

248. Kaiser PK, Offerman JT, Lipton SA: Neuronal injury due to HIV-1 envelope protein is blocked by anti-gp120 antibodies but not by anti-CD4 antibodies. Neurology 40:1757, 1990
249. Schuitemaker H, Kootstra NA, Groenink M et al: Viral and cellular requirements for replication of HIV in primary monocytes, abstracted. p. 100. VII International Conference on AIDS, Vol. 1, Florence, Italy, June 16–21, 1991
250. Nong Y, Kandil O, Tobin EH et al: The HIV core protein p24 inhibits IFN γ induced increase of HLA-DR and cytochrome b heavy chain mRNA levels in the human monocyte-like cell line THP-1. Cell Immunol 132:10, 1991
251. Miller MA, Garry RF, Jaynes JM et al: A structural correlation between lentivirus membrane proteins and natural cytolytic peptides. AIDS Res Hum Retroviruses 7:511, 1991
252. Frankel AD, Pabo CO: Cellular uptake of the tat protein from human immunodeficiency virus. Cell 55:1189, 1988
253. Ensoli B, Buonaguro L, Barillari G et al: Release, uptake, and effects of extracellular human immunodeficiency virus type 1 tat protein on cell growth and viral transactivation. J Virol 67:277, 1993
254. Zauli G, Re MC, Davis B et al: Tat protein stimulates production of TGF-β 1 by bone marrow macrophages: potential mechanism for HIV-1-induced hematopoietic suppression. Blood 80:3036, 1992
255. Vogel J, Hinrichs SH, Reynolds RK et al: The HIV-1 tat gene induces dermal lesions resembling Kaposi's sarcoma in transgenic mice. Nature 335:606, 1988
256. Bodi I, Abraham AA, Kimmel PL: Macrophages in HIV-associated kidney diseases. Am J Kid Dis, 24:762, 1994
257. Bodi I, Kimmel PL, Abraham AA et al: Increased TGF-β expression in human HIVAN, abstracted. J Am Soc Nephrol 4:461, 1993
258. Neilson EG, McCafferty E, Feldman A et al: Spontaneous interstitial nephritis in kd/kd mice. An experimental model of autoimmune disease. J Immunol 133:2560, 1984
259. Wolf G, Neilson EG: Molecular mechanisms of tubulointerstitial hypertrophy and hyperplasia. Kidney Int 39:401, 1991
260. Main IW, Nikolic-Paterson DJ, Atkins RC: T cells and macrophages and their role in renal injury. Sem Nephrol 12:395, 1992
261. Schainuck LI, Striker GE, Luther RE, Benditt EP: Structural-functional correlations in renal disease. Hum Pathol 1:631, 1970
262. Risdon RA, Sloper JAC, de Wardener HE: Relationship between renal function and histologic changes in renal biopsy specimens from patients with persistent glomerulonephritis. Lancet 2:363, 1968
263. Bohle A, Mackensen-Haen S, Gise HV: Significance of tubulointerstitial changes in the renal cortex for the function and concentration ability of the kidney. Am J Nephrol 7:421, 1987
264. D'Agati V, Suh JI, Carbone L et al: Pathology of HIV-associated nephropathy. A detailed morphologic and comparative study. Kidney Int 35:1358, 1989
265. Koyama A, Fujisaki M, Kobayashi M et al: A glomerular permeability factor produced by human T cell hybridomas. Kidney Int 40:453, 1990
266. Markovic-Lipkovski J, Muller CA, Risler T et al: Mononuclear leukocytes, expression of HLA/Class II antigens and ICAM 1 in FGS. Nephron 59:286, 1991
267. Embretson J, Zupancic M, Ribas JL et al: Massive covert infection of helper T lymphocytes and macrophages by HIV during incubation of AIDS. Nature 362:359, 1993

268. Schreiner GF: Role of macrophages in glomerular injury. Sem Nephrol 11:268, 1991
269. Cattell V: Macrophages in acute glomerular inflammation. Kidney Int 45:945, 1994
270. Mann R, Zakheim B, Clayman M et al: Murine interstitial nephritis. IV. Long-term cultured L3T4+ T cell lines transfer delayed expression of disease as I-A-restricted inductors of the effector T cell repertoire. J Immunol 135:286, 1985
271. Neilson EG, Sun MJ, Kelly CJ et al: Molecular characterization of a major nephritogenic domain in the autoantigen of anti-tubular basement membrane disease. Proc Natl Acad Sci USA 88:2006, 1991
272. Clerici M, Shearer GM: A TH1-TH2 switch is a critical step in the etiology of HIV infection. Immunol Today 14:107, 1993
273. Clerici M, Hakim F, Venzon DJ et al: Changes in interleukin-2 and interleukin-4 production in asymptomatic human immunodeficiency virus-seropositive individuals. J Clin Invest 91:759, 1993
274. Modlin RL, Bloom BR: Immune regulation: learning from leprosy. Hosp Pract 28:71, 1993
275. Strutz F, Neilson EG: The role of lymphocytes in the progression of interstitial disease. Kidney Int 45:S45, S106, 1994
276. Nakajima K, Martinez-Maza O, Hirano T et al: Induction of IL-6 (B cell stimulatory factor-2/IFN-beta 2) production by HIV. Immunology 142:531, 1989
277. Zangerle R, Gallati H, Sarcletti M et al: Increased serum concentrations of soluble tumor necrosis factor receptors in HIV-infected individuals are associated with immune activation. J AIDS 7:79, 1994
278. Allen JB, Wong HL, Guyre PM et al: Association of circulating receptor FCYRIII+ monocytes in AIDS patients with elevated TGF-β levels. J Clin Invest 87:1773, 1991
279. Eyster ME, Goedert JJ, Poon M et al: Acid-labile alpha interferon: a possible preclinical marker for AIDS in hemophilia. N Engl J Med 309:583, 1983
280. Schattner A: Interferons and autoimmunity. Am J Med Sci 295:532, 1988
281. Sharma K, Ziyadeh F: Transforming growth factor-beta system and the kidney. Semin Nephrol 13:116, 1993
282. Veis JH, Yamashita W, Liu YJ et al: The biology of mesangial cells in glomerulonephritis. Proc Soc Exp Biol Med 199:199, 1990
283. Warde EN: Cytokine growth factors and glomerulonephritis. Nephron 57:257, 1991
284. Border WA, Okuda S, Languino LR et al: Suppression of experimental glomerulonephritis by antiserum against transforming growth factor β. Nature 346:371, 1990
285. Kakizaki Y, Kraft N, Atkins RC: Differential control of mesangial cell proliferation by interferon-gamma. Clin Exp Immunol 85:157, 1991
286. Martin M, Schwinzer R, Schellekens H et al: Glomerular mesangial cells in local inflammation. Induction of expression of MHC class II antigens by IFN-gamma. J Immunol 142:1887, 1989
287. Bockus D, Remington F, Luu J et al: Induction of cylindrical confronting cisternae in Daudi lymphoblastoid cells by recombinant alpha-interferon. Hum Pathol 19:78, 1988
288. Border W, Yamamoto T, Gold L et al: HIVAN is linked to TGF-β and matrix protein expression in human kidney, abstracted. J Am Soc Nephrol 4:675, 1993
289. Mattana J, Abramovici M, Singhal P: Effects of HIV sera and macrophage

supernatants on mesangial cell proliferation and matrix synthesis. Am J Pathol 143:814, 1993
290. Miller MD, Krangel MS: Biology and biochemistry of chemokines: a family of chemotactic and inflammatory cytokines. Crit Rev Immunol 12:17, 1992
291. Larsen CG, Anderson AO, Apella E et al: The neutrophil activating protein NAP-1 is also chemotactic for T lymphocytes. Science 246:1464, 1989
292. Schmouder RL, Strieter RM, Wiggins RC et al: In vitro and in vivo interleukin 8 production in human renal cortical epithelia. Kidney Int 41:191, 1992
293. Kusner DJ, Luebbers EL, Nowinski RJ et al: Cytokine and LPS induced synthesis of interleukin-8 from human mesangial cells. Kidney Int 39:1240, 1991
294. Schall TJ, Bacon K, Toy KJ et al: Selective attraction of monocytes and T lymphocytes of the memory phenotype by cytokine RANTES. Nature 347:669, 1990
295. Schall TJ, Jongstra J, Dyer BJ et al: A human T cell specific molecule is a member of a new gene family. J Immunol 141:1018, 1988
296. Heeger P, Wolf G, Meyers C et al: Isolation and characterization of cDNA from renal tubular epithelium encoding murine RANTES. Kidney Int 41:220, 1992
297. Rovin BH, Yoshiumura T, Tan L: Cytokine-induced production of monocyte chemoattractant protein-1 by cultured human mesangial cells. J Immunol 148: 2148, 1992
298. Yoshimura T, Yuhki N, Moore SK et al: Human monocyte chemoattractant protein-1 (MCP-1): full length cDNA cloning, expression in mitogen-stimulated blood mononuclear leukocytes, and sequence similarity to mouse competence gene JE. FEBS Lett 244:487, 1989
299. Rot A, Krieger M, Brunner T et al: RANTES and macrophage inflammatory protein 1 alpha induce the migration and activation of normal human eosinophil granulocytes. J Exp Med 176:1489, 1992
300. Wolpe SD, Cerami A: MIP-1 & 2: members of a novel cytokine superfamily. FASEB J 3:2565, 1989
301. Satriano JA, Hora K, Shan Z et al: Regulation of MCP-1 and macrophage CSF-1 by IFN-γ, TNF-α, IgG aggregates, and cAMP in mouse mesangial cells. J Immunol 150:1971, 1993
302. Kimmel PL, Bodi I, Abraham AA et al: Increased renal tissue cytokines in human HIV nephropathy, abstracted. J Am Soc Nephrol 4:279, 1993
303. Rubin-Kelley VE, Jevnikar AM: Antigen presentation by renal tubular epithelial cells. J Am Soc Nephrol 2:13, 1991
304. Diaz Gallo C, Jevnikar AM, Brennan DC et al: Autoreactive kidney infiltrating T cell clones in murine lupus nephritis. Kidney Int 42:851, 1992
305. Jenkins MK, De Silva DR, Johnson JG et al: Costimulating factors and signals relevant for antigen presenting cell function. Adv Exp Med Biol 329:87, 1993
306. Puppo F, Brenci S, Lanza L et al: Major histocompatibility gene products and HIV infection. J Lab Clin Med 117:91, 1991
307. Choppin J, Morinon F, Gomard E et al: Analysis of physical interactions between peptides and HLA molecules and application to the detection of HIV-1 antigenic peptides. J Exp Med 172:889, 1990
308. Choppin J, Mortinon F, Connan F et al: HLA-binding regions of HIV-1 proteins II. A systemic study of viral proteins. J Immunol 147:575, 1991
309. Zagury JF, Bernard J, Achour A et al: Identification of CD4 and major histocompatibility complex functional peptide sites and their homology with oligopeptides from HIV-1 glycoprotein gp120: role in AIDS pathogenesis. Proc Natl Acad Sci 90:7573, 1993

310. Callahan KM, Fort MM, Obah EA et al: Genetic variability in HIV-1 gp120 affects interactions with HLA molecules and T cell receptor. J Immunol 144:3341, 1990
311. Banda NK, Bernier J, Kurahara DK et al: Cross linking CD4 by HIV gp120 primes T cells for activation induced apoptosis. J Exp Med 176:1099, 1992
312. Mann DL, Read-Connole E, Arthur LO et al: HLA-DR is involved in the HIV-1 binding site on cells expressing MHC class II antigens. J Immunol 141:1131, 1988
313. Lopalco L, De-Santis C, Meneveri R et al: HIV-1 gp120 C5 region mimics the HLA class I a1 peptide-binding domain. Eur J Immunol 23:2016, 1993
314. Blackburn R, Clerici M, Mann D et al: Common sequence in HIV gp41 and HLA class II b chains can generate crossreactive antibodies with immunosuppressive potential. Adv Exp Med Biol 303:63, 1991
315. Golding M, Robey FA, Gates FT III et al: Identification of homologous regions in HIV-1 gp41 and human MHC Class II b 1 domain. J Exp Med 167:914, 1988
316. Pantaleo G, Graziosi C, Fauci AS: New concepts in the pathogenesis of HIV infection. N Engl J Med 328:327, 1993
317. Acha-Orbea H: Bacterial and viral superantigens: Role in autoimmunity? Ann Rheum Dis 52:S6, 1993
318. Imberti L, Sottini A, Bettinardi A et al: Selective depletion in HIV infection of T cells that bear specific T cell receptor Vb sequences. Science 254:860, 1992
319. Laurence J, Hodtsev AS, Posnett DN: Superantigen implicated in dependence of HIV-1 replication in T cells on TCR Vb expression. Nature 358:255, 1992
320. Oravecz T, Norcross MA: Costimulatory properties of human CD4 molecule: enhancement of CD3-induced T-cell activation by HIV-1 through glycoprotein gp120. First National Conference on Human Retroviruses and Related Infections, 1993. Abstract, p. 70.
321. Kimmel PL, Phillips TM, Ferreira-Centeno A et al: Idiotypic IgA nephropathy in patients with HIV infection. N Engl J Med 327:702, 1992

16

Animal Models of Lentivirus-Associated Renal Disease

Jeffrey B. Kopp
Paul E. Klotman

INTRODUCTION

EIAV: IMMUNE COMPLEX RENAL DISEASE

FIV: FOCAL AND SEGMENTAL GLOMERULOSCLEROSIS

SIMIAN IMMUNODEFICIENCY VIRUS

HIV-TRANSGENIC MICE

CONCLUSIONS

INTRODUCTION

The clinical and pathologic syndromes of human immunodeficiency virus (HIV)-associated renal disease have been delineated elsewhere. Studies of pathogenic mechanisms of these syndromes have been limited by the extremely restricted host range characteristic of HIV-1.[1] HIV-1 infects chimpanzees and pig-tailed macaques[2] but does not cause immunologic or renal disease in these animals. Baboons and rhesus macaques can be infected by HIV-2,[3] but renal disease has not been associated with HIV-2 infection of either humans or nonhuman primates. A chimeric mouse model has been developed, the severe combined immunodeficiency defect (SCID)-hu mouse, a mouse homozygous for the severe combined immunodeficiency defect that has been immunologically reconstituted with fetal human immunologic cells or adult human peripheral lymphocytes.[4,5] This chimeric human-mouse system is susceptible to infection with HIV-1; renal disease has not been reported. Two alternate approaches have exploited animal models to explore mechanisms of HIV-associated nephropathy. First, renal involvement has been characterized in animals infected, both naturally and experimentally, by lentiviruses other than HIV-1. Second, renal disease has been assessed in mice transgenic for HIV-1 genes. This chapter examines the results of these two approaches.

The viral family *Retroviridae* is traditionally divided into three subfamilies, *Oncovirinae, Spumavirinae,* and *Lentivirinae.* Classification is based on pathogenicity and virion structure rather than genomic structure.[6] Thus the oncoviruses include retroviruses that are known to induce tumors. Oncoviruses have been identified in range of animal hosts, including birds (e.g., Rous sarcoma virus), mice (e.g., Moloney murine leukemia virus, mouse mammary tumor virus), and cats (e.g., feline leukemia virus, FeLV). These viruses possess structural genes *gag* and *env,* the enzymatic genes encoded within *pol,* and in some cases oncogenes as well. Among the mouse oncoviral-associated syndromes is murine acquired immunodeficiency syndrome (MAIDS), which is caused by a complex of a defective murine leukemia virus and an intact helper virus. This viral complex induces immune cell proliferation and consequent immunodeficiency.[7] Renal disease has not been reported in MAIDS. In murine models of lupus nephritis, immune complexes eluted from nephritic kidneys contain gp70, an acute phase reactant protein produced in liver that is similar but not identical to envelope gp70 proteins derived from several different murine retroviruses.[8,9] Serum levels of gp70, however, are similar in lupus-susceptible and nonsusceptible strains. Although levels of gp70/anti-gp70 immune complexes are correlated with glomerulonephritis in susceptible mice, a direct pathologic role for gp70 or for retroviral gene products remains to be demonstrated. In cats, FeLV infection has been associated with glomerulonephritis. Renal pathology is notable for thickening of glomerular basement membrane and Bowman's capsule, subepithelial spikes, and FeLV structural antigens complexed with IgG and complement deposited in glomeruli.[10,11] Oncoviruses that affect humans include human T-cell lymphoma virus type I (HTLV-I, which in addition to lymphoma is associated with myelopathy, myositis, retinitis, and dermatitis but not with renal disease) and HTLV-II (possibly associated with hairy cell leukemia). In additional to *gag, pol,* and *env,* these viruses possess at least two additional open reading frames that encode regulatory proteins (Tax, Rex). A second subfamily of retroviruses, the spumaviruses or "foamy" viruses, have not been associated with disease in man.

Lentiviruses possess a complex genome, encoding many regulatory and accessory genes. These viruses produce multinucleated syncytia and cytolytic changes in cell culture and do not induce tumors in vivo. (Although an increased incidence of several tumors is a characteristic of HIV-1 infection, it appears that tumorigenesis is not due to a direct cellular transformation by the virus, as is the case with the oncoviruses. Although the mechanisms of HIV-associated tumorigenesis are unknown, altered cytokine regulation or other factors may contribute.) As their name implies, lentiviruses cause lifelong persistent infections characterized by the delayed onset of disease. A wide variety of clinical syndromes have been associated with lentiviral

Table 16-1. Lentiviral Pathology[a]

Virus	Host	Nonrenal Disease	Renal Disease
HIV-1	Human	AIDS	FSGS, glomerulonephritis
HIV-2	Human	Immun. abnormalities	—
FIV	Cat	AIDS	FSGS
SIV	Macaque	AIDS	FSGS
EIAV	Horse	Anemia	Glomerulonephritis
BIV	Bovine	AIDS	—
CAEV	Goat	Arthritis, encephalitis	—
Maedi-visna	Sheep	Encephalitis, pneumonia	—

Abbreviations: FIV, feline immunodeficiency virus; SIV, simian immunodeficiency virus; BIV, bovine immunodeficiency virus; EIAV, equine infectious anemia virus; CAEV, caprine arthritis–encephalitis virus.

[a] Among the lentiviruses, HIV-1 is associated with both FSGS and immune complex glomerulonephritis. SIV and FIV are associated with FSGS, whereas EIAV has been associated with immune complex glomerulonephritis.

infection (Table 16-1). Renal disease has been associated with HIV-1, equine infectious anemia virus (EIAV), feline immunodeficiency virus (FIV), and simian immunodeficiency virus (SIV).

EIAV: IMMUNE COMPLEX RENAL DISEASE

Horses infected with EIAV experience an acute, self-limited viral syndrome, followed by a chronic syndrome characterized by febrile episodes and anemia due to a combination of suppressed erythropoiesis and accelerated erythrocyte destruction.[12] The predominant infected cell is the macrophage. During the acute phase, EIAV antigen is present in monocyte/macrophages throughout the body. In the chronic phase of the disease, macrophage infection is most prominent in the spleen, lymph nodes, lung, bone marrow, liver, and kidney. Banks et al.[13] infected horses and performed serial renal biopsies over a period lasting up to 3 months. Glomerulonephritis characterized by cellular proliferation and thickened glomerular basement membranes was present in 75 percent of horses; immunoglobulin and complement were present in a granular distribution along the basement membrane and within the mesangium. Immunoglobulin eluted from glomeruli was shown to contain EIAV antigen, suggesting that immune complexes may be present within glomeruli and could play a pathogenic role.[13]

FIV: FOCAL AND SEGMENTAL GLOMERULOSCLEROSIS

FIV, discovered in 1987, causes an acquired immunodeficiency syndrome (AIDS)-like syndrome in cats.[14] As in human patients infected with HIV-1, cats infected with FIV manifest a decline in the number of CD4+ T cells and hypergammaglobulinemia. Clinical syndromes associated with FIV infection include lymphadenopathy, myeloproliferative disorders, anemia, stomatitis, dermatitis, and diarrhea. In vitro, FIV infects feline peripheral blood mononuclear cells, peritoneal macrophages, astrocytes, and kidney cells.[15]

Renal disease occurs frequently in FIV-infected cats, affecting 9 percent of 700 cats infected with FIV and 32 percent of 103 cats dying with FIV.[16] Recently, the FIV-associated renal syndrome has been characterized in some detail.[17] FIV-infected cats manifest azotemia and proteinuria with varying degrees of glomerular selectivity. Histologically, kidneys are remarkable for expansion of the mesangial matrix, segmental glomerulosclerosis, and interstitial inflammatory infiltrates (Fig. 16-1). Tubular alterations, including flattening of epithelial cells, microcystic tubular dilatation, and the presence of proteinaceous casts, correlate with the severity of glomerular involvement. Glomerular immune deposits are limited to coarsely granular segmental accumulations of IgM and C3, with lesser amounts of IgG and no IgA. Ultrastructural features include an increase in mesangial matrix and basement membrane folding. Glomerular endothelial cells show abundant rough endoplasmic reticulum, but tubuloreticular structures similar to those associated with HIV-1 infection have not been reported. Glomerular visceral epithelial cells are hypertrophic, with occasional electron-dense protein droplets. Budding retroviral particles are not observed. Immunostaining reveals p24 antigen localized to tubular epithelial cells, as well as to scattered interstitial cells and glomerular cells.[17a,17b] Whether this cellular p24 derives from viral replication within these cells remains to be demonstrated.

FIV infects cultured peripheral blood mononuclear cells, primary macrophages, and lymphocytic cell lines, in a fashion similar to that of HIV-1.[14] FIV is capable of infecting Crandall feline kidney cells (CRFK), a cell line with an epithelial morphology that produces high titers of virus without cytopathic effect. When these cells are serum deprived, FIV induces syncytium formation and cytopathic changes.[15,18] Treatment of FIV-infected CRFK cells with tumor necrosis factor-α (TNF-α) induces apoptosis,[19] which has been implicated in the pathogenesis of HIV-induced lymphocytic cell depletion.[20] These studies lend support to in vivo studies cited above which indicate that renal epithelial cells may be an important target for FIV.

Thus, the pathologic features of FIV-associated nephropathy bear a striking resemblance to those of HIV-associated focal and segmental glomerulosclerosis (FSGS). The mechanisms by which FIV induces renal disease are not known. The histologic features of immune complex nephritis are lacking. Although there is no proof of direct viral infection of renal cells in vivo, low-level retroviral replication may be difficult to detect by electron microscopy. Possible mechanisms for FIV-associated nephropathy, like those of HIV-associated nephropathy, include direct infection of renal cells, infection of passenger lymphocytes and monocytes, and paracrine effects of viral pro-

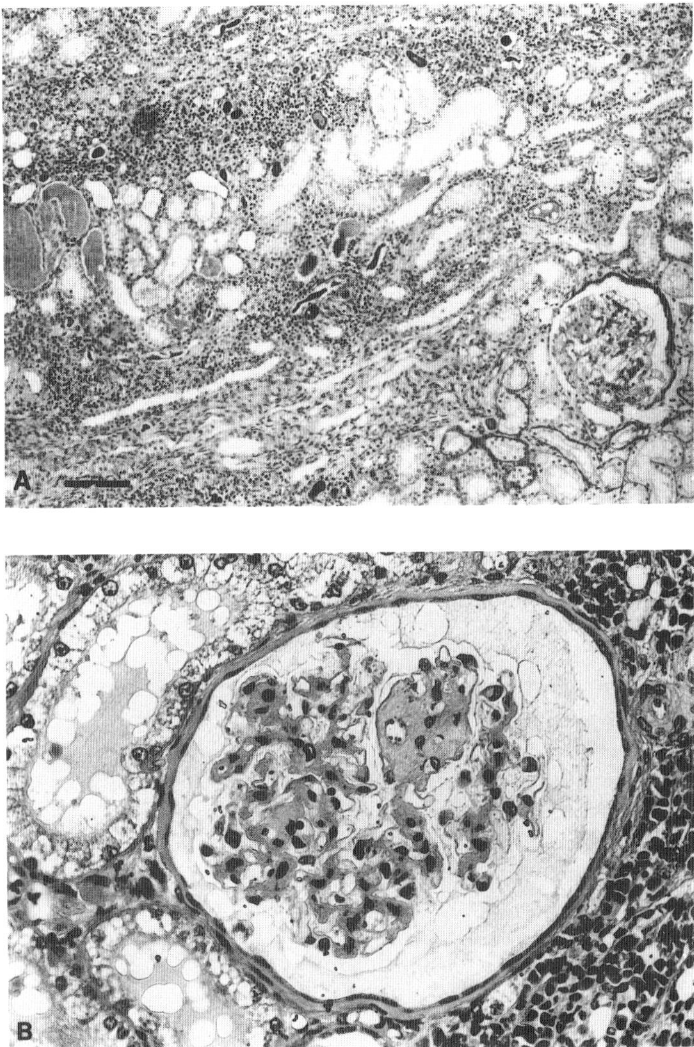

Fig. 16-1. Renal pathology in FIV-infected cats. (**A**) Dilatation of Bowman space, presence of interstitial infiltration, and dilated tubules forming microcysts containing proteinaceous deposits. (H&E, bar = 125 μM) (**B**) Severe segmental glomerulosclerosis with narrowing of capillary lumens. (Jones periodic acid-silver methanamine stain.) (From Poli et al.,[17] with permission.)

teins and cytokines. FIV-associated nephropathy may provide a useful small animal model to investigate mechanisms of lentiviral-induced renal disease.

SIMIAN IMMUNODEFICIENCY VIRUS

SIV is related to HIV-2 and, more distantly, to HIV-1. Multiple strains of SIV have been isolated; they are named according to the original simian species from which each was isolated, for example, SIV_{mac} from rhesus macaques (*Macaca mulatta*), SIV_{cyn} from cynomolgus macaques (*Macaca fasicularis*), and SIV_{sm} from sooty mangabeys (*Cercocebus atys*). SIV strains are capable of infecting macaques in the laboratory, including rhesus, cynomolgus, and pigtail (*Macaca nemestrina*) macaques, and induce syndromes that include simian AIDS.[21] Significant strain differences exist, such that not all strains are infectious in all species and infectious strains do not induce AIDS in all species. Like human AIDS, simian AIDS is characterized by a progressive decline in CD4+ T cells and disturbed macrophage function. In addition, there is widespread dissemination of SIV to virtually all organs, including lymphoid tissue, brain, lung, gut, and kidney.[22] In both lymphoid and nonlymphoid organs, the macrophage is the predominant cell type infected.

Renal disease is seen in macaques infected with SIV.[23,24] The pathology is that of FSGS, with enlarged glomeruli, mesangial expansion, modest cellular proliferation, and thickening and duplication of glomerular basement membranes. In addition, mesangial hyperplasia without glomerulosclerosis is seen. The renal interstitium is characterized by focal inflammation and tubular dilatation. Electron microscopy shows endothelial tubuloreticular structures, but these are also present in normal monkeys; viral particles and immune deposits are lacking.

The mechanisms by which SIV induces renal disease are of great interest. SIV proteins have been localized to kidney by immunohistochemistry. In tissue taken from terminally ill rhesus monkeys, SIV antigen expression was localized to mononuclear cells within the renal interstitium in three of four cases.[22] Presumably this represents infection of renal interstitial macrophages, although in situ hybridization studies to document viral RNA within these cells have not been reported. Proviral DNA (representing the DNA copy of the lentiviral RNA genome) can be shown by Southern blot analysis to be present within renal tissue, as it is within many other tissues from SIV-infected macaques.[22] In all tissues studied, including lymph node, spleen, liver, ileum, and brain, 85 percent to 100 percent of proviral SIV DNA is present in an unintegrated, extrachromosomal form. Proviral DNA can exist within the host cell in both integrated and unintegrated forms. Integration into the host genome is required for productive infection of lymphocytes in cell culture, for both HIV and SIV. On the other hand, unintegrated DNA dominates in brain macrophages in HIV-infected patients.[25] The biologic significance of unintegrated DNA is unknown, but it can serve as a template for RNA synthesis and thereby generate lentiviral proteins,[26] with the potential for toxicity in the infected cell or, if these proteins are exported, in neighboring cells. Thus the presence of SIV protein and proviral SIV DNA within the kidney suggests that local expression of SIV genes could contribute to renal pathology. As in HIV-associated nephropathy, it will be critical to identify which renal parenchymal cells or inflammatory cells, if any, are actively transcribing SIV RNAs.

Because not all patients with HIV-1 develop renal disease, it has been proposed that infection of the kidney by other pathogens may contribute to the development of HIV-associated nephropathy. In this regard, the SIV model provides an instructive parallel. SIV-infected monkeys are prone to infection with SV40, an oncogenic DNA virus of the family *Papovaviridae.* SV40 infects normal monkeys without evident pathology, although it induces tumors after inoculation into baby rodents. Horvath et al.[27] described four rhesus macaques infected with SIV who developed SV40-related disease. Central nervous system (CNS) disease occurred in three monkeys, all with apparent reactivation of latent SV40 infection, and renal disease occurred in a fourth monkey after SV40 seroconversion.[27] This latter monkey manifested diffuse tubulointerstitial fibrosis with mononuclear cell infiltrates, focal glomerulosclerosis, and glomerular atrophy. Tubular epithelial cells contained enlarged nuclei with intranuclear inclusions, which were particularly prominent in sloughed epithelial cells contained within tubular casts. Electron microscopy demonstrated abundant polyoma viral particles in the nuclei of degenerating epithelial cells, and SV40 infection of these cells was confirmed by in situ hybridization using DNA probes encoding the SV40 large T antigen. These findings suggest that SV40 may act as a cofactor to induce renal disease in SIV-infected monkeys.

Papovaviruses that infect humans include JC virus and BK virus (the names derive from the index cases); like SV40, they are oncogenic in newborn hamsters and transform cells in vitro. Infection with JC and BK viruses appears to be widespread in man, with approximately half of the population having antibodies to JC virus and over 75 percent having antibodies to BK virus. Subclinical persistent infections are common, particularly in the urinary tract, from which virus may be shed intermittently for many years. Pathologic findings within the urinary tract are few, but may include nuclear inclusions within ureteral epithelial cells. Periodic, asymptomatic reactivation of latent renal infection may occur with pregnancy, diabetes, or old age. In immunosuppressed hosts, both viruses are associated with disease. JC virus is associated with progressive multifocal leukoencephalopathy, and this virus has been implicated in increased incidence of this disorder in HIV-infected patients.[28] BK virus has been implicated in hemorrhagic cystitis in bone marrow transplant recipients[29,30] and in tubulointerstitial nephritis in a child with hyperimmunoglobulinemia M immunodeficiency.[31] There is serologic evidence of BK virus reactivation in patients with AIDS,[32] and recently BK virus has been associated with interstitial nephritis in two patients infected with HIV-1.[18,33] Thus in both HIV-infected patients and SIV-infected macaques, polyoma viruses are associated with tubulointerstitial nephritis. Significantly, these infections lack the typical features of HIV-associated nephropathy (heavy proteinuria, FSGS, microcystic tubular dilatation), suggesting that polyoma viruses are unlikely to be implicated in the pathogenesis of HIV-associated FSGS. Nevertheless, polyoma viruses may cause interstitial nephritis in some individuals with HIV-1 infection.

HIV-TRANSGENIC MICE

Transgenic animals have emerged in the past years as valuable model systems with which to dissect the role of particular gene products in vivo.[34,35] HIV-transgenic mice in particular have been useful in delineating the actions of HIV-1 gene products on host cells. A wide range of HIV-transgenic mice have been reported to date (Table 16-2). In considering the data in this table, several points are worth bearing in mind.

First, the promoter selected (e.g., the HIV-1 long terminal repeat [LTR] versus promoters with greater tissue specificity) influences which tissues express the transgene. The LTR sequences differ among different HIV-1 strains; mice transgenic for the LTRs from CNS-derived strains (HIV-1$_{JR-CSF}$ and HIV-1$_{JR-FL}$) express a reporter gene in brain whereas mice transgenic for the LTR from HIV-1$_{IIIB}$ do not.[36] Even when the same construct is used, expression may occur in different tissues in lines derived from different founder animals, as will be discussed in detail below. These differences are likely due to features of the particular genomic integration site in any given line, such as adjacent promoters, enhancers, and silencers, and chromosomal structure that influences the relative accessibility of regulatory factors to the transgene.

Second, the HIV-1 clone used to derive the transgene may influence the phenotype of the transgenic mouse. HIV-1 clones exhibit considerable sequence heterogeneity, and some of these differences have been correlated with differences in biologic behavior, both in vitro and in vivo. Thus the HIV-1$_{IIIB}$ strain grows well in immortalized T-cell lines and primary human T cells, whereas HIV-1$_{BaL}$ grows well in macrophages and primary human T cells but grows poorly in immortalized T-cell lines. Variation in HIV-1 envelope sequences correlate with the ability to induce syncytia in vitro,[37] which in turn correlates with disease progression.[38] Furthermore, envelope sequences from within the V3 loop are responsible for cell tropism: V3 sequences derived from HIV-1$_{BaL}$ are sufficient to confer macrophage tropism to HIV-1$_{IIIB}$.[39,40] The Tat protein derived from HIV-1 clones NL4-3 and HxB2 are each composed of 86 amino acid residues, whereas Tat derived from SF2 and BaL are composed of 101 amino acid residues. It remains unclear what functional consequences, if any, are associated with these differences.[41]

Third, the mouse strain selected may influence the phenotype, just as genetic influences likely underlie the predisposition of black patients to develop HIV-associated nephropathy. For example, Mehtali et al.[42] report that the *rev* gene is associated with immune disorders and skin abnormalities on the CD1 background but not on the C57B1/6 or SJL background.[42] This

Table 16-2. HIV-1 Transgenic Mice[a]

Reference	HIV-1 Clone	Genes or (Deletion)	Promoter	Mouse Strain	Renal Expression	Renal Disease
Promoter + reporter gene						
Leonard et al.[55]	LAV	CAT	HIV-1	FVB/N	0/4	NS
Skowronski[56]	HxB2	SV40 T	HIV-1	C3HeB/FeJ	1/3	NS
Cavard et al.[57]	LAI	β-gal	HIV-1	NS	0/3	NS
Morrey et al.[58,59]	HxB2	luciferase	HIV-1	FVB/N	NS	NS
Mehtali et al.[60]	LAI	α1-AT	HIV-1	C57Bl/6 × SJL	0/5	NS
Corboy et al.[36]	JR-CSF	β-gal	HIV-1	CD1	0/2	NS
Corboy et al.[36]	JR-FL	β-gal	HIV-1	CD1	0/4	NS
Single HIV gene						
Khillan et al.[61]	HxB2	*tat*	αA-Cry	FVB/N	NS	NS
Vogel et al.[44]	SF2	*tat*	HIV-1	CD1	0/3	0/3
Mehtali and Kieny[42]	LAI	*tat*	HMG	C57Bl/6 × SJL	1/1	0/1
Mehtali and Kieny[42]	LAI	*rev*	HMG	C57Bl/6,SJL,CD1	1/1	0/1
Skowronski et al.[62]	NL4-3	*nef*	CD3-δ	C3HeB/FeJ	ND	ND
Skowronski et al.[62]	HxB3	*nef*	CD3-δ	C3HeB/FeJ	ND	ND
Dickie et al.[45]	NL4-3	*nef*	HIV-1	FVB/N	0/6	0/6
Dickie et al.[45]	NL4-3	*nef*	MMTV	FVB/N	0/7	0/7
Toggas et al.[63]	LAV	*env* (gp120)	GFAP	C57Bl/6 × SJL	NS	NS
Multiple HIV genes						
Leonard et al.[46]	NL4-3	provirus	HIV-1	FVB/N	0/3	0/3
Iwakura et al.[47]	NL4-3	(*pol*)	HIV-1	C3H/HeN	0/4	0/4
Dickie et al.[43]	NL4-3	(*gag-pol*)	HIV-1	FVB/N	3/8	3/8
Dickie, personal communication	NL4-3	(*gag-pol-nef*)	HIV-1	FVB/N	1/8	1/8

[a] The viral strain from which the transgene was derived is shown. The HIV-1 genes included in the transgene are shown; in the case of deletions, the absent genes are given in parentheses and the remaining HIV-1 genes are present in the transgene. In cases where HIV-1 clones have been renamed, the current name is given; LAI has replaced BRU and SF2 has replaced ARV-2. Reporter genes used include SV40 T antigen (SV40 T), β-galactosidase (β-gal), chloramphenicol acetyl transferase (CAT), luciferase, and α1-antitrypsin (α1-AT). The promoter present in the transgene is listed: the murine αA-crystallin (αA-cry) promoter, the HIV-1 LTR, the murine HMG (hydroxymethyl glutaryl CoA reductase) promoter, the CD3-δ chain promoter, the mouse mammary tumor virus (MMTV) LTR, or the glial fibrillary acidic protein (GFAP). The mouse strain or strains in which the transgene has been placed or bred are listed. The number of lines in which the transgene is expressed in kidney, as assessed by Northern analysis or reporter gene analysis, and the total number of lines characterized are shown. The number of lines manifesting renal disease and the total number of lines are shown. ND denotes data not determined; NS denotes data not stated in the reference.

is likely due to differences in host response genes between different inbred mouse strains, although other mechanisms such as interaction with endogenous retroviruses have not been ruled out.

Fourth, renal disease is a distinctly unusual complication developing in HIV-transgenic mice, occurring with two different transgenic constructs (three mouse lines containing one cDNA construct[43] and one mouse line containing a second cDNA construct) (P. Dickie, personal communication, 1993). The majority of transgenic mice do not develop renal disease. This is true both of HIV-1 transgenic mice in particular and transgenic mice in general. Significantly, all transgenic lines that develop nephropathy express viral mRNA in kidney (Table 16-2, *gag-pol* deleted proviral genomes of Dickie et al.[43]). Furthermore, single-gene transgenic lines (Table 16-2, *tat* and *nef* lines of Mehtali et al.[42]) that express viral mRNA in kidney do not develop renal disease, although the number of lines available for analysis is small. These data suggest that certain HIV-1 genes induce renal disease in transgenic mice, and that local viral gene expression within the kidney is required.

Fifth, as will be described below, the similarities in renal histopathology among these lines and between the mouse and human HIV-associated nephropathy argues that this syndrome may be due to the effects of HIV gene products.

Individual HIV-1 genes have been used to generate HIV-transgenic mice, and to examine the effects on the host of local expression of HIV-1 gene products in a noninfectious animal model. Vogel et al.[44] reported that mice bearing Tat under the control of the HIV-1 LTR express viral RNA only in skin and develop subcutaneous tumors that have been suggested as a model for Kaposi sarcoma.[44] (Interestingly, expression in murine skin is a common feature of mice transgenic for genes under the control of the HIV-1 LTR, which has been exploited to develop convenient in vivo test systems using the reporter genes driven by the HIV-1 LTR [Table 16-2].) These LTR-Tat-transgenic mice did not express transgene RNA in kidney and did not develop renal disease. Mehtali et al.[42] have made numerous single-gene transgenic mice; among these are mice bearing, separately, the *tat* and *rev* genes derived from HIV-1$_{LAI}$ (formerly named HIV-1$_{BRU}$) and driven by hydroxymethyl glutaryl CoA (HMG-CoA) reductase promoter, which was selected for its widely distributed activity. Viral RNA encoding Tat and Rev were expressed in kidney but no renal disease was noted (M. Mehtali, personal communication, 1994). Mice transgenic for *nef* derived from HIV-1$_{NL4-3}$ under the control of either the homologous LTR or the Maloney murine tumor virus LTR do not express HIV-1 RNA in kidney and do not develop renal disease.[45]

An alternate approach to developing transgenic mice as a model for HIV pathogenesis is to use multiple HIV-1 genes. Leonard et al.[46] used an intact, infectious proviral genome from HIV-1$_{NL4-3}$ to generate transgenic mice. In this mouse, HIV-1 could be recovered using a permissive cell line and measuring reverse transcriptase activity. NL4-3 is an infectious hybrid clone in which the 5′ portion of the NY5 clone and the 3′ portion of the LAV clone were combined. It also contains approximately 2 kb of human flanking sequences. Importantly, NL4-3 contains open reading frames encoding all six of the regulatory and accessory genes *tat, rev, nef, vif, vpr,* and *vpu,* which makes possible the expression of these gene products in transgenic mice. (By contrast, in HxB2, *vpr* is truncated, *vif* lacks an initiation codon, and *nef* has a premature stop codon.) Kidney disease did not occur in these proviral transgenic mice. Two factors may have played a role. First, there was no expression of the transgene in kidney. Second, all mice died by 25 days, a time when renal disease first appears in the d1443 mouse to be discussed below. Finally, Iwakura et al.[47] developed mice transgenic for an HIV-1 construct derived from pNL4-3 by deleting 2.37 kb of sequence within the *pol* gene. Four lines of mice were established, and three developed cataracts with varying degrees of penetrance. None of the lines were found to express viral RNA in kidney and none developed renal disease. In summary, renal disease has only occurred in an HIV-transgenic mouse in which multiple HIV-1 genes were present, although renal disease has not occurred in every HIV-transgenic mouse with multiple HIV-1 genes.

We have characterized in some detail the renal disease that occurs in another multigene transgenic mouse, which bears a *gag-pol* deleted HIV-1 construct, pNL4-3:d1443 (Fig. 16-2). This construct was created from pNL4-

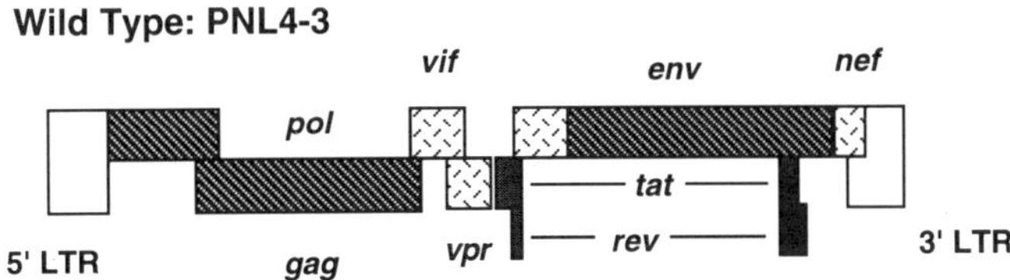

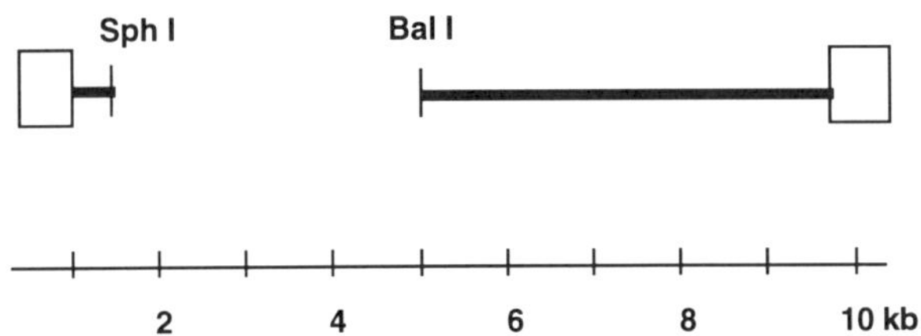

Fig. 16-2. The full-length HIV-1 proviral genome (shown for the clone pNL4-3) is comprised of the structural genes *gag* and *env,* the enzymatic genes encoded in *pol,* and the six regulatory/accessory genes *tat, rev, nef, vif, vpr,* and *vpu,* in addition to the 5′ and 3′ LTRs. Below is shown the pNL4-3:d1443 *gag-pol* deleted cDNA used to generate transgenic mice that develop nephropathy.

3 by a deletion of 3.1 kb of sequence within the *gag-pol* region. Thus, the deletion construct d1443 includes the 5' and 3' LTRs and the entire coding sequences of *env, tat, rev, nef, vif, vpr,* and *vpu.* Dickie et al. obtained nine founder mice, and all but one gave rise to lines when mated with normal FVB/N mice. None of the founder mice developed renal disease or other phenotypic abnormalities, suggesting that they may have been chimeric for the transgene. Three of eight lines manifested nephropathy beginning in the F1 generation; all lines showed similar histopathology, including FSGS and microcystic tubular dilatation.[43,48] In two of these lines, all mice succumbed to uremia in the F1 generation. The third line, Tg26, has survived and continues to breed successfully.[43,48,49] These mice have no evidence of infection with opportunistic pathogens. Homozygous Tg26 mice die prematurely with a wasting syndrome, with an increased number of CD8+ T cells in lymph node.[50] By contrast, heterozygous Tg26 mice develop normally and have normal numbers of CD4+ and CD8+ T cells in lymph node (N. Dorfmann, J. Kopp, unpublished observations, 1992).

Heterozygous transgenic mice develop proteinuria beginning at 22 to 25 days of age, as assessed by an elevation in urine protein to creatinine ratio

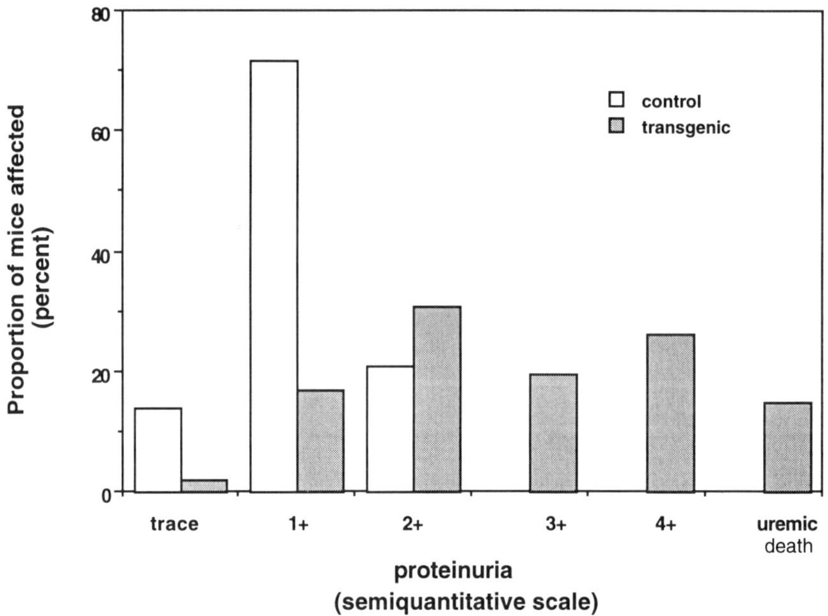

Fig. 16-3. Prevalence of proteinuria in HIV-transgenic mice. Heterozygous transgenic mice bearing the pNL4-3:d1443 construct were evaluated for proteinuria at 100 days by urinary protein dipstick. Urine from 249 transgenic mice and 272 normal mice from 89 litters was tested by semiquantitative dipstick, and the proportion of each group testing positive for each level of proteinuria is shown. At 100 days, 15 percent of transgenic mice had already died with uremia.

measured on a spot specimen. We have determined the prevalence of renal functional abnormalities in a large population of HIV-transgenic mice. We followed 89 litters prospectively, including 530 heterozygous transgenic mice and 364 normal littermates. By 100 days of age, 81 transgenic mice (15 percent) had died of uremia. We measured proteinuria using semiquantitative dipstick in the remaining mice. All of the normal mice had proteinuria of 2+ or less (Fig. 16-3). By contrast, 183 (35 percent of the original transgenic cohort) had 3 or 4+ proteinuria, whereas 266 (50 percent) had levels of proteinuria indistinguishable from those of normal mice. This indicates phenotypic heterogeneity within line Tg26 of the d1443 mouse, due to either reduced penetrance or expressivity or both. Further studies investigating this heterogeneity are discussed below.

The other features of nephrotic syndrome, including edema, hypoalbuminemia, and hypercholesterolemia, appeared in Tg26 mice between 60 and 300 days of age. When edema was manifest, blood urea nitrogen concentration was usually in excess of 100 mg/dl and death occurred within 5 to 10 days. In addition, approximately 5 to 10 percent of uremic mice did not develop edema, but instead developed wasting. The cumulative prevalence of uremic death was 18 percent at 100 days of age, 30 percent at 200 days of age, and 37 percent at 300 days of age (Fig. 16-4). Mice that had not developed uremia by the age of 300 days of age in general did not develop

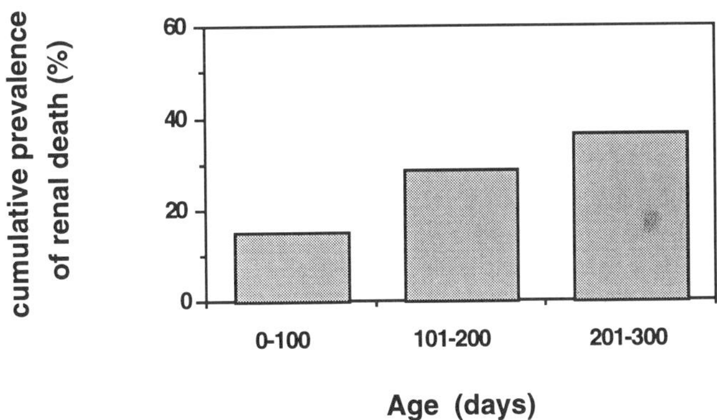

Fig. 16-4. Prevalence of uremic death in HIV-transgenic mice. The survival of HIV-transgenic mice was determined in 89 litters followed over 300 days (litters in which 100 percent follow-up data to 300 days was unavailable were excluded). A total of 303 mice were identified as transgenic at the time of weaning. At 100 days, 55 mice had died with uremia and 248 remained alive, representing an 18 percent mortality rate. By 200 days of age, another 35 mice had died with uremia and 213 mice remained alive, representing a cumulative mortality of 30 percent. By 300 days of age, another 23 mice had died with uremia and 190 remained alive, representing a cumulative mortality of 37 percent. Uremic death after 300 days was an infrequent occurrence (data not shown).

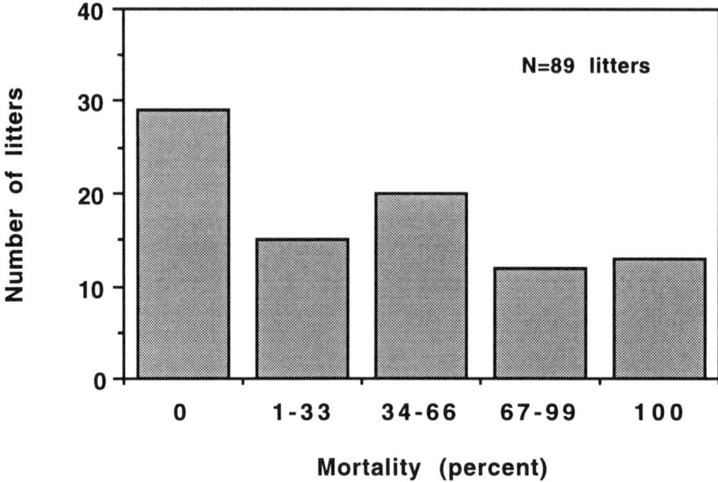

Fig. 16-5. Distribution of mortality rates in HIV-transgenic mice. The per-litter uremic mortality rates were calculated for HIV-transgenic mice from 89 litters, whose overall mortality rate was 37 percent. The data are presented above as the number of litters within tertiles of mortality, with litters having 0 percent or 100 percent mortality shown separately. This reveals a homogenous distribution of litter mortality rates, ranging from 42 litters with 0 percent to 33 percent mortality, 21 litters with 34 percent to 66 percent mortality, and 26 litters with 67 to 100 percent mortality.

uremia and lived out a normal life span of approximately 2 years, despite bearing the transgene and having minor renal histologic abnormalities.

We were interested in defining more precisely the reasons for this variable expression of the end-stage renal disease phenotype. Analysis of 89 litters revealed a per-litter renal mortality rate that ranged from 0 to 100 percent (Fig. 16-5). We next investigated whether this variable penetrance of severe renal disease was a heritable characteristic. We analyzed all breeding pairs for which we had at least three litters, and considered the average mortality rates among litters derived from each breeding pair (both heterozygote crossed with heterozygote and heterozygote crossed with homozygote). In 70 litters from 20 breeding pairs, mortality rates in the offspring of each breeding pair were normally distributed (Fig. 16-6). These data would tend to argue against a genetic basis for variability in renal disease expression.

Taking a different approach, we considered whether differences in the state of DNA methylation might contribute to variable HIV gene expression among different litters. Approximately 4 percent of the cytosines in vertebrate genomes are methylated, and all occurrences of 5-methylcytosine are associated with the dinucleotide CpG (this terminology defines the orientation as 5′ CG 3′). CpG islands, or regions of the vertebrate genome that possess an abundance of unmethylated CpG residues, are associated with the promoters of actively transcribed genes.[51] Although the mechanisms

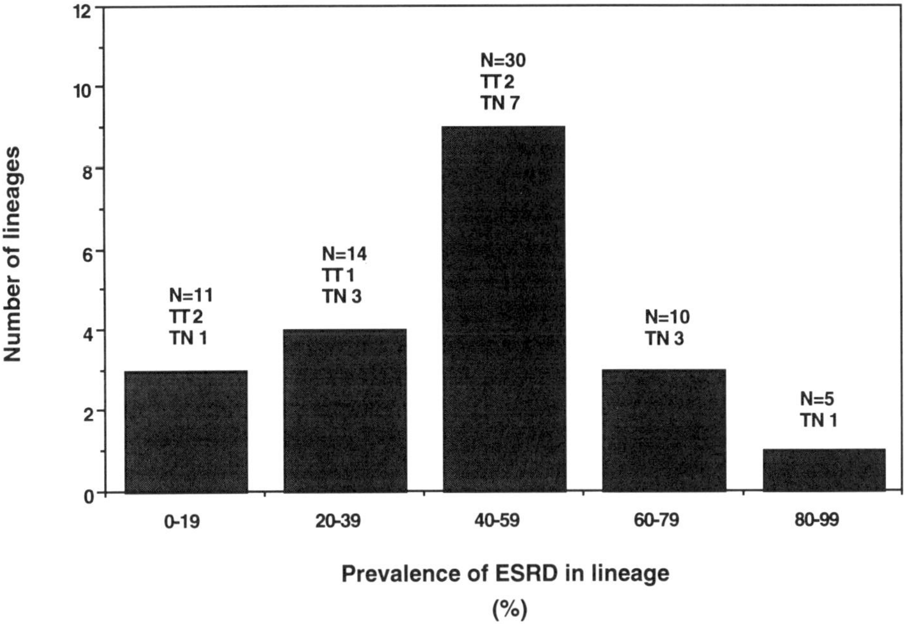

Fig. 16-6. Distribution of mortality rates among lineages. In order to examine whether the differential expression of end-stage renal disease in different litters was genetically based, we analyzed mortality rates among 70 litters, representing all litters for which data were available from at least 3 litters from each breeding pair. The average uremic mortality was calculated for each lineage, defined as all offspring from a breeding pair, and is displayed by quintile. The data above each bar includes the number of litters (N) in each quintile and the genotype of the parents in the breeding pair (a heterozygous transgenic mouse mated with another transgenic mouse is denoted TT and a heterozygous transgenic mouse mated with a normal mouse is denoted TN). For example, three lineages had mortality rates from 0 to 19 percent; there were a total of 11 litters in these three lineages, and the breeding pairs were composed of two heterozygous-heterozygous crosses and one heterozygous-normal cross.

involved are not fully understood, it is believed that CpG islands have the characteristics of active chromatin, including a nucleosome-free gap, which facilitates the binding of RNA polymerase II. Patterns of CpG methylation are heritable, tissue-specific, and correlated with gene expression. Retroviral sequences are susceptible to CpG methylation following integration into the host genome. The murine leukemia virus LTR has been shown to undergo hypermethylation, with consequent inactivation of viral transcription and expression.[52] Studies of the HIV-1 LTR suggest that methylation of a CpG sequence within the consensus nuclear factor of the kappa light chain in B cells (NF-κB) site inhibits binding of the NF-κB protein to the DNA and transcriptional activation of the LTR.[53] To investigate the role of CpG methylation, we digested tail DNA from high and low prevalence litters with the restriction enzyme *Msp* I (which cuts at CCGG regardless of methylation; this site is present at three locations within the pNL4-3 LTR) and *Hpa* II (which cuts at CCGG only in the absence of methylation). Restriction fragment length polymorphisms of the transgene were not detected by Southern analysis (data not shown), indicating that methylation of these sequences were not different in mice with varying prevalence of end-stage renal disease. Further studies using DNA from various tissues, in particular kidney, and using methylation interference footprinting are required to evaluate the role of methylation in this transgenic line.

In conclusion, the mechanisms responsible for phenotypic variability in the d1443 mouse remain unknown but appear to occur in a stochastic fashion. Similar variable disease expressions are commonly seen in human disease, where they are often attributed to genetic variability. That explanation is obviously not applicable in the setting of inbred mouse lines. It has long been recognized that diseases affecting inbred mouse lines frequently also show variable expression; the reason for this remains obscure. Those designing and analyzing experiments with HIV-transgenic mice and with other transgenic mice must bear in mind the variations in penetrance, expressivity, time of onset, and rate of progression of the phenotype that occur, despite the fact that all mice may have been derived from a single founder animal and have been maintained on one genetic background. Furthermore, frequently F1 hybrid females are used to provide oocytes for microinjection, as shown in Table 16-2, due to the increased numbers of oocytes available from hybrids and increased tolerance of these oocytes to experimental manipulation. When F1 hybrids are used as donors, the transgenic founder mice will have a mixed genetic background, and subsequent generations will have various genetic mixture until an inbred transgenic strain is developed.

Abnormal renal histology is noted beginning about 35 to 45 days of age in d1443 mice. Both heterozygotes and homozygotes develop disease, with approximately equal frequency. Although most homozygotes die of a runting and wasting syndrome by day 30,[50] occasional mice survive to 100 days and exhibit renal disease identical to that of the heterozygotes. The earliest changes are FSGS and abnormalities of parietal glomerular epithelial cells, which are dysplastic, enlarged, and exhibit nuclear atypia. Tubules show dilatation and eosinophilic casts, with occasional tubular profiles showing flattened, atrophic epithelium. Mice with more advanced lesions show increasingly diffuse glomerulosclerosis, with a progressively larger fraction of glomeruli appearing globally sclerosed and senescent (Fig. 16-7). Similarly, tubular dilatation is progressively more marked, with some tubules attaining a size of 2 to 3 glomerular diameters. Mononuclear cell infiltrates are present, most prominently around blood vessels, but also scattered within the interstitium. The interstitium is also notable for an increase in fibroblastic cells and matrix. Examination for immune deposits shows mild to moderate accumulation of IgM and IgA within sclerotic portions of glomeruli, whereas IgG and C3 are largely absent. Ultrastructural changes within the glomerulus include podocyte foot process fusion, mesangial expansion, and

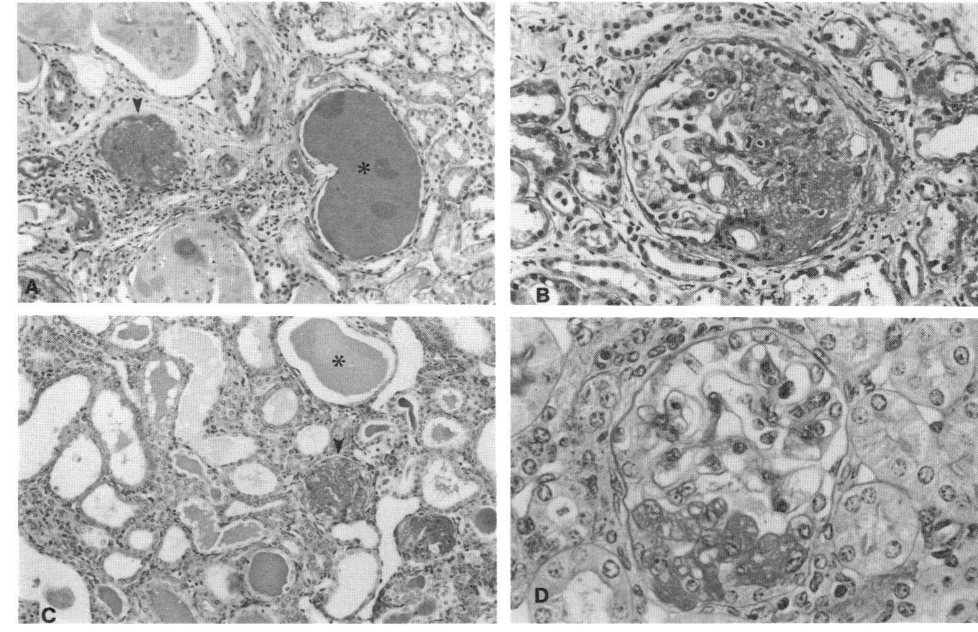

Fig. 16-7. Renal pathology of human HIV-associated nephropathy and the HIV-transgenic mice. **(A)** Kidney from patient with HIVAN, showing obsolescent glomerulus (*arrowhead*), dilated tubule occupied by proteinaceous cast (*asterisk*), and mononuclear cell infiltrate. **(B)** Kidney from same patient, showing segmental glomerulosclerosis, reactive glomerular epithelial cells, and interstitial fibrosis. **(C)** Kidney from HIV-transgenic mouse, with glomerulosclerosis (*arrowhead*) and dilated tubules, some of which contain proteinaceous casts (*asterisk*). **(D)** Kidney from HIV-transgenic mouse, with segmental glomerulosclerosis and reactive glomerular epithelial cells. (All slides stained with PAS; original magnification: **(A)** 50, **(B)** 125, **(C)** 50, and **(D)** 200.) (From Rappaport et al.,[64] with permission.)

Table 16-3. Expression of HIV-1 RNA in Mice Bearing pNL4-3:d1443[a]

Line	Skin	Muscle	Lymphoid	Intestine	Kidney	Brain
5	–	–	–	–	–	–
10	–	–	–	–	–	–
21	–	–	–	–	–	–
22	–	–	–	–	+	–
25	+	+	+	+	+	+
26	+	+	+	+	+	+
31	+	–	+	+	–	–
32	+	–	+	+	–	–

[a] Expression of HIV-1 mRNA in mice transgenic for a *gag-pol* deleted HIV-1 construct (pNL4-3:d1443) was determined by Northern analysis (data from Dickie et al.[43]). Renal disease was observed only in lines 22, 25, and 26, which, it should be noted, were also the only lines to express HIV-1 mRNA in kidney.

wrinkling of the glomerular basement membranes, whereas electron-dense deposits are absent.

The eight lines derived from the pNL4-3:d1443 construct showed differences in the tissues that transcribe viral mRNA, as assessed by Northern blot analysis (Table 16-3). Three lines (5, 10, 21) did not express viral mRNA in any tissue examined. Four lines (25, 26, 31, 32) expressed viral mRNA in skin, intestine, and lymphoid tissue. Three lines (22, 25, 26) expressed viral mRNA in kidney, and all developed renal disease as discussed above. In line 26, mRNA was expressed in muscle and skin at high levels throughout life, and is associated with focal myositis and epidermal papillomas.[54] By contrast, renal transgene expression in line 26 was absent in newborn mice, appeared at approximately 18 days of age, and subsided after approximately day 40.[43,48] Thus the expression of viral genes, as assessed by steady-state levels of RNA observed on Northern blots, preceded the appearance of proteinuria by a few days. Renal histologic abnormalities became apparent around day 40, just as viral RNA was becoming undetectable in kidney. In view of the fact that all three lines that demonstrated renal transgene expression also developed renal disease, and the temporal association of renal transgene expression with proteinuria, it appears that renal transgene expression is associated with renal damage. As is the case for other renal diseases, progression of histologic and functional abnormalities in this model may occur even after the initiating stimulus is removed, if the initial insult is of sufficient severity.

Immunostaining of glomeruli from transgenic mice revealed increased accumulation of collagen IV, laminin, and heparan sulfate proteoglycan. Northern blot analysis showed an increase with age in steady-state levels of $\alpha1(IV)$ collagen mRNA from whole kidneys taken from transgenic mice, compared with normal mice.[48] These data were derived from single mice harvested at days 28, 50, 100, and 200 days of age. In order to characterize this further, we sacrificed a litter of mice at 60 days of age, a time point at which one transgenic mouse had edema. Kidneys were scored for the pres-

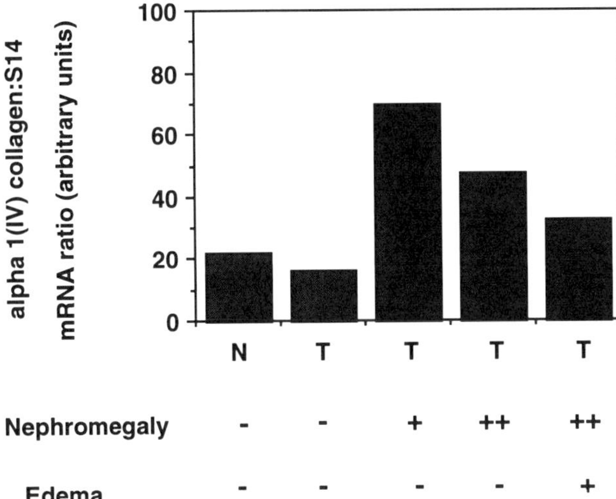

Fig. 16-8. Expression of α1(IV) collagen mRNA in whole kidney by Northern analysis. A litter composed of one normal mouse (N) and four transgenic mice (T) was sacrificed at 60 days of age. One transgenic mouse had edema, and at autopsy mild nephromegaly (+) was noted in one transgenic mouse and severe nephromegaly (++) was noted in two transgenic mice. Total kidney RNA was prepared by guanidine-thiocyanate solubilization and cesium chloride centrifugation, and Northern analysis was performed using cDNA probes encoding α1(IV) collagen and S14 ribosomal protein RNA. The signal intensity was quantitated using a phosphorimager and the ratio of collagen type IV to the normalizing mRNA S14 is shown in arbitrary units.

ence and severity of nephromegaly, and total kidney RNA was subjected to Northern analysis. The ratios of α1(IV) collagen mRNA to the mRNA for a normalizing gene, S14 ribosomal protein, are presented in Fig. 16-8. Expression of α1(IV) collagen mRNA was similar in a normal mouse littermate and a transgenic mouse without nephromegaly, whereas expression increased approximately fivefold in a mouse showing early nephromegaly. With further disease progression, as judged by more severe degrees of nephromegaly and ultimately by the onset of edema and nephrotic syndrome, the accumulation of α1(IV) collagen mRNA becomes less marked. The use of total renal RNA does not allow us to determine the location of increased α1(IV) collagen mRNA expression, which may occur in the glomeruli, tubules, or renal vasculature. Nevertheless, these data are quite consistent with similar studies of matrix accumulation in other rodent models of progressive glomerulosclerosis, indicating enhanced expression of α1(IV) collagen mRNA.

In the d1443 mouse, HIV proteins are localized to the glomerulus. Immunostaining using HIV-seropositive patient serum shows evidence of viral protein.[43] Similarly, an antibody directed against a peptide derived from rev protein detects rev in sclerotic glomeruli, whereas immunostaining using antibodies directed against gp41, gp120, Tat, Nef, and Vif has been negative.[48] Western blots using an antiserum to gp160 suggest that a 40-kDa protein is expressed in transgenic mouse kidney, although its identity as gp41 has not been established, whereas antisera against p17, Tat, Rev, Nef, and Vpu were negative.[43,48] These somewhat conflicting data suggest the possibility that an envelope protein, possibly gp41, and Rev may be present within glomeruli, particularly with the onset of glomerulosclerosis. It remains uncertain whether these proteins are produced locally within the glomerulus or are deposited from the circulation, although Western blots of serum have been negative (B. Weeks, J. Kopp, unpublished observations).

More recently, mice transgenic for another HIV-1 partial construct, NL4-3 deleted of *gag, pol,* and *nef,* have been found to manifest renal disease essentially identical to that seen in the d1443 mouse (P. Dickie, personal communication, 1993). This report further supports the observation that HIV-1 gene products are linked to the appearance of a renal histologic pattern characterized by FSGS and microcystic tubular dilatation. Together with the data from the d1443 mouse, they suggest that renal expression of viral RNA is required in the transgenic mouse model for the appearance of renal disease, and they narrow the list of candidate genes involved in the pathogenesis of this renal syndrome to *env, tat, rev, vif, vpr,* and *vpu.* It is likely, however, that HIV-associated FSGS is a multifactorial disease and may require the renal expression of one or more viral proteins, and possibly host response factors as well.

CONCLUSIONS

There is now widespread consensus that HIV-associated nephropathy is a consequence of HIV-1 infection, although the mechanisms of pathogenesis remain an enigma. The animal models of lentiviral-associated nephropathy suggest that the particular histopathologic syndrome comprised of FSGS, microcystic tubular dilatation, and mononuclear interstitial infiltrate is present in several lentiviral infections. Furthermore, abnormalities of the glomerular epithelial and tubular epithelial cells are particularly prominent. Although many HIV-transgenic mice have been reported, only two constructs (in a total of four lines) have been associated with a renal disease that shares functional histologic features with HIV-associated nephropathy. These findings suggest that renal expression of HIV-1 genes is closely linked to the appearance of renal disease. Further, the findings in transgenic mice suggest that some or all of the viral genes *env, tat, rev, vif, vpr,* and *vpu* are required for renal injury. Thus these animal models have provided important insights into the pathogenesis of HIV-associated nephropathy, and provide systems for future investigations into more effective therapies.

ACKNOWLEDGMENTS

The authors wish to thank Dr. Peter Dickie, Dr. Paul Luciw, Dr. Majid Mehtali, Dr. Alessandro Poli, and Dr. Jacek Skowronski for their generosity in sharing unpublished data concerning their HIV-transgenic mouse lines, and Dr. Alessandro Poli for giving permission to reproduce photomicrographs. The authors also wish to thank Dr. Jay Rappaport and Dr. William Schnaper for critical review of the manuscript.

REFERENCES

1. Letvin NL: Animal models for the study of HIV infections. Curr Opin Immunol 4:481, 1992
2. Agy MB, Frumkin LR, Corey L et al: Infection of Macaca nemestrina by human immunodeficiency virus type-1. Science 257:103, 1992
3. Castro BA, Nepomuceno M, Lerche NW et al: Persistent infection of baboons and rhesus monkeys with different strains of HIV-2. Virology 184:219, 1991
4. Mosier DE, Gulizia RJ, Baird SM et al: HIV infection of human-PBL-SCID mice. Science 251:791, 1991
5. Ruprecht RM, Koch JA, Sharma PL et al: Development of antiviral treatment strategies in murine models. AIDS Res Human Retroviruses 8:997, 1992
6. Coffin JM: Retroviridae and their replication. p. 645. In Fields BN, Knipe DM (eds): Fundamental Virology. Raven Press, New York, 1991
7. Jolicoeur P: Murine acquired immunodeficiency syndrome: an animal model to study the AIDS pathogenesis. FASEB J 5:2398, 1992
8. Theophilus AN, Dixon FJ: Murine models of systemic lupus erythematosus. Adv Immunol 37:269, 1985
9. Austin HI: Murine models. In: Balow JE, moderator. Lupus nephritis. Ann Intern Med 106:79, 1987
10. Jakowski RM, Essex M, Hardy WD et al: Membranous glomerulonephritis in a household cluster of cats persistently viremic with feline leukemia virus. p. 141. In Hardy WD, Essex M, McClelland AJ (eds): Feline Leukemia Virus. Elsevier North Holland, Amsterdam, 1980
11. Hardy WD: Immunopathology induced by feline leukemia virus. Springer Semin Immunpathol 5:75, 1982
12. McGuire TC, O'Rourke KI, Perryman LE: Immunopathogenesis of equine infectious anemia lentivirus disease. Dev Biol Stand 72:31, 1989
13. Banks KL, McGuire TC, Henson JB: Immunologically mediated glomerulitis of horses. Lab Invest 26:701, 1972
14. Pedersen NC, Ho EW, Brown ML et al: Isolation of a T-lymphotropic virus from domestic cats with an immunodeficiency-like syndrome. Science 235:790, 1987
15. Tozzini F, Matteucci D, Bandecchi P et al: Simple in vitro methods for titrating feline immunodeficiency virus (FIV) and FIV antibodies. J Virol Methods 37: 241, 1992
16. Ishida T, Washizu T, Toriyabe K et al: Feline immunodeficiency virus infection in cats in Japan. J Am Vet Med Assoc 194:221, 1989
17. Poli A, Abramo F, Taccini E et al: Renal involvement in feline immunodeficiency virus infection: a clinicopathologic study. Nephron 64:282, 1993

17a. Lombardi S, Poli A, Massi C et al: Detection of feline immunodeficiency virus p24 antigen and p24-specific antibodies by monoclonal antibody-based assays. J Virol Meth 46:287, 1994

17b. Poli A, Abramo F, Matteucci D et al: Renal involvement in feline immunodeficiency virus infection: p24 antigen detection, virus isolation, and PCR analysis. Vet Immunol Immunopathol, in press

18. Smith RD, Linnemann C, Anderson P et al: ESRD due to polyoma virus interstitial nephritis in an HIV(+) patient. J Am Soc Nephrol 4:287, 1993

19. Ohno K, Nakano T, Matusumoto Y et al: Apoptosis induced by tumor necrosis factor in cells chronically infected with feline immunodeficiency virus. J Virol 67:2429, 1993

20. Ameisen JC, Capron A: Cell dysfunction and depletion in AIDS: the programmed cell death hypothesis. Immunol Today 12:102, 1991

21. Kestler H, Kodama T, Ringler D et al: Induction of AIDS in rhesus monkeys by molecularly clone simian immunodeficiency virus. Science 248:1109, 1990

22. Hirsch VM, Zack PM, Vogel AP et al: Simian immunodeficiency virus infection of macaques: end-stage disease is characterized by widespread distribution of proviral DNA in tissues. J Infect Dis 163:976, 1991

23. Alpers CE, Baskin GB: Sclerosing glomerulopathy in rhesus monkeys with simian AIDS, abstracted. Kidney Int 35:339, 1989

24. Baskerville A, Ramsay A, Cranage MP et al: Histopathological changes in simian immunodeficiency virus infection. J Pathol 162:67, 1990

25. Pang S, Koyanagi Y, Miles S et al: High levels of unintegrated HIV-1 DNA in brain tissue of AIDS dementia patients. Nature 343:85, 1990

26. Stevenson M, Haggerty S, Lamonica CA et al: Integration is not necessary for expression of HIV-1 protein products. J Virol 64:2421, 1990

27. Horvath CJ, Simon MA, Bergsagel DJ et al: Simian virus 40-induced disease in rhesus monkeys with simian acquired immunodeficiency syndrome. Am J Pathol 140:1431, 1992

28. von Einsiedel RW, Fife TD, Aksamit AJ et al: Progressive multifocal leukoencephalopathy in AIDS: a clinicopathologic study and review of the literature. J Neurol 240:391, 1993

29. Arthur RR, Shah KV, Baust SJ et al: Association of BK viruria with hemorrhagic cystitis in recipients of bone marrow transplants. N Engl J Med 315:230, 1986

30. Apperley JF, Rice SJ, Bishop JA et al: Late-onset hemorrhagic cystitis associated with urinary excretion of polyoma viruses after bone marrow transplantation. Transplantation 43:108, 1987

31. Rosen S, Harmon W, Krensky AM et al: Tubulo-interstitial nephritis associated with polyomavirus (BK type) infection. N Engl J Med 308:1192, 1983

32. Flaegstad T, Permin H, Husebekk A et al: BK virus infection in patients with AIDS. Scand J Infect Dis 20:145, 1988

33. Vallbracht A, Löhler J, Gossman J et al: Disseminated BK type polyomavirus infection in an AIDS patient associated with central nervous system disease. Am J Pathol 143:29, 1993

34. Merlino GT: Transgenic animals in biomedical research. FASEB J 5:2996, 1991

35. Striker LJ, Doi T, Striker GE: Transgenic mice in renal research. Adv Nephrol (Necker) 20:91, 1991

36. Corboy JR, Buzy RM, Zink MC et al: Expression directed from HIV long terminal repeats in the central nervous system of transgenic mice. Science 258:1804, 1992

37. Groenink M, Fouchier RAM, Broersen S et al: Relation of phenotype evolution of HIV-1 to envelope V2 configuration. Science 260:1513, 1993

38. Koot M, Keet IPM, Vos AHV et al: Prognostic value of HIV-1 syncytium-inducing phenotype for rate of CD4+ cell depletion and progression to AIDS. Ann Intern Med 118:681, 1993

39. Hwang SS, Boyle TJ, Lyerly HK et al: Identification of the envelope V3 loop as the primary determinant of cell tropism in HIV-1. Science 253:71, 1991

40. Shioda T, Levy JA, Cheng-Major C: Macrophage and T cell-line tropisms of HIV-1 are determined by specific regions of the envelope gp120 gene. Nature 349:167, 1991

41. Gartenhaus R, Michaels F, Hall L et al: Relative activities of HIV-1-IIIB and HIV-1-BAL LTR and tat in primary monocytes and lymphocytes. AIDS Res Human Retroviruses 7:681, 1991

42. Mehtali M, Kieny MP: HIV-1 tat and rev-related pathologies in transgenic mice. AIDS Res Human Retroviruses 8:901, 1992

43. Dickie P, Felser M, Eckhaus M et al: HIV-associated nephropathy in transgenic mice expressing HIV-1 genes. Virology 185:109, 1991

44. Vogel J, Hinrichs SH, Reynolds RK et al: The HIV tat gene induces dermal lesions resembling Kaposi's sarcoma in transgenic mice. Nature 335:606, 1988

45. Dickie P, Ramsdell F, Notkins AL et al: Spontaneous and inducible epidermal hyperplasia in transgenic mice expressing HIV-1 nef. Virology 197:431, 1993

46. Leonard JM, Abramczuk JW, Pezen DS et al: Development of disease and virus recovery in transgenic mice containing HIV proviral DNA. Science 242:1665, 1988

47. Iwakura Y, Shioda T, Tosu M et al: The induction of cataracts by HIV-1 in transgenic mice. AIDS 6:1069, 1992

48. Kopp JB, Klotman ME, Adler SH et al: Progressive glomerulosclerosis and enhanced renal accumulation of basement membrane components in mice transgenic for HIV-1 genes. Proc Natl Acad Sci USA 89:1577, 1992

49. Kopp JB, Ray PE, Adler SH et al: Nephropathy in HIV-transgenic mice. p. 194. In Koide H, Hayashi T (eds): Extracellular Matrix in the Kidney. Contributions in Nephrology. Vol. 107. Karger, Basel, 1994

50. Santoro TJ, Bryant JL, Pellicoro J et al: Growth failure and AIDS-like cachexia syndrome in HIV-1 transgenic mice. Virology. In press

51. Antequera F, Bird A: CpG islands. p. 169. In Jost JP, Saluz HP (eds): DNA Methylation: Molecular Biology and Biological Significance. Birkhäuser Verlag, Basel, 1993

52. Harbers K, Schieke N, Stuhlmann H et al: DNA methylation and gene expression: endogenous retroviral genome becomes infectious after molecular cloning. Proc Natl Acad Sci USA 78:7609, 1981

53. Bednarik DP: DNA methylation and retrovirus expression. p. 300. In Jost JP, Saluz HP (eds): DNA Methylation: Molecular Biology and Biologic Significance. Birkhaüser Verlag, Basel, 1993

54. Kopp JB, Rooney JF, Wohlenberg C et al: Cutaneous disorders and viral gene expression in HIV-1 transgenic mice. AIDS Res Human Retroviruses 9:267, 1993

55. Leonard J, Khillan JS, Gendelman HE et al: The human immunodeficiency virus long terminal repeat is preferentially expressed in Langerhans cells in transgenic mice. AIDS Res Human Retroviruses 5:421, 1989

56. Skowronski J: Expression of a human immunodeficiency virus type 1 long terminal repeat/simian virus 40 early region fusion gene in transgenic mice. J Virol 65:754, 1991

57. Cavard D, Zider A, Vernet M et al: In vivo activation by ultraviolet rays of the

human immunodeficiency virus type 1 long terminal repeat. J Clin Invest 86: 1369, 1990
58. Morrey JD, Bourn SM, Bunch RD et al: In vivo activation of human immunodeficiency virus type 1 long terminal repeat by UV type A light plus psoralen and UV-B light in the skin of transgenic mice. J Virol 65:5045, 1991
59. Morrey JD, Bourn SM, Bunch TD et al: HIV-1 LTR activation model: evaluation of various agents in skin of transgenic mice. J AIDS 5:1195, 1992
60. Mehtali M, Munschy M, Ali-Hadji D et al: A novel transgenic mouse model for the in vivo evaluation of anti-human immunodeficiency virus type 1 drugs. AIDS Res Human Retroviruses 8:1959, 1992
61. Khillan JS, Deen DC, Yu S et al: Gene transactivation by the TAT gene of HIV in transgenic mice. Nucl Acids Res 16:1423, 1988
62. Skowronski J, Parks D, Mariani R: Altered T cell activation and development in transgenic mice expressing the HIV-1 nef gene. EMBO J 12:703, 1993
63. Toggas SM, Masliah E, Rockenstein EM et al: Central nervous system damage produced by expression of the HIV-1 coat protein gp120 in transgenic mice. Nature 367:188, 1994
64. Rappaport J, Kopp JB, Klotman PE: Host-virus interactions and the molecular regulation of HIV-1: role in the pathogenesis of HIV-associated nephropathy. Kid Int 46:16, 1994

Index

Page numbers followed by f *represent figures; those followed by* t *represent tables.*